CW00403228

Jinsil Seong

Editor

Radiotherapy of Liver Cancer

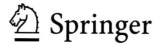 Springer

Editor
Jinsil Seong
Department of Radiation Oncology
Yonsei Cancer Center
Yonsei University College of Medicine
Seoul
Korea

ISBN 978-981-16-1817-8   ISBN 978-981-16-1815-4   (eBook)
https://doi.org/10.1007/978-981-16-1815-4

This Springer imprint is published by the registered company Springer Nature Singapore Pte Ltd.
The registered company address is: 152 Beach Road, #21-01/04 Gateway East, Singapore
189721, Singapore

Preface

Liver cancer is the world's leading cancer not only in incidence but also in lethality. Considering its age prevalence in 4th to 6th decades, which are the main axis of socioeconomic activity, liver cancer needs special attention to overcome. During the past decades, efforts have been focused on how to improve therapeutic outcome in parallel with how to detect early cancer. Actually there has been remarkable development particularly in the therapeutic aspect.

Radiotherapy is one of the major cancer therapy modalities. However, it has long been underestimated in the management of liver cancer. It could be attributable to the old concept that required the whole liver as a volume to be irradiated while radiation dose tolerance of the whole liver is far less than that for tumor control. Now, we have gone through two big changes: first, a conceptual change of a focal but not whole liver as a radiation volume and, second, more importantly, emergence of modern radiotherapy technology to deliver therapeutic dose precisely to the tumor while avoiding radiosensitive adjacent organ. Consequently, we have witnessed a rapid increase in clinical application of radiotherapy for liver cancer, followed by numerous reports of excellent outcomes.

Despite clinical demand, the guidance available to clinicians has remained limited on radiotherapy of liver cancer. This book was intended to address this deficit on the basis of the best available evidence by providing up-to-date information on all aspects of radiotherapy for liver cancer, from the basic science to clinical practice. The first two sections explain the relevant basic science and present detailed information on the available technologies and techniques, including the most recent advances. The radiotherapy strategies appropriate in different patient groups are then fully described, covering the use of ablative, adjuvant, neoadjuvant, definitive radiotherapy, radiotherapy as a bridge to liver transplantation, and palliative radiotherapy. The final section addresses a range of specific issues of concern to the clinician.

As an editor, I am very honored to invite world-class experts in liver cancer as contributors to this book. Thank you so much for your time and dedication! I am quite sure that *Radiotherapy of Liver Cancer* will be an ideal reference for clinical radiation oncologists, radiation oncology residents, oncologists, and hepatologists.

Seoul, Korea   Jinsil Seong

Contents

Part I

Basic Science in Radiotherapy of Liver Cancer

Principle of Cancer Radiotherapy

1

Victor Ho-Fun Lee and Anne Wing-Mui Lee

Abstract

Radiotherapy is one of the most common types of nonsurgical anticancer treatment modality, employed in more than 50% of cases. Almost half of cancer patients are cured of their cancer by radiotherapy as part of their anticancer treatment. Radiotherapy kills cancer by the use of ionizing radiation which causes permanent and irreversible double-strand DNA breaks in cancer cells leading to cell death. Unfortunately, it can also kill normal cells leading to acute and chronic treatment-related complications. Traditionally, radiotherapy was seldom employed in the treatment of hepatocellular carcinoma (HCC) because of the risk of severe and sometimes irreversible radiation-induced liver injury (RILD), since a large volume of normal liver which took into account the physiological movement of the liver and the tumors inside during breathing might be irradiated. However, with the advent of new radiation technologies and motion management devices, radiation therapy can now be safely delivered to liver tumors. Further radiation dose escalation in the form of hypofractionated stereotactic body radiation therapy (SBRT) is also now feasible, which delivers a high dose of radiation to the tumors while sparing the adjacent normal organs from unnecessary irradiation, leading to a much better tumor response and favorable safety profile. Furthermore, endovascular radioembolization with radioisotope also produced encouraging results in the treatment of unresectable HCC. In this chapter, we will describe how radiotherapy works in cancer cells and elucidate different types of radiation therapy for HCC.

Keywords

Radiotherapy · External beam radiotherapy · Charged particle therapy · Radioembolization · Radiation-induced liver injury

1.1 Introduction

Radiotherapy is an effective and commonly used treatment modality in the treatment of many cancer types. The treatment objective can be either radical (aiming at cure) or palliative (aiming at symptom relief). Forty percent of patients cured of their cancer have received radiotherapy as a part of their therapy, either on its own or in combination with surgery or chemotherapy or more recently targeted therapy and immunotherapy

V. H.-F. Lee · A. W.-M. Lee (✉)
Department of Clinical Oncology, LKS Faculty of Medicine, The University of Hong Kong, Hong Kong, Hong Kong

Clinical Oncology Center, The University of Hong Kong-Shenzhen Hospital, Shenzhen, China
e-mail: awmlee@hku.hk

[1]. Radical treatment can be as the definitive therapy (e.g., for head and neck, skin or prostate cancers), neoadjuvant prior to surgery (e.g., chemoradiotherapy for esophageal or rectal cancer), or adjuvant following definitive treatment (e.g., for head and neck and breast cancers).

Different histological cancer types possess different inherent radiation sensitivities, which determine whether radiotherapy should be considered as part of anticancer treatment and also the dose essential to achieve the treatment objective as mentioned above. HCC is considered moderately sensitive to radiation, when compared to the more sensitive types including small-cell carcinoma, seminoma, and lymphoma, and the less sensitive types like sarcoma and melanoma.

Radiation therapy can be broadly classified and delivered in four main ways: (1) external beam radiotherapy in which the radiation (photons, electrons, and charged particle) is emitted by an external machine passing through the skin before reaching the tumors, (2) implanted radioisotopes in the form of brachytherapy, (3) internal radiation therapy in which the radioisotopes through injection or ingestion are preferentially taken up by specific body tissues, and (4) selective internal radiation therapy or endovascular radiation therapy in which radioisotopes are injected into the tributaries of the feeding vessels which offer blood supply to the tumors (Table 1.1). External beam radiotherapy and more recently selective internal radiation therapy, also known as radioembolization, are the most commonly used radiation modalities for HCC.

1.2 External Beam Radiotherapy

This is the most common type of radiotherapy employed to treat HCC. The high-energy (6–20 megavoltage) photons generated are able to penetrate deep enough to reach and kill the tumor cells. In general, high-energy fast moving electrons are first produced by the powerful electron gun which accelerate through the electromagnet in the linear accelerator and ultimately collide with the target to generate X-rays. The linear accelerator is housed in a specially-made bunker surrounded by thick concrete and lead walls which offer radiation protection and safety (Fig. 1.1). The international unit to describe radiation prescription and absorption is Gray (Gy), which is defined as 1 Gy = 1 J/Kg. Conventional radical radiotherapy is usually given in multiple sessions (fractions) every day, 5 days per week, lasting for 5–7 weeks, depending on the dose to be prescribed. The concept of fractionation is to enhance the therapeutic ratio or therapeutic window so that a high radiation dose can be delivered to the tumor cells while adequate time is allowed for repair and repopulation of the adjacent normal cells (Fig. 1.2).

Table 1.1 Types and clinical indications of radiotherapy used

Types	Clinical indications
Photons	Capable of penetrating into the deeper structures of the body while relatively sparing the skin. Suitable for deep-seated tumors, for example, bladder and rectal cancers.
Electrons	Capable of delivering high radiation dose up to a few centimeters depth from the skin surface with little dose beyond. Most suitable as superficial treatment for skin cancers.
Charged particle therapy	Capable of depositing most of its energy at a specific and characteristic depth after tissue penetration with high precision. Most suitable for pediatric tumors, brain tumors, and spinal tumors.
Radioisotopes	
Interstitial, implanted, or intracavitary	Radioisotopes placed inside the tumors, or the lumens or cavities of the patient's body. Examples include iodine-125 interstitial brachytherapy for prostate cancer and iridium-192 intracavitary brachytherapy for cervical cancer.
Ingested or injected	Radioisotopes ingested or injected which are preferentially taken up by specific body tissues/cells with preferential avidity with these radioisotopes. Examples include iodine-131 for thyroid cancer and Radium-223 for bone metastasis of prostate cancer.
Endovascular	Radioisotopes injected intravascularly into the feeding vessels supplying the tumors. An example is transarterial radioembolization with yttrium-90 microspheres for liver cancer.

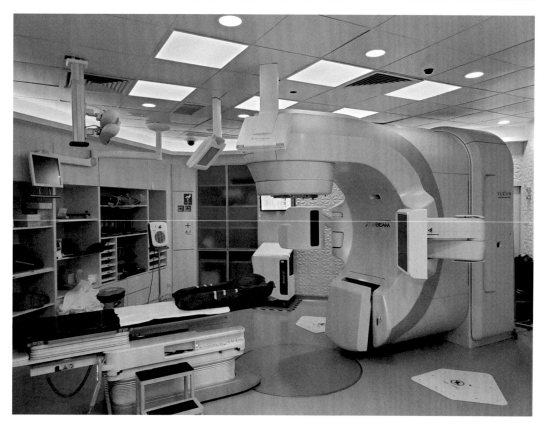

Fig. 1.1 A linear accelerator equipped with a cone-beam CT scanner and ExacTrac Adaptive Gating System housed in a thick-walled bunker

Fig. 1.2 Diagram illustrating the concept of therapeutic ratio of differential responses of tumor cells and normal cells to radiation therapy

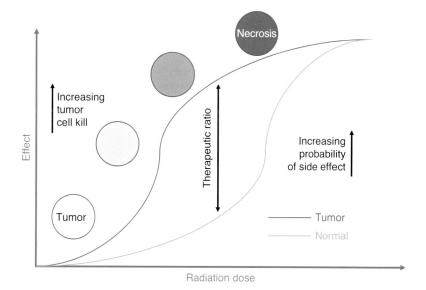

1.3 Mechanisms and Effects of Radiotherapy on Cancer and Normal Cells

The paths and effects of radiation on tissue can be divided into four phases, namely the physical, chemical, biological, and clinical phases. The physical phase relates to the absorption of radiation in tissues leading to secondary ionization with the ejection of orbital electrons and the subsequent excitation of these electrons to reach a higher energy level. It is followed by the chemical phase in which these damaged atoms or molecules react with other cellular components giving rise to chemical bond breakage and the generation of free radicals. The subsequent biological phase following the precedent chemical damage with chains of enzymatic reactions results in DNA damage and subsequent cell death. Finally, the clinical phase is the clinical effect on the tissues/cells after radiation. For tumor cells, they will die primarily as a result of direct and permanent DNA damage or indirectly by reduction of tumor vascularity or enhanced host immune response against them. Normal cells also die because of direct cell death similar to tumor cells, or indirectly because of reduced stem cell capacity to repair, regenerate and replace the damaged normal cells, or limited blood supply as a result of radiation damage of the vasculature.

1.4 Preparatory Process Before Radiotherapy

The treating radiation oncologists have to, first of all, decide if the tumors of their HCC patients are amenable to radiotherapy, and the treatment objective is radical or palliative. With the recent advances of radiation techniques (to be further described in subsequent chapters), those tumors (e.g., multiple bilobar tumors, tumors >5 cm, or those close to abutting the adjacent critical normal structures) originally considered only feasible for palliative radiotherapy in the old era may now be deemed feasible for radical high-dose radiotherapy. All cases must be discussed in multidisciplinary tumor board with other specialists including surgeons, radiologists, interventionalists, medical oncologists, and pathologists for the most appropriate and tailor-made treatment approach. This is followed by the complex process in which the radiation oncologists, together with medical physicists, dosimetrists, and radiation therapists have to devise the most suitable radiation treatment plans for their patients based on the patients' inherent medical fitness, tumor location, radiobiology, radiation safety, radiation dosimetry, treatment planning, and potential interactions with other treatment modalities their patients have received or subsequently receive after radiotherapy.

1.5 Immobilization, Motion Management, Image Acquisition, and Target Volume Delineation

Once the treating oncologist and the patients have agreed upon radiotherapy, a series of pretreatment preparatory work has to be performed. First of all, rigid immobilization has to be implemented to ensure accurate patient and tumor positioning during the whole course of radiotherapy. In general, body fix or vacuum bed are used to provide a comfortable patient position and ensure accurate body alignment on the treatment couch (Fig. 1.3). For high-dose radiotherapy, especially stereotactic body radiation therapy (SBRT) (described in the subsequent chapters), reliable and reproducible motion management of the patients and their tumors are of paramount importance to ensure safe and precise radiotherapy delivery. In general, motion management can be achieved by active breathing control (ABC) or voluntarily by self-initiated breath holds, respiratory gating, and abdominal compression. For breath-holding, patients are requested to hold their breaths (usually after expiration) during radiotherapy delivery. The ABC apparatus is a modified spirometer consisting of two pairs of flow monitors and scissor valves to control inspiration and expiration, respectively (Fig. 1.4). The radiation therapist activates ABC at a predefined lung volume by closing both valves to immobilize the breathing motion for about 15–20 s while the radiation

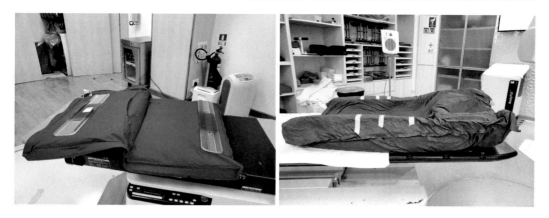

Fig. 1.3 BodyFIX® (Elekta) and Vac-Lok™ (CIVCO® Radiotherapy) commonly used as immobilization devices in stereotactic body radiation therapy for liver cancer

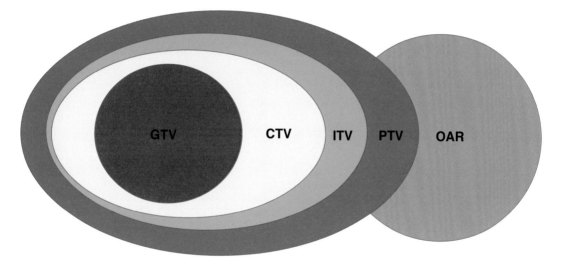

Fig. 1.4 Diagram illustrating the relative concepts of gross tumor volume, clinical target volume, internal target volume, planning target volume, and organ-at-risk.

Abbreviations: GTV, gross tumor volume; CTV, clinical target volume; ITV, internal target volume; OAR, organ-at-risk; PTV, planning target volume

machine is switched on to deliver radiation at the same time. The patient is then allowed to relax and breathe freely until the next ABC activation. The cycle is repeated until complete delivery of a treatment fraction, which typically takes 30–45 min. Voluntary inspiratory breath hold technique can be considered in those who can hold the breath for at least 15 s but unable to hold the mouthpiece of the ABC apparatus without air leakage. Pretreatment chest physiotherapy and breath hold training may be indicated to improve patient compliance and reduce fatigue after repeated breath-holding. Respiratory gating techniques involve radiation delivery in a certain phase of respiratory cycles (usually toward end-expiration during which the liver position is relatively stagnant when compared to end-inspiratory phase). A four-dimensional computed tomography (4D-CT) for radiotherapy planning purposes is done with the Real-time Patient Management (RPM) system (Varian Medical Systems, Palo Alto, CA, USA), which consists of an infrared reflective block and an infrared tracking camera in the radiation treatment bunker. The reflective block is placed on the skin surface of the anterior abdomen about midway between the xiphisternum and umbilicus, acting as a surrogate to monitor the motion of the liver, while the infrared

Table 1.2 Comparison of different motion management techniques used in radiotherapy for liver cancers

Technique	Advantage	Disadvantage
Breath-holding	Shorter treatment time	Not suitable for patients with limited pulmonary function
	Smallest radiation treated volume	Causes fatigue in patients as at least 15–20 breath holds are needed for 1 fraction of radiotherapy
Respiratory gating	Feasible for patients with limited pulmonary function	Longer treatment time
	More comfortable to patients	Not suitable for patients with irregular and unsteady respiratory cycles
		Larger radiation treated volume
Abdominal compression	Probably shortest treatment time	Discomfort and trauma to patients
	Feasible for patients with limited pulmonary function	Inconsistent deformation of the liver in between fractions of radiotherapy

camera tracks the movement of the reflective block. The up-and-down breathing movement of the abdominal wall and thus position of the reflective block now reflects the respiratory phase during which CT images are acquired for position monitoring. As a result, positions of the tumor in various respiratory phases can be displayed on the 4D-CT images. Respiratory gating can be executed with either the RPM or the ExacTrac Adaptive Gating systems (BrainLab AG, Germany). Abdominal compression in which the anterior abdominal wall and thus the liver and its tumors are compressed mechanically can be achieved by placing a board/device on the anterior abdominal wall surface limiting their movements during respiration [2]. Occasionally, metallic fiducial markers are placed in the vicinity of the tumors to aid tumor positional tracking during radiation therapy, in particular SBRT [3]. Comparisons among these motion management measures are shown in Table 1.2.

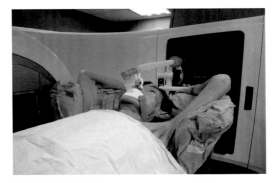

Fig. 1.5 An active breathing control apparatus to control and monitor breathing holds for a patient's liver cancer treated with stereotactic body radiation therapy

1.6   Simulation and Image Acquisition

After the most suitable radiation technique and motion management modality is determined, CT images will be acquired for target volume delineation. This set of planning CT images are often co-registered with other modalities of images for instance magnetic resonance imaging (MRI) and positron emission tomography for more accurate gross tumor volume (GTV) delineation. GTV refers to the tumor volumes grossly observed in the planning CT images, aided by other co-registered images (Fig. 1.5). A margin created around the GTV to account for the microscopic spread of the disease may be needed to become the clinical target volume (CTV). An extra eccentric volume based on CTV to become internal target volume (ITV) is often required to encompass the physiological movement of the tumor, though no additional margin is needed if the patient can take reliable active or voluntary breath holds during radiotherapy which eliminates any physiological tumor motion. ITV must be verified with either 4D-CT or fluoroscopy. Finally, the planning target volume (PTV) is created around CTV/ITV with usually a 3–5 mm margin to take machine and patient setup errors into account, which is also the ultimate volume treated with the prescribed radiation dose.

1.7 Treatment Planning and Optimization

After target volume delineation by the treating oncologists, the next step will be optimizing the radiation beam arrangement and modulation of radiation beam intensity so that the desired radiation dose can precisely cover the PTV, while the adjacent normal critical structures known as organs-at-risk (OARs) can be effectively spared from unnecessary radiation. OARs in liver cancer radiotherapy include liver, heart, esophagus, stomach, duodenum, small bowel, large bowel, gallbladder, common bile duct (or biliary tract), kidneys, spinal cord, and skin, for which a maximum dose (or dose to the maximum 0.5 cc or 0.1 cc) is usually determined by radiation oncologists and dosimetrists during treatment optimization. Several international and institutional guidelines have recommended dose constraints for each OAR, which is dependent on the prescribed dose to the PTV and the number of fractions of radiotherapy [4–8]. The final radiotherapy plan must meet the predefined acceptance criteria before it can be executed to patients (Fig. 1.6).

1.8 Pretreatment Setup Verification and Radiotherapy Delivery

Prior to every fraction of radiotherapy, all patients must be set up in the same manner and the same position as they were for the simulation and planning CT scanning to ensure treatment accuracy and safety. Various forms of imaging techniques to verify patient treatment position and tumor location are available (Table 1.3). On-board imaging with orthogonal X-ray simulation is the simplest method to align the patient position according to the anatomical bony landmarks and the location of fiducial markers if implanted. However, it is not so accurate since the liver cannot be visualized and it cannot verify the treatment position when radiation is delivered. Nevertheless, it is often used as the first tool to grossly align the patient position before further fine-tuning with translational and rotational correction with cone-beam CT scan and other devices. It is also commonly used for palliative liver radiotherapy since it is much easier to perform. Kilovoltage cone-beam CT scanner mounted on modern linear accelerators provides more accurate image-guided positional verification as the real-time liver position can be compared and matched with the liver position in the planning CT images so that more precise and finer on-couch correction of treatment position can be made. However, real-time positional monitoring cannot be achieved when the radiation beam is on. RPM and ExacTrac Adaptive Gating system can provide real-time positional monitoring. The infrared camera mounted on the ceiling of the treatment room can track movements of the reflective block placed on the anterior abdominal wall skin surface to turn the radiation beam on and off during respiratory gating. That said, intrafraction

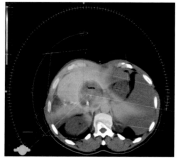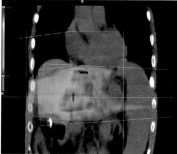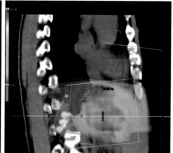

Fig. 1.6 A radiation treatment plan in transverse, coronal, and sagittal planes of a patient's solitary liver cancer optimized by volumetric arc modulated therapy. The prescribed dose was 40 Gy in 5 fractions and the color wash threshold was set at 10 Gy

Table 1.3 Various forms of positional verification techniques used in radiotherapy for liver cancer

Technique	Advantage	Disadvantage
On-board imaging	Simple and easy to perform	Less accurate
	Applicable in both breath-holding and respiratory gating techniques	Tumors cannot be visualized and verified
	Fluoroscopic mode available	
Cone-beam computed tomography	More accurate than on-board imaging	More time consuming for image acquisition which may not be applicable for breath-holding technique
	Three-dimensional verification of the liver and the tumor position	Unable to verify the tumor position when radiation is delivered
ExacTrac adaptive gating system	Real-time tumor position can be performed even when radiation is delivered	For respiratory gating only
		Fiducial markers required
Fiducial marker placement	Accurate tumor location	Marker dislodgement or migration
		Bleeding
		Interventionalist required for marker placement

deformations of the liver can still occur during respiration, which cannot be easily detected by the trajectory of the skin motion [9].

1.9 Recent Advances in Radiotherapy for Liver Cancer

Radiotherapy was once very rarely employed as a radical treatment for liver cancer, owing to the risk of RILD (characterized by central veno-occlusive disease caused by fibrin deposition, thrombosis, congestion, and hemorrhage under microscopy) following a large radiation field covering a large proportion of normal liver throughout the whole respiratory cycles. A retrospective study of 40 patients who received total liver irradiation for metastatic disease revealed that no patients who received <30 Gy suffered from RILD, rising to 12.5% (1 of 8) who received 30–35 Gy over 3–4 weeks, 55.6% (5 of 9) who received 35–40 Gy, and 38.9% who received >40 Gy [10]. The pioneer work done by the Michigan group suggested that the mean liver dose using the Lyman normal tissue complication probability model is a reliable metric when evaluating the radiotherapy plans and RILD [11]. With the recent employment of image co-registration with more contemporary imaging modalities like MRI and PET, as well as more precise and accurate patient positioning and motion management devices as mentioned above, a better defined GTV, a narrower margin around the GTV, and hence a smaller PTV can be more readily achieved. In parallel, more sophisticated treatment optimization tools and treatment delivery provide superior tumor coverage and conformity and better dose sparing of OARs. The traditional three-dimensional conformal radiotherapy (3DCRT) employing a fixed number of static beams without dose modulation has been gradually replaced by intensity-modulated radiation therapy (IMRT) and volumetric modulated arc therapy (VMAT) [12–16]. Both IMRT and VMAT can constantly regulate and modulate the dose intensity by computerized movement of the small multileaf collimators (MLC) during radiation, which facilitates radiation delivery as SBRT. Volumetric arc modulated therapy especially delivered by flattening filter-free (FFF) beams offers both highly conformal and much swifter radiation delivery compared to treatment without FFF [16]. More recently, highly conformal and precision radiotherapy to liver lesions can also be delivered by a robotic radiosurgery/radiotherapy system. A recent dosimetric study showed that the quality of the radiotherapy plans generated by the robotic CyberKnife M6 radiosurgery system equipped with MLC (CyberKnife®, Accuray®, USA) is comparable to IMRT plans generated by linear accelerators [17].

1.10 Transarterial Radioembolization

Transarterial radioembolization (TARE) or selective internal radiation therapy (SIRT) refers to the endovascular injection of tiny microspheres made of glass or resin conjugated with the pure β-emitting yttrium-90 into the feeding arteries of liver tumors. Similar to other types of embolization, TARE exploits the differential–difference of blood supply to the tumors (mainly from arteries) and the normal liver parenchyma (mainly from the portal venous system). β-emissions contributed by yttrium-90 have a very high energy of 2.3 MeV, but only a maximum penetration of 11 mm and a physical half-life of 64 hours, making them suitable for TARE with limited toxicities to the surrounding normal hepatic parenchymal cells [18]. Before actual treatment with yttrium-90 microspheres, hepatic angiography to identify the anatomy of the hepatic arterial vasculature and the injection of technetium-99 m macroaggregated albumin (MAA) followed by ^{99m}Tc-MAA scanning to assess the potential for shunting microspheres to the lungs as well as the potential for the deposition of microspheres to the gastrointestinal tract. Yttrium-90 injection cannot be considered to a patient if (1) deposition of microspheres to the gastrointestinal tract that cannot be corrected by placement of the catheter distal to collateral vessels or the application of standard angiographic techniques, such as coil embolization to prevent deposition of microspheres elsewhere in the gastrointestinal tract, of (2) exposure of radiation to the lungs of 30 Gy for a single injection. The interventionalists have to determine the exact location of placement of the catheter based on the hepatic vascular anatomy in the angiographic findings. Coil embolization may be required to allow safe injection of microspheres into the arteries supplying the tumors but not the other non-tumor supplying vessels, so as to minimize the risk of radiation damage to other organs/structures.

In a retrospective study, TARE produced complete pathological necrosis in 61% of treated lesions and 89% of lesions of <3 cm) [19]. However, the two recently published phase 3 randomized-controlled trials (SIRveNIB SARAH) on TARE for locally advanced inoperable HCC did not improve overall survival compared to sorafenib [20, 21].

1.11 Further Technological Advances of Radiotherapy for Liver Cancer

As mentioned before, technological advances in radiation techniques and improved clinical and radiobiological understanding of liver cancers have made the classical type of RILD rare. However, there might still be occasions where nonfatal but persistent nonclassical RILD could occur after SBRT or 3DCRT. It was previously reported that the nonclassical RILD can be observed in 3–46% of patients after radiation therapy [22–30]. The discovery and emergence of charged particle therapy (CPT) which involves entirely different principles of cancer radiobiology have made a tremendous paradigm shift in radiotherapy for liver cancer. Currently, proton beam therapy and carbon ion radiotherapy as the most clinically applicable types of CPT have been extensively explored and evaluated in liver cancer treatment.

The obvious advantage of CPT over photon therapy with X-ray or gamma-rays lies in its characteristic pathway when penetrating into the tissues. Instead of following the inverse square law for photons in which the radiation dose was progressively deposited along the beam path, CPT dissipates a very small amount of energy until at a certain depth where most of the energy is deposited within a very short distance known as the Bragg peak. Every type of CPT has an inherently and characteristically distinct Bragg peak which can be slightly modified manually by contemporary technologies. In clinical practice, multiple Bragg peaks of different energies are conglomerated with each other to create a spread-out Bragg peak, so that very minimal radiation exit dose will be deposited beyond the tumor target. Besides, the relative biological effectiveness (RBE) for CPT is also higher than that of the photon. For protons, the RBE is approximately 1.1 in the clinical setting though it is dependent on various factors including tissue-specific radiosensitivity, biological endpoint, dose level, and oxygen concentration [31–33]. Therefore, the benefits of protons over photons are contributed by its characteristic energy deposition rather than the biological advantage.

Compared to protons, carbon ions provide comparable physical characteristics of energy deposition but with a slightly less entrance dose. However, their RBEs are substantially higher than the RBEs of protons. Depending on the types of tissue, biological endpoint, depth, and other factors, the RBE for carbon ions ranged between 2 and 5 [34, 35]. Such higher RBEs for carbon ions are attributed to the higher linear energy transfer produced by heavier ions leading to greater radiobiological damage [36–38]. Such radiobiological characteristics render carbon ions particularly suited for treating radioresistant tumors, for example, sarcoma, chordoma, and also probably HCC [39]. Preclinical studies revealed that RBE values vary between 2 and 4 depending on the HCC subtypes, which may be further potentiated when given in combination with other systemic therapies like chemotherapy and targeted therapy [34, 40].

1.12 Conclusion

Radiotherapy has been gaining popularity and acceptability as a nonsurgical treatment modality for HCC. The recent advances in precise radiotherapy machines and treatment planning algorithms which produce highly conformal radiation plans allow for safe, swift, and effective delivery of high-dose ablative radiotherapy leading to promising local control and manageable toxicities. Further randomized-controlled trials on radiotherapy, with or without additional therapeutics, will help better define the role of radiotherapy in HCC management.

References

1. Delaney G, Jacob S, Featherstone C, et al. The role of radiotherapy in cancer treatment: estimating optimal utilisation from a review of evidence-based clinical guidelines. Cancer. 2005;104:1129–37.
2. Eccles CL, Dawson LA, Moseley JL, Brock KK. Interfraction liver shape variability and impact on GTV position during liver stereotactic radiotherapy using abdominal compression. Int J Radiat Oncol Biol Phys. 2011;80(3):938–46.
3. Shimohigashi Y, Toya R, Saito T, et al. Tumor motion changes in stereotactic body radiotherapy for liver tumors: an evaluation based on four-dimensional cone-beam computed tomography and fiducial markers. Radiat Oncol. 2017;12(1):61.
4. RTOG-1112 Randomized phase III study of sorafenib versus stereotactic body radiation therapy followed by sorafenib in hepatocellular carcinoma. NRG Oncol. https://www.nrgoncology.org/Clinical-Trials/Protocol/rtog-1112?filter=rtog-1112
5. Hanna GG, Murray L, Patel R, et al. UK consensus on normal tissue dose constraints for stereotactic radiotherapy. Clin Oncol (R Coll Radiol). 2018;30(1):5–14.
6. Pollom EL, Chin AL, Diehn M, Loo BW, Chang DT. Normal tissue constraints for abdominal and thoracic stereotactic body radiotherapy. Semin Radiat Oncol. 2017;27:197–208.
7. Thomas TO, Hasan S, Small W Jr, et al. The tolerance of gastrointestinal organs to stereotactic body radiation therapy: what do we know so far? J Gastrointest Oncol. 2014;5:236–46.
8. Milano MT, Katz AW, Schell MC, Phillip A, Okunieff P. Descriptive analysis of oligometastatic lesions treated with curative-intent stereotactic body radiotherapy. Int J Radiat Oncol Biol Phys. 2008;72:1516–22.
9. von Siebenthal M, Székely G, Lomax AJ, Cattin PC. Systematic errors in respiratory gating due to intrafraction deformations of the liver. Med Phys. 2007;34(9):3620–9.
10. Ingold JA, Reed GB, Kaplan HS, Bagshaw MA. Radiation hepatitis. Am J Roentgenol Radium Therapy Nucl Med. 1965;93:200–8.
11. Dawson LA, Normolle D, Balter JM, McGinn CJ, Lawrence TS, Ten Haken RK. Analysis of radiation-induced liver disease using the Lyman NTCP model. Int J Radiat Oncol Biol Phys. 2002;53:810–21.
12. Hou JZ, Zeng ZC, Wang BL, Yang P, Zhang JY, Mo HF. High dose radiotherapy with image-guided hypo-IMRT for hepatocellular carcinoma with portal vein and/or inferior vena cava tumor thrombi is more feasible and efficacious than conventional 3D-CRT. Jpn J Clin Oncol. 2016;46(4):357–62.
13. Wang PM, Hsu WC, Chung NN, et al. Feasibility of stereotactic body radiation therapy with volumetric modulated arc therapy and high intensity photon beams for hepatocellular carcinoma patients. Radiat Oncol. 2014;9:18.

14. Bae SH, Jang WI, Park HC. Intensity-modulated radiotherapy for hepatocellular carcinoma: dosimetric and clinical results. Oncotarget. 2017;8(35):59965–76.
15. Kim JW, Kim DY, Han KH, Seong J. Phase I/II trial of helical IMRT-based stereotactic body radiotherapy for hepatocellular carcinoma. Dig Liver Dis. 2019;51(3):445–51.
16. Scorsetti M, Comito T, Cozzi L, et al. The challenge of inoperable hepatocellular carcinoma (HCC): results of a single-institutional experience on stereotactic body radiation therapy (SBRT). J Cancer Res Clin Oncol. 2015;141(7):1301–9.
17. Jin L, Price RA, Wang L, et al. Dosimetric and delivery efficiency investigation for treating hepatic lesions with a MLC-equipped robotic radiosurgery-radiotherapy combined system. Med Phys. 2016;43(2):727–33.
18. Venkatanarasimha N, Gogna A, Tong KTA, et al. Radioembolisation of hepatocellular carcinoma: a primer. Clin Radiol. 2017;72:1002–13.
19. Riaz A, Kulik L, Lewandowski RJ, et al. Radiologic-pathologic correlation of hepatocellular carcinoma treated with internal radiation using yttrium-90 microspheres. Hepatology. 2009;49:1185–93.
20. Chow PKH, Gandhi M, Tan SB, et al. SIRveNIB: selective internal radiation therapy versus sorafenib in Asia-Pacific patients with hepatocellular carcinoma. J Clin Oncol. 2018;36(19):1913–21.
21. Vilgrain V, Pereira H, Assenat E, et al. Efficacy and safety of selective internal radiotherapy with yttrium-90 resin microspheres compared with sorafenib in locally advanced and inoperable hepatocellular carcinoma (SARAH): an open-label randomised controlled phase 3 trial. Lancet Oncol. 2017;18(12):1624–36.
22. Bujold A, Massey CA, Kim JJ, et al. Sequential phase I and II trials of stereotactic body radiotherapy for locally advanced hepatocellular carcinoma. J Clin Oncol. 2013;31:1631–9.
23. Chapman TR, Bowen SR, Schaub SK, et al. Toward consensus reporting of radiation-induced liver toxicity in the treatment of primary liver malignancies: defining clinically relevant endpoints. Pract Radiat Oncol. 2017;8(3):157–66.
24. Culleton S, Jiang H, Haddad CR, et al. Outcomes following definitive stereotactic body radiotherapy for patients with Child-Pugh B or C hepatocellular carcinoma. Radiother Oncol. 2014;111:412–7.
25. Lasley FD, Mannina EM, Johnson CS, et al. Treatment variables related to liver toxicity in patients with hepatocellular carcinoma, Child-Pugh class A and B enrolled in a phase1-2 trial of stereotactic body radiation therapy. Pract Radiat Oncol. 2015;5:e443–9.
26. Que J, Kuo HT, Lin LC, et al. Clinical outcomes and prognostic factors of cyberknife stereotactic body radiation therapy for unresectable hepatocellular carcinoma. BMC Cancer. 2016;16:451.
27. Sanuki N, Takeda A, Oku Y, et al. Influence of liver toxicities on prognosis after stereotactic body radiation therapy for hepatocellular carcinoma. Hepatol Res. 2015;45:540–7.
28. Sanuki N, Takeda A, Oku Y, et al. Stereotactic body radiotherapy for small hepatocellular carcinoma: a retrospective outcome analysis in 185 patients. Acta Oncol. 2014;53:399–404.
29. Song JH, Jeong BK, Choi HS, et al. Defining radiation-induced hepatic toxicity in hepatocellular carcinoma patients treated with stereotactic body radiotherapy. J Cancer. 2017;8:4155–61.
30. Velec M, Haddad CR, Craig T, et al. Predictors of liver toxicity following stereotactic body radiation therapy for hepatocellular carcinoma. Int J Radiat Oncol Biol Phys. 2017;97:939–46.
31. Giovannini G, Bohlen T, Cabal G, et al. Variable RBE in proton therapy: comparison of different model predictions and their influence on clinical-like scenarios. Radiat Oncol. 2016;11:68.
32. Paganetti H. Relative biological effectiveness (RBE) values for proton beam therapy. Variations as a function of biological endpoint, dose, and linear energy transfer. Phys Med Biol. 2014;59:R419–72.
33. Paganetti H, Niemierko A, Ancukiewicz M, et al. Relative biological effectiveness (RBE) values for proton beam therapy. Int J Radiat Oncol Biol Phys. 2002;53:407–21.
34. Habermehl D, Ilicic K, Dehne S, et al. The relative biological effectiveness for carbon and oxygen ion beams using theraster-scanning technique in hepatocellular carcinoma cell lines. PLoS One. 2014;9:e113591.
35. Habermehl D, Debus J, Ganten T, et al. Hypofractionated carbon ion therapy delivered with scanned ion beams for patients with hepatocellular carcinoma -feasibility and clinical response. Radiat Oncol. 2013;l8:59.
36. El Shafie RA, Habermehl D, Rieken S, et al. In vitro evaluation of photon and raster-scanned carbon ion radiotherapy in combination with gemcitabine in pancreatic cancer cell lines. J Radiat Res. 2013;54(Suppl 1):i113–9.
37. Dreher C, Habermehl D, Ecker S, et al. Optimization of carbon ion and proton treatment plans using the raster-scanning technique for patients with unresectable pancreatic cancer. Radiat Oncol. 2015;10:237.
38. Combs SE, Zipp L, Rieken S, et al. In vitro evaluation of photon and carbon ion radiotherapy in combination with chemotherapy in glioblastoma cells. Radiat Oncol. 2012;7:9.
39. Kamada T, Tsujii H, Blakely EA, et al. Carbon ion radiotherapy in Japan: an assessment of 20 years of clinical experience. Lancet Oncol. 2015;16:e93–e100.
40. Dehne S, Fritz C, Rieken S, et al. Combination of photon and carbon ion irradiation with targeted therapy substances temsirolimus and gemcitabine in hepatocellular carcinoma cell lines. Front Oncol. 2017;7:35.

Radiobiology of the Liver

Rafi Kabarriti and Chandan Guha

Abstract

Advancements in imaging and radiation treatment planning have resulted in the increasing use of radiation therapy (RT) for liver cancer. However, Radiation-induced liver disease (RILD) remains a major limitation of RT. The pathophysiology, diagnosis, and treatment of RILD are discussed in this chapter. Classic RILD manifests with hepatomegaly, anicteric ascites, and thrombocytopenia, and alkaline phosphatase elevated out of proportion to other liver enzymes, 1–3 months after liver RT. The pathological hallmark is that of veno-occlusive disease (VOD) and sinusoidal obstructive syndrome (SOS). In addition to endothelial cell damage, hepatic stellate cell activation is noted in patients with severe congestive changes of classic RILD. There are multiple clinically useful tools, such as Model for End-Stage Liver Disease (MELD), Child–Turcotte–Pugh (CTP) classification, ALBI and PALBI grades to quantify liver function changes following RT. Other more interventional laboratory measures that have been investigated to measure liver function include Indocyanine green (ICG) and HepQuant SHUNT test that require administration of ICG or cholate and measuring their clearance rates. Potential biomarkers of liver toxicity include those related to endothelial injury and increased expression of adhesion molecules, pro-inflammatory and procoagulant cytokines. In patients suspected of developing classic RILD, early diagnosis and intervention can potentially improve outcomes. Baseline and serial imaging using ultrasound, portal venous perfusion imaging by dynamic contrast-enhanced computed tomography (CT) or magnetic resonance imaging (MRI) may help detect early signs suggestive of VOD/SOS and more importantly to exclude diagnoses other than VOD/SOS. The current management of RILD is mostly supportive with no approved pharmacologic therapy to date. Strategies to potentially treat RILD including TGFβ inhibition, Hedgehog inhibition, CXCR4 inhibition, hepatocyte transplantation, and bone marrow-derived stromal cell therapy are currently under investigation. Taking advantage of radiation as an immunomodulatory drug for in situ tumor vaccination provides the rationale for combining SBRT with immunotherapy for the treatment of liver cancer.

R. Kabarriti
Departments of Radiation Oncology, Montefiore Medical Center, Albert Einstein College of Medicine, Bronx, NY, USA

C. Guha (✉)
Departments of Radiation Oncology, Montefiore Medical Center, Albert Einstein College of Medicine, Bronx, NY, USA

Department of Pathology, Montefiore Medical Center, Albert Einstein College of Medicine, Bronx, NY, USA

Keywords

Liver radiobiology · Radiation-induced liver disease · RILD · Biomarkers · Liver functional imaging

2.1 Whole Liver Radiation Therapy (RT)

Prior to the availability of megavoltage RT, the liver was thought to be a relatively radioresistant organ based on the limited reports of liver toxicity in the era where 200–250 kV X-ray was the only available external beam treatment modality with poor penetration of the beam and the limiting skin dose [1]. As it became feasible to treat the whole liver with higher radiation doses using megavoltage RT, it quickly became clear that liver toxicity was dose dependent. In 1965, Ingold et al. reported on the radiation effects on the liver where 13 of 40 patients receiving whole liver irradiation developed a clinical syndrome which they termed as "radiation hepatitis" [2]. More specifically, they reported on the dose–complication relationship for whole liver RT where "radiation hepatitis" occurred in 1/8 (12.5%) patients who received 30–35 Gy over 3–4 weeks and 12/27 (44%) patients who received >35 Gy. This "radiation hepatitis" was characterized by the development of abnormal liver function tests, hepatomegaly, and ascites, progressing to a fatal outcome. Serum alkaline phosphatase was the most reliable laboratory index of radiation damage and radiation hepatitis.

In 1976, the Radiation Therapy Oncology Group (RTOG) initiated a pilot study (RTOG 7605) using whole liver RT for palliation of hepatic metastasis in 109 patients using various dosing schemas including 21 Gy in 7 fractions, 20 Gy in 10 fractions, 25.60 Gy in 16 fractions and 30 Gy in 15 fractions. While these relatively low doses were safe and offered palliation with some symptomatic improvement and no documented cases of RILD, there was no impact on overall survival with a median survival of 11 weeks [3].

In the 1980s, there was interest in testing accelerated hyperfractionated whole liver RT utilizing 1.2–1.5 Gy fractions twice daily to total doses of 24–33 Gy as well as addition of chemotherapy to improve response rates and decrease toxicity rates in patients with HCC and liver metastasis [4, 5]. By shortening overall treatment time and reducing inter-treatment interval using accelerated RT, the goal was to reduce the likelihood for tumor repopulation by rapidly proliferating tumor cells. This was thought to be especially important for HCC given the rapid doubling time for HCC cells. At the same time, hyperfractionation can increase the opportunity for proliferating tumor clonogens to redistribute into more sensitive portions of the cell cycle, allowing for more efficient cell killing with each ensuing fraction. By reducing fraction size, hyperfractionation may also permit delivery of higher total doses with equivalent or potentially lesser late effects as late effects are dependent on fraction size. Unfortunately, despite the use of hyperfractionated RT even when combined with radiosensitizing chemotherapy, total radiation doses remained relatively low and did not demonstrate a significant benefit over standard daily radiation, but acute toxicity appeared to be higher. In addition, the arm with total doses of 33 Gy in 1.5 Gy BID fractions carried a substantial risk of delayed radiation injury with 5 of 51 patients developing severe (grade 3) "radiation hepatitis" [4]. In 1991, Emami et al. described the whole liver tolerances where whole liver irradiation of 30 and 40 Gy had an estimated 5% and 50% risk of RILD, respectively [6].

2.2 Partial Liver RT

Advancements in imaging and radiation delivery, to better visualize and treat liver tumors using three-dimensional conformal RT (3D-CRT), allowed for dose escalation studies where only part of the liver was treated. Studies at the University of Michigan, which collected quantitative dose-volume data, showed that dose escalation with partial liver RT was safe and feasible. Interestingly, while the irradiated liver lobes atrophied, the unirradiated liver lobes showed compensatory hypertrophy. Using data from 203 patients, treated by 3D-CRT technique with a median dose of 60.75 Gy combined with concurrent Floxuridine (FUdR) or BUdR via hepatic artery infusion, Dawson et al. reported on the dose-volume tolerance for radiation-induced liver disease (RILD) using the Lyman–Kutcher–Burman normal tissue complication probability (NTCP) model [7]. They demonstrated that the liver exhibits a large volume effect for RILD and the mean liver dose was a relatively simple parameter that was found to be strongly associated with the development of RILD. Radiation dose was limited by the volume of liver irradiated where the radiation dose needs to be decreased as the volume of treated liver increases in larger tumors as radiation liver injury was still a concern. The revised models also showed that patients with primary hepatobiliary malignancies that had underlying liver dysfunction had a lower tolerance to liver radiation than patients with liver metastases. The published Quantitative Normal Tissue Effects in The Clinic (QUANTEC) report on radiation-associated liver injury confirmed that the risk of RILD in the treatment of primary liver tumors increases rapidly as the mean liver dose becomes greater than 30 Gy in 2-Gy fractions [8]. However, with advanced treatment planning very high doses (up to 90 Gy) can be administered if the radiation volume is small enough (~1/3 of the total liver volume) and mean normal liver dose (liver minus gross tumor volume) can be kept under 28 Gy in 2 Gy fractions for primary liver cancer and <32 Gy in 2 Gy fractions for liver metastasis [8].

2.3 Hypofractionation/ Stereotactic Body Radiation Therapy (SBRT)

The advent of image-guided RT, respiratory motion management, and use of multiple coplanar and non-coplanar radiation fields allowed for the introduction of stereotactic body RT (SBRT) or stereotactic ablative radiotherapy (SABR) to deliver high ablative doses of radiation to well-defined targets in the liver with high accuracy and steep dose gradients. This highly conformal type of RT with steep dose gradients between the target and normal tissues allows for delivery of high and potentially ablative doses of radiation to the tumor while minimizing dose to the uninvolved liver and surrounding organs at risk. Several clinical studies have recently demonstrated excellent local control of the irradiated liver tumor using short courses (1–5 fractions) of hypofractionated RT [9–19].

The cytocidal effects of ionizing radiation are primarily mediated by dose-dependent generation of oxidative free radicals that cause cellular DNA damage, resulting in cell cycle arrest and senescence, as well as cell death via mitotic catastrophe, apoptosis, necrosis, and necroptosis of irradiated cells. Conventional radiotherapy fractionation schedules take advantage of reoxygenation and redistribution of cancer cells to more radiosensitive points of the cell cycle. However, fractionation with a lower dose fraction also allows for the survival of cancer stem cells, enabling repopulation and tumor regrowth. The radiobiological mechanisms that govern SBRT remain under investigation, although the interplay of a highly ablative dose of radiation and tumor vasculature has been identified as a promising explanation for its effect. SBRT allows for the ablation of the tumor endothelium due to acid sphingomyelinase-mediated generation of ceramide in cell surface lipid rafts that signals the induction of apoptosis in the microvascular endothelium of the irradiated stromal tissues [20]. Although SBRT is used primarily to achieve local control of liver tumors, there is emerging data that antitumor immunity may be enhanced through the delivery of highly ablative doses of radiation. Ablative radiation promotes the release of tumor antigens and damage-associated molecular pattern (DAMP) molecules from irradiated tumor cells for activation of dendritic cells (DC). DCs engulf, process, and cross-present tumor antigens on class I MHC for activating CD8+ cytotoxic T cells (CTLs) that are responsible for eradicating surviving clonogens in the irradiated tumor. In murine models of melanoma [21], colorectal cancer [22] and hepatocellular cancer [23, 24], ablation of immune effector cells, especially CD8+ T cells abrogated control of both local and systemic disease and cure. These studies suggest that RT can induce local and systemic anti-tumoral immunity that contributes to the high rates of tumor control, usually seen after SBRT. Furthermore, SBRT can be applied to convert an immunologically "cold" tumor to immune effector cell-rich "hot" tumors by promoting antigen and DAMP release and infiltration and activation of CD8+ CTLs in irradiated tumors, thereby generating an autologous in situ tumor vaccine.

2.4 Radiation-Induced Liver Disease (RILD)

RILD remains a major limitation of RT even when using SBRT for the treatment of liver cancer. A critical volume from the uninvolved liver of at least 700 cm^3 in patients with liver metastasis should receive <15 Gy in 3 fractions to reduce the likelihood of RILD [8]. Patients with underlying liver cirrhosis need to spare larger volumes of the uninvolved liver and use more fractions (5 fractions) in advanced cirrhosis to lower the risk of RILD [8].

Classic RILD manifests with hepatomegaly, anicteric ascites, and thrombocytopenia, and alkaline phosphatase elevated out of proportion to other liver enzymes [25], 1–3 months after liver RT. Symptoms can include fatigue, abdominal pain, and increased abdominal girth as a result of portal hypertension and ascites. The pathological hallmark is that of veno-occlusive disease (VOD) of the central and sublobular veins and centrilobular sinusoids [26, 27]. Morphologically, VOD is characterized by occlusion of the central vein lumen by erythrocytes trapped in a dense meshwork of reticulin and collagen fibers, with atrophy of centrilobular liver plates and loss of acinar zone 3 hepatocytes typically observed [26, 27]. The term sinusoidal obstructive syndrome (SOS) has been proposed as a better description of the pathology of liver injury seen after the administration of chemotherapy with or without RT [28]. In addition to endothelial cell damage, hepatic stellate cell activation is noted in patients with severe RILD [29]. Hepatic stellate cells have multiple functions,

including modulating liver regeneration, secretion of lipoproteins, growth factors, and cytokines that play a key role in regulating inflammation and fibrosis. Of these cytokines, transforming growth factor-β (TGF-β) has been implicated in the perisinusoidal and hepatic fibrosis in RILD [30, 31] (Fig. 2.1).

2.5 Non-classic RILD

Other RT-induced liver toxicities have been termed "non-classic RILD" that presents with markedly elevated serum transaminases (>5X upper limit of normal), a general decline in liver function seen as worsening of Child–Pugh Score by 2 or more points, and reactivation of viral hepatitis. Non-classic RILD also may have elevated total bilirubin and low albumin levels and lacks the hepatomegaly, ascites, and elevated alkaline phosphatase seen in classic RILD. Patients with underlying liver disease, such as patients with hepatitis B, nonalcoholic fatty liver disease, cirrhosis of varying etiologies, limited post-resection normal liver volumes, prior hepatotoxic chemotherapy, and tumor-related dysfunction from vascular or biliary involvement are at increased risk for non-classic RILD [32].

In the non-classic RILD syndromes, hepatocellular loss and dysfunction along with hepatic sinusoidal endothelial death and stellate cell activation have also been noted. In livers with regenerating hepatocytes as in cirrhotic livers, radiation can induce mitotic catastrophe and cell death of the regenerating hepatocytes, thereby causing hepatocyte injury which manifests itself with markedly elevated serum transaminases (> 5 times the upper limit of normal) within 3 months of completion of hepatic RT [33]. Additionally, loss of hepatocellular regeneration capacity has been noted to be a consequence of hepatic irradiation and may render the irradiated liver incapable of compensatory hypertrophy that prevents irreversible hepatic failure [34]. Similarly, patients with Hepatitis B Virus carrier status have been shown to have an increased risk of this toxicity, compared to the noncarrier group. HBV reactivation is usually defined as an increase in

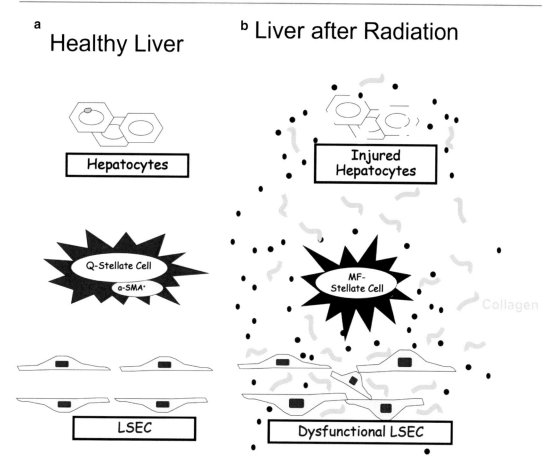

Fig. 2.1 (**a**) Unirradiated liver with healthy hepatocytes, quiescent stellate cell (Q-Stellate Cell), and liver sinusoidal endothelial (LSEC) cells. (**b**) Hepatic irradiation results in endothelial cell damage, hepatic stellate cell activation to activated myofibroblastic Stellate Cell (MF-Stellate Cell), hepatocyte dysfunction, and secretion of lipoproteins, growth factors, and cytokines resulting in perisinusoidal and hepatic fibrosis and modulation of liver regeneration

HBV DNA levels to more than 10 times the baseline level [35], and clinical presentation ranges from mild aminotransferase elevations to acute liver failure. Chou et al. demonstrated that the HBV reactivation is due to a bystander effect, whereby IL-6 is released from endothelial cells after irradiation, which acts upon infected hepatocytes to stimulate HBV replication [36].

While clinical data shows that liver SBRT is relatively safe with no overt liver toxicities in patients with cirrhosis and primary liver cancer, 10–30% of them will experience a decline in liver function, 3 months after SBRT, even without disease progression [37]. Investigators at the Princess Margaret Hospital showed that in Child–Pugh A patients, 29% had a progression in Child–Pugh class, 3 months after SBRT [38]. Similarly, investigators at the Indiana University reported 20% of Child–Pugh A patients experienced a decline in Child–Pugh class, 3 months after SBRT [39]. Pretreatment Child–Pugh status and the dose-volume constraints for the liver, including the absolute normal liver volume spared from at least 15 Gy (VS15) >700 mL and/or the percentage (%) of normal liver volume receiving more than 15 Gy (V15) <1/3 normal liver volume were critical determinants of RILD [40]. In addition, the tumor volume is also a significant predictor of liver function decline after SBRT [41]. Patients with Child–Pugh B or C and primary HCC are more likely to experience liver toxicities as defined by worsening liver function [42].

2.6 Laboratory Investigations

Currently, there are multiple clinically useful tools to quantify liver function which can be used to monitor liver changes related to RT and their association with baseline liver function and radiation dose (Table 2.1). Some of these include Model for End-Stage Liver Disease (MELD), Child–Turcotte–Pugh (CTP) classification, Albumin-Bilirubin (ALBI) and Platelet-albumin-bilirubin (PALBI) grades.

Table 2.1 Clinical tools to monitor liver function following radiotherapy

Clinical data	
Subjective	Fatigue, right upper quadrant pain, weight gain, increased abdominal girth, bleeding, decreased alertness, encephalopathy
Physical examination	Hepatomegaly, ascites, right upper quadrant tenderness, leg edema, anasarca
Laboratory data	
Model for End-Stage Liver Disease (MELD)	Serum bilirubin, creatinine, international normalized ratio (INR), and sodium
Child–Turcotte–Pugh (CTP) classification	Serum albumin, bilirubin and INR. Clinical assessments of ascites and encephalopathy
ALBI grade	Serum bilirubin and albumin
PALBI grade	Serum bilirubin, albumin and platelet count
Indocyanine green (ICG)	Serum clearance rate of ICG after intravenous administration
HepQuant SHUNT test	Measures liver function and blood flow using systemic and portal clearances of cholate and calculates disease severity index (DSI)
Imaging data	
Ultrasound	Hepatomegaly, splenomegaly, ascites, gallbladder wall thickening, portal vein dilation, decrease or reversal of the portal venous flow

Table 2.1 (continued)

Ultrasound transient Elastography	Liver stiffness, hepatic venous pressure gradient (HVPG)
Dynamic contrast-enhanced CT	Cross-sectional visualization of tumor, portal venous system and abdominal solid organs as well as demarcated region of reduced enhancement in radiation treatment zone. Atrophy of irradiated lobe with hypertrophy of non-irradiated lobes
Multiparametric dynamic gadoxetate disodium contrast-enhanced MRI	Cross-sectional imaging, blood flow dynamics, and spatial hepatocellular function
Asialoglycoprotein receptor (ASGPR) SPECT uptake scans	Functional hepatocyte mass by measuring the number of functional cell surface receptors on hepatocytes
Sulfur colloid SPECT uptake scans	Kupffer cell mass and function
PET/CT using [Nmethyl-11C] cholylsarcosine (^{11}C-CSar)	Bile acid biomarker to quantify hepatic excretory function
Wedged hepatic venous pressure gradient (WHVPG)	Measures the difference in pressure between the portal vein and the inferior vena cava which is elevated in patients with sinusoidal portal hypertension.
Biomarkers	
Inflammatory	TNFalpha and IL1β, IL8, sIL2R, VEGF
Endothelial	von Willebrand factor (vWF), thrombomodulin, and soluble intercellular adhesion molecule-1 (sICAM-1), PAI-1 (plasminogen activation inhibitor 1), endothelin 1, SDF-1 and CXCL12
Fibrosis	N-terminal propeptide for type III procollagen (P-III-P), TGF-β
Coagulation	Protein C, Antithrombin III, plasminogen
Circulating	Serum hyaluronic acid
Metabolomics	Plasma metabolites, regulation of amino acid and lipid metabolism, change in energy metabolism, calcium signaling, choline metabolism, pentose and purine metabolism and microbiome

MELD was originally developed to provide an assessment of mortality for patients undergoing transjugular intrahepatic portosystemic shunts [43]. It is based on three laboratory values including serum bilirubin, creatinine, and international normalized ratio (INR). It is used for the evaluation of hepatic reserve and was adopted by the United Network for Organ Sharing (UNOS) to stratify patients on the liver transplantation waiting list based on their risk of death within 3 months [44]. One of the advantages of MELD is that it includes creatinine which takes into account renal function and relies on objective laboratory tests. However, it has not been validated as a predictor of survival in patients with cirrhosis who are not on the transplantation waiting list.

Child–Turcotte–Pugh (CTP) classification was initially developed to predict mortality in patients with cirrhosis undergoing surgery for portal hypertension especially variceal bleeding [45]. It incorporates both laboratory measurements including serum albumin, bilirubin, and INR as well as clinical assessments of ascites and encephalopathy. It has routinely been used to estimate functional liver reserve and predict survival in patients with HCC [46, 47].

Albumin-Bilirubin (ALBI) grade is derived from serum bilirubin and albumin levels and has been used as a surrogate for liver function in patients with HCC. This was initially developed using a cohort of over 6000 patients from Japan, Europe, the United States, and China and was shown to provide objective and discriminatory measures of liver function in patients with HCC [48]. It performed as well as CTP score and was able to further categorize CTP A patients into either ALBI grade 1 or 2. Another advantage of ALBI grade is that it does not require the use of subjective variables such as ascites and encephalopathy which are needed for Child–Pugh grades.

Platelet-albumin-bilirubin (PALBI) grade was derived by adding platelet counts to ALBI score as a surrogate for portal hypertension [49]. A cohort of 6669 patients with HCC from a national cohort of the Korean Central Cancer Registry comparing CTP class, MELD score, and ALBI and PALBI grades as predictors for overall survival showed that PALBI and ALBI grades were more reliable for accessing liver function and predicting OS [50].

Both CTP and ALBI scores have been used to assess liver function in patients undergoing SBRT and a recent study looking at outcomes of SBRT for hepatocellular carcinoma without macrovascular invasion showed that 15.9% out of 214 evaluable patients experienced a worsening CP score and 21.2% of 241 evaluable patients had a worsening in ALBI grade, 3 months after SBRT [51].

Another laboratory measure that has been investigated to measure liver function is Indocyanine green (ICG). ICG uptake and metabolism can correlate with dynamic liver function but requires intravenous administration and collection of multiple serum samples after administration to measure clearance. After intravenous administration, ICG is taken up from the plasma almost exclusively by the hepatic parenchymal cells and is secreted into the bile. A serum clearance rate of ICG, as a result, can potentially serve as a reliable index of liver function. To measure ICG clearance, patients are given ICG intravenously via catheter and then serum samples are collected at approximately 5, 10, 15, and 20 min after injecting the dye. ICG clearance has been used extensively in Asia to assess the safety of liver resections for HCC and to predict survival in critically ill patients. Investigators at the University of Michigan have used ICG to predict liver injury after treatment and have also used it to adapt the radiation dose to minimize the risk of toxicity. Using this technique, 69 patients achieved 95% 2-year local control and only 7% of patients had liver deterioration (as determined by an increase in Child–Pugh Score by 2 points) [52].

A more recent laboratory measure that is being investigated to measure liver function is the HepQuant SHUNT test that measures cholate hepatic uptake from both systemic and portal circulations to calculate the degree of portosystemic shunting as well as hepatic function using disease severe index (DSI). Both of these measures have been shown to correlate with the severity of chronic liver disease and in studies detected and measured the severity and progression of disease and the response to treatments [53, 54]. The HepQuant SHUNT test requires intravenous and oral administration of cholate and collection of multiple serum samples up to 90 minutes after administration which may make its routine clinical use difficult.

A metabolomic approach has been used to determine metabolic signatures that could serve as biomarkers for early detection of RILD [55]. In mice receiving 0, 10, or 50 Gy whole liver irradiation in 1 fraction, there was a change in energy metabolism, calcium signaling, choline metabolism, pentose and purine metabolism, and microbiome in response to liver irradiation. The plasma metabolites showed radiation dose dependence, and a dependence on the microbiome, allowing for the potential use of these metabolites as a biomarker for identifying patients at risk of developing RILD [55]. In patients undergoing liver SBRT, dysregulation of amino acid and lipid metabolism after only one to two of the planned six fractions of SBRT was associated with radiation-induced liver injury at 3 months post treatment in HCC patients. Specifically, there was differential upregulation of serine, alanine, taurine, and lipid metabolites early during SBRT compared to baseline, suggesting that high protein and lipid turnover early during SBRT may portend for greater liver toxicity [56].

Other potential biomarkers of liver toxicity, while not specifically studied after liver irradiation, have been investigated to predict sinusoidal endothelial cell injury and VOD in patients with bone marrow transplantation. These include biomarkers of endothelial injury and increased expression of adhesion molecules, proinflammatory cytokines, and procoagulant factors [32]. Biomarkers of endothelial injury including von Willebrand Factor (vWF), thrombomodulin, and soluble intercellular adhesion molecule-1 (sICAM-1) were significantly elevated in patients with VOD and were able to predict the development of VOD/SOS with high sensitivity and specificity in patients treated with sirolimus [57]. Elevated serum levels of plasminogen activator inhibitor type 1 (PAI-1), probably produced by activated stellate cells and damaged endothelial cells, can potentially distinguish liver injury of SOS from other common forms of liver dysfunction, such as hepatitis and graft-versus-host disease. Particularly when associated with hyperbilirubinemia [58, 59]. Serum levels of hyaluronic acid have been shown to be a marker of sinusoidal endothelial injury in rodents after liver irradiation [60] and are also elevated in patients with SOS/VOD [61]. Low levels of antithrombin (AT) and protein C, reflecting a hypercoagulable state, have also been noted in patients with SOS [62]. Platelet refractoriness has been well described in pediatric VOD/SOS literature and is presumably due to endothelial activation [63]. Because stellate cell-mediated hepatic subendothelial fibrosis is ongoing in RILD and VOD, markers of fibrosis such as TGF-β, collagen propeptide, and N-terminal peptide of type III procollagen remain elevated [32, 64, 65].

2.6.1 Imaging of Liver Injury

Following liver irradiation, the irradiated liver atrophies and the non-irradiated liver undergoes hypertrophy to compensate and maintain fixed physiologic organ size. Computed tomography findings following conventionally fractionated radiotherapy and SBRT demonstrate a reversible region of reduced enhancement within the irradiation region compared with the corresponding liver, possibly representing increased water or fat content in the irradiated liver. Depending on the volume of irradiated liver and baseline liver function, there can be eventual atrophy of the irradiated segment and compensatory hypertrophy of the untreated liver [32]. However, these radiographic findings do not correlate with the clinical manifestation of RILD. Using portal venous perfusion imaging by dynamic contrast-enhanced (DCE) computed tomography (CT) [66] or magnetic resonance imaging (MRI) [67], Cao et al. showed a decrease in portal perfusion after RT, likely indicating radiation-induced SOS. There was substantial variability in the individual sensitivity to hepatic radiation injury, and there was a significant correlation between the mean liver portal venous perfusion and liver function as measured by ICG-R15 retention. While these studies provide information on blood flow, they provide little if any information regarding hepatocellular function [32].

Asialoglycoprotein receptor (ASGPR) uptake scans using noninvasive single-photon emission computed tomography scans can be used for hepatocellular function. ASGPRs are receptors found on the sinusoidal surface of hepatocytes that mediate the removal of serum glycoproteins, lipoproteins, fibronectin, and apoptotic cells. Liver-directed hypofractionated RT in cynomolgus monkeys resulted in a significant time-dependent reduction in hepatocyte receptor function as determined by ASGPR-mediated imaging studies [68]. The alteration in the modified ASGPR index persisted for more than a year after RT and was associated with a corresponding rise in ASGPR ligand clearance indices, likely reflecting impaired expression of this receptor. Hepatic ASGPR function decreased to 40–60% of pretreatment values after a single course of RT [68]. Therefore, the uptake and subsequent endocytosis of labeled asialoglycoproteins can be imaged to distinguish functional regions of hepatocytes from nonfunctional zones.

In addition to impacting hepatocellular function, hepatic irradiation inhibits the phagocytic capacity of Kupffer cells in rodents [60]. ^{99m}Tc-labeled Sulfur Colloid SPECT/CT in a mouse model of liver irradiation showed decreased uptake of the radionuclide in the irradiated region of the mouse liver [69]. Similar to sulfur colloid, superparamagnetic iron oxide is a particulate magnetic resonance contrast agent that is selectively taken up by the Kupffer cells. Superparamagnetic iron oxide (SPIO) –enhanced T2-weighted gradient echo (GRE) imaging was also able to detect subclinical SOS in patients with chemotherapy-treated colorectal liver metastases [70].

Other SPECT tracers that may have utility in assessing liver function include ^{99m}Tc-labeled diethylene triamine penta-acetate–galactosyl human serum albumin (^{99m}Tc-GSA) which has been used clinically and may offer complimentary advantages as it would not be dependent on liver blood flow and other biochemical processes

[71]. ^{99m}Tc-mebrofenin could also be used as another alternative to measure total or regional liver function [72].

Dynamic gadoxetate disodium contrast-enhanced MRI imaging has the potential to not only provide information on blood flow but also to provide information regarding hepatocellular function. Approximately 50% of an injected dose of gadoxetate disodium is taken up by the liver. Gadoxetic acid distributes into the vascular and extravascular spaces during the arterial, portal venous, and late dynamic phases, and then progressively into the hepatocytes and bile ducts during the hepatobiliary phase. Analysis of this imaging for liver function assessments has not been fully established yet. A solution suggested by a group from Japan assigned any part of the liver with a signal ≥ 1.5 times that of the spleen on delayed post-contrast imaging as functional liver based on contrast-enhanced MRI scans acquired in the hepatobiliary phase [73]. Strategies to generate functional liver maps using multiparametric contrast-enhanced MRI scans have the potential to risk-stratify and monitor patients at risk of radiation-induced liver injury and develop RT plans that optimally spare functional liver uninvolved by tumor.

In patients suspected of developing classic RILD, early diagnosis and intervention can potentially improve outcomes. Baseline and serial ultrasound may help detect early signs suggestive of VOD/SOS and more importantly to exclude diagnoses other than VOD/SOS. Findings on ultrasound that are more specific for SOS/VOD include a decrease or reversal of the portal venous flow [74]. However, this is generally believed to be a late finding. Other less specific findings on ultrasound can include hepatomegaly, splenomegaly, ascites, gallbladder wall thickening, and portal vein dilation [74]. Newer ultrasound technologies, including shear wave elastography [75] and contrast enhancement [76] are promising strategies for the early detection and monitoring of SOS/VOD. Liver stiffness measurements assessed by transient elastography (FibroScan; Echosens, Paris, France) can be used to identify clinically significant portal hypertension, and clinical studies have shown a good correlation between liver stiffness and the hepatic venous pressure gradient (HVPG), the gold standard in the evaluation of portal pressure [74, 77]. MRI and CT imaging provide excellent cross-sectional visualization of the portal venous system and abdominal solid organs but do not clearly offer major advantages over ultrasound, especially in patients suspected to have SOS/VOD. However, advanced MR imaging such as magnetic resonance elastography and superparamagnetic iron oxide (SPIO)-enhanced T2-weighted gradient echo (GRE) imaging may have a role in risk-stratification before treatment. Superparamagnetic iron oxide (SPIO)-enhanced T2-weighted gradient echo (GRE) imaging was also able to detect subclinical SOS in patients with chemotherapy-treated colorectal liver metastases [70].

2.6.2 Therapeutic Approaches for RILD

Current management of radiation-induced liver toxicity is mostly supportive with the use of diuretics to relieve fluid retention, analgesics for pain, paracentesis for tense ascites, correction of coagulopathy, and steroids to prevent hepatic congestion are used as supportive care. Given the pathophysiology behind RILD involves VOD with the presence of clots in central veins, tissue plasminogen activator (tPA) with or without heparin anticoagulation has been used as treatments. In a large anticoagulation study, although 12 out of 42 patients (29%) with severe VOD who received tPA and concomitant heparin responded to the therapy, it was also associated with a significant risk of life-threatening hemorrhage. Therefore, the authors concluded that tPA/heparin should be given early during the course of VOD and be avoided in patients with multi-organ failure [78]. Defibrotide (Defitelio®) is a bovine and porcine oligonucleotide that has fibrinolytic antithrombotic properties and is currently approved for the treatment of adult and pediatric patients with hepatic VOD, also known as sinusoidal obstruction syndrome (SOS), with

renal or pulmonary dysfunction following hematopoietic stem-cell transplantation (HSCT). Defibrotide has been used in RILD with some success [79].

The main approach to RILD is prevention or risk minimization; however, there is currently no approved radioprotective agent. Radioprotective agents for RILD are currently being investigated. In one study, classic RILD occurred in only 4 of 23 patients treated with amifostine in combination with whole liver radiation for diffuse metastatic liver disease despite treating to doses of 40 Gy or more to the whole liver [80]. Amifostine is currently approved to prevent renal toxicity in patients receiving repeated cycles of cisplatin for advanced ovarian cancer, and xerostomia in patients receiving radiation after surgery for some head and neck cancers. In another study, low molecular weight heparin, pentoxifylline, and ursodeoxycholic acid were found to be protective when MR changes were used as an indication of early RILD [81]. Other strategies to potentially treat RILD include TGFβ inhibition, Hedgehog inhibition, CXCR4 inhibition, hepatocyte transplantation, and bone marrow-derived stromal cell therapy, and are currently under investigation [79].

Regarding HBV reactivation, guidelines for the treatment of chronic hepatitis B infection from the American Association for the Study of Liver Diseases [82] recommend HBsAg and anti-HBc (total or immunoglobulin G) testing be performed in all persons before initiation of any immunosuppressive, cytotoxic, or immunomodulatory therapy. More specifically, anti-HBV prophylaxis should be initiated in patients who are HBsAg-positive and anti-HBc-positive, while patients who are HBsAg-negative, anti-HBc-positive patients could be carefully monitored with ALT, HBV DNA, and HBsAg with the intent for on-demand therapy, with some exceptions. The preferred anti-HBV drugs are ones with a high resistance barrier as follows: pegylated interferon-alpha, entecavir, and tenofovir versus the less preferred low resistance barrier agents: lamivudine, adefovir, and telbivudine.

2.6.3 Future Directions

2.6.3.1 Cell Transplantation to Ameliorate RILD

Hepatocyte transplantation has been considered an alternative to orthotopic liver transplantation for the treatment of end-stage metabolic disorders for decades. However, one major hurdle that has prevented large-scale clinical application is the low engraftment and repopulation efficiency of transplanted cells. Using preparative hepatic irradiation, transplanted hepatocytes engraft and repopulate in the irradiated livers in mice and rats [83]. Furthermore, hepatocyte transplantation after preparative HIR completely ameliorated inherited liver-based metabolic disorder in rodent and murine models of Crigler–Najjar syndrome, primary hyperoxaluria, and hypercholesterolemia [60, 83]. Extrapolating this concept to RILD, transplantation of unirradiated hepatocytes into irradiated livers ameliorated RILD and improved survival of rats treated with partial hepatic resection and RT [34]. Second, intraportal transplantation of LSEC, in combination with HGF, induced engraftment and gradual regeneration of the radiation-damaged hepatic sinusoidal endothelium by the donor cells, thereby ameliorating RT-induced sinusoidal obstruction syndrome [34, 84]. Given the scarcity of liver organs, strategies using cell transplantation to treat patients with RILD may offer a novel way to regenerate the liver [85].

2.6.3.2 Radiation as an Immunomodulatory Drug *for* In Situ Tumor Vaccination

Radiotherapy improves tumor-specific immune responses in many preclinical studies by inducing necrotic cell death. As a result, SBRT can elicit an abscopal effect which is an immune process that eliminates tumors outside the RT field. This abscopal effect is likely due to promoting effector T cells at the tumor site and induce expression of molecules that enhances tumor cell recognition by T cells. Indeed, in a correlative study, SBRT increased peripheral memory CD4+ and CD8+ T cells after irradiation to parenchymal sites [86]. However, the abscopal effect is rare and RT alone was insufficient to generate a robust concentration of CD8 T cells to effectively inhibit tumor growth. Conversely, high-dose hypofractionation radiation can potentially induce an immune-mediated abscopal effect when combined with immunotherapy [87]. It was also shown that DNA double-strand damages (main form of ionizing radiation damage) up-regulate PD-L1 expression in cancer cells and thereby contributing to an immunotolerant environment [88]. These attributes taken together provide the rationale for combining SBRT with immunotherapy to increase the immunogenicity of the tumor cells by decreasing immunotolerance and decrease cancer progression.

Not all radiation fractionation is equal with respect to its immunomodulatory effects. The scheduling, dosing, and the total time of treatment of radiation on tumors have been shown to have differing immunomodulatory effects. Ablative fractionation causes immunogenic cell death with >90% local control of the irradiated tumors. Conventional fractionation, on the other hand, using lower dose daily fractions delivered over weeks is typically considered immunosuppressive, repeatedly killing any radiosensitive infiltrating immune cells [89]. Sub-ablative RT increases the expression of immunomodulatory molecules on the tumor cell surface, thereby increasing the susceptibility of the surviving tumor cells to CTL attack. However, subablative RT also increases the recruitment of bone marrow-derived CD11b + myeloid cells that promote vasculogenesis and tumor regrowth [90, 91]. For an in situ vaccine approach, sub-ablative doses of RT could fail to provide an immune-activating tumor microenvironment, in part because of the post-ablation recruitment of myeloid cells and vasculogenesis, mediated by HIF-1-dependent stromal cell-derived factor-1 (SDF-1) and its receptor, CXCR4 [90, 92].

For in situ tumor vaccination using RT to be effective, an intact cancer immunity cycle with each step working in cohort with the next is required [93]. The steps include the release and engulfment of tumor-associated antigens by antigen-presenting cells, especially DCs, DC activation and maturation, cross-presentation of antigen to T cells, T cell activation, and accessibility into the tumor. Combination treatments that target these various steps to augment the radiation-immunity cycle improve the likelihood of robust effector cell response within the tumor and thus, favorable clinical outcome after RT. Classifying tumor microenvironments by their immunogenic potential would allow for the personalization of the most efficacious combination treatments. A roadmap has been suggested for designing combination trials of immunotherapy with SBRT, based upon the radiation-immunity cycle and the immune landscape of the tumors.

Immunologically, "hot" inflamed tumors favor infiltration of lymphocytes and typically have high mutagenic loads. These tumors have all components needed for effective immune responses; however, the immune machinery is suppressed due to adaptive immune resistance from the expression of immune checkpoint molecules, and/or tumor infiltration of Treg and TAM. Targetable candidates for immune checkpoints, such as PD-L1, PD-L2, TIM3, and LAG3 are ever increasing, as new pathways of adaptive resistance are being discovered. Tumors, expressing high levels of PD-L1 may respond well to anti-PD1/PD-L1 immune checkpoint blockade (ICB), but may lose efficacy through compensatory mechanisms [94, 95]. Blocking alternative targets for ICB therapy should then be considered for PDL-1 negative tumors. If ablative fractionation is possible, SBRT followed by Flt3L can be combined with concomitant ICB in these patients for adequate in situ vaccination. When dose constraints for organs at risk preclude the use of ablative fractionation, sub-ablative immunomodulatory RT can be combined with ICB along with other therapies, such as activating anti-CD40 antibodies. Since RT induces the expression of cell death receptors on the tumor cell surface, adoptive cell transfer with cytokine-activated T cells or chimeric antigen receptor-expressing T (CAR-T) cells can be added after RT to increase the efficiency of immunotherapy for these tumors. Alternatively, tumor-associated macrophages (TAMs) can be targeted by blocking antibodies to CSF-1 receptor or IDO inhibitors.

Immunologically, "Cold" tumors have low lymphocyte infiltration can be participating in immune exclusion or immune escape, limiting accessibility or limiting visibility to immune responses, respectively. The best therapies for this tumor immunophenotype would be anti-angiogenic, anti-stromal therapies, non-ablative focused ultrasound and RT to modulate the tumor microenvironment using relatively low doses of radiation typically using 0.5–2 Gy. The low dose radiation can normalize the tortuous tumor vascular network which could allow for more efficient perfusion and increase accessibility [96, 97]. Such treatments can be combined with ablative RT to induce a tumor-targeted response, synergistically. Combinations of RT, Flt3L, and anti-CD40 could mature and activate APCs sufficiently to induce antigen presentation and T cell activation. In murine models of hepatocellular cancer, combining RT with Flt3L and anti-CD40 was able to overcome the immunosuppressive environment of HCC, induce a strong cytotoxic T lymphocyte immune response and memory that resulted in high rates of tumor control and improved survival [23, 24].

As shown above, the goal of combination therapies is therefore to enhance the beneficial aspects of each therapy for synergistic effects. These strategies could augment tumor-specific immune responses for each individual patient using this roadmap with careful consideration of dose and fractionation of RT, types of immunotherapeutic agents, and the baseline immunophenotype of the tumor.Conflict of InterestThe authors report no conflict of interest.

References

1. Kaplan HS, Bagshaw MA. Radiation hepatitis: possible prevention by combined isotopic and external radiation therapy. Radiology. 1968;91(6):1214–20.
2. Ingold JA, Reed GB, Kaplan HS, Bagshaw MA. Radiation hepatitis. Am J Roentgenol Radium Therapy, Nucl Med. 1965;93:200–8.
3. Borgelt BB, Gelber R, Brady LW, Griffin T, Hendrickson FR. The palliation of hepatic metastases: results of the radiation therapy oncology group pilot study. Int J Radiat Oncol Biol Phys. 1981;7(5):587–91.

4. Russell AH, Clyde C, Wasserman TH, Turner SS, Rotman M. Accelerated hyperfractionated hepatic irradiation in the management of patients with liver metastases: results of the RTOG dose escalating protocol. Int J Radiat Oncol Biol Phys. 1993;27(1):117–23.

5. Stillwagon GB, Order SE, Guse C, Klein JL, Leichner PK, Leibel SA, et al. 194 hepatocellular cancers treated by radiation and chemotherapy combinations: toxicity and response: a radiation therapy oncology group study. Int J Radiat Oncol Biol Phys. 1989;17(6):1223–9.

6. Emami B, Lyman J, Brown A, Coia L, Goitein M, Munzenrider JE, et al. Tolerance of normal tissue to therapeutic irradiation. Int J Radiat Oncol Biol Phys. 1991;21(1):109–22.

7. Dawson LA, Normolle D, Balter JM, McGinn CJ, Lawrence TS, Ten Haken RK. Analysis of radiation-induced liver disease using the Lyman NTCP model. Int J Radiat Oncol Biol Phys. 2002;53(4):810–21.

8. Pan CC, Kavanagh BD, Dawson LA, Li XA, Das SK, Miften M, et al. Radiation-associated liver injury. Int J Radiat Oncol Biol Phys. 2010;76(3 Suppl):S94–100.

9. Ohri N, Tome WA, Mendez Romero A, Miften M, Ten Haken RK, Dawson LA, et al. Local control after stereotactic body radiation therapy for liver tumors. Int J Radiat Oncol Biol Phys. 2018; https://doi.org/10.1016/j.ijrobp.2017.12.288.

10. Mahadevan A, Blanck O, Lanciano R, Peddada A, Sundararaman S, D'Ambrosio D, et al. Stereotactic body radiotherapy (SBRT) for liver metastasis - clinical outcomes from the international multi-institutional RSSearch® patient registry. Radiat Oncol. 2018;13(1):26.

11. Herfarth KK, Debus J, Lohr F, Bahner ML, Rhein B, Fritz P, et al. Stereotactic single-dose radiation therapy of liver tumors: results of a phase I/II trial. J Clin Oncol. 2001;19(1):164–70.

12. Hoyer M, Roed H, Traberg Hansen A, Ohlhuis L, Petersen J, Nellemann H, et al. Phase II study on stereotactic body radiotherapy of colorectal metastases. Acta Oncol. 2006;45(7):823–30.

13. Mendez Romero A, Wunderink W, Hussain SM, De Pooter JA, Heijmen BJ, Nowak PC, et al. Stereotactic body radiation therapy for primary and metastatic liver tumors: a single institution phase i-ii study. Acta Oncol. 2006;45(7):831–7.

14. Schefter TE, Kavanagh BD, Timmerman RD, Cardenes HR, Baron A, Gaspar LE. A phase I trial of stereotactic body radiation therapy (SBRT) for liver metastases. Int J Radiat Oncol Biol Phys. 2005;62(5):1371–8.

15. Rusthoven KE, Kavanagh BD, Cardenes H, Stieber VW, Burri SH, Feigenberg SJ, et al. Multi-institutional phase I/II trial of stereotactic body radiation therapy for liver metastases. J Clin Oncol. 2009;27(10):1572–8.

16. Lee MT, Kim JJ, Dinniwell R, Brierley J, Lockwood G, Wong R, et al. Phase I study of individualized stereotactic body radiotherapy of liver metastases. J Clin Oncol. 2009;27(10):1585–91.

17. Goodman KA, Wiegner EA, Maturen KE, Zhang Z, Mo Q, Yang G, et al. Dose-escalation study of single-fraction stereotactic body radiotherapy for liver malignancies. Int J Radiat Oncol Biol Phys. 2010;78(2):486–93.

18. Scorsetti M, Arcangeli S, Tozzi A, Comito T, Alongi F, Navarria P, et al. Is stereotactic body radiation therapy an attractive option for unresectable liver metastases? A preliminary report from a phase 2 trial. Int J Radiat Oncol Biol Phys. 2013;86(2):336–42.

19. Ambrosino G, Polistina F, Costantin G, Francescon P, Guglielmi R, Zanco P, et al. Image-guided robotic stereotactic radiosurgery for unresectable liver metastases: preliminary results. Anticancer Res. 2009;29(8):3381–4.

20. Garcia-Barros M, Paris F, Cordon-Cardo C, Lyden D, Rafii S, Haimovitz-Friedman A, et al. Tumor response to radiotherapy regulated by endothelial cell apoptosis. Science. 2003;300(5622):1155–9.

21. Lee Y, Auh SL, Wang Y, Burnette B, Meng Y, Beckett M, et al. Therapeutic effects of ablative radiation on local tumor require CD8+ T cells: changing strategies for cancer treatment. Blood. 2009;114(3):589–95.

22. Filatenkov A, Baker J, Mueller AM, Kenkel J, Ahn GO, Dutt S, et al. Ablative tumor radiation can change the tumor immune cell microenvironment to induce durable complete remissions. Clin Cancer Res. 2015;21(16):3727–39.

23. Kawashita Y, Deb NJ, Garg M, Kabarriti R, Alfieri A, Takahashi M, et al. An autologous in situ tumor vaccination approach for hepatocellular carcinoma. 1. Flt3 ligand gene transfer increases antitumor effects of a radio-inducible suicide gene therapy in an ectopic tumor model. Radiat Res. 2014;182(2):191–200.

24. Kawashita Y, Deb NJ, Garg MK, Kabarriti R, Fan Z, Alfieri AA, et al. An autologous in situ tumor vaccination approach for hepatocellular carcinoma. 2. Tumor-specific immunity and cure after radio-inducible suicide gene therapy and systemic CD40-ligand and Flt3-ligand gene therapy in an orthotopic tumor model. Radiat Res. 2014;182(2):201–10.

25. Lawrence TS, Robertson JM, Anscher MS, Jirtle RL, Ensminger WD, Fajardo LF. Hepatic toxicity resulting from cancer treatment. Int J Radiat Oncol Biol Phys. 1995;31(5):1237–48.

26. Ogata K, Hizawa K, Yoshida M, Kitamuro T, Akagi G, Kagawa K, et al. Hepatic injury following irradiation: a morphologic study. Tokushima J Exp Med. 1963;43:240–51.

27. Reed GB Jr, Cox AJ Jr. The human liver after radiation injury. A form of veno-occlusive disease. Am J Pathol. 1966;48(4):597–611.

28. DeLeve LD, Shulman HM, McDonald GB. Toxic injury to hepatic sinusoids: sinusoidal obstruction syndrome (veno-occlusive disease). Semin Liver Dis. 2002;22(1):27–42.

29. Sempoux C, Horsmans Y, Geubel A, Fraikin J, Van Beers BE, Gigot JF, et al. Severe radiation-induced liver disease following localized radiation therapy for biliopancreatic carcinoma: activation of

hepatic stellate cells as an early event. Hepatology. 1997;26(1):128–34.

30. Anscher MS, Crocker IR, Jirtle RL. Transforming growth factor-beta 1 expression in irradiated liver. Radiat Res. 1990;122(1):77–85.

31. Anscher MS, Peters WP, Reisenbichler H, Petros WP, Jirtle RL. Transforming growth factor beta as a predictor of liver and lung fibrosis after autologous bone marrow transplantation for advanced breast cancer. N Engl J Med. 1993;328(22):1592–8.

32. Guha C, Kavanagh BD. Hepatic radiation toxicity: avoidance and amelioration. Semin Radiat Oncol. 2011;21(4):256–63.

33. Cheng JC, Wu JK, Lee PC, Liu HS, Jian JJ, Lin YM, et al. Biologic susceptibility of hepatocellular carcinoma patients treated with radiotherapy to radiation-induced liver disease. Int J Radiat Oncol Biol Phys. 2004;60(5):1502–9.

34. Guha C, Sharma A, Gupta S, Alfieri A, Gorla GR, Gagandeep S, et al. Amelioration of radiation-induced liver damage in partially hepatectomized rats by hepatocyte transplantation. Cancer Res. 1999;59(23):5871–4.

35. Kim JH, Park JW, Kim TH, Koh DW, Lee WJ, Kim CM. Hepatitis B virus reactivation after three-dimensional conformal radiotherapy in patients with hepatitis B virus-related hepatocellular carcinoma. Int J Radiat Oncol Biol Phys. 2007;69(3):813–9.

36. Chou CH, Chen PJ, Lee PH, Cheng AL, Hsu HC, Cheng JC. Radiation-induced hepatitis B virus reactivation in liver mediated by the bystander effect from irradiated endothelial cells. Clin Cancer Res. 2007;13(3):851–7.

37. Miften M, Vinogradskiy Y, Moiseenko V, Grimm J, Yorke E, Jackson A, et al. Radiation dose-volume effects for liver SBRT. Int J Radiat Oncol Biol Phys. 2018; https://doi.org/10.1016/j.ijrobp.2017.12.290.

38. Bujold A, Massey CA, Kim JJ, Brierley J, Cho C, Wong RK, et al. Sequential phase I and II trials of stereotactic body radiotherapy for locally advanced hepatocellular carcinoma. J Clin Oncol. 2013;31(13):1631–9.

39. Andolino DL, Johnson CS, Maluccio M, Kwo P, Tector AJ, Zook J, et al. Stereotactic body radiotherapy for primary hepatocellular carcinoma. Int J Radiat Oncol Biol Phys. 2011;81(4):e447–53.

40. Su TS, Luo R, Liang P, Cheng T, Zhou Y, Huang Y. A prospective cohort study of hepatic toxicity after stereotactic body radiation therapy for hepatocellular carcinoma. Radiother Oncol. 2018;129(1):136–42.

41. Hasan S, Thai N, Uemura T, Kudithipudi V, Renz P, Abel S, et al. Hepatocellular carcinoma with child Pugh-a cirrhosis treated with stereotactic body radiotherapy. World J Gastrointest Surg. 2017;9(12):256–63.

42. Nabavizadeh N, Waller JG, Fain R 3rd, Chen Y, Degnin CR, Elliott DA, et al. Safety and efficacy of accelerated hypofractionation and stereotactic body radiation therapy for hepatocellular carcinoma patients with varying degrees of hepatic impairment. Int J Radiat Oncol Biol Phys. 2018;100(3):577–85.

43. Malinchoc M, Kamath PS, Gordon FD, Peine CJ, Rank J, ter Borg PC. A model to predict poor survival in patients undergoing transjugular intrahepatic porto-systemic shunts. Hepatology. 2000;31(4):864–71.

44. Martin AP, Bartels M, Hauss J, Fangmann J. Overview of the MELD score and the UNOS adult liver allocation system. Transplant Proc. 2007;39(10):3169–74.

45. Trey C, Burns DG, Saunders SJ. Treatment of hepatic coma by exchange blood transfusion. N Engl J Med. 1966;274(9):473–81.

46. Bruix J, Castells A, Bosch J, Feu F, Fuster J, Garcia-Pagan JC, et al. Surgical resection of hepatocellular carcinoma in cirrhotic patients: prognostic value of preoperative portal pressure. Gastroenterology. 1996;111(4):1018–22.

47. Groszmann RJ, Wongcharatrawee S. The hepatic venous pressure gradient: anything worth doing should be done right. Hepatology. 2004;39(2):280–2.

48. Johnson PJ, Berhane S, Kagebayashi C, Satomura S, Teng M, Reeves HL, et al. Assessment of liver function in patients with hepatocellular carcinoma: a new evidence-based approach-the ALBI grade. J Clin Oncol. 2015;33(6):550–8.

49. Liu PH, Hsu CY, Hsia CY, Lee YH, Chiou YY, Huang YH, et al. ALBI and PALBI grade predict survival for HCC across treatment modalities and BCLC stages in the MELD era. J Gastroenterol Hepatol. 2017;32(4):879–86.

50. Lee SK, Song MJ, Kim SH, Park M. Comparing various scoring system for predicting overall survival according to treatment modalities in hepatocellular carcinoma focused on platelet-albumin-bilirubin (PALBI) and albumin-bilirubin (ALBI) grade: a nationwide cohort study. PLoS One. 2019;14(5):e0216173.

51. Mathew AS, Atenafu EG, Owen D, Maurino C, Brade A, Brierley J, et al. Long term outcomes of stereotactic body radiation therapy for hepatocellular carcinoma without macrovascular invasion. Eur J Cancer. 2020;134:41–51.

52. Feng M, Suresh K, Schipper MJ, Bazzi L, Ben-Josef E, Matuszak MM, et al. Individualized adaptive stereotactic body radiotherapy for liver tumors in patients at high risk for liver damage: a phase 2 clinical trial. JAMA Oncol. 2018;4(1):40–7.

53. Everson GT, Shiffman ML, Hoefs JC, Morgan TR, Sterling RK, Wagner DA, et al. Quantitative liver function tests improve the prediction of clinical outcomes in chronic hepatitis C: results from the hepatitis C antiviral long-term treatment against cirrhosis trial. Hepatology. 2012;55(4):1019–29.

54. Burton JR, Helmke S, Lauriski S, Kittelson J, Everson GT. The within-individual reproducibility of the disease severity index from the HepQuant SHUNT test of liver function and physiology. Transl Res. 2021; https://doi.org/10.1016/j.trsl.2020.12.010.

55. Kurland IJ, Broin P, Golden A, Su G, Meng F, Liu L, et al. Integrative metabolic signatures for hepatic radiation injury. PLoS One. 2015;10(6):e0124795.

56. Ng SSW, Jang GH, Kurland IJ, Qiu Y, Guha C, Dawson LA. Plasma metabolomic profiles in liver cancer patients following stereotactic body radiotherapy. EBioMedicine. 2020;59:102973.

57. Cutler C, Kim HT, Ayanian S, Bradwin G, Revta C, Aldridge J, et al. Prediction of veno-occlusive disease using biomarkers of endothelial injury. Biol Blood Marrow Transplant. 2010;16(8):1180–5.

58. Lee JH, Lee KH, Kim S, Seol M, Park CJ, Chi HS, et al. Plasminogen activator inhibitor-1 is an independent diagnostic marker as well as severity predictor of hepatic veno-occlusive disease after allogeneic bone marrow transplantation in adults conditioned with busulphan and cyclophosphamide. Br J Haematol. 2002;118(4):1087–94.

59. Salat C, Holler E, Kolb HJ, Reinhardt B, Pihusch R, Wilmanns W, et al. Plasminogen activator inhibitor-1 confirms the diagnosis of hepatic veno-occlusive disease in patients with hyperbilirubinemia after bone marrow transplantation. Blood. 1997;89(6):2184–8.

60. Yamanouchi K, Zhou H, Roy-Chowdhury N, Macaluso F, Liu L, Yamamoto T, et al. Hepatic irradiation augments engraftment of donor cells following hepatocyte transplantation. Hepatology. 2009;49(1):258–67.

61. Fried MW, Duncan A, Soroka S, Connaghan DG, Farrand A, Peter J, et al. Serum hyaluronic acid in patients with veno-occlusive disease following bone marrow transplantation. Bone Marrow Transplant. 2001;27(6):635–9.

62. Tabbara IA, Ghazal CD, Ghazal HH. Early drop in protein C and antithrombin III is a predictor for the development of venoocclusive disease in patients undergoing hematopoietic stem cell transplantation. J Hematother. 1996;5(1):79–84.

63. Roeker LE, Kim HT, Glotzbecker B, Nageshwar P, Nikiforow S, Koreth J, et al. Early clinical predictors of hepatic veno-occlusive disease/sinusoidal obstruction syndrome after myeloablative stem cell transplantation. Biol Blood Marrow Transplant. 2019;25(1):137–44.

64. Eltumi M, Trivedi P, Hobbs JR, Portmann B, Cheeseman P, Downie C, et al. Monitoring of venoocclusive disease after bone marrow transplantation by serum aminopropeptide of type III procollagen. Lancet. 1993;342(8870):518–21.

65. Rio B, Bauduer F, Arrago JP, Zittoun R. N-terminal peptide of type III procollagen: a marker for the development of hepatic veno-occlusive disease after BMT and a basis for determining the timing of prophylactic heparin. Bone Marrow Transplant. 1993;11(6):471–2.

66. Cao Y, Pan C, Balter JM, Platt JF, Francis IR, Knol JA, et al. Liver function after irradiation based on computed tomographic portal vein perfusion imaging. Int J Radiat Oncol Biol Phys. 2008;70(1):154–60.

67. Cao Y, Wang H, Johnson TD, Pan C, Hussain H, Balter JM, et al. Prediction of liver function by using magnetic resonance-based portal venous perfusion imaging. Int J Radiat Oncol Biol Phys. 2013;85(1):258–63.

68. Yannam GR, Han B, Setoyama K, Yamamoto T, Ito R, Brooks JM, et al. A nonhuman primate model of human radiation-induced venocclusive liver disease and hepatocyte injury. Int J Radiat Oncol Biol Phys. 2014;88(2):404–11.

69. Kabarriti R, Brodin NP, Yaffe H, Barahman M, Koba WR, Liu L, et al. Non-invasive targeted hepatic irradiation and SPECT/CT functional imaging to study radiation-induced liver damage in small animal models. Cancers (Basel). 2019;11(11):1796.

70. Ward J, Guthrie JA, Sheridan MB, Boyes S, Smith JT, Wilson D, et al. Sinusoidal obstructive syndrome diagnosed with superparamagnetic iron oxide-enhanced magnetic resonance imaging in patients with chemotherapy-treated colorectal liver metastases. J Clin Oncol. 2008;26(26):4304–10.

71. Kwon AH, Ha-Kawa SK, Uetsuji S, Inoue T, Matsui Y, Kamiyama Y. Preoperative determination of the surgical procedure for hepatectomy using technetium-99m-galactosyl human serum albumin (99mTc-GSA) liver scintigraphy. Hepatology. 1997;25(2):426–9.

72. de Graaf W, van Lienden KP, van Gulik TM, Bennink RJ. (99m)Tc-mebrofenin hepatobiliary scintigraphy with SPECT for the assessment of hepatic function and liver functional volume before partial hepatectomy. J Nucl Med. 2010;51(2):229–36.

73. Tsegmed U, Kimura T, Nakashima T, Nakamura Y, Higaki T, Imano N, et al. Functional image-guided stereotactic body radiation therapy planning for patients with hepatocellular carcinoma. Med Dosim. 2017;42(2):97–103.

74. Chan SS, Colecchia A, Duarte RF, Bonifazi F, Ravaioli F, Bourhis JH. Imaging in hepatic veno-occlusive disease/sinusoidal obstruction syndrome. Biol Blood Marrow Transplant. 2020;26(10):1770–9.

75. Reddivalla N, Robinson AL, Reid KJ, Radhi MA, Dalal J, Opfer EK, et al. Using liver elastography to diagnose sinusoidal obstruction syndrome in pediatric patients undergoing hematopoetic stem cell transplant. Bone Marrow Transplant. 2020;55(3):523–30.

76. Trenker C, Sohlbach K, Dietrich CF, Görg C. Clinical diagnosis of veno-occlusive disease using contrast enhanced ultrasound. Bone Marrow Transplant. 2018;53(10):1369–71.

77. Berzigotti A. Non-invasive evaluation of portal hypertension using ultrasound elastography. J Hepatol. 2017;67(2):399–411.

78. Bearman SI, Lee JL, Baron AE, McDonald GB. Treatment of hepatic venocclusive disease with recombinant human tissue plasminogen activator and heparin in 42 marrow transplant patients. Blood. 1997;89(5):1501–6.

79. Koay EJ, Owen D, Das P. Radiation-induced liver disease and modern radiotherapy. Semin Radiat Oncol. 2018;28(4):321–31.

80. Feng M, Smith DE, Normolle DP, Knol JA, Pan CC, Ben-Josef E, et al. A phase I clinical and pharmacology study using amifostine as a radioprotector in dose-escalated whole liver radiation therapy. Int J Radiat Oncol Biol Phys. 2012;83(5):1441–7.

81. Seidensticker M, Seidensticker R, Damm R, Mohnike K, Pech M, Sangro B, et al. Prospective randomized trial of enoxaparin, pentoxifylline and ursodeoxycholic acid for prevention of radiation-induced liver toxicity. PLoS One. 2014;9(11):e112731.

82. Terrault NA, Lok ASF, McMahon BJ, Chang KM, Hwang JP, Jonas MM, et al. Update on prevention, diagnosis, and treatment of chronic hepatitis B: AASLD 2018 hepatitis B guidance. Hepatology. 2018;67(4):1560–99.

83. Zhou H, Dong X, Kabarriti R, Chen Y, Avsar Y, Wang X, et al. Single liver lobe repopulation with wildtype hepatocytes using regional hepatic irradiation cures jaundice in Gunn rats. PLoS One. 2012;7(10):e46775.

84. Kabarriti RZH, Vainshtein JV, Saha S, Hannan R, Thawani N, Alfieri A, Kalnicki S, Guha C. Transplantation of liver sinusoidal endothelial cells repairs HIR induced hepatic endothelial cell damage. Int J Radiat Oncol Biol Phys. 2010;78(3):S41.

85. Barahman M, Asp P, Roy-Chowdhury N, Kinkhabwala M, Roy-Chowdhury J, Kabarriti R, et al. Hepatocyte transplantation: Quo Vadis? Int J Radiat Oncol Biol Phys. 2019;103(4):922–34.

86. McGee HM, Daly ME, Azghadi S, Stewart SL, Oesterich L, Schlom J, et al. Stereotactic ablative radiation therapy induces systemic differences in peripheral blood immunophenotype dependent on irradiated site. Int J Radiat Oncol Biol Phys. 2018;101(5):1259–70.

87. Dewan MZ, Galloway AE, Kawashima N, Dewyngaert JK, Babb JS, Formenti SC, et al. Fractionated but not single-dose radiotherapy induces an immune-mediated abscopal effect when combined with anti-CTLA-4 antibody. Clin Cancer Res. 2009;15(17):5379–88.

88. Sato H, Niimi A, Yasuhara T, Permata TBM, Hagiwara Y, Isono M, et al. DNA double-strand break repair pathway regulates PD-L1 expression in cancer cells. Nat Commun. 2017;8(1):1751.

89. MacLennan I, Kay H. Analysis of treatment in childhood leukemia. IV. The critical association between dose fractionation and immunosuppression induced by cranial irradiation. Cancer. 1978;41(1):108–11.

90. Kioi M, Vogel H, Schultz G, Hoffman RM, Harsh GR, Brown JM. Inhibition of vasculogenesis, but not angiogenesis, prevents the recurrence of glioblastoma after irradiation in mice. J Clin Invest. 2010;120(3):694–705.

91. Brown JM. Vasculogenesis: a crucial player in the resistance of solid tumours to radiotherapy. Br J Radiol. 2014;87(1035):20130686.

92. Kozin SV, Kamoun WS, Huang Y, Dawson MR, Jain RK, Duda DG. Recruitment of myeloid but not endothelial precursor cells facilitates tumor regrowth after local irradiation. Cancer Res. 2010;70(14):5679–85.

93. Chen DS, Mellman I. Oncology meets immunology: the cancer-immunity cycle. Immunity. 2013;39(1):1–10.

94. Benci JL, Xu B, Qiu Y, Wu TJ, Dada H, Twyman-Saint Victor C, et al. Tumor interferon signaling regulates a multigenic resistance program to immune checkpoint blockade. Cell. 2016;167(6):1540–54. e12

95. Minn AJ, Wherry EJ. Combination cancer therapies with immune checkpoint blockade: convergence on interferon signaling. Cell. 2016;165(2):272–5.

96. Ministro A, de Oliveira P, Nunes RJ, dos Santos RA, Correia A, Carvalho T, et al. Low-dose ionizing radiation induces therapeutic neovascularization in a preclinical model of hindlimb ischemia. Cardiovasc Res. 2017;113(7):783–94.

97. Potiron VA, Abderrahmani R, Clément-Colmou K, Marionneau-Lambot S, Oullier T, Paris F, et al. Improved functionality of the vasculature during conventionally fractionated radiation therapy of prostate cancer. PLoS One. 2013;8(12):e84076.

Imaging Anatomy for the Radiation Oncologist

3

Yeun-Yoon Kim and Jin-Young Choi

Abstract

To facilitate comprehension on cross-sectional imaging, we introduce appropriate imaging protocols for computed tomography (CT) and magnetic resonance imaging (MRI). On cross-sectional images of CT and MRI, hepatic segments can be located by several anatomical indices and portal vein branching. The majority of hepatic lymph drains into the portal lymphatic system, and regional lymph nodes for hepatocellular carcinoma include the hepatic hilar, hepatoduodenal ligament, inferior phrenic, and caval lymph nodes. Intrahepatic bile ducts are not usually seen on CT due to their small caliber, but bilateral hepatic ducts and the common hepatic duct can be identified at the hepatic hilum and need to be delineated to avoid potential biliary stricture after radiotherapy. For luminal organs at risk, an external surface contouring is recommended, and the drawn contour needs to include partial volume artifacts to ensure that the entire wall is included. Imaging features of the arterioportal shunt, malignant portal vein thrombosis, intraductal growing hepatocellular carcinoma, intrahepatic metastasis, and viable tumor after locoregional treatment are also summarized in this chapter because they can aid in the exact evaluation of tumor extent.

Keywords

Cross-sectional anatomy · Computed tomography · Magnetic resonance imaging · Liver · Organs at risk · Hepatocellular carcinoma

3.1 Cross-Sectional Imaging Protocol

3.1.1 Computed Tomography (CT)

The dynamic liver CT protocol is a multiphase imaging protocol that optimally demonstrates the enhancement of hepatic vasculatures, liver parenchyma, and focal liver lesions while taking into consideration the dual blood supply from the hepatic artery and portal vein to the liver. Unenhanced scans are useful for visualizing calcifications or Lipiodol after transarterial chemoembolization (TACE) [1]. The early arterial phase can be scanned 15–25 s after contrast injection to visualize the anatomy of arterial vasculatures. However, the optimal timing for the arterial phase hyperenhancement (APHE) of hepatocellular carcinoma (HCC) is the late arterial phase scanned 30–45 s after contrast injection in which portal veins are also enhanced [2].

Y.-Y. Kim · J.-Y. Choi (✉)
Department of Radiology, Severance Hospital, Yonsei University College of Medicine, Seoul, South Korea
e-mail: GAFIELD2@yuhs.ac

© Springer Nature Singapore Pte Ltd. 2021
J. Seong (ed.), *Radiotherapy of Liver Cancer*, https://doi.org/10.1007/978-981-16-1815-4_3

In the portal venous phase scanned 60–70 s after contrast injection, hepatic veins are also opacified. As blood returns from the bowel loops to the portal veins, liver parenchymal enhancement is maximized, and hypovascular tumors are well appreciated as hypoenhancing findings in the portal venous phase. Washout may be visualized in the portal venous phase, but the use of the delayed phase scanned 2–5 min after contrast injection increases the visualization rate of washout in HCC [3]. Multiphase liver imaging with arterial, particularly late arterial, portal venous, and delayed phases are required for the diagnosis of HCC [4, 5] (Table 3.1).

3.1.2 Magnetic Resonance Imaging (MRI)

Like liver dynamic CT, multiphase, fat-suppressed T1-weighted imaging in liver dynamic MRI is used to evaluate the enhancement pattern of tumors (Table 3.1). If a hepatobiliary agent, such as gadoxetic acid, is used, the delayed phase scanned at 2–5 min is referred to as the transitional phase; in the transitional phase, the liver parenchyma gradually enhances due to hepatocellular uptake of the contrast agent and vasculatures become hypointense as the contrast agent clears from the vasculatures [6]. In the hepatobiliary phase obtained approximately 20 min after contrast injection, the contrast between the tumor and the liver is maximized, and the biliary tree is well visualized due to the biliary excretion of contrast materials.

In T2-weighted images, fluid or cystic structures appear markedly hyperintense. Therefore, the biliary tree and bowel loops may be easier to identify using this sequence [7]. Also, lesions can be characterized as solid when they demonstrate intermediate T2 hyperintensity. In diffusion-weighted imaging (DWI), solid lesions with restricted diffusion of water molecules appear hyperintense on high b-value images, and the apparent diffusion coefficient (ADC) map shows low ADC values. On the other hand, cystic lesions without restricted diffusion of water molecules show signal loss on high b-value images, and consequently have high ADC values.

3.2 Imaging Anatomy of the Liver

3.2.1 Liver Segmental Anatomy

Understanding hepatic segmental anatomy is essential for the identification of the exact location and extent of hepatic tumors. The Brisbane 2000 system is the most recent nomenclature system for hepatic anatomy proposed by the International Hepato-Pancreato-Biliary Association. In this system, the term *hemiliver* is used for first-order division (i.e., right and left

Table 3.1 CT and MRI protocol for liver imaging

Imaging modality	Comments
CT	• Multiphasic imaging is required for diagnostic liver imaging. • Early arterial phase (scan timing, 15–25 s after contrast injection) is used to visualize arterial vasculatures. • Late arterial phase (30–45 s) is the optimal phase for the visualization of hypervascular tumors. • Portal venous phase (60–70 s) is essential for the visualization of hypovascular tumors. • Delayed phase (2–5 min) increases the visualization rate of HCC washout.
MRI	• Fat-suppressed multiphase T1-weighted imaging is required to evaluate the vascular profile of tumors. • T2-weighted imaging helps characterize cystic and solid lesions. • DWI helps detect and characterize cystic and solid lesions. • HBP (20 min after gadoxetic acid contrast injection) helps detect tumors and evaluate the biliary tree.

CT computed tomography; *DWI* diffusion-weighted imaging; *HBP* hepatobiliary phase; *HCC* hepatocellular carcinoma; *MRI* magnetic resonance imaging

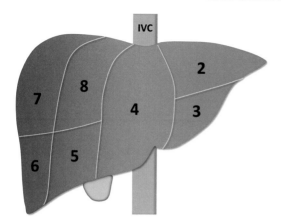

Fig. 3.1 Diagram of hepatic segmentation. Hepatic segments are numbered clockwise as seen in the frontal projection. Segment 1 (not seen), or the caudate lobe, is located at the posterior aspect of segment 4, surrounding the inferior vena cava (IVC)

hemilivers), *section* for second-order division, and *segment* for third-order division [8]. As in the commonly used Couinaud classification, the liver is divided into eight functional segments in the Brisbane 2000 system based on the ramification of the portal vein, and hepatic segments are numbered clockwise as seen in the frontal projection (Fig. 3.1). While the Couinaud classification refers to segment 2 as the left lateral sector and segments 3 and 4 as the left paramedian sector, the Brisbane 2000 system combines segments 2 and 3 into the left lateral section, and refers to segment 4 as the left medial section.

On cross-sectional images of CT and MRI, hepatic segments can be located by anatomical indices and portal vein branching. Instead of early arterial phase images in which portal veins are not yet opacified, portal venous phase images are the appropriate choice for identifying hepatic segmental anatomy as portal veins and hepatic veins are well opacified on these images.

Segment 1 (or the caudate lobe) functions autonomously, apart from both hemilivers in terms of vascular and biliary systems. The caudate lobe is supplied by small portal vein branches originating directly from portal bifurcation or bilateral portal veins, and separate emissary caudate veins drain directly to the inferior vena cava (IVC) (Fig. 3.2) [9]. The caudate lobe is separated from segment 2 by the fissure for ligamentum venosum (Fig. 3.3). Among the three portions of the caudate lobe, the caudate process connects the caudate lobe to the right hemiliver; the paracaval portion is bordered posteriorly by the intrahepatic IVC; and the papillary process (or Spigel's lobe) is a prominence protruding into the lesser sac, which can sometimes be mistaken for a lymph node or extrahepatic mass on the axial images of CT or MRI (Fig. 3.2) [10].

The left portal vein can be divided into the transverse portion and umbilical portion, marked by the attachment of the ligamentum venosum. The umbilical portion is then divided into branches supplying segments 2 (the left lateral superior segment), 3 (the left lateral inferior segment), and 4 (the left medial segment), and the ligamentum teres is attached at its end (Fig. 3.3). Therefore, the left lateral and medial sections are marked by the umbilical portion of the left portal vein. Segment 4 can be further divided into subsegments 4a (the left medial superior segment) and 4b (the left medial inferior segment) with the left portal vein dividing the cranial and caudal subsegments [11]. Last but not least, segment 2 sometimes extends to the perisplenic area, and the radiation oncologist needs to look out for tumors in the left lateral tip of the liver (Fig. 3.3).

The right portal vein splits into the right anterior and right posterior sectional portal veins, which further branch into the superior and inferior segmental branches. The right anterior section of the liver consists of segments 5 (the right anterior inferior segment) and 8 (the right anterior superior segment), and the right posterior section consists of segments 6 (the right posterior inferior segment) and 7 (the right posterior superior segment) (Fig. 3.4).

The separating planes can also be identified with hepatic veins, but this can sometimes be difficult to do owing to anatomic variations in the hepatic veins. The plane passing through the fossa for the gallbladder and IVC divides the liver into the right hemiliver and left hemiliver (i.e., Cantlie's line), and the middle hepatic vein usually lines on this plane (Fig. 3.3). The right hepatic vein separates the right anterior and pos-

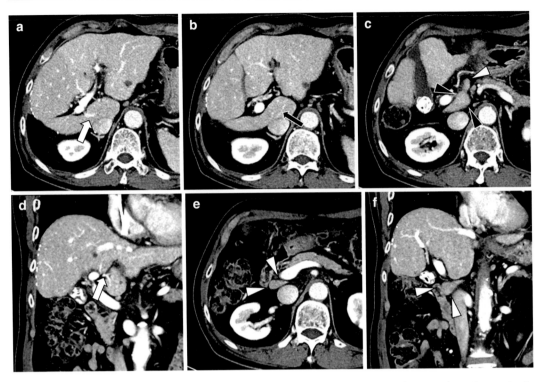

Fig. 3.2 Cross-sectional anatomy of the caudate lobe. (**a**) A portal vein branch (white arrow) which originates directly from the right main portal vein supplies blood to the caudate lobe, and (**b**) an emissary caudate vein (black arrow) drains directly to the IVC. The caudate lobe is functionally independent from other hepatic segments. (**c**) The papillary process of the caudate lobe (black arrow-heads) is seen in the space between the main portal vein and inferior vena cava (i.e., portocaval space). Note similar attenuation of the papillary process and an adjacent common hepatic lymph node (white arrowhead). (**d**) The coronal image also visualizes a portal vein branch supplying the caudate lobe. (**e, f**) A portocaval lymph node (white arrowheads) is located inferior to the caudate lobe

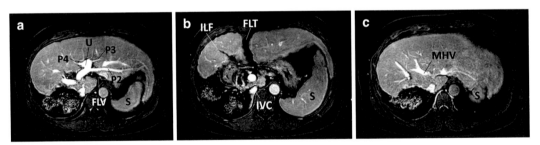

Fig. 3.3 Anatomy of the left hemiliver in a patient who underwent right posterior sectionectomy. (**a**) The left portal vein can be divided into the transverse portion and umbilical portion, marked by the attachment of ligamentum venosum. The umbilical portion (U) is then divided into branches supplying segments 2 (P2), 3 (P3), and 4 (P4), and the ligamentum teres is attached at its end. Note, segment 2 extends to the left subphrenic space surrounding the spleen (S). (**b**) The plane passing through the fossa for the gallbladder (or interlobar fissure, ILF) and IVC corresponds to Cantlie's line, in which the (**c**) middle hepatic vein (MHV) lies. FLV = fissure for ligamentum venosum, FLT = fissure for ligamentum teres

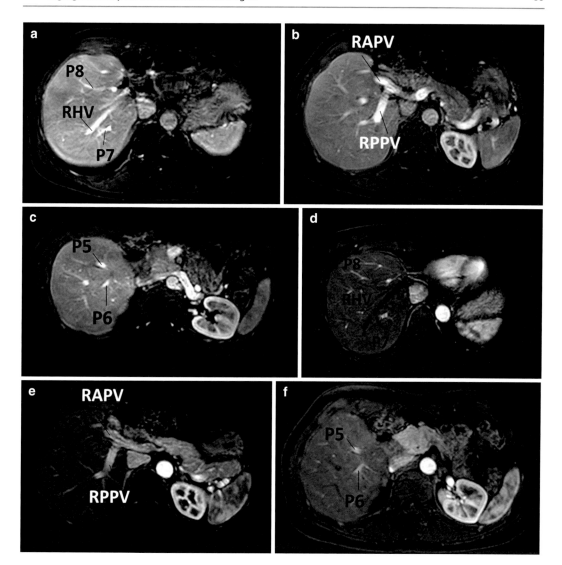

Fig. 3.4 Anatomy of the right hemiliver in a patient who underwent left hemihepatectomy. (**a–c**) On the portal venous phase images, the right portal vein divides into the right anterior and right posterior sectional portal veins (RAPV and RPPV, respectively), which further branches into the superior and inferior segmental branches. The right anterior section of the liver consists of segments 5 (P5) and 8 (P8), and the right posterior section consists of segments 6 (P6) and 7 (P7). (**d–f**) On the late arterial phase images in the corresponding slices, portal veins are opacified, but hepatic veins remain unenhanced. Note (**a, d**) that the right hepatic vein (RHV) separates the right anterior and posterior sections

terior sections, and the left hepatic vein separates the left medial and lateral sections.

3.2.2 Lymphatic Drainage of the Liver

Approximately one-fourth to one-half of the lymph drained by the thoracic duct is produced in the liver [12]. The majority of hepatic lymph (i.e., deep lymphatics and superficial lymphatics from the hepatic concave surface) drains into the portal lymphatic system, which consists of lymph nodes (LNs) in the hepatic hilum and lesser omentum, and then flows to celiac LNs and LNs between the aorta and infrarenal IVC, and subsequently to the cisterna chyli (Fig. 3.5) [13–15]. Superficial lymphatics from the hepatic convex surface drain

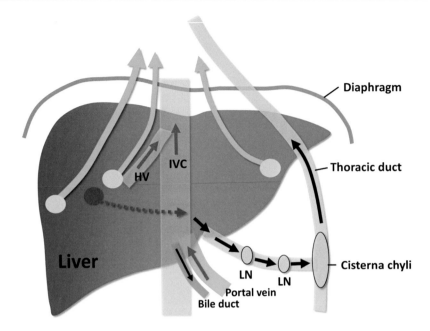

Fig. 3.5 Diagram of hepatic lymph drainage. The deep lymphatics and superficial lymphatics from the hepatic concave surface drain into lymph nodes (LNs) in the hepatic hilum and lesser omentum, such as the portocaval, retropancreatic, and common hepatic LNs. The lymph then drains to celiac LNs and retroperitoneal LNs, and subsequently to the cisterna chyli. The superficial lymphatics from the hepatic convex surface and other deep lymphatics drain through the diaphragm and reach the mediastinal LNs

through coronary ligaments, and other deep lymphatic vessels course along the hepatic veins and IVC, both of which penetrate the diaphragm and reach the mediastinal chains (Figs. 3.5 and 3.6). Therefore, regional LNs for HCC include the hepatic hilar, hepatoduodenal ligament, inferior phrenic, and caval LNs (Fig. 3.6) [16]. The incidence of LN metastasis in HCC ranges from 5% in operable patients to 25% in autopsy cases [17, 18]. In a HCC patient cohort with extrahepatic metastasis, lymph node metastasis was found in up to 55% of patients, with the most common locations for the metastasis being the retroperitoneal, porta hepatis, and mediastinal LNs, in that order [19].

hepatic duct (CHD) (Fig. 3.7) [20]. Intrahepatic bile ducts are not usually seen on CT due to their small caliber, but bilateral hepatic ducts and CHD can be identified at the hepatic hilum. In the hepatoduodenal ligament, the cystic duct and CHD combine to become the common bile duct (CBD) with a diameter measuring approximately 0.5–0.6 cm. CBD courses into the pancreatic head, meets the pancreatic duct, and forms the ampulla of Vater at the medial wall of the second portion of the duodenum. When planning radiotherapy for tumors in the caudate lobe or near the hepatic hilum, bilateral hepatic ducts, CHD, and CBD need to be delineated to avoid potential biliary stricture after treatment [7, 21].

3.2.3 Anatomy of the Bile Duct

The intrahepatic bile duct frequently shows anatomic variations. Nonetheless, the right posterior bile duct most commonly joins the right anterior bile duct to form the right hepatic duct, which makes hilar confluence with the left hepatic duct at the porta hepatis and becomes the common

3.2.4 Luminal Organs at Risk: Hollow Viscus

Guidelines recommend contouring the external surface of luminal organs at risk, and recommend the inclusion of partial volume artifacts (i.e., averaging of attenuation or signals in the same pixel or voxel containing two different tissues) to

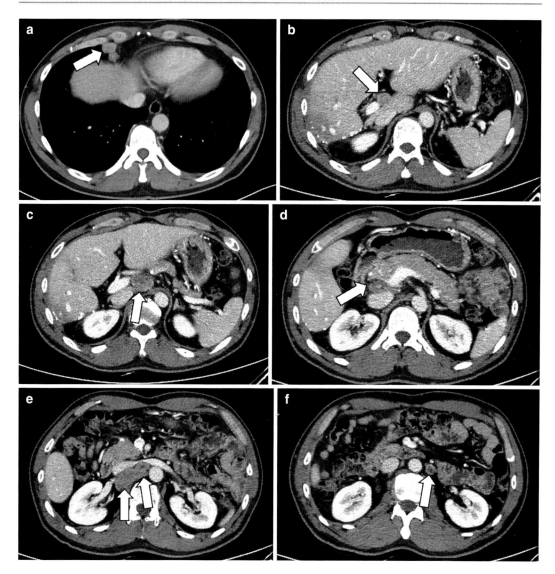

Fig. 3.6 Common locations of LN metastases are shown in a patient with hepatocellular carcinoma (HCC). (**a**) Enlarged, metastatic LNs in the anterior cardiophrenic angle (arrow) were treated with radiotherapy. (**b–f**) After 5 months, LN metastases (arrows) were found in the (**b**) hepatic hilar, (**c**) common hepatic, (**d**) portocaval, (**e**) retrocaval and aortocaval, and (**f**) left paraaortic chains

ensure that the entire wall is included in the contour [7]. The stomach is characterized by thick mucosal folds called gastric rugae, which are well visualized when the lumen is collapsed (Fig. 3.8). The gastric cardia connects the esophagogastric junction and gastric body; the gastric fundus is a dome-shaped portion underneath the left hemidiaphragm; the gastric body is the main part of the stomach; the gastric antrum is the lowermost, prepyloric portion; and the gastric pylorus is the sphincter between the gastric antrum and duodenal bulb.

The duodenal bulb or the first portion is the only intraperitoneal portion of the duodenum that is suspended by the hepatoduodenal ligament; the second portion is a descending portion where the CBD and main pancreatic duct enter the lumen via the ampulla of Vater; the third portion is a transverse portion that courses between the aorta and superior mesenteric vessels at the level

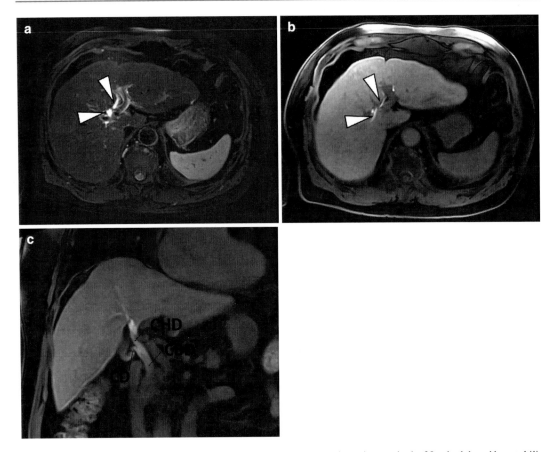

Fig. 3.7 Visualization of intrahepatic and extrahepatic bile ducts on gadoxetic acid-enhanced MRI. (**a**) Bilateral hepatic ducts (arrowheads) are shown in the hepatic hilum with markedly high signals of bile fluid on T2-weighted image. (**b**, **c**) As the hepatobiliary contrast agent is excreted into the bile ducts, contrast media in the biliary tree appear hyperintense in the 20-min delayed hepatobiliary phase (HBP). Bilateral hepatic ducts (arrowheads) visualized in the (**b**) axial image combine to become the common hepatic duct (CHD) which meets the cystic duct (CD) to form the common bile duct (CBD) as shown in the (**c**) 20-min delayed coronal image

of L3; the fourth portion is an ascending portion that ends at the same level as the duodenal bulb or the level of T12, and forms a sharp, anteroinferior angulation that connects to the proximal jejunum (Fig. 3.8).

The jejunum and ileum are suspended to the posterior abdominal wall by the mesentery, and characterized by circular mucosal folds. The jejunum is located mainly in the left upper quadrant, starting from the duodenojejunal junction, and comprises approximately 40% of the small bowel. The ileum is located mainly in the right abdomen and pelvic cavity, ending in the ileocecal valve, and comprises approximately 60% of the small bowel.

The colon is characterized by sacculations or haustra caused by longitudinal contractions of the taenia coli. The transverse colon is mobile due to its intraperitoneal location, with the hepatic and splenic flexures defining its beginning and end, respectively. The colon, especially the hepatic flexure, is rarely interposed between the liver and diaphragm (i.e., Chilaiditi sign) [22], which may require particular attention when planning radiotherapy (Fig. 3.8).

3.3   Practical Considerations in the Evaluation of Tumor Extent

Table 3.2 summarizes characteristic imaging features used to evaluate tumor extent for radiotherapy.

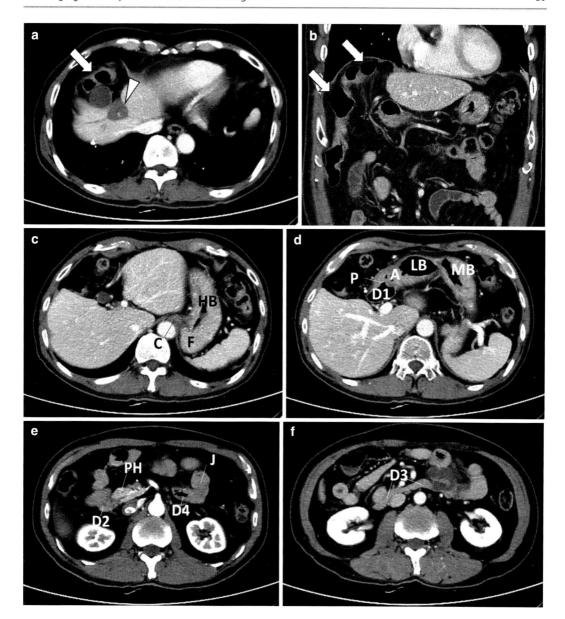

Fig. 3.8 Anatomy of the hepatic flexure of the colon, stomach, and duodenum. (**a, b**) The redundant hepatic flexure of the colon (arrows) appears just below the right hemidiaphragm and courses adjacent to the liver. The colon can be identified by its haustra, and is easily traced on the (**b**) coronal image. Note, a tumor (arrowhead) in hepatic segment 4 previously treated with radiofrequency ablation is shown on the (**a**) axial image. (**c, d**) The gastric cardia (C) connects the esophagogastric junction and gas-

tric body (HB = high body, MB = mid body, LB = lower body); the gastric fundus (F) is a dome-shaped portion underneath the left hemidiaphragm. (**d**) The gastric pylorus (P) is a sphincter between the gastric antrum (A) and duodenal bulb (D1). (**e, f**) The second portion of the duodenum (D2) descends, the third portion (D3) lies transversely, and the fourth portion (D4) ascends before the duodenum makes a sharp, anteroinferior turn into the proximal jejunum (J). PH = pancreatic head

Table 3.2 Characteristic imaging features used to evaluate tumor extent for radiotherapy

Entity	Important imaging features on CT or MRI
Arterioportal shunt	• Wedge-shaped, irregular, or linear APHE in the subcapsular or peripheral location of the liver • Absence of delayed washout • Isointensity on unenhanced T1- and T2-weighted images, DWI, or HBP images
Malignant tumor thrombosis	• Direct extension of a parenchymal tumor into an adjacent vessel • Presence of thin linear or punctate, arterially enhancing vessels within the portal venous or hepatic venous thrombosis • Expansion of the main portal vein to a diameter of 23 mm or greater
Intraductal growing HCC	• Hypo- or isointensity on T1-weighted images • Mildly hyper- or isointense on T2-weighted images • APHE and washout
Intrahepatic metastasis	• APHE, washout, intermediate T2 hyperintensity, diffusion restriction, and transitional phase or HBP hypointensity, even in subcentimeter lesions
Post-locoregional treatment viability	• Nodular, mass-like, or thick and irregular APHE contained within or along the margin. • Gradual increase in size and extent during imaging follow-up • Atypical, hypovascular tumor similar to pretreatment appearance

APHE arterial phase hyperenhancement; *CT* computed tomography; *DWI* diffusion-weighted imaging; *HBP* hepatobiliary phase; *HCC* hepatocellular carcinoma; *MRI* magnetic resonance imaging

3.3.1 Arterioportal Shunt

An arterioportal shunt (APS), or hypervascular pseudolesion, refers to an area of hepatic parenchymal hyperenhancement in the arterial phase of CT or MRI due to perfusion alteration. APS is a major mimicker of HCC and can sometimes create problems for differential diagnosis. APS can be classified as either tumorous or non-tumorous. Tumorous APS is caused by portal venous or portal venular obstruction due to the tumor, which causes a compensatory increase in arterial supply. Non-tumorous APS is caused by an alteration in flow dynamics due to liver cirrhosis; fibrotic distortion of the liver parenchyma narrows the hepatic sinusoids and hepatic venules, and subsequently increases arterial perfusion [23].

APS has the following clinical implications: (a) it can be mistaken for hypervascular tumors, such as HCC; (b) it can lead to overestimation of tumor size and extent; (c) hypervascular tumors can be masked by large APS; (d) the presence of massive tumorous APS can decrease the efficacy of locoregional treatment, such as transarterial chemoembolization, and alternative management plans will have to be considered [24].

The appearance of APS on CT and MRI is dependent on the pressure gradient of arterioportal perfusion and the imaging plane (axial vs. coronal plane) [25, 26]. Wedge-shaped, irregular, or linear APS in the typical subcapsular or peripheral location is easy to diagnose. However, nodular APS frequently mimics HCC. As APS has a three-dimensional cone shape, nodular APS may appear wedge-shaped on another orthogonal plane (Fig. 3.9).

Washout in delayed phases of CT or MRI is considered as one of the most reliable findings to suggest HCC instead of APS (Fig. 3.9) [23]. However, the absence of delayed washout does not completely exclude the possibility of HCC, especially on CT. At MRI, APS usually does not show signal changes on unenhanced T1- and T2-weighted images or DWI [27, 28]. In addition, non-tumorous APS does not usually show signal alteration on hepatobiliary phase (HBP) images of gadoxetic acid-enhanced MRI because the hepatobiliary uptake of contrast is not much affected by perfusion alteration; while most HCCs are hypointense in the HBP, APS is isointense in the HBP [27, 28].

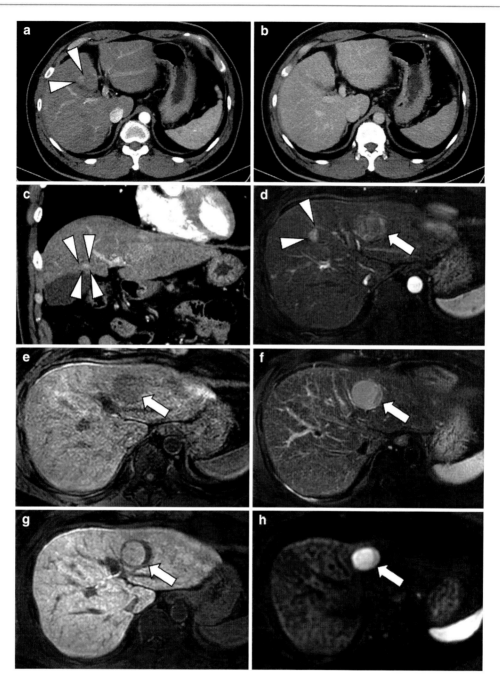

Fig. 3.9 An arterioportal shunt (APS) in hepatic segment 4. (**a**, **b**) On the axial images of CT, a nodular APS (arrowheads) in the medial subcapsular surface of segment 4 shows (**a**) arterial phase hyperenhancement (APHE) but is not delineated in the (**b**) delayed phase due to its isoattenuation to the liver. (**c**) On the coronal image of CT, the APS (arrowheads) is less voluminous than on the axial image because of its wedged shape. (**d**–**h**) On the axial images of MRI, (**d**) the nodular APS (arrowheads) is isointense on the (**e**) unenhanced T1- and (**f**) T2-weighted images, (**g**) hepatobiliary phase (HBP) image, and (**h**) diffusion-weighted image. In contrast, an HCC (arrows) in hepatic segment 3 shows (**d**) APHE, (**e**) T1 hypointensity, (**f**) intermediate T2 hyperintensity, (**e**) a nonenhancing capsule in the HBP, and (**f**) restricted diffusion

3.3.2 Malignant Portal Vein Thrombosis

Portal vein tumor thrombosis is common in patients with HCC [5]. HCC more commonly invades portal veins than hepatic veins [29], and rarely invades hepatic arteries [30]. If a malignant tumor thrombosis is present, patients are considered unsuitable for curative treatment, such as surgical resection or liver transplantation [31].

Bland thrombosis in the cirrhotic liver needs to be differentiated from malignant tumor thrombosis associated with HCC. Tumor thrombosis can be diagnosed by the following features: (a) direct extension of a parenchymal tumor into an adjacent vessel (Fig. 3.10) [32]; (b) the presence of thin linear or punctate, arterially enhancing vessels within the portal venous or hepatic venous thrombosis (i.e., threads and streaks sign) (Fig. 3.11) [33]; (c) expansion of the main portal vein to a diameter of

23 mm or greater (sensitivity and specificity, 63% and 100%, respectively) [34].

Some investigators have found that DWI of MRI can aid differentiation as well [35], but others have not [36]. Meanwhile, dual-energy CT that enables quantification of iodine density in the portal vein thrombosis is an emerging technique with the reported sensitivity and specificity being as high as 100% and 91%, respectively, for tumor thrombosis [37]. Further studies are needed to validate the utility of DWI and dual-energy CT for differential diagnosis.

3.3.3 Intraductal Growing HCC

HCC rarely causes obstructive jaundice due to bile duct tumor thrombosis [38]. Therefore, HCC with bile duct tumor thrombosis can often be mistaken for intraductal growing cholangiocarci-

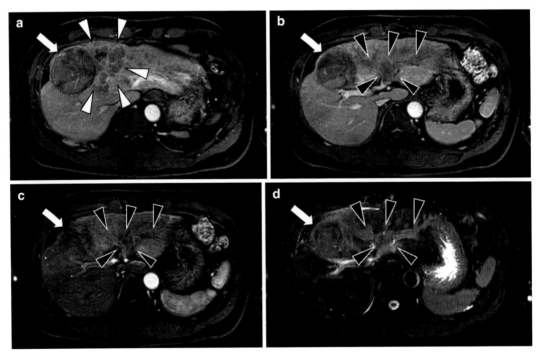

Fig. 3.10 HCC with portal vein invasion and extensive malignant portal vein tumor thrombosis (PVTT) on MRI. (**a**, **b**) In the portal venous phase, (**a**) a 7-cm encapsulated mass (arrow) in segment 8 of the liver and adjacent, infiltrative mass (white arrowheads) in segment 4 directly invade the portal vein branch of segment 4. (**b**) Diffuse expansile thrombosis in the left portal vein and its seg-

mental branches (black arrowheads) shows washout, similar to the main mass (arrow). (**c**) In the arterial phase, the left hemiliver shows diffuse APHE due to APS formed secondary to PVTT (black arrowheads). (**d**) Diffuse HCC in the left hemiliver with PVTT (black arrowheads) as well as the encapsulated HCC in segment 8 (arrow) are of intermediate hyperintensity on the T2-weighted image

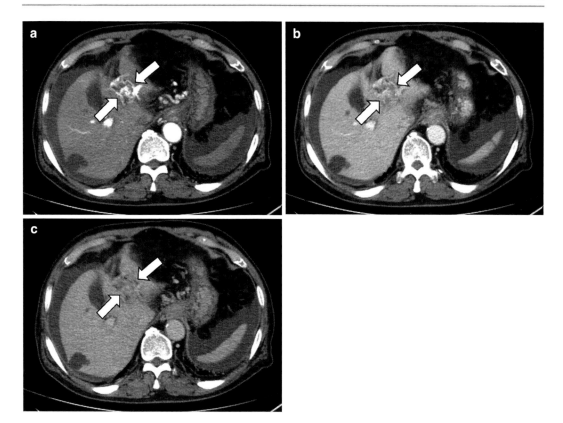

Fig. 3.11 Malignant PVTT on CT. (**a–c**) The umbilical portion of the left portal vein has widened to a diameter of 2 cm due to the tumor thrombosis (arrows). (**a**) There are punctate, arterial enhancing foci within the thrombosis, which are referred to as the "thread and streak sign"

noma or biliary stones [39]. Nonetheless, HCC can invade the bile duct and form intraductal tumor thrombosis, or even present as an isolated intraductal mass.

Similar to HCCs in the liver, HCC with bile duct tumor thrombosis is hypointense or isointense on T1-weighted images, mildly hyperintense or isointense on T2-weighted images, and shows APHE and washout (Fig. 3.12) [40]. This enhancement pattern can help differentiate it from cholangiocarcinoma, which usually shows progressive contrast enhancement in the delayed phase, and from biliary stones, which do not show contrast enhancement [41, 42]. The proportion of tumor cells within the bile duct tumor thrombosis determines the degree of enhancement [43]. For example, a tumor thrombosis that consists mainly of cancer cell clusters and contains little necrotic tissue or few blood clots

hyperenhances in the arterial phase of CT or MRI. On the other hand, when a tumor thrombosis mainly consists of necrotic tissue or blood clots, it may not show contrast enhancement.

As the portal vein and bile duct are located near each other within Glisson's capsule, HCC with bile duct tumor thrombosis may be accompanied by portal vein tumor thrombosis [40, 44–47]. Therefore, portal veins should also be carefully examined in HCC with bile duct tumor thrombosis.

3.3.4 Intrahepatic Metastasis

Identifying the exact number and location of multiple tumors is essential for accurate tumor staging. Intrahepatic metastasis is an important cause of early recurrence after curative treatment

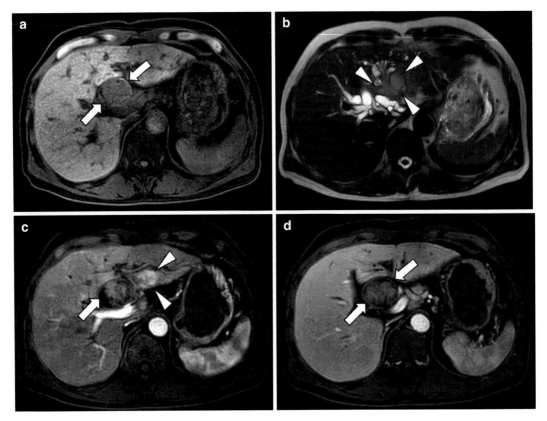

Fig. 3.12 Intraductal growing HCC on MRI. (**a**) There is an expansile, intraductal growing mass (arrows) in the common hepatic duct with T1 hypointensity. (**b**) An intermediate T2 hyperintense mass in hepatic segment 3 (arrowheads) encases the left portal vein and directly invades the left hepatic duct. Due to hilar bile duct inva- sion, intrahepatic bile ducts of the right hemiliver and the caudate lobe show obstructive dilatation. (**c**) The mass in segment 3 (arrowheads) shows APHE, and the intraductal growing mass (arrow) also shows a milder degree of APHE. (**d**) The intraductal growing mass (arrow) shows washout in the portal venous phase

for HCC, and timely detection and treatment of intrahepatic metastasis at the initial HCC diagnosis can improve patient survival [48, 49]. Detection of intrahepatic metastasis at the time of radiation therapy may also optimize treatment plans.

Compared to CT alone, performing MRI with CT increases the detection of additional HCC nodules, particularly small-sized lesions [48, 50]. With the help of diffusion restriction and HBP hypointensity features, DWI and HBP images of gadoxetic acid-enhanced MRI become key sequences for improving the detectability of small metastases [48, 50–53]. Importantly, the presence of MRI features, including APHE, washout, intermediate T2 hyperintensity, diffusion restriction, and transi-

tional phase or HBP hypointensity, are considered to indicate HCC for subcentimeter lesions (Fig. 3.13) [54–56].

3.3.5 Post-Locoregional Treatment Imaging

Tumor viability after locoregional treatment can be assessed by CT and MRI. As suggested by the European Association for the Study of the Liver criteria and modified Response Evaluation Criteria in Solid Tumors, APHE is the primary feature to suggest a viable tumor in the treated site [5, 57]. Thin perilesional hyperemia after locoregional treatment needs to be differentiated from viable tumors, and the criterion for

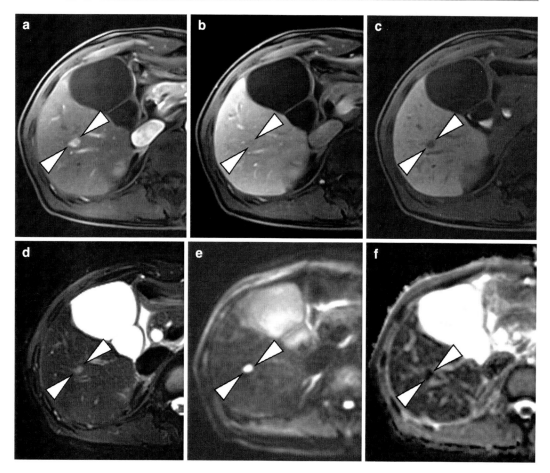

Fig. 3.13 Intrahepatic metastasis in a patient with a history of cryoablation for HCC. A 1.2 cm-sized nodule (arrowheads) in segment 5/6 of the liver shows (**a**) APHE, (**b**) mild portal venous phase washout, (**c**) HBP hypointensity, (**d**) intermediate T2 hyperintensity, (**e**) high signal intensity on the diffusion-weighted image ($b = 800$), and (**f**) low apparent diffusion coefficient value (i.e., diffusion restriction). Imaging features are compatible with an intrahepatic metastasis of HCC

this differentiation is well described in the Liver Imaging Reporting and Data System treatment response algorithm as follows: Nodular, mass-like, or thick and irregular APHE contained within or along the margin suggests a viable tumor (Fig. 3.14) [4]. Although compact Lipiodol accumulation in the treated lesion after TACE suggests a low probability of residual tumor [58], the Lipiodol itself, containing iodine content, may hamper the evaluation of APHE after treatment due to its innate hyperattenuation on CT. Therefore, unenhanced CT scans are necessary to evaluate treatment response after TACE [1]. In addition, coagulation necrosis after ablation therapy appears hyperintense on T1-weighted images, and subtraction imaging between arterial phase scans and unenhanced scans may better demonstrate the presence or absence of APHE within the ablation zone [59]. Gradual increase in size and extent during imaging follow-up also suggests tumor viability. Of note, pretreatment imaging should be taken into consideration when assessing treatment response, because atypical, hypovascular HCC can look similar to its pre-treatment appearance even after treatment.

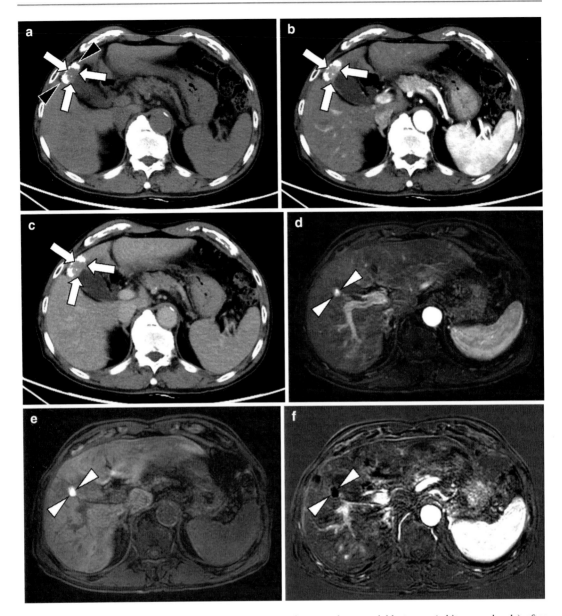

Fig. 3.14 Viable and nonviable tumors after TACE in a patient with HCC. (**a–c**) The axial images of CT show a viable tumor (arrows) after TACE. Heterogeneous Lipiodol uptake (black arrowheads) in a tumor located in segment 4 of the liver appears hyperattenuated on the (**a**) unenhanced image. The Lipiodol defective area (arrows) shows (**b**) mass-like APHE and (**c**) delayed washout, suggesting a viable tumor. (**d–f**) The axial images of MRI show another nonviable tumor (white arrowheads) after TACE. (**d**) The treated tumor in segment 5 of the liver demonstrates hyperintensity in the arterial phase. (**e**) Note that the same lesion is also hyperintense on the unenhanced T1-weighted image. (**f**) Subtraction between the arterial phase image and unenhanced image shows dark signals within the lesion, suggesting no contrast enhancement and non-viability

References

1. Chiu RY, Yap WW, Patel R, Liu D, Klass D, Harris AC. Hepatocellular carcinoma post embolotherapy: imaging appearances and pitfalls on computed tomography and magnetic resonance imaging. Can Assoc Radiol J. 2016;67(2):158–72. https://doi.org/10.1016/j.carj.2015.09.006.

2. Murakami T, Kim T, Kawata S, Kanematsu M, Federle MP, Hori M, et al. Evaluation of optimal timing of arterial phase imaging for the detection of hypervascular hepatocellular carcinoma by using triple arterial phase imaging with multidetector-row helical computed tomography. Invest Radiol. 2003;38(8):497–503. https://doi.org/10.1097/01.rli.0000074584.12494.e3.

3. Monzawa S, Ichikawa T, Nakajima H, Kitanaka Y, Omata K, Araki T. Dynamic CT for detecting small hepatocellular carcinoma: usefulness of delayed phase imaging. AJR Am J Roentgenol. 2007;188(1):147–53. https://doi.org/10.2214/ajr.05.0512.

4. Chernyak V, Fowler KJ, Kamaya A, Kielar AZ, Elsayes KM, Bashir MR, et al. Liver imaging reporting and data system (LI-RADS) version 2018: imaging of hepatocellular carcinoma in at-risk patients. Radiology. 2018;289(3):816–30. https://doi.org/10.1148/radiol.2018181494.

5. European Association for the Study of the Liver. EASL clinical practice guidelines: management of hepatocellular carcinoma. J Hepatol. 2018;69(1):182–236. https://doi.org/10.1016/j.jhep.2018.03.019.

6. Hope TA, Fowler KJ, Sirlin CB, Costa EA, Yee J, Yeh BM, et al. Hepatobiliary agents and their role in LI-RADS. Abdom Imaging. 2015;40(3):613–25. https://doi.org/10.1007/s00261-014-0227-5.

7. Lukovic J, Henke L, Gani C, Kim TK, Stanescu T, Hosni A, et al. MRI-based upper abdominal organs-at-risk atlas for radiation oncology. Int J Radiat Oncol Biol Phys. 2020;106(4):743–53. https://doi.org/10.1016/j.ijrobp.2019.12.003.

8. Strasberg SM. Nomenclature of hepatic anatomy and resections: a review of the Brisbane 2000 system. J Hepatobiliary Pancreat Surg. 2005;12(5):351–5. https://doi.org/10.1007/s00534-005-0999-7.

9. Murakami G, Hata F. Human liver caudate lobe and liver segment. Anat Sci Int. 2002;77(4):211–24. https://doi.org/10.1046/j.0022-7722.2002.00033.x.

10. Auh YH, Rosen A, Rubenstein WA, Engel IA, Whalen JP, Kazam E. CT of the papillary process of the caudate lobe of the liver. AJR Am J Roentgenol. 1984;142(3):535–8. https://doi.org/10.2214/ajr.142.3.535.

11. Majno P, Mentha G, Toso C, Morel P, Peitgen HO, Fasel JH. Anatomy of the liver: an outline with three levels of complexity - a further step towards tailored territorial liver resections. J Hepatol. 2014;60(3):654–62. https://doi.org/10.1016/j.jhep.2013.10.026.

12. Ohtani O, Ohtani Y. Lymph circulation in the liver. Anat Rec (Hoboken). 2008;291(6):643–52. https://doi.org/10.1002/ar.20681.

13. Tanaka M, Iwakiri Y. The hepatic lymphatic vascular system: structure, function, markers, and lymphangiogenesis. Cell Mol Gastroenterol Hepatol. 2016;2(6):733–49. https://doi.org/10.1016/j.jcmgh.2016.09.002.

14. Lupinacci RM, Paye F, Coelho FF, Kruger JA, Herman P. Lymphatic drainage of the liver and its implications in the management of colorectal cancer liver metastases. Updat Surg. 2014;66(4):239–45. https://doi.org/10.1007/s13304-014-0265-0.

15. Ercolani G, Grazi GL, Ravaioli M, Grigioni WF, Cescon M, Gardini A, et al. The role of lymphadenectomy for liver tumors: further considerations on the appropriateness of treatment strategy. Ann Surg. 2004;239(2):202–9. https://doi.org/10.1097/01.sla.0000109154.00020.e0.

16. Xiaohong S, Huikai L, Feng W, Ti Z, Yunlong C, Qiang L. Clinical significance of lymph node metastasis in patients undergoing partial hepatectomy for hepatocellular carcinoma. World J Surg. 2010;34(5):1028–33. https://doi.org/10.1007/s00268-010-0400-0.

17. Sun HC, Zhuang PY, Qin LX, Ye QH, Wang L, Ren N, et al. Incidence and prognostic values of lymph node metastasis in operable hepatocellular carcinoma and evaluation of routine complete lymphadenectomy. J Surg Oncol. 2007;96(1):37–45. https://doi.org/10.1002/jso.20772.

18. Watanabe J, Nakashima O, Kojiro M. Clinicopathologic study on lymph node metastasis of hepatocellular carcinoma: a retrospective study of 660 consecutive autopsy cases. Jpn J Clin Oncol. 1994;24(1):37–41. https://doi.org/10.1093/oxfordjournals.jjco.a039672.

19. Xia F, Wu L, Lau WY, Li G, Huan H, Qian C, et al. Positive lymph node metastasis has a marked impact on the long-term survival of patients with hepatocellular carcinoma with extrahepatic metastasis. PLoS One. 2014;9(4):e95889. https://doi.org/10.1371/journal.pone.0095889.

20. Choi JW, Kim TK, Kim KW, Kim AY, Kim PN, Ha HK, et al. Anatomic variation in intrahepatic bile ducts: an analysis of intraoperative cholangiograms in 300 consecutive donors for living donor liver transplantation. Korean J Radiol. 2003;4(2):85–90. https://doi.org/10.3348/kjr.2003.4.2.85.

21. Jabbour SK, Hashem SA, Bosch W, Kim TK, Finkelstein SE, Anderson BM, et al. Upper abdominal normal organ contouring guidelines and atlas: a Radiation Therapy Oncology Group consensus. Pract Radiat Oncol. 2014;4(2):82–9. https://doi.org/10.1016/j.prro.2013.06.004.

22. Kamiyoshihara M, Ibe T, Takeyoshi I. Chilaiditi's sign mimicking a traumatic diaphragmatic hernia. Ann Thorac Surg. 2009;87(3):959–61. https://doi.org/10.1016/j.athoracsur.2008.07.033.

23. Ahn JH, Yu JS, Hwang SH, Chung JJ, Kim JH, Kim KW. Nontumorous arterioportal shunts in the liver: CT and MRI findings considering mechanisms and fate. Eur Radiol. 2010;20(2):385–94. https://doi.org/10.1007/s00330-009-1542-z.

24. Xiao YD, Ma C, Zhang ZS, Liu J. Safety and efficacy assessment of transarterial chemoembolization using drug-eluting beads in patients with hepatocellular carcinoma and arterioportal shunt: a single-center experience. Cancer Manag Res. 2019;11:1551–7. https://doi.org/10.2147/CMAR.S193948.

25. Choi BI, Lee KH, Han JK, Lee JM. Hepatic arterioportal shunts: dynamic CT and MR features. Korean J Radiol. 2002;3(1):1–15. https://doi.org/10.3348/kjr.2002.3.1.1.

26. Jang HJ, Khalili K, Yu H, Kim TK. Perfusion and parenchymal changes related to vascular alterations of the liver. Abdom Imaging. 2012;37(3):404–21. https://doi.org/10.1007/s00261-011-9767-0.

27. Choi JY, Lee JM, Sirlin CB. CT and MR imaging diagnosis and staging of hepatocellular carcinoma: part II. Extracellular agents, hepatobiliary agents, and ancillary imaging features. Radiology. 2014;273(1):30–50. https://doi.org/10.1148/radiol.14132362.

28. Motosugi U, Ichikawa T, Sou H, Sano K, Tominaga L, Muhi A, et al. Distinguishing hypervascular pseudolesions of the liver from hypervascular hepatocellular carcinomas with gadoxetic acid-enhanced MR imaging. Radiology. 2010;256(1):151–8. https://doi.org/10.1148/radiol.10091885.

29. Choi JY, Lee JM, Sirlin CB. CT and MR imaging diagnosis and staging of hepatocellular carcinoma: part I. Development, growth, and spread: key pathologic and imaging aspects. Radiology. 2014;272(3):635–54. https://doi.org/10.1148/radiol.14132361.

30. Edmondson HA, Steiner PE. Primary carcinoma of the liver. A study of 100 cases among 48,900 necropsies. Cancer. 1954;7(3):462–503. https://doi.org/10.1002/1097-0142(195405)7:3<462::AID-CNCR2820070308>3.0.CO;2-E.

31. Llovet JM, Fuster J, Bruix J, Barcelona-Clinic Liver Cancer Group. The Barcelona approach: diagnosis, staging, and treatment of hepatocellular carcinoma. Liver Transpl. 2004;10(2 Suppl 1):S115–20. https://doi.org/10.1002/lt.20034.

32. Cannella R, Taibbi A, Porrello G, Dioguardi Burgio M, Cabibbo G, Bartolotta TV. Hepatocellular carcinoma with macrovascular invasion: multimodality imaging features for the diagnosis. Diagn Interv Radiol. 2020;26(6):531–40. https://doi.org/10.5152/dir.2020.19569.

33. Raab BW. The thread and streak sign. Radiology. 2005;236(1):284–5. https://doi.org/10.1148/radiol.2361030114.

34. Tublin ME, Dodd GD 3rd, Baron RL. Benign and malignant portal vein thrombosis: differentiation by CT characteristics. AJR Am J Roentgenol. 1997;168(3):719–23. https://doi.org/10.2214/ajr.168.3.9057522.

35. Catalano OA, Choy G, Zhu A, Hahn PF, Sahani DV. Differentiation of malignant thrombus from bland thrombus of the portal vein in patients with hepatocellular carcinoma: application of diffusion-weighted MR imaging. Radiology. 2010;254(1):154–62. https://doi.org/10.1148/radiol.09090304.

36. Sandrasegaran K, Tahir B, Nutakki K, Akisik FM, Bodanapally U, Tann M, et al. Usefulness of conventional MRI sequences and diffusion-weighted imaging in differentiating malignant from benign portal vein thrombus in cirrhotic patients. AJR Am J Roentgenol. 2013;201(6):1211–9. https://doi.org/10.2214/AJR.12.10171.

37. Ascenti G, Sofia C, Mazziotti S, Silipigni S, D'Angelo T, Pergolizzi S, et al. Dual-energy CT with iodine quantification in distinguishing between bland and neoplastic portal vein thrombosis in patients with hepatocellular carcinoma. Clin Radiol. 2016;71(9):938.e1–9. https://doi.org/10.1016/j.crad.2016.05.002.

38. Kojiro M, Kawabata K, Kawano Y, Shirai F, Takemoto N, Nakashima T. Hepatocellular carcinoma presenting as intrabile duct tumor growth: a clinicopathologic study of 24 cases. Cancer. 1982;49(10):2144–7. https://doi.org/10.1002/1097-0142(19820515)49:10<2144::aid-cncr2820491026>3.0.co;2-o.

39. Zeng H, Xu LB, Wen JM, Zhang R, Zhu MS, Shi XD, et al. Hepatocellular carcinoma with bile duct tumor thrombus: a clinicopathological analysis of factors predictive of recurrence and outcome after surgery. Medicine (Baltimore). 2015;94(1):e364. https://doi.org/10.1097/MD.0000000000000364.

40. Tseng JH, Hung CF, Ng KK, Wan YL, Yeh TS, Chiu CT. Icteric-type hepatoma: magnetic resonance imaging and magnetic resonance cholangiographic features. Abdom Imaging. 2001;26(2):171–7. https://doi.org/10.1007/s002610000136.

41. Seo N, Kim DY, Choi JY. Cross-sectional imaging of intrahepatic cholangiocarcinoma: development, growth, spread, and prognosis. AJR Am J Roentgenol. 2017;209(2):W64–75. https://doi.org/10.2214/AJR.16.16923.

42. Jung AY, Lee JM, Choi SH, Kim SH, Lee JY, Kim SW, et al. Computed tomography features of an intraductal polypoid mass: differentiation between hepatocellular carcinoma with bile duct tumor invasion and intraductal papillary cholangiocarcinoma. J Comput Assist Tomogr. 2006;30(1):18–24. https://doi.org/10.1097/01.rct.0000188837.71136.fe.

43. Liu Q, Chen J, Li H, Liang B, Zhang L, Hu T. Hepatocellular carcinoma with bile duct tumor thrombi: correlation of magnetic resonance imaging features to histopathologic manifestations. Eur J Radiol. 2010;76(1):103–9. https://doi.org/10.1016/j.ejrad.2009.05.020.

44. Shiomi M, Kamiya J, Nagino M, Uesaka K, Sano T, Hayakawa N, et al. Hepatocellular carcinoma with biliary tumor thrombi: aggressive operative approach after appropriate preoperative management. Surgery. 2001;129(6):692–8. https://doi.org/10.1067/msy.2001.113889.

45. Qin LX, Ma ZC, Wu ZQ, Fan J, Zhou XD, Sun HC, et al. Diagnosis and surgical treatments of hepatocellular carcinoma with tumor thrombosis in bile duct: experience of 34 patients. World J Gastroenterol. 2004;10(10):1397–401. https://doi.org/10.3748/wjg.v10.i10.1397.

46. Peng BG, Liang LJ, Li SQ, Zhou F, Hua YP, Luo SM. Surgical treatment of hepatocellular carcinoma with bile duct tumor thrombi. World J Gastroenterol. 2005;11(25):3966–9. https://doi.org/10.3748/wjg.v11.i25.3966.

47. Gabata T, Terayama N, Kobayashi S, Sanada J, Kadoya M, Matsui O. MR imaging of hepatocellular carcinomas with biliary tumor thrombi. Abdom Imaging. 2007;32(4):470–4. https://doi.org/10.1007/s00261-006-9154-4.

48. Kim HD, Lim YS, Han S, An J, Kim GA, Kim SY, et al. Evaluation of early stage hepatocellular carcinoma by magnetic resonance imaging with gadoxetic acid detects additional lesions and increases overall survival. Gastroenterology. 2015;148(7):1371–82. https://doi.org/10.1053/j.gastro.2015.02.051.

49. Yang SL, Luo YY, Chen M, Zhou YP, Lu FR, Deng DF, et al. A systematic review and meta-analysis comparing the prognosis of multicentric occurrence and vs. intrahepatic metastasis in patients with recurrent hepatocellular carcinoma after hepatectomy. HPB (Oxford). 2017;19(10):835–42. https://doi.org/10.1016/j.hpb.2017.06.002.

50. Yu JS, Chung JJ, Kim JH, Cho ES, Kim DJ, Ahn JH, et al. Detection of small intrahepatic metastases of hepatocellular carcinomas using diffusion-weighted imaging: comparison with conventional dynamic MRI. Magn Reson Imaging. 2011;29(7):985–92. https://doi.org/10.1016/j.mri.2011.04.010.

51. Holzapfel K, Eiber MJ, Fingerle AA, Bruegel M, Rummeny EJ, Gaa J. Detection, classification, and characterization of focal liver lesions: value of diffusion-weighted MR imaging, gadoxetic acid-enhanced MR imaging and the combination of both methods. Abdom Imaging. 2012;37(1):74–82. https://doi.org/10.1007/s00261-011-9758-1.

52. Lowenthal D, Zeile M, Lim WY, Wybranski C, Fischbach F, Wieners G, et al. Detection and characterisation of focal liver lesions in colorectal carcinoma patients: comparison of diffusion-weighted and Gd-EOB-DTPA enhanced MR imaging. Eur Radiol. 2011;21(4):832–40. https://doi.org/10.1007/s00330-010-1977-2.

53. Kim YK, Kim YK, Park HJ, Park MJ, Lee WJ, Choi D. Noncontrast MRI with diffusion-weighted imaging as the sole imaging modality for detecting liver malignancy in patients with high risk for hepatocellular carcinoma. Magn Reson Imaging. 2014;32(6):610–8. https://doi.org/10.1016/j.mri.2013.12.021.

54. Lee MW, Lim HK. Management of sub-centimeter recurrent hepatocellular carcinoma after curative treatment: current status and future. World J Gastroenterol. 2018;24(46):5215–22. https://doi.org/10.3748/wjg.v24.i46.5215.

55. Park CJ, An C, Park S, Choi JY, Kim MJ. Management of subcentimetre arterially enhancing and hepatobiliary hypointense lesions on gadoxetic acid-enhanced MRI in patients at risk for HCC. Eur Radiol. 2018;28(4):1476–84. https://doi.org/10.1007/s00330-017-5088-1.

56. Yu MH, Kim JH, Yoon JH, Kim HC, Chung JW, Han JK, et al. Small (≤1-cm) hepatocellular carcinoma: diagnostic performance and imaging features at gadoxetic acid-enhanced MR imaging. Radiology. 2014;271(3):748–60. https://doi.org/10.1148/radiol.14131996.

57. Lencioni R, Llovet JM. Modified RECIST (mRECIST) assessment for hepatocellular carcinoma. Semin Liver Dis. 2010;30(1):52–60. https://doi.org/10.1055/s-0030-1247132.

58. Dioguardi Burgio M, Sartoris R, Libotean C, Zappa M, Sibert A, Vilgrain V, et al. Lipiodol retention pattern after TACE for HCC is a predictor for local progression in lesions with complete response. Cancer Imaging. 2019;19(1):75. https://doi.org/10.1186/s40644-019-0260-2.

59. Hussein RS, Tantawy W, Abbas YA. MRI assessment of hepatocellular carcinoma after locoregional therapy. Insights Imaging. 2019;10(1):8. https://doi.org/10.1186/s13244-019-0690-1.

Functional Assessment of Liver for Radiation Oncologist

4

Jun Yong Park

Abstract

Improvement of short- and long-term prognosis after radiation therapy (RT) has been the main focus of radiation oncologists over the last two decades. Most patients with liver cancer have underlying liver disease, and a pre-RT hepatic functional reserve evaluation is important to avoid post-RT hepatic failure and death. Better selection of patients based on hepatic functional reserve can be the most important contributing factor to the success of RT for liver cancer. However, liver function involves a spectrum of metabolic functions, so there is no single test that can accurately and practically measure all functions at the same time. This chapter introduces what radiation oncologists need to know in order to evaluate hepatic functional reserves and several scoring systems to evaluate them.

Keywords

Radiation therapy · Radiotherapy-induced liver disease · Hepatic functional reserve · Scoring system · Indocyanine green clearance

J. Y. Park (✉)
Department of Internal Medicine, Institute of Gastroenterology, Yonsei University College of Medicine, Seoul, South Korea
e-mail: DRPJY@yuhs.ac

Traditionally, the liver has been believed to have a relatively low radiation tolerance. This is a major limitation for radiation therapy (RT) in liver cancer treatment [1]. Technological advances with improvement in target localization, image guidance, patient immobilization, and delivery of conformal radiation have allowed the use of high doses of radiation to conform to the target volume while sparing surrounding non-tumorous liver parenchyma [2, 3]. However, most patients with primary liver cancer, especially hepatocellular carcinoma (HCC), have chronic active hepatitis B, C, or alcoholic cirrhosis with subsequent impaired liver function, and they are considered to have an even lower tolerance of radiation to the liver. Also, radiation to the liver may result in radiotherapy-induced liver disease (RILD) [4, 5]. A mean dose of 30 Gy is usually considered safe, but the liver's tolerance of radiation is lower in patients with known liver function impairment. These patients are more susceptible to developing RILD. RILD occurs as an acute response during or within a few weeks of RT or as a late-response months to years after RT, and is associated with a high mortality rate in patients with liver cancer [6, 7] Predictors of RILD have not yet been established and depend on the exact definition used, radiation method, and type of liver cancer; therefore, the assessment of liver function, which can predict the risk of liver failure and mortality, is absolutely necessary for safe RT. The goals of hepatic functional assessment when implementing RT in liver can-

J. Seong (ed.), *Radiotherapy of Liver Cancer*, https://doi.org/10.1007/978-981-16-1815-4_4

cer is to select appropriate patients and predict safety margins. Accurate assessment of hepatic functional reserve and toxicity measurements can lead to safer dose recommendations for patients with liver cancer and could improve local control. However, the liver is a multi-functioned organ and there is no single comprehensive liver function test.

4.1 Radiotherapy-Induced Liver Disease (RILD)

In the case of liver tumors, the therapeutic ratio is narrowed because of concerns relating to RILD, particularly in a population with known liver function impairment. Post-irradiation liver damage ranges from asymptomatic conditions with or without biochemical abnormalities to fatal hepatic failure. RILD, which was originally described by Ingold et al. [8], is a serious condition and death due to RT has been reported in the literature after conventional RT as well as after stereotactic body radiation therapy (SBRT) [9, 10]. It is also a very challenging condition, as there are few or no clinical characteristics related to its early phase; once the clinical signs appear, it is most often too late to intervene. Historically, the risk of hepatic decompensation due to RILD has discouraged the use of RT to treat liver cancer. RILD triggers a fibrotic process leading to the obliteration of central veins and widespread venous congestion.

There are two types of RILD: classic RILD and non-classic RILD. Classic RILD was historically the dose-limiting complication of post-whole hepatic radiation to 30–35 Gy using conventionally fractionated radiotherapy [7]. Patients with classic RILD usually have symptoms of fatigue, ascites, anicteric hepatomegaly, and an isolated elevation in alkaline phosphatase (ALP) disproportionate to that of other liver enzymes. Pathophysiologically veno-occlusive disease, characterized by complete obliteration of the central vein lumina by erythrocytes trapped in a network of reticulin and collagen fibers, is highly associated with the clinical syndromes of subacute radiation injury of liver [11]. Risk factors for the occurrence of classic RILD included high mean liver dose, primary liver cancer, male, and hepatic arterial chemotherapy [12]. With the increased precision of modern radiotherapy techniques, classic RILD is very rare. Patients with underlying chronic liver disease may present with liver function abnormalities including markedly elevated serum alanine aminotransferase (ALT) and aspartate aminotransferase (AST) (more than 5 times the upper limit of normal), and jaundice within 3 months of radiation therapy [1, 6, 7]. Compared with classic RILD due to dose-limiting complications, non-classic RILD, which occurs with RT using CT-based planning, causes increases in transaminase and bilirubin. Vulnerable populations affected by non-classical RILD are those with underlying chronic liver disease, such as patients with hepatitis B or C and cirrhosis due to a variety of causes. Hepatic non-parenchymal cells, such as Kupffer cells, sinusoidal endothelial cells, and hepatic stellate cells, are known to be radiosensitive. These cells release various substances that promote liver fibrosis, contributing to distorted liver structure and function during radiation [13–15]. This radiation-induced hepatic fibrosis is becoming an increasingly serious problem in patients with underlying liver disease. Once a patient has developed classic or non-classic RILD, best supportive care is generally the only management that can be done.

4.2 General Liver Biochemical and Function Test

ALT, AST, ALP, and bilirubin are biochemical markers of liver injury. Albumin, bilirubin, and prothrombin time are markers of hepatocellular function. These reflect different functions of the liver—that is, to excrete anions (bilirubin), hepatocellular integrity (transaminases), formation and the subsequent free flow of bile (bilirubin and ALP), and protein synthesis (albumin). Elevations of liver enzymes often reflect damage to the liver or biliary obstruction, whereas an abnormal serum albumin or prothrombin time may be seen in the setting of impaired hepatic synthetic function. The serum bilirubin in part measures the hepatic ability to detoxify metabolites and transport organic anions into bile. These tests can be helpful in determining the area of hepatic injury, and the pattern of elevation can help organize a differential diagnosis. However, none of these parameters provide quantitative information on the hepatic functional reserve as a single indicator. To overcome this limitation, scoring systems were introduced (Table 4.1). Traditionally, general scores, including the Child-Turcotte-Pugh (CTP) score and the Model for End-Stage Liver Disease (MELD) score, are useful for estimating integrated liver function and disease severity, and can serve as helpful medical decision-making tools for guiding patient care.

4.3 Child-Turcotte-Pugh (CTP) Score

In 1964, Child and Turcotte proposed a grading system for liver function to predict postoperative mortality of cirrhotic patients undergoing a portocaval shunt surgery [16]. The initial version of the Child-Turcotte score included two continuous variables (bilirubin and albumin) and three quantitative variables (ascites, encephalopathy, and nutritional status). This grading system was modified by Pugh et al. almost 10 years later, and the system has subsequently been known as the CTP score [17]. In this modified version, nutritional status is replaced by prothrombin time. The CTP score is a simple system for grading liver function based on these five easily measured parameters: (i) the presence or absence of encephalopathy; (ii) the presence or absence of ascites; (iii) the serum total bilirubin level; (iv) the serum albumin level, and (v) the prothrombin time. The score, corresponding to the sum of individual points, allows categorization of patients in CTP grades A (5–6 points), B (7–9 points) and C (10–15 points): A—good hepatic function, B—moderately impaired hepatic function, and C—advanced hepatic dysfunction. The CTP score is widely known not only to predict short-term and long-term outcomes in cirrhotic patients, but also to predict hepatic toxicity after several treatment modalities in liver cancer patients with hepatic dysfunction. Therefore, the CTP score has been used extensively in assessing liver function and plays an important role in most common scoring systems that guide treatment decisions and treatment options for patients with liver cancer. For example, CTP A patients are generally considered safe candidates for elective surgery. CTP B patients can proceed with surgery after medical optimization but still have increased risk. Elective surgery is contraindicated in CTP C patients. Similarly, with liver RT, many studies have reported that CTP scores can predict the prognosis such as liver toxicity and treatment outcomes [12, 18–21]. However, the application of the CTP score has several limitations: (i) the assessment of ascites and encephalopathy is subjective; it therefore can be difficult for clinical assessment and scoring of these factors to be consistent among different evaluators; (ii) all five parameters have the same weight; (iii) there are only ten different scores (based on points) available; and (iv) this scoring system does not account for renal function, which is a reliable prognostic marker in cirrhosis.

Table 4.1 Prognostic scoring system for evaluating liver function

Score	Parameter
Child-Turcotte-Pugh (CTP) score	Serum bilirubin, albumin, prothrombin time, ascites, encephalopathy
Model for End-Stage Liver Disease (MELD) Score (= $3.78 \times \log_e[\text{serum bilirubin (mg/dL)}] + 11.2 \times \log_e[\text{INR}] + 9.57 \times \log_e[\text{serum creatinine (mg/dL)}] + 6.43$)	Serum bilirubin, creatinine, and prothrombin time; range 6–40
Albumin-Bilirubin (ALBI) score (= $\log_{10}$ bilirubin $\times 0.66$) + (albumin $\times -0.085$).)	Serum bilirubin, albumin; ≤ -2.60 (ALBI grade 1), > -2.60 to ≤ -1.39 (ALBI grade 2), > -1.39 (ALBI grade 3)

4.4 Model for End-Stage Liver Disease (MELD) Score

The MELD score was first reported to predict three-month mortality following elective transjugular intrahepatic portosystemic shunt placement [22]. The original model included serum bilirubin, serum creatinine, prothrombin time, and etiology of the liver disease (cholestatic or alcoholic versus other etiologies). The etiology of liver disease was subsequently removed from the model for reasons such as the difficulty of classifying patients with multiple causes of chronic liver disease. In addition, this modification of the MELD score, by excluding the etiology of liver disease, did not significantly affect the accuracy of the model in predicting three-month survival [23]. The MELD score is widely used to predict the mortality risk of patients with end-stage liver disease and is applied for the allocation of deceased donor liver transplantation [24]. In patients with cirrhosis, an increasing MELD score is associated with increasing severity of hepatic dysfunction and increasing 3-month mortality risk. In addition, recently, there are many reports that the MELD score can be used to predict the severity and prognosis of diseases after liver transplantation, as well as to apply it to other liver cancer treatments such as hepatic resection surgery, trans-arterial chemoembolization (TACE), and RT. These prognostic predictions are also known to be more useful than CTP scores [25–27]. The MELD scoring system has prognostic value in a variety of clinical settings for cirrhotic patients beyond those applied to the deceased donor liver transplant allocation, and is particularly useful for predicting the prognosis after various treatments in patients of liver cancer. However, the MELD score has a limitation in that there is no clearly defined cutoff value, so different cutoff values of the MELD score must be determined for different situations.

4.5 Albumin-Bilirubin (ALBI) Score

Recently, a simple and objective method for the evaluation of hepatic functional reserve has introduced a new model for assessing the severity of liver dysfunction, and some have reported its usefulness for HCC treatment planning in different tumor stages [28–31]. Termed albumin-bilirubin (ALBI) score, it is calculated using only serum albumin and total bilirubin. The ALBI grade is a prognostic nomogram emerging from the multivariate screen of routine clinic-pathologic variables in a large, international cohort of patients with HCC, further validated in a separate group of cirrhotic patients without liver cancer. Also, this scoring system was later validated for HCC patients receiving resection, TACE, sorafenib, and SBRT [32–36]. The ALBI scoring system has especially been shown to be more discriminatory than the CTP score (A5 vs A6) in determining overall survival, and the baseline ALBI score has been shown to predict toxicity after RT [35, 37, 38].

Calculating with only two objective factors (albumin and total bilirubin) is one of advantages because these can be readily obtained from a routine blood test and lack of data is infrequent, especially in retrospective analyses. The ALBI score reduced the number of variables from the MELD score and eliminated the subjective components, including ascites and encephalopathy, from the CTP score. The ALBI nomogram has also been useful in further prognostically stratifying patients within each Barcelona Clinic Liver Cancer stage and Child-Pugh class of HCC. However, the weakness of this scoring system is that grade 2 covers a wide range and fails to assess portal hypertension. Care should also be taken when interpreting the results of hepatic functional reserve in patients with constitutional jaundice with elevated bilirubin levels, such as in Gilbert's syndrome.

In addition, scoring systems for measuring hepatic functional reserve modified by ALBI score, such as a modified ALBI score and platelet-albumin-bilirubin score, have been proposed.

4.6 Indocyanine Green (ICG) Clearance Test

ICG clearance measurement is a dynamic method of measuring hepatic functional reserve that consists of evaluating the hepatic clearance of ICG

15 min after its intravenous administration (ICG R15). ICG is a nontoxic, anionic water-soluble tricarbocyanine dye. When injected into the systemic circulation, ICG goes through a significant first pass effect in the normal liver. ICG has a relatively high intrinsic clearance. ICG R15 represents hepatic perfusion and thus is a direct measurement of dynamic liver function [39]. Normal values of ICG-R15 are around 10%, and the extent of the increases in ICG R15 reflects the degree of liver dysfunction. ICG R15 most likely increases in patients with cirrhosis because of intrahepatic shunt and sinusoidal capillarization [40]. This test has been used extensively in Asia and parts of Europe to assess post-hepatic resection functional reserve and to predict survival in critically ill patients [41]. Also, the addition of the ICG R15 to traditional liver metrics such as CTP and ALBI scores can improve the assessment of hepatic functional reserve in HCC patients [42, 43]. Even in RT for liver cancer, several studies have reported that baseline ICG R15 values can be a useful factor in predicting the prognosis and toxicity after RT [44, 45]. Additionally, there are many reports that the change in this value after RT is the most important [43, 46]. During RT, ICG measurements can be used to adjust the patient's RT treatment plan. If the estimated risk of toxicity is high, the dose may be reduced or a potentially higher dose may be given to patients who need an addition to achieve local control [43, 47].

There are, however, several drawbacks to determining the hepatic functional reserve through ICG R15 measurement. One of the confounding factors in measuring ICG clearance is its flow dependency. Change in hepatic blood flow such as that caused by intrahepatic shunting may affect the ICG clearance rate, making the test less predictable. Another point is that the ICG clearance test reflects the overall hepatic functional reserve but does not take into account regional variations that may occur within the liver, obscuring a possible functional disadvantage of the segments to be preserved [39, 48]. The transportation of ICG competes with that of bilirubin, so the ICG test is not suitable for patients with jaundice. In order to avoid these shortcomings, the ICG test should be interpreted with caution.

References

1. Pan CC, Kavanagh BD, Dawson LA, Li XA, Das SK, Miften M, et al. Radiation-associated liver injury. Int J Radiat Oncol. 2010;76:S94–100.
2. Bujold A, Massey CA, Kim JJ, Brierley J, Cho C, Wong RK, et al. Sequential phase I and II trials of stereotactic body radiotherapy for locally advanced hepatocellular carcinoma. J Clin Oncol. 2013;31:1631–9.
3. Choi SH, Seong J. Strategic application of radiotherapy for hepatocellular carcinoma. Clin Mol Hepatol. 2018;24:114–34.
4. Khozouz RF, Huq SZ, Perry MC. Radiation-induced liver disease. J Clin Oncol. 2008;26:4844–5.
5. Kim J, Jung Y. Radiation-induced liver disease: current understanding and future perspective. Exp Mol Med. 2017;49:e359.
6. Guha C, Kavanagh BD. Hepatic radiation toxicity: avoidance and amelioration. Semin Radiat Oncol. 2011;21:256–63.
7. Koay EJ, Owen D, Das P. Radiation-induced liver disease and modern radiotherapy. Semen Radiat Oncol. 2018;28:321–31.
8. Ingold JA, Reed GB, Kaplan HS, Bagshaw MA. Radiation hepatitis. Am J Roentgenol Radium Therapy, Nucl Med. 1965;93:200–8.
9. Cheng JC, Wu JK, Huang CM, Liu HS, Huang DY, Cheng SH, et al. Radiation-induced liver disease after three-dimensional conformal radiotherapy for patients with hepatocellular carcinoma: dosimetric analysis and implication. Int J Radiat Oncol. 2002;54:156–62.
10. Jung J, Yoon SM, Kim SY, Cho B, Park JH, Kim SS, et al. Radiation induced liver disease after stereotactic body radiotherapy for small hepatocellular carcinoma: clinical and dose-volumetric parameters. Radiat Oncol. 2013;8:249.
11. Lawrence TS, Robertson JM, Anscher MS, Jirtle RL, Ensminger WD, Fajardo LF. Hepatic toxicity resulting from cancer treatment. Int J Radiat Oncol Biol Phys. 1995;31:1237–48.
12. Dawson LA, Normolle D, Balter JM, McGinn CJ, Lawrence TS, Ten Haken RK. Analysis of radiation-induced liver disease using the Lyman NTCP model. Int J Radiat Oncol Biol Phys. 2002;53:810–21.
13. Christiansen H, Saile B, Neubauer-Saile K, Tippelt S, Rave-Frank M, Hermann RM, et al. Irradiation leads to susceptibility of hepatocytes to TNF-alpha mediated apoptosis. Radiother Oncol. 2004;72:291–6.
14. Yamanouchi K, Zhou H, Roy-Chowdhury N, Macaluso F, Liu L, Yamamoto T, et al. Hepatic irradiation augments engraftment of donor cells following hepatocyte transplantation. Hepatology. 2009;49:258–67.
15. Du SS, Qiang M, Zeng ZC, Ke AW, Ji Y, Zhang ZY, et al. Inactivation of Kupffer cells by gadolinium chloride protects murine liver from radiation-induced apoptosis. Int J Radiat Oncol Biol Phys. 2010;76:1225–34.
16. Child CG, Turcotte JG. Surgery and portal hypertension. Major Probl Clin Surg. 1964;1:1–85.

17. Pugh RN, Murray-Lyon IM, Dawson JL, Pietroni MC, Williams R. Transection of the oesophagus for bleeding oesophageal varices. Br J Surg. 1973;60:646–9.

18. Cheng JC, Wu JK, Lee PC, Liu H, Jian JJ, Lin Y, et al. Biologic susceptibility of hepatocellular carcinoma patients treated with radiotherapy to radiation-induced liver disease. Int J Radiat Oncol Biol Phys. 2004;60:1502–9.

19. Cardenes HR, Price TR, Perkins SM, Maluccio M, Kwo P, Breen TE, et al. Phase I feasibility trial of stereotactic body radiation therapy for primary hepatocellular carcinoma. Clin Transl Oncol. 2010;12:218–25.

20. Chino F, Stephens SJ, Choi SS, Marin D, Kim CY, Morse MA, et al. The role of external beam radiotherapy in the treatment of hepatocellular cancer. Cancer. 2018;124:3476–89.

21. Bae SH, Park HC, Yoon WS, Yoon SM, Jung I, Lee IJ, et al. Treatment outcome after fractionated conformal radiotherapy for hepatocellular carcinoma in patients with Child-Pugh classification B in Korea (KROG 16-05). Cancer Res Treat. 2019;51:1589–99.

22. Malinchoc M, Kamath PS, Gordon FD, Peine CJ, Rank J, ter Borg PC. A model to predict poor survival in patients undergoing transjugular intrahepatic portosystemic shunts. Hepatology. 2000;31:864–71.

23. Wiesner RH, McDiarmid SV, Kamath PS, Edwards EB, Malinchoc M, Kremers WK, et al. MELD and PELD: application of survival models to liver allocation. Liver Transpl. 2001;7:567–80.

24. Wiesner R, Edwards E, Freeman R, Harper A, Kim R, Kamath P, et al. Model for end-stage liver disease (MELD) and allocation of donor livers. Gastroenterology. 2003;124:91–6.

25. Klein KB, Stafinski TD, Menon D. Predicting survival after liver transplantation based on pre-transplant MELD score: a systematic review of the literature. PLoS One. 2013;8:e80661.

26. Teh SH, Christein J, Donohue J, Que F, Kendrick M, Farnell M, et al. Hepatic resection of hepatocellular carcinoma in patients with cirrhosis: model of End-Stage Liver Disease (MELD) score predicts perioperative mortality. J Gastrointest Surg. 2005;9:1207–15.

27. Okazaki E, Yamamoto A, Nishida N, Hamuro M, Ogino R, Hosono M, et al. Three-dimensional conformal radiotherapy for locally advanced hepatocellular carcinoma with portal vein tumour thrombosis: evaluating effectiveness of the model for end-stage liver disease (MELD) score compared with the Child-Pugh classification. Br J Radiol. 2016;89:20150945.

28. Johnson PJ, Berhane S, Kagebayashi C, Satomura S, Teng M, Reeves HL, et al. Assessment of liver function in patients with hepatocellular carcinoma: a new evidence-based approach-the ALBI grade. J Clin Oncol. 2015;33:550–8.

29. Hiraoka A, Kumada T, Kudo M, Hirooka M, Tsuji K, Itobayashi E, et al. Albumin-Bilirubin (ALBI) grade as part of the evidence-based clinical practice guideline for HCC of the Japan Society of Hepatology: a comparison with the liver damage and Child-Pugh classifications. Liver Cancer. 2017;6:204–15.

30. Chan AW, Kumada T, Toyoda H, Tada T, Chong CC, Mo FK, et al. Integration of albumin-bilirubin (ALBI) score into Barcelona Clinic Liver Cancer (BCLC) system for hepatocellular carcinoma. J Gastroenterol Hepatol. 2016;31:1300–6.

31. Pinato DJ, Sharma R, Allara E, Yen C, Arizumi T, Kubota K, et al. The ALBI grade provides objective hepatic reserve estimation across each BCLC stage of hepatocellular carcinoma. J Hepatol. 2017;66:338–46.

32. Toyoda H, Lai PB, O'Beirne J, Chong CC, Berhane S, Reeves H, et al. Long-term impact of liver function on curative therapy for hepatocellular carcinoma: application of the ALBI grade. Br J Cancer. 2016;114:744–50.

33. Hickey R, Mouli S, Kulik L, Desai K, Thornburg B, Ganger D, et al. Independent analysis of albumin-bilirubin grade in a 765-patient cohort treated with transarterial locoregional therapy for hepatocellular carcinoma. J Vasc Interv Radiol. 2016;27:795–802.

34. Edeline J, Blanc JF, Johnson P, Campillo-Gimenez B, Ross P, Ma YT, et al. A multicentre comparison between Child Pugh and albumin-bilirubin scores in patients treated with sorafenib for hepatocellular carcinoma. Liver Int. 2016;36:1821–8.

35. Lo CH, Liu MY, Lee MS, Yang JF, Jen YM, Lin CS, et al. Comparison between Child-Turcotte-Pugh and albumin-bilirubin scores in assessing the prognosis of hepatocellular carcinoma after stereotactic ablative radiotherapy. Int J Radiat Oncol Biol Phys. 2017;99:145–52.

36. Mathew AS, Atenafu EG, Owen D, Maurino C, Brade A, Brierley J, et al. Long term outcomes of stereotactic body radiation therapy for hepatocellular carcinoma without macrovascular invasion. Eur J Cancer. 2020;134:41–51.

37. Velec M, Haddad CR, Craig T, Wang L, Lindsay P, Brierley J, et al. Predictors of liver toxicity following stereotactic body radiation therapy for hepatocellular carcinoma. Int J Radiat Oncol Biol Phys. 2017;97:939–46.

38. Murray LJ, Sykes J, Brierley J, Kim JJ, Wong RKS, Ringash J, et al. Baseline albumin-bilirubin (ALBI) score in western patients with hepatocellular carcinoma treated with stereotactic body radiation therapy (SBRT). Int J Radiat Oncol Biol Phys. 2018;101:900–9.

39. Leevy CM, Smith F, Longueville J, Paumgartner G, Howard MM. Indocyanine green clearance as a test for hepatic function. Evaluation by dichromatic ear densitometry. JAMA. 1967;200:236–40.

40. Seyama Y, Kokudo N. Assessment of liver function for safe hepatic resection. Hepatol Res. 2009;39:107–16.

41. Yamamoto Y, Ikoma H, Morimura R, Konishi H, Murayama Y, Komatsu S, et al. Clinical analysis of anatomical resection for the treatment of hepatocellular carcinoma based on the stratification of liver function. World J Surg. 2014;38:1154–63.

42. Hiraoka A, Kumada T, Tsuji K, Takaguchi K, Itobayashi E, Kariyama K, et al. Validation of modi-

fied ALBI grade for more detailed assessment of hepatic function in hepatocellular carcinoma patients: a multicenter analysis. Liver Cancer. 2019;8:121–9.

43. Suresh K, Owen D, Bazzi L, Jackson W, Ten Haken RK, Cuneo K, et al. Using indocyanine green extraction to predict liver function after stereotactic body radiation therapy for hepatocellular carcinoma. Int J Radiat Oncol Biol Phys. 2018;100:131–7.

44. Cheng SH, Lin YM, Chuang VP, Yang PS, Cheng JC, Huang AT, et al. A pilot study of three-dimensional conformal radiotherapy in unresectable hepatocellular carcinoma. J Gastroenterol Hepatol. 1999;14:1025–33.

45. Yoon HI, Koom WS, Lee IJ, Jeong K, Chung Y, Kim JK, et al. The significance of ICG-R15 in predicting hepatic toxicity in patients receiving radio-

therapy for hepatocellular carcinoma. Liver Int. 2012;32:1165–71.

46. Stenmark MH, Cao Y, Wang H, Jackson A, Ben-Josef E, Ten Haken RK, et al. Estimating functional liver reserve following hepatic irradiation: adaptive normal tissue response models. Radiother Oncol. 2014;111:418–23.

47. Feng M, Suresh K, Schipper MJ, Bazzi L, Ben-Josef E, Matuszak MM, et al. Individualized adaptive stereotactic body radiotherapy for liver tumors in patients at high risk for liver damage: a phase 2 clinical trial. JAMA Oncol. 2018;4:40–7.

48. Rassam F, Olthof PB, Bennink RJ, van Gulik TM. Current modalities for the assessment of future remnant liver function. Visc Med. 2017;33:442–8.

Bo Hyun Kim ⓘ and Joong-Won Park ⓘ

Abstract

Approximately 50% and 30% of hepatocellular carcinoma (HCC) cases worldwide are attributed to hepatitis B virus (HBV) and hepatitis C virus (HCV) infection, respectively. Antiviral therapy using nucleos(t)ide analogs (NA) reduces HCC occurrence and recurrence in HBV-related HCC. NA therapy also improves overall survival by preventing liver function deterioration and decompensation. Indefinite antiviral therapy is recommended for most patients with HBV-related HCC. For HCV-related HCC, antiviral therapy using an interferon-based or interferon-free regimen reduces the risk of HCC. Despite an earlier debate, there is no convincing long-term data regarding direct-acting antiviral (DAA) therapy increasing HCC recurrence, whereas interferon-based antiviral therapy decreased HCC recurrence after curative treatment. However, DAA therapy improves the overall and liver-related mortality, especially in patients with complete response after curative treatment. Patients with HCV-related HCC who are eligible for curative treatment should receive DAA therapy after the completion of HCC treatment.

B. H. Kim · J.-W. Park (✉)
Center for Liver and Pancreatobiliary Cancer,
National Cancer Center,
Goyang, Gyeonggi-do, Republic of Korea
e-mail: jwpark@ncc.re.kr

Keywords

Antiviral therapy · Hepatitis B virus ·
Hepatitis C virus · Hepatocellular carcinoma ·
Occurrence · Recurrence · Prognosis

5.1 Introduction

Hepatocellular carcinoma (HCC) is the most common histological type of cancer and accounts for 70–85% of primary liver cancer [1]. Most HCCs have underlying etiology such as chronic viral hepatitis B and C virus (HBV and HCV, respectively) infection, alcohol intake, and aflatoxin exposure. Among them, approximately 50% and 30% of HCC cases worldwide are attributed to HBV and HCV infection, respectively [1, 2].

5.2 Hepatitis B Virus

5.2.1 Antiviral Agents for HBV

The ultimate goal of antiviral therapy for patients with chronic HBV infection is to improve survival and quality of life by preventing disease progression (fibrosis progression) and, consequently, cirrhosis and HCC [3, 4]. In patients with HBV-related HCC, the goals of antiviral therapy are to suppress HBV replication to induce the stabilization of HBV-induced liver disease, prevent disease progression, and reduce the risk of HCC recurrence after potentially curative treatment [3, 4]. Stabilizing HBV-induced liver disease enables patients to receive more effective treatment for HCC [3, 4].

Generally, antiviral treatment is recommended for patients with HBeAg-positive chronic HBV infection, HBV DNA ≥20,000 IU/mL, and serum alanine aminotransferase (ALT) levels ≥2 * upper limit of normal (ULN) or for patients with HBeAg-negative chronic hepatitis HBV infection, HBV DNA ≥2000 IU/mL, and serum ALT levels ≥2 * ULN [3–5]. For patients with decompensated cirrhosis, all international guidelines recommend antiviral therapy if serum HBV is detectable, regardless of HBeAg positivity or ALT levels [3–5]. Antiviral therapy should also be initiated in patients with compensated cirrhosis if serum HBV DNA is ≥2000 IU/mL. Even if patients with compensated cirrhosis have lower levels of HBV DNA (<2000 IU/mL), they should be closely monitored or treated with antiviral therapy [3–6]. Antiviral therapy is also recommended for patients with HBV-related HCC if serum HBV DNA is detectable [4].

Currently, there are two main classes of drugs for the treatment of chronic HBV infection: pegylated interferon alpha and nucleos(t)ide analogs (NAs). Although a finite duration of treatment with pegylated interferon alpha could induce immunological control, its use is quite limited in patients with cirrhosis or HCC because of low response rates, undesirable adverse events, and inconvenience of subcutaneous injection.

Although NAs have some advantages of oral administration and good tolerability, they have a potential risk of resistance. However, resistance is very rare if newer NAs such as entecavir or tenofovir are used in treatment-naïve patients with chronic HBV infection (CHB). In recent times, NAs are widely used in most patients with chronic HBV infection, including HBV-related HCC. Among various NAs, those with a high genetic barrier to resistance, such as entecavir, tenofovir disoproxil fumarate, tenofovir alafenamide, and besiforvir are preferred over those with the low genetic barriers such as lamivudine, telbivudine, clevudine, and adefovir [3–5]. NAs with low genetic barriers are no longer recommended as an initial therapy. During antiviral therapy, serum HBV DNA should be measured every 3–6 months even after a virological response.

Drug safety is an important issue as most patients require antiviral therapy indefinitely. Entecavir, tenofovir disoproxil fumarate, or tenofovir alafenamide can be safely used in most patients with chronic HBV infection. Since tenofovir disoproxil fumarate has been associated with the risk of developing mild renal and bone impairment, entecavir or tenofovir alafenamide is preferred in patients with underlying renal or bone disease [3, 4, 7]. However, data on the long-term outcome or safety of tenofovir alafenamide is lacking in patients with decompensated cirrhosis or HCC.

5.2.2 Role of Antiviral Therapy to Reduce Risk of Developing Liver Cancer

Several HBV-related factors contribute to the development of HCC in patients with CHB. High serum HBV DNA (>2000 IU/mL), high serum HBsAg, genotype C, delayed HBeAg seroconversion, and basal core promoter mutation have been identified as predictors of HCC [4].

A prospective cohort study of 3653 participants revealed high HBV DNA titer as a strong risk predictor of HCC independent of HBeAg positivity, serum ALT level, and the presence of liver cirrhosis [8]. The incidence of HCC increased with baseline HBV DNA level in a dose-dependent manner, and a decline of viremia was associated with a reduced risk of HCC [8]. Continuous treatment with lamivudine reduced the incidence of hepatic decompensation and the risk of HCC in patients with CHB compared to placebo [9, 10]. Entecavir or tenofovir also decrease the risk of developing HCC significantly [11–14]. A retrospective study of 5374 patients with CHB comparing lamivudine and entecavir, low and high genetic barrier NA, respectively, demonstrated that entecavir was associated with a lower risk of mortality or transplantation; however, no significant differences were observed regarding the risk of HCC [15]. Another retrospective study revealed that entecavir significantly reduced the incidence of HCC compared to lamivudine, and the suppression effect was greater in patients with HBV-related cirrhosis [12]. A recent meta-analysis also supports the superiority of entecavir over lamivudine with regard to the risk of developing HCC [16].

There is a debate about the potency of the two representative potent high genetic barrier NAs, entecavir and tenofovir, in the prevention of HCC. A retrospective cohort study using a large administrative dataset and a tertiary hospital-based cohort demonstrated that tenofovir was associated with a lower risk of HCC than entecavir [17]. On the contrary, multiple studies have shown no significant differences between entecavir and tenofovir in terms of the risk of HCC [18–21]. Another retrospective cohort study and meta-analysis showed a better effect of tenofovir in reducing the risk of developing HCC than entecavir [22, 23]. Unidentified confounders or the slightly different mechanism of nucleotide analogs (tenofovir) over nucleoside analogs (entecavir) may contribute to the different effects of lowering the risk of developing HCC, but further studies are needed to clarify this [24].

Although NAs significantly reduce the incidence of HCC, they do not eliminate the risk and HCC still develops. A meta-analysis demonstrated that HCC develops at a rate of 1.3 per 100 person-years in patients with CHB receiving NAs [10]. The risk of HCC persists even for patients receiving potent NAs for 5 years or more [25]. Even under effective NA therapy, careful long-term HCC surveillance should be continued.

5.2.3 Role of Antiviral Therapy to Prevent Recurrence in Liver Cancer

HCC is well known for its high recurrence rate even after curative surgical resection [26]. Overall, the 5-year recurrence rate of HCC after curative resection is 60–70% [27]. Even for single nodular HCC measuring <3 cm, the 5-year recurrence rate after surgical resection was 44%

[28]. Typically, recurrence within 2 years after resection is classified as early recurrence, recurrence after 2 years is classified as late recurrence, and late recurrence of more than 2 years after resection is considered de novo HCC [29]. Tumor-related factors contribute to early recurrence. In contrast, underlying disease-related factors influence late recurrence [26, 29, 30]. For patients with HBV infection, HBV affects recurrence. High HBV DNA load is an independent risk factor for HCC recurrence after surgical resection [30–32].

A randomized controlled study found that antiviral treatment significantly improved recurrence-free survival in patients whose HBV DNA of more than 500 copies/mL after curative resection [32]. A retrospective cohort study of 4569 patients who received curative liver resection also supported the association between NA therapy and the lower risk of HCC recurrence [33]. Another small randomized controlled study also reported that antiviral therapy improved recurrence-free survival and was an independent protective factor of late tumor recurrence [34]. A meta-analysis demonstrated that NA therapy was associated with better recurrence-free survival and overall survival in HBV-related patients treated with curative treatment such as ablation or resection [35].

A retrospective analysis showed that NAs with a high genetic barrier to resistance, such as tenofovir or entecavir, reduced the risk of recurrence compared with NAs with a low genetic barrier or no antiviral treatment in patients treated with surgical resection or ablation [36]. Although a recent single-center study reported that tenofovir was significantly associated with a lower risk of recurrence and better survival than entecavir among patients who underwent curative surgical resection for HCC, this conclusion is debatable [37].

5.2.4 Effect of Antiviral Therapy on Prognosis of Liver Cancer

Antiviral therapy also improves the prognosis of patients with HBV-related HCC. The efficacy of antiviral therapy was comparable in patients with or without HCC, and antiviral therapy improved liver function in patients with HBV-related HCC [38, 39]. Receiving antiviral treatment was an independent predictor for overall survival in patients treated with surgical resection [32, 34]. Antiviral therapy significantly improved liver function 6 months after surgery compared to the control and improved overall survival [32]. Moreover, patients receiving antiviral therapy had better liver function, and a significantly greater proportion of patients could receive curative treatment at the time of recurrence after surgical resection [40]. Antiviral therapy also improved the overall survival in patients with advanced HCC treated with sorafenib [41, 42].

A Korean nationwide cohort study reported that the survival of HCC was significantly improved over time, and it was remarkable in patients with HBV-related HCC [43]. Exponential use of antiviral agents for HBV might contribute to improved survival and recent advances in cancer diagnosis and treatment [43]. Antiviral agents can prolong the life expectancy of patients with HBV-related HCC by preventing decompensation since liver function and tumor stage affect the survival outcome of liver cancer [9, 44, 45].

5.2.5 Prophylactic Antiviral Therapy

In patients with HBV-related HCC, HBV reactivation is frequently observed after treatment such as surgical resection (14%–32%) [46, 47], radiofrequency ablation (5.6–9.1%) [48, 49], transcatheter arterial chemoembolization (TACE) (4–40%) [50–53], hepatic arterial infusion chemotherapy (24–67%) [54, 55], external beam radiation therapy (12.7–24.6%) [56–58], and cytotoxic chemotherapy (30–60%) [59]. Molecular targeted therapy also increased the risk of HBV reactivation [60], which may further lead to liver function deterioration and hepatic decompensation. Hence, it is conceivable that antiviral therapy can prevent liver function deterioration, thereby improving the prognosis of

patients with HCC undergoing antitumor treatment. Prophylactic antiviral therapy reduces the risk of HBV reactivation, prevents acute liver function deterioration following surgical resection and TACE, and improves long-term survival [50, 52, 61, 62].

5.3 Hepatitis C Virus

5.3.1 Antiviral Agents for HCV

The goal of antiviral therapy for patients with HCV infection is to cure the infection, thereby preventing complications of HCV-related liver diseases, including fibrosis, cirrhosis, and HCC [63, 64]. The endpoint of therapy is a sustained virological response (SVR), defined by undetectable HCV RNA after 12 weeks (SVR12) or 24 weeks (SVR24) after a finite duration treatment [63, 64]. Achieving SVR is regarded as a definite cure of HCV infection in most cases because HCV does not relapse in 99% of patients achieving SVR [65].

All patients with chronic HCV infection who do not have contraindications for treatment should be treated [63, 64, 66]. Interferon-alpha-based therapy was the standard therapy for HCV; however, it could not be recommended for all patients with HCV infection due to low efficacy and poor tolerability. With the introduction of direct-acting antivirals (DAAs), the treatment of HCV has dramatically improved in the last decade. Most patients can be treated with the new DAAs with favorable safety profiles and excellent success rates. DAAs have shown SVR rates of more than 95% in most patients with chronic HCV infection, although treatment regimens and durations differ depending on the experience of prior treatment, HCV genotype, and the presence of compensated or decompensated liver cirrhosis [67]. Previously, HCV genotype was determined before antiviral therapy. In recent times, pangenotypic DAA-based regimens such as glecaprevir/pibrentasvir or sofosbuvir/velpatasvir are preferred because of their virologic efficacy, convenience, and tolerability [66, 68].

SVR rates were lower for patients with HCC than for those without HCC [69–71]. Among patients with HCC, a higher SVR rate was observed in those who received curative treatment [72]. Untreated or partially treated HCC may further decrease SVR rates [71, 73–75]. Patients with HCC who are eligible for curative treatment should receive DAA therapy after completion of HCC treatment [66]. DAA therapy can be deferred for a period of 4–6 months to confirm complete response to HCC therapy [76]. For patients with HCC who do not show complete response to anti-tumor treatment, decisions regarding DAA therapy should consider the degree of liver function, tumor burden, and life expectancy [76].

5.3.2 Role of Antiviral Therapy to Reduce Risk of Developing Liver Cancer

Interferon-based therapy has demonstrated that achieving SVR significantly decreases the risk of developing HCC in patients with chronic HCV infection compared with those untreated, irrespective of the degree of fibrosis or cirrhosis [77, 78]. The risk of HCC did not differ between interferon-based or DAA therapy, although the short-term observation period for DAA-treated patients may limit the findings [79]. HCC risk reduction was observed in patients who achieved SVR following DAA therapy regardless of the presence of cirrhosis [80]. SVR achieved by DAAs also decreased the incidence of HCC in patients with compensated or decompensated cirrhosis [81]. While patients with cirrhosis who achieved SVR 1 remained at a high risk of developing HCC, the risk declined afterwards [80–83].

SVR reduces the rate of decompensation and the risk of HCC; however, it does not abolish the risk of HCC [84, 85]. In patients with HCV-related cirrhosis or advanced fibrosis, the risk of HCC persists even 10 years after SVR [86]. One of the postulated reasons is that epigenetic and gene expression changes persist after successful DAA therapy [87, 88]. Therefore, surveillance for HCC should be continued.

5.3.3 Role of Antiviral Therapy to Prevent Recurrence in Liver Cancer

Interferon-based therapy has consistently been shown to decrease the recurrence of HCC after curative treatment [89]. Some earlier reports raised concerns that DAA therapy may increase the recurrence of HCC following curative treatment. However, there are no conclusive data to support the increase or decrease in the risk of HCC recurrence [90–92]. Multiple studies demonstrated that the recurrence rate of DAA-treated patients was not significantly high compared with untreated control patients and that the recurrence rate did not differ between those who received interferon-based and DAA therapy after successful curative treatment for HCC [79, 93–95]. Furthermore, a multicenter cohort study reported that SVR achieved either by interferon-based or interferon-free regimens reduced tumor recurrence after curative treatment for HCC [96].

5.3.4 Effect of Antiviral Therapy on Prognosis of Liver Cancer

In patients with HCV-related HCC who have shown complete response to HCC therapy, DAA therapy improved overall survival and reduced the risk of hepatic decompensation and liver-related mortality [95, 97]. DAA therapy and achieving SVR12 is associated with increased overall survival in HCV patients with HCC [98]. In patients with early-stage HCC who had shown complete response after curative treatment, DAA therapy significantly reduced hepatic decompensation and improved overall survival [95]. Successful DAA therapy may also improve overall survival even for patients who receive palliative treatment for HCC, which implies that antiviral therapy should be considered for patients ineligible for curative treatment; however, it warrants further investigation [99].

5.3.5   Prophylactic Antiviral Therapy

The data on HCV reactivation in patients with HCV-related HCC undergoing antitumor treatment are scarce. A retrospective study comparing the rate of viral reactivation, hepatitis flare, and liver failure between HBV- and HCV-related HCC reported that the risk of hepatitis and liver failure was significantly lower in patients with HCV-related HCC [100].

5.4   Conclusion

HBV and HCV undermine the liver function and cause HCC. Appropriate antiviral therapy can decrease the risk of HCC occurrence and recurrence and improve the overall prognosis of patients with HCC.

Conflict of Interest J-WP has served in a consulting or advisory role for Roche, Genetech, BMS, Bayer, Eisai, Ipsen, and AstraZeneca; received honoraria from Bayer and Eisai; and participated in research sponsored by Ono-BMS, AstraZeneca, Blueprint, Roche, Eisai, Exelixis, Kowa, and Merk.

BHK has served in an advisory role for Eisai and Roche; received honoraria from Abbvie; and participated in research sponsored by Ono-BMS.

References

1. Perz JF, Armstrong GL, Farrington LA, Hutin YJ, Bell BP. The contributions of hepatitis B virus and hepatitis C virus infections to cirrhosis and primary liver cancer worldwide. J Hepatol. 2006;45(4):529–38. https://doi.org/10.1016/j.jhep.2006.05.013.
2. Global Burden of Disease Liver Cancer Collabration, Akinyemiju T, Abera S, Ahmed M, Alam N, Alemayohu MA, et al. The burden of primary liver cancer and underlying etiologies from 1990 to 2015 at the global, regional, and national level: results from the Global Burden of Disease Study 2015. JAMA Oncol. 2017;3(12):1683–91. https://doi.org/10.1001/jamaoncol.2017.3055.
3. European Association for the Study of the Liver. EASL 2017 clinical practice guidelines on the management of hepatitis B virus infection. J Hepatol. 2017;67(2):370–98. https://doi.org/10.1016/j.jhep.2017.03.021.
4. Korean Association for the Study of the Liver. KASL clinical practice guidelines for management of chronic hepatitis B. Clin Mol Hepatol. 2019;25(2):93–159. https://doi.org/10.3350/cmh.2019.1002.
5. Terrault NA, Lok ASF, McMahon BJ, Chang KM, Hwang JP, Jonas MM, et al. Update on prevention, diagnosis, and treatment of chronic hepatitis B: AASLD 2018 hepatitis B guidance. Hepatology. 2018;67(4):1560–99. https://doi.org/10.1002/hep.29800.
6. Yim HJ, Kim JH, Park JY, Yoon EL, Park H, Kwon JH, et al. Comparison of clinical practice guidelines for the management of chronic hepatitis B: when to start, when to change, and when to stop. Clin Mol Hepatol. 2020; https://doi.org/10.3350/cmh.2020.0049.
7. Agarwal K, Brunetto M, Seto WK, Lim Y-S, Fung S, Marcellin P, et al. 96 weeks treatment of tenofovir alafenamide vs. tenofovir disoproxil fumarate for hepatitis B virus infection. J Hepatol. 2018;68(4):672–81. https://doi.org/10.1016/j.jhep.2017.11.039.
8. Chen CJ, Yang HI, Su J, Jen CL, You SL, Lu SN, et al. Risk of hepatocellular carcinoma across a biological gradient of serum hepatitis B virus DNA level. JAMA. 2006;295(1):65–73. https://doi.org/10.1001/jama.295.1.65.
9. Liaw YF, Sung JJ, Chow WC, Farrell G, Lee CZ, Yuen H, et al. Lamivudine for patients with chronic hepatitis B and advanced liver disease. N Engl J Med. 2004;351(15):1521–31. https://doi.org/10.1056/NEJMoa033364.
10. Singal AK, Salameh H, Kuo YF, Fontana RJ. Meta-analysis: the impact of oral anti-viral agents on the incidence of hepatocellular carcinoma in chronic hepatitis B. Aliment Pharmacol Ther. 2013;38(2):98–106. https://doi.org/10.1111/apt.12344.
11. Wong GL, Chan HL, Mak CW, Lee SK, Ip ZM, Lam AT, et al. Entecavir treatment reduces hepatic events and deaths in chronic hepatitis B patients with liver cirrhosis. Hepatology. 2013;58(5):1537–47. https://doi.org/10.1002/hep.26301.
12. Hosaka T, Suzuki F, Kobayashi M, Seko Y, Kawamura Y, Sezaki H, et al. Long-term entecavir treatment reduces hepatocellular carcinoma incidence in patients with hepatitis B virus infection. Hepatology. 2013;58(1):98–107. https://doi.org/10.1002/hep.26180.
13. Ahn J, Lim JK, Lee HM, Lok AS, Nguyen M, Pan CQ, et al. Lower observed hepatocellular carcinoma incidence in chronic hepatitis B patients treated with Entecavir: results of the ENUMERATE study. Am J Gastroenterol. 2016;111(9):1297–304. https://doi.org/10.1038/ajg.2016.257.
14. Kim WR, Loomba R, Berg T, Aguilar Schall RE, Yee LJ, Dinh PV, et al. Impact of long-term tenofovir disoproxil fumarate on incidence of hepatocellular carcinoma in patients with chronic

hepatitis B. Cancer. 2015;121(20):3631–8. https://doi.org/10.1002/cncr.29537.

15. Lim YS, Han S, Heo NY, Shim JH, Lee HC, Suh DJ. Mortality, liver transplantation, and hepatocellular carcinoma among patients with chronic hepatitis B treated with entecavir vs lamivudine. Gastroenterology. 2014;147(1):152–61. https://doi.org/10.1053/j.gastro.2014.02.033.

16. Wang X, Liu X, Dang Z, Yu L, Jiang Y, Wang X, et al. Nucleos(t)ide analogues for reducing hepatocellular carcinoma in chronic hepatitis B patients: a systematic review and meta-analysis. Gut Liver. 2020;14(2):232–47. https://doi.org/10.5009/gnl18546.

17. Choi J, Kim HJ, Lee J, Cho S, Ko MJ, Lim YS. Risk of hepatocellular carcinoma in patients treated with Entecavir vs Tenofovir for chronic hepatitis B: a Korean Nationwide Cohort Study. JAMA Oncol. 2019;5(1):30–6. https://doi.org/10.1001/jamaoncol.2018.4070.

18. Kim SU, Seo YS, Lee HA, Kim MN, Lee YR, Lee HW, et al. A multicenter study of entecavir vs. tenofovir on prognosis of treatment-naive chronic hepatitis B in South Korea. J Hepatol. 2019;71(3):456–64. https://doi.org/10.1016/j.jhep.2019.03.028.

19. Lee SW, Kwon JH, Lee HL, Yoo SH, Nam HC, Sung PS, et al. Comparison of tenofovir and entecavir on the risk of hepatocellular carcinoma and mortality in treatment-naive patients with chronic hepatitis B in Korea: a large-scale, propensity score analysis. Gut. 2020;69(7):1301–8. https://doi.org/10.1136/gutjnl-2019-318947.

20. Hsu YC, Wong GL, Chen CH, Peng CY, Yeh ML, Cheung KS, et al. Tenofovir versus entecavir for hepatocellular carcinoma prevention in an international consortium of chronic hepatitis B. Am J Gastroenterol. 2020;115(2):271–80. https://doi.org/10.14309/ajg.0000000000000428.

21. Papatheodoridis GV, Dalekos GN, Idilman R, Sypsa V, Van Boemmel F, Buti M, et al. Similar risk of hepatocellular carcinoma during long-term entecavir or tenofovir therapy in Caucasian patients with chronic hepatitis B. J Hepatol. 2020; https://doi.org/10.1016/j.jhep.2020.06.011.

22. Yip TC, Wong VW, Chan HL, Tse YK, Lui GC, Wong GL. Tenofovir is associated with lower risk of hepatocellular carcinoma than entecavir in patients with chronic HBV infection in China. Gastroenterology. 2020;158(1):215–25. https://doi.org/10.1053/j.gastro.2019.09.025.

23. Gu L, Yao Q, Shen Z, He Y, Ng DM, Yang T, et al. Comparison of tenofovir versus entecavir on reducing incidence of hepatocellular carcinoma in chronic hepatitis B patients: a systematic review and meta-analysis. J Gastroenterol Hepatol. 2020; https://doi.org/10.1111/jgh.15036.

24. Murata K, Asano M, Matsumoto A, Sugiyama M, Nishida N, Tanaka E, et al. Induction of IFN-lambda3 as an additional effect of nucleotide, not nucleoside, analogues: a new potential target for HBV infection.

Gut. 2018;67(2):362–71. https://doi.org/10.1136/gutjnl-2016-312653.

25. Kim SU, Seo YS, Lee HA, Kim MN, Lee EJ, Shin HJ, et al. Hepatocellular carcinoma risk steadily persists over time despite long-term antiviral therapy for hepatitis B: a multicenter study. Cancer Epidemiol Biomark Prev. 2020;29(4):832–7. https://doi.org/10.1158/1055-9965.EPI-19-0614.

26. Korean Liver Cancer Association, National Cancer Center. 2018 Korean Liver Cancer Association-National Cancer Center Korea practice guidelines for the management of hepatocellular carcinoma. Gut Liver. 2019;13(3):227–99. https://doi.org/10.5009/gnl19024.

27. Lee EC, Kim SH, Park H, Lee SD, Lee SA, Park SJ. Survival analysis after liver resection for hepatocellular carcinoma: a consecutive cohort of 1002 patients. J Gastroenterol Hepatol. 2017;32(5):1055–63. https://doi.org/10.1111/jgh.13632.

28. Yang HJ, Lee JH, Lee DH, Yu SJ, Kim YJ, Yoon JH, et al. Small single-nodule hepatocellular carcinoma: comparison of transarterial chemoembolization, radiofrequency ablation, and hepatic resection by using inverse probability weighting. Radiology. 2014;271(3):909–18. https://doi.org/10.1148/radiol.13131760.

29. Imamura H, Matsuyama Y, Tanaka E, Ohkubo T, Hasegawa K, Miyagawa S, et al. Risk factors contributing to early and late phase intrahepatic recurrence of hepatocellular carcinoma after hepatectomy. J Hepatol. 2003;38(2):200–7. https://doi.org/10.1016/s0168-8278(02)00360-4.

30. Wu JC, Huang YH, Chau GY, Su CW, Lai CR, Lee PC, et al. Risk factors for early and late recurrence in hepatitis B-related hepatocellular carcinoma. J Hepatol. 2009;51(5):890–7. https://doi.org/10.1016/j.jhep.2009.07.009.

31. Sohn W, Paik YH, Kim JM, Kwon CH, Joh JW, Cho JY, et al. HBV DNA and HBsAg levels as risk predictors of early and late recurrence after curative resection of HBV-related hepatocellular carcinoma. Ann Surg Oncol. 2014;21(7):2429–35. https://doi.org/10.1245/s10434-014-3621-x.

32. Yin J, Li N, Han Y, Xue J, Deng Y, Shi J, et al. Effect of antiviral treatment with nucleotide/nucleoside analogs on postoperative prognosis of hepatitis B virus-related hepatocellular carcinoma: a two-stage longitudinal clinical study. J Clin Oncol. 2013;31(29):3647–55. https://doi.org/10.1200/JCO.2012.48.5896.

33. Wu C-Y, Chen Y-J, Ho HJ, Hsu Y-C, Kuo KN, Wu M-S, et al. Association between nucleoside analogues and risk of hepatitis B virus-related hepatocellular carcinoma recurrence following liver resection. JAMA. 2012;308(18):1906–13. https://doi.org/10.1001/2012.jama.11975.

34. Huang G, Lau WY, Wang ZG, Pan ZY, Yuan SX, Shen F, et al. Antiviral therapy improves postoperative survival in patients with hepatocellular carcinoma: a randomized controlled trial. Ann

Surg. 2015;261(1):56–66. https://doi.org/10.1097/SLA.0000000000000858.

35. Sun P, Dong X, Cheng X, Hu Q, Zheng Q. Nucleot(s) ide analogues for hepatitis B virus-related hepatocellular carcinoma after curative treatment: a systematic review and meta-analysis. PLoS One. 2014;9(7):e102761. https://doi.org/10.1371/journal.pone.0102761.

36. Cho H, Ahn H, Lee DH, Lee JH, Jung YJ, Chang Y, et al. Entecavir and tenofovir reduce hepatitis B virus-related hepatocellular carcinoma recurrence more effectively than other antivirals. J Viral Hepat. 2018;25(6):707–17. https://doi.org/10.1111/jvh.12855.

37. Choi J, Jo C, Lim YS. Tenofovir vs. entecavir on recurrence of hepatitis B virus-related hepatocellular carcinoma after surgical resection. Hepatology. 2020; https://doi.org/10.1002/hep.31289.

38. Kim JH, Park JW, Koh DW, Lee WJ, Kim CM. Efficacy of lamivudine on hepatitis B viral status and liver function in patients with hepatitis B virus-related hepatocellular carcinoma. Liver Int. 2009;29(2):203–7. https://doi.org/10.1111/j.1478-3231.2008.01828.x.

39. Jin YJ, Shim JH, Lee HC, Yoo DJ, Kim KM, Lim YS, et al. Suppressive effects of entecavir on hepatitis B virus and hepatocellular carcinoma. J Gastroenterol Hepatol. 2011;26(9):1380–8. https://doi.org/10.1111/j.1440-1746.2011.06776.x.

40. Chong CC, Wong GL, Wong VW, Ip PC, Cheung YS, Wong J, et al. Antiviral therapy improves post-hepatectomy survival in patients with hepatitis B virus-related hepatocellular carcinoma: a prospective-retrospective study. Aliment Pharmacol Ther. 2015;41(2):199–208. https://doi.org/10.1111/apt.13034.

41. Xu L, Gao H, Huang J, Wang H, Zhou Z, Zhang Y, et al. Antiviral therapy in the improvement of survival of patients with hepatitis B virus-related hepatocellular carcinoma treated with sorafenib. J Gastroenterol Hepatol. 2015;30(6):1032–9. https://doi.org/10.1111/jgh.12910.

42. Yang Y, Wen F, Li J, Zhang P, Yan W, Hao P, et al. A high baseline HBV load and antiviral therapy affect the survival of patients with advanced HBV-related HCC treated with sorafenib. Liver Int. 2015;35(9):2147–54. https://doi.org/10.1111/liv.12805.

43. Kim BH, Lim YS, Kim EY, Kong HJ, Won YJ, Han S, et al. Temporal improvement in survival of patients with hepatocellular carcinoma in a hepatitis B virus-endemic population. J Gastroenterol Hepatol. 2017; https://doi.org/10.1111/jgh.13848.

44. Forner A, Llovet JM, Bruix J. Hepatocellular carcinoma. Lancet. 2012;379(9822):1245–55. https://doi.org/10.1016/S0140-6736(11)61347-0.

45. Choi J, Han S, Kim N, Lim YS. Increasing burden of liver cancer despite extensive use of antiviral agents in a hepatitis B virus-endemic population. Hepatology. 2017; https://doi.org/10.1002/hep.29321.

46. Kubo S, Nishiguchi S, Hamba H, Hirohashi K, Tanaka H, Shuto T, et al. Reactivation of viral replication after liver resection in patients infected with hepatitis B virus. Ann Surg. 2001;233(1):139–45. https://doi.org/10.1097/00000658-200101000-00020.

47. Huang L, Li J, Yan J, Sun J, Zhang X, Wu M, et al. Antiviral therapy decreases viral reactivation in patients with hepatitis B virus-related hepatocellular carcinoma undergoing hepatectomy: a randomized controlled trial. J Viral Hepat. 2013;20(5):336–42. https://doi.org/10.1111/jvh.12036.

48. Dan JQ, Zhang YJ, Huang JT, Chen MS, Gao HJ, Peng ZW, et al. Hepatitis B virus reactivation after radiofrequency ablation or hepatic resection for HBV-related small hepatocellular carcinoma: a retrospective study. Eur J Surg Oncol. 2013;39(8):865–72. https://doi.org/10.1016/j.ejso.2013.03.020.

49. Yoshida H, Yoshida H, Goto E, Sato T, Ohki T, Masuzaki R, et al. Safety and efficacy of lamivudine after radiofrequency ablation in patients with hepatitis B virus-related hepatocellular carcinoma. Hepatol Int. 2008;2(1):89–94. https://doi.org/10.1007/s12072-007-9020-7.

50. Lao XM, Luo G, Ye LT, Luo C, Shi M, Wang D, et al. Effects of antiviral therapy on hepatitis B virus reactivation and liver function after resection or chemoembolization for hepatocellular carcinoma. Liver Int. 2013;33(4):595–604. https://doi.org/10.1111/liv.12112.

51. Lao XM, Wang D, Shi M, Liu G, Li S, Guo R, et al. Changes in hepatitis B virus DNA levels and liver function after transcatheter arterial chemoembolization of hepatocellular carcinoma. Hepatol Res. 2011;41(6):553–63. https://doi.org/10.1111/j.1872-034X.2011.00796.x.

52. Jang JW, Choi JY, Bae SH, Yoon SK, Chang UI, Kim CW, et al. A randomized controlled study of preemptive lamivudine in patients receiving transarterial chemo-lipiodolization. Hepatology. 2006;43(2):233–40. https://doi.org/10.1002/hep.21024.

53. Park JW, Park KW, Cho SH, Park HS, Lee WJ, Lee DH, et al. Risk of hepatitis B exacerbation is low after transcatheter arterial chemoembolization therapy for patients with HBV-related hepatocellular carcinoma: report of a prospective study. Am J Gastroenterol. 2005;100(10):2194–200. https://doi.org/10.1111/j.1572-0241.2005.00232.x.

54. Nagamatsu H, Itano S, Nagaoka S, Akiyoshi J, Matsugaki S, Kurogi J, et al. Prophylactic lamivudine administration prevents exacerbation of liver damage in HBe antigen positive patients with hepatocellular carcinoma undergoing transhepatic arterial infusion chemotherapy. Am J Gastroenterol. 2004;99(12):2369–75. https://doi.org/10.1111/j.1572-0241.2004.40069.x.

55. Tamori A, Nishiguchi S, Tanaka M, Kurooka H, Fujimoto S, Nakamura K, et al. Lamivudine therapy for hepatitis B virus reactivation in a patient receiv-

ing intra-arterial chemotherapy for advanced hepato-cellular carcinoma. Hepatol Res. 2003;26(1):77–80. https://doi.org/10.1016/s1386-6346(03)00002-0.

56. Kim JH, Park JW, Kim TH, Koh DW, Lee WJ, Kim CM. Hepatitis B virus reactivation after three-dimensional conformal radiotherapy in patients with hepatitis B virus-related hepatocellular carcinoma. Int J Radiat Oncol Biol Phys. 2007;69(3):813–9. https://doi.org/10.1016/j.ijrobp.2007.04.005.

57. Huang W, Zhang W, Fan M, Lu Y, Zhang J, Li H, et al. Risk factors for hepatitis B virus reactivation after conformal radiotherapy in patients with hepatocellular carcinoma. Cancer Sci. 2014;105(6):697–703. https://doi.org/10.1111/cas.12400.

58. Jun BG, Kim YD, Kim SG, Kim YS, Jeong SW, Jang JY, et al. Hepatitis B virus reactivation after radiotherapy for hepatocellular carcinoma and efficacy of antiviral treatment: a multicenter study. PLoS One. 2018;13(7):e0201316. https://doi.org/10.1371/journal.pone.0201316.

59. Yeo W, Lam KC, Zee B, Chan PS, Mo FK, Ho WM, et al. Hepatitis B reactivation in patients with hepatocellular carcinoma undergoing systemic chemotherapy. Ann Oncol. 2004;15(11):1661–6. https://doi.org/10.1093/annonc/mdh430.

60. Lim S, Han J, Kim GM, Han KH, Choi HJ. Hepatitis B viral load predicts survival in hepatocellular carcinoma patients treated with sorafenib. J Gastroenterol Hepatol. 2015;30(6):1024–31. https://doi.org/10.1111/jgh.12898.

61. Yoo SH, Jang JW, Kwon JH, Jung SM, Jang B, Choi JY. Preemptive antiviral therapy with entecavir can reduce acute deterioration of hepatic function following transarterial chemoembolization. Clin Mol Hepatol. 2016;22(4):458–65. https://doi.org/10.3350/cmh.2016.0054.

62. Jang JW, Yoo SH, Nam HC, Jang BH, Sung Sung PS, Lee W, et al. Association of prophylactic anti-hepatitis B virus therapy with improved long-term survival in patients with hepatocellular carcinoma undergoing transarterial therapy. Clin Infect Dis. 2020;71(3):546–55. https://doi.org/10.1093/cid/ciz860.

63. European Association for the Study of the Liver. EASL recommendations on treatment of hepatitis C 2018. J Hepatol. 2018;69(2):461–511. https://doi.org/10.1016/j.jhep.2018.03.026.

64. Korean Association for the Study of the Liver. KASL clinical practice guidelines: management of hepatitis C. Clin Mol Hepatol. 2014;20(2):89–136. https://doi.org/10.3350/cmh.2014.20.2.89.

65. Swain MG, Lai MY, Shiffman ML, Cooksley WG, Zeuzem S, Dieterich DT, et al. A sustained virologic response is durable in patients with chronic hepatitis C treated with peginterferon alfa-2a and ribavirin. Gastroenterology. 2010;139(5):1593–601. https://doi.org/10.1053/j.gastro.2010.07.009.

66. European Association for the Study of the Liver. EASL recommendations on treatment of hepatitis C:

final update of the series☆. J Hepatol. 2020; https://doi.org/10.1016/j.jhep.2020.08.018.

67. Korean Association for the Study of the Liver. 2017 KASL clinical practice guidelines management of hepatitis C: treatment of chronic hepatitis C. Clin Mol Hepatol. 2018;24(3):169–229. https://doi.org/10.3350/cmh.2018.1004.

68. Ghany MG, Morgan TR, Panel A-IHCG. Hepatitis C guidance 2019 update: American Association for the Study of Liver Diseases-Infectious Diseases Society of America recommendations for testing, managing, and treating hepatitis C virus infection. Hepatology. 2020;71(2):686–721. https://doi.org/10.1002/hep.31060.

69. Beste LA, Green PK, Berry K, Kogut MJ, Allison SK, Ioannou GN. Effectiveness of hepatitis C antiviral treatment in a USA cohort of veteran patients with hepatocellular carcinoma. J Hepatol. 2017;67(1):32–9. https://doi.org/10.1016/j.jhep.2017.02.027.

70. Prenner SB, VanWagner LB, Flamm SL, Salem R, Lewandowski RJ, Kulik L. Hepatocellular carcinoma decreases the chance of successful hepatitis C virus therapy with direct-acting antivirals. J Hepatol. 2017;66(6):1173–81. https://doi.org/10.1016/j.jhep.2017.01.020.

71. Ji F, Yeo YH, Wei MT, Ogawa E, Enomoto M, Lee DH, et al. Sustained virologic response to direct-acting antiviral therapy in patients with chronic hepatitis C and hepatocellular carcinoma: a systematic review and meta-analysis. J Hepatol. 2019;71(3):473–85. https://doi.org/10.1016/j.jhep.2019.04.017.

72. He S, Lockart I, Alavi M, Danta M, Hajarizadeh B, Dore GJ. Systematic review with meta-analysis: effectiveness of direct-acting antiviral treatment for hepatitis C in patients with hepatocellular carcinoma. Aliment Pharmacol Ther. 2020;51(1):34–52. https://doi.org/10.1111/apt.15598.

73. Yen YH, Chen CH, Hung CH, Wang JH, Lu SN, Kee KM, et al. Active hepatocellular carcinoma is an independent risk factor of direct-acting antiviral treatment failure: a retrospective study with prospectively collected data. PLoS One. 2019;14(10):e0222605. https://doi.org/10.1371/journal.pone.0222605.

74. Ogawa E, Toyoda H, Iio E, Jun DW, Huang CF, Enomoto M, et al. HCV cure rates are reduced in patients with active but not inactive hepatocellular carcinoma: a practice implication. Clin Infect Dis. 2019; https://doi.org/10.1093/cid/ciz1160.

75. Huang CF, Yeh ML, Huang CI, Liang PC, Lin YH, Hsieh MY, et al. Equal treatment efficacy of direct-acting antivirals in patients with chronic hepatitis C and hepatocellular carcinoma? A prospective cohort study. BMJ Open. 2019;9(5):e026703. https://doi.org/10.1136/bmjopen-2018-026703.

76. Singal AG, Lim JK, Kanwal F. AGA clinical practice update on interaction between oral direct-acting antivirals for chronic hepatitis C infection and hepatocellular carcinoma: expert review. Gastroenterology.

2019;156(8):2149–57. https://doi.org/10.1053/j.gastro.2019.02.046.

77. Morgan RL, Baack B, Smith BD, Yartel A, Pitasi M, Falck-Ytter Y. Eradication of hepatitis C virus infection and the development of hepatocellular carcinoma: a meta-analysis of observational studies. Ann Intern Med. 2013;158(5 Pt 1):329–37. https://doi.org/10.7326/0003-4819-158-5-201303050-00005.

78. Singal AG, Volk ML, Jensen D, Di Bisceglie AM, Schoenfeld PS. A sustained viral response is associated with reduced liver-related morbidity and mortality in patients with hepatitis C virus. Clin Gastroenterol Hepatol. 2010;8(3) https://doi.org/10.1016/j.cgh.2009.11.018.

79. Waziry R, Hajarizadeh B, Grebely J, Amin J, Law M, Danta M, et al. Hepatocellular carcinoma risk following direct-acting antiviral HCV therapy: a systematic review, meta-analyses, and meta-regression. J Hepatol. 2017;67(6):1204–12. https://doi.org/10.1016/j.jhep.2017.07.025.

80. Ioannou GN, Green PK, Berry K. HCV eradication induced by direct-acting antiviral agents reduces the risk of hepatocellular carcinoma. J Hepatol. 2018;68(1):25–32. https://doi.org/10.1016/j.jhep.2017.08.030.

81. Calvaruso V, Cabibbo G, Cacciola I, Petta S, Madonia S, Bellia A, et al. Incidence of hepatocellular carcinoma in patients with HCV-associated cirrhosis treated with direct-acting antiviral agents. Gastroenterology. 2018;155(2):411–21. https://doi.org/10.1053/j.gastro.2018.04.008.

82. Kanwal F, Kramer J, Asch SM, Chayanupatkul M, Cao Y, El-Serag HB. Risk of hepatocellular cancer in HCV patients treated with direct-acting antiviral agents. Gastroenterology. 2017;153(4):996–1005. https://doi.org/10.1053/j.gastro.2017.06.012.

83. Romano A, Angeli P, Piovesan S, Noventa F, Anastassopoulos G, Chemello L, et al. Newly diagnosed hepatocellular carcinoma in patients with advanced hepatitis C treated with DAAs: a prospective population study. J Hepatol. 2018;69(2):345–52. https://doi.org/10.1016/j.jhep.2018.03.009.

84. Nahon P, Bourcier V, Layese R, Audureau E, Cagnot C, Marcellin P, et al. Eradication of hepatitis C virus infection in patients with cirrhosis reduces risk of liver and non-liver complications. Gastroenterology. 2017;152(1):142–56. https://doi.org/10.1053/j.gastro.2016.09.009.

85. El-Serag HB, Kanwal F, Richardson P, Kramer J. Risk of hepatocellular carcinoma after sustained virological response in veterans with hepatitis C virus infection. Hepatology. 2016;64(1):130–7. https://doi.org/10.1002/hep.28535.

86. Ioannou GN, Beste LA, Green PK, Singal AG, Tapper EB, Waljee AK, et al. Increased risk for hepatocellular carcinoma persists up to 10 years after HCV eradication in patients with baseline cirrhosis or high FIB-4 scores. Gastroenterology. 2019;157(5):1264–78. https://doi.org/10.1053/j.gastro.2019.07.033.

87. Hamdane N, Juhling F, Crouchet E, El Saghire H, Thumann C, Oudot MA, et al. HCV-induced epigenetic changes associated with liver cancer risk persist after sustained virologic response. Gastroenterology. 2019;156(8):2313–29. https://doi.org/10.1053/j.gastro.2019.02.038.

88. Perez S, Kaspi A, Domovitz T, Davidovich A, Lavi-Itzkovitz A, Meirson T, et al. Hepatitis C virus leaves an epigenetic signature post cure of infection by direct-acting antivirals. PLoS Genet. 2019;15(6):e1008181. https://doi.org/10.1371/journal.pgen.1008181.

89. Singal AK, Freeman DH Jr, Anand BS. Meta-analysis: interferon improves outcomes following ablation or resection of hepatocellular carcinoma. Aliment Pharmacol Ther. 2010;32(7):851–8. https://doi.org/10.1111/j.1365-2036.2010.04414.x.

90. Reig M, Marino Z, Perello C, Inarrairaegui M, Ribeiro A, Lens S, et al. Unexpected high rate of early tumor recurrence in patients with HCV-related HCC undergoing interferon-free therapy. J Hepatol. 2016;65(4):719–26. https://doi.org/10.1016/j.jhep.2016.04.008.

91. ANRS collaborative study group on hepatocellular carcinoma. Lack of evidence of an effect of direct-acting antivirals on the recurrence of hepatocellular carcinoma: data from three ANRS cohorts. J Hepatol. 2016;65(4):734–40. https://doi.org/10.1016/j.jhep.2016.05.045.

92. Singal AG, Rich NE, Mehta N, Branch A, Pillai A, Hoteit M, et al. Direct-acting antiviral therapy not associated with recurrence of hepatocellular carcinoma in a multicenter north American Cohort Study. Gastroenterology. 2019;156(6):1683–92. https://doi.org/10.1053/j.gastro.2019.01.027.

93. Cabibbo G, Petta S, Calvaruso V, Cacciola I, Cannavò MR, Madonia S, et al. Is early recurrence of hepatocellular carcinoma in HCV cirrhotic patients affected by treatment with direct-acting antivirals? A prospective multicentre study. Aliment Pharmacol Ther. 2017;46(7):688–95. https://doi.org/10.1111/apt.14256.

94. Nishibatake Kinoshita M, Minami T, Tateishi R, Wake T, Nakagomi R, Fujiwara N, et al. Impact of direct-acting antivirals on early recurrence of HCV-related HCC: comparison with interferon-based therapy. J Hepatol. 2019;70(1):78–86. https://doi.org/10.1016/j.jhep.2018.09.029.

95. Cabibbo G, Celsa C, Calvaruso V, Petta S, Cacciola I, Cannavo MR, et al. Direct-acting antivirals after successful treatment of early hepatocellular carcinoma improve survival in HCV-cirrhotic patients. J Hepatol. 2019;71(2):265–73. https://doi.org/10.1016/j.jhep.2019.03.027.

96. Petta S, Cabibbo G, Barbara M, Attardo S, Bucci L, Farinati F, et al. Hepatocellular carcinoma recurrence in patients with curative resection or ablation: impact of HCV eradication does not depend on the use of interferon. Aliment Pharmacol

Ther. 2017;45(1):160–8. https://doi.org/10.1111/apt.13821.

97. Singal AG, Rich NE, Mehta N, Branch AD, Pillai A, Hoteit M, et al. Direct-acting antiviral therapy for hepatitis C virus infection is associated with increased survival in patients with a history of hepatocellular carcinoma. Gastroenterology. 2019;157(5):1253–63. https://doi.org/10.1053/j.gastro.2019.07.040.

98. Kamp WM, Sellers CM, Stein S, Lim JK, Kim HS. Impact of direct acting antivirals on survival in patients with chronic hepatitis C and hepatocellular carcinoma. Sci Rep. 2019;9(1):17081. https://doi.org/10.1038/s41598-019-53051-2.

99. Dang H, Yeo YH, Yasuda S, Huang CF, Iio E, Landis C, et al. Cure with interferon-free direct-acting antiviral is associated with increased survival in patients with hepatitis C virus-related hepatocellular carcinoma from both east and west. Hepatology. 2020;71(6):1910–22. https://doi.org/10.1002/hep.30988.

100. Sung PS, Bae SH, Jang JW, Song DS, Kim HY, Yoo SH, et al. Differences in the patterns and outcomes of enhanced viral replication between hepatitis C virus and hepatitis B virus in patients with hepatocellular carcinoma during transarterial chemolipiodolization. Korean J Hepatol. 2011;17(4):299–306. https://doi.org/10.3350/kjhep.2011.17.4.299.

Part II

Technologies and Techniques in Radiotherapy of Liver Cancer

Technological Advances in Radiotherapy

6

Belal Abousaida, Cheng-en Hsieh, Bhanu P. Venkatesulu, and Sunil Krishnan

Abstract

Radiation therapy, a highly effective treatment modality for hepatocellular carcinoma, is underutilized due to challenges posed by radiosensitivity of the non-tumor-bearing liver, movement of the liver with respiration, and the poor definition of the tumor edge on many occasions. Nonetheless, technological advances have improved our ability to safely target tumors in the liver while sparing adjacent normal liver and gastrointestinal mucosa, thereby making increasing numbers of patients with liver tumors amenable to radiation therapy with curative intent. This transition from the era of two- and three-dimensional radiation therapy to the modern era of radiotherapy was catalyzed by the advent of intensity-modulated radiation therapy (IMRT), stereotactic body radiation therapy (SBRT), image-guided radiation therapy (IGRT), and charged particle therapy resulting in a resurgence of interest in radiation therapy for liver tumors. We outline the technological advances that are at the vanguard of this renewed interest and the associated improved outcomes seen with radiation therapy for liver tumors.

Keywords

Radiation therapy · Hepatocellular carcinoma · Stereotactic · Proton · Image-guided · Carbon ion · Motion management

Belal Abousaida, Cheng-en Hsieh and Bhanu P. Venkatesulu contributed equally with all other contributors.

B. Abousaida · S. Krishnan (✉)
Department of Radiation Oncology, Mayo Clinic Florida, Jacksonville, FL, USA
e-mail: krishnan.sunil@mayo.edu

C.-e. Hsieh
Department of Immunology, MD Anderson Cancer Center, Houston, TX, USA

Department of Radiation Oncology, Chang Gung Memorial Hospital at Linkou, Taoyuan, Taiwan

B. P. Venkatesulu
Department of Radiation Oncology, Loyola University Stritch School of Medicine, Chicago, IL, USA

6.1 Introduction

Liver cancer is the sixth most common cause of cancer and the fourth leading cause of cancer-specific mortality worldwide as reported in 2018. Primary liver cancer includes hepatocellular carcinoma (HCC) as well as intrahepatic cholangiocarcinoma (IHC) which accounts for 75–85% and 10–15% of cases, respectively. The main risk factors for HCC include hepatitis-C, hepatitis-B, alcoholism, smoking, aflatoxin exposure and others. The advent of hepatitis-B vaccine has resulted in a dramatic reduction in incidence of hepatitis-B associated HCC with hepatitis-C being the most common cause in the eastern world and alcohol being the most important cause in the western world [1]. Surgical resection or liver transplant remains the gold standard for primary liver cancers with excellent outcomes though only 30% of patients are able to undergo resection for liver limited disease [2]. Local control is one of the most important predictors of survival outcomes with more than two-thirds of mortality being attributed to local progression leading to liver decompensation [3]. Many patients are deemed surgically unresectable in view of poor performance status, coexisting comorbidities, and poor functional liver reserve. Numerous liver-directed therapies have been undertaken in patients not amenable for surgical interventions such as radiofrequency ablation, external beam radiation therapy (EBRT), transcatheter arterial chemoembolization (TACE), and microsphere brachytherapy with Yttrium-90 (90Y). EBRT has been historically used as a palliative option for whole liver radiation and less commonly as an ablative therapy in view of concern for radiation-induced liver disease. The transition from the two-dimensional radiation therapy era to the modern radiotherapy era with 3D conformal radiotherapy, intensity modulated radiation therapy (IMRT), stereotactic body radiation therapy (SBRT), and charged particle therapy has resulted in a resurgence of interest of this noninvasive option. We outline some of the technological advances that have made increasing numbers of patients with liver tumors amenable to radiation therapy with curative intent.

6.2 Conformal Radiotherapy

The historical approach was to use whole liver irradiation (WLI) to a dose of 30–35 Gy via two-dimensional planning predominately as a means of providing symptom relief with the intent of palliation [4]. Technological prowess with EBRT such as CT-based planning, dose volume histograms, cone beam computed tomography (CBCT), motion management, and standardization of metrics via Quantitative Analysis of Normal Tissue Effects in the Clinic (QUANTEC) has resulted in the ability to sculpt the radiation

beams to conform delivery of a higher therapeutic dose to the tumor while reducing normal tissue complication probability. The majority of the data for EBRT has been on Child–Pugh class A patients and very few patients with Child–Pugh class B.

Some of the early prospective reports on the use of 3D-CRT were from the University of Michigan. In a phase 2 clinical trial of 128 patients receiving twice daily radiation (1.5 Gy per fraction) to a focal median radiation dose of 60.75 Gy with concurrent administration of intra-arterial hepatic (IAH) fluorodeoxyuridine (FdUrd), patients who received biologically equivalent doses higher than 75 Gy had superior survival outcomes of 23.9 versus 14.9 months. Four percent of patients experienced radiation-induced liver disease and 38% experienced grade 3 or 4 toxicity [5]. The logistical issues with delivering twice daily fraction as well as concern for the increased acute toxicities paved the way for conventional fractionation. The French phase II RTF-1 trial assessed 3DCRT in 27 patients with small-size HCC not amenable for surgical resection to a dose of 66 Gy in 33 fractions. Complete response was observed in 80% of patients with a reported grade 4 toxicity rate of 22% [6]. The toxicity rates were high with 3DCRT which limited the ability to potentially escalate the radiation dose safely for better tumor control outcomes.

The advent of intensity-modulated radiotherapy (IMRT) and dynamic multileaf collimators (MLCs) revolutionized the way radiation is delivered in the clinic. IMRT enhances the conformality that could be achieved by 3DCRT with multiple beam angles and also provides an opportunity to escalate the radiation dose to the liver tumor without the downside of radiation-induced liver disease. Studies by Yoon and Hou et al. showed that with IMRT higher radiation doses were delivered compared to 3D-CRT with superior overall survival, progression-free survival, and with no differences in the incidence of radiation-induced liver disease. These reports were in patients with Child–Pugh A and B disease, less than 3 tumor nodules, tumor size >3 cm, with/without portal venous thrombosis [7,

8]. The delivery of higher radiation doses requires better definition of the tumor target and also better accounting of liver motion during various phases of respiration.

6.3 Image-Guided Radiotherapy Technology

6.3.1 Target Delineation

Delineating the hepatocellular carcinoma or intrahepatic cholangiocarcinoma is the most important step in the radiation treatment planning workflow. The normal liver has similar enhancement in comparison to an HCC without contrast imaging. While the diagnostic scan is typically a multi-phase CT scan including arterial (up to 20–30 s after contrast injection), venous (50–60 s), and late delayed phase (>180 s), the simulation scan typically seeks to identify the tumor in the later phases since the arterial phase may be missed while attempting to obtain multiple breathholds. Primary HCCs demonstrate a brisk early arterial enhancement phase with a rapid washout in the venous phase [9]. For patients with contraindications to iodinated contrast use, MR imaging has utility in delineation of the liver tumor volume. The MR imaging should be ideally obtained in the same simulation position as the planning CT scan and effort should be made to obtain the MR in a single breath hold with a slice thickness of less than 5 mm to account for the respiratory motion [10]. FDG PET does not provide added information in the treatment planning process of HCC. Image co-registration of a planning CT scan with the MRI often requires deformable registration. The accuracy of co-registration may influence the choice of the planning target volume margins [11].

6.3.2 Respiratory Motion Management

The simplest techniques to account for motion management include slow CT scanning, inhalation and exhalation breath-hold CT, 4D/ respiration-correlated CT, and respiratory-gated treatment. Slow CT scanning is not recommended for liver tumors in view of motion blurring. The inhalation and exhalation breath-hold CT has the main shortcoming of the tumor lag relative to normal tissue. On the contrary, 4D CT scans incorporate information from the various phases of respiration and a maximum/minimum intensity projection (MIP) image generated from these scans can be used to create an internal target volume. Unlike its use for lung cancers where the tumor stands out elegantly in contrast to the surrounding lung, the use of MIP images is less helpful for liver tumors. The American Association of Physicists in Medicine (AAPM) Task Group on the management of respiratory motion in radiation oncology (TG-76) recommends that motion management techniques be utilized for the radiation planning process whenever the breathing motion exceeds 5 mm [12]. In a study that assessed the respiration-induced motion of each liver segment of a 4D scan, the average motion of the entire liver was 0.6 ± 3.0 mm in the left-right (LR) direction, 2.3 ± 2.4 mm in the anterior-posterior (AP) direction, and 5.7 ± 3.4 mm in the superior-inferior (SI) direction with segment 7 and segments on the lateral side having the highest motion in the SI direction [13].

There are a multitude of ways to account for excess respiratory motion which include breath-hold methods (deep-inspiration breath hold, active-breathing control, self-held breath hold without respiratory monitoring, self-held breath hold with respiratory monitoring, and end-expiratory breath hold); forced shallow breathing with abdominal compression; gating with external respiratory control as well as internal fiducial markers, and tumor tracking methods. The breath hold-based techniques are noninvasive and convenient ways to essentially freeze the normal organs and tumor in a daily reproducible treatment position based on a specific phase of respiration. The deep inspiratory or end-expiratory breath holds are the most commonly used for liver tumors [14]. The active breathing control (ABC) is a device that is used to freeze the breathing at a prespecified phase which consists of a digital spirometer connected to a balloon valve. The patient is advised to inhale to a specific volume, and at a specific phase of breathing and lung volume, the balloon valve is closed. The valve is inflated by an air compressor that holds the patient's breath. This is more commonly used for lung cancer than liver cancer and liver tumor patients with good pulmonary reserve do well too [15]. Respiratory gating techniques that have been described above are highly dependent on patient compliance and a good pulmonary reserve. In scenarios wherein respiratory gating is not possible, an abdominal compression strategy can be used to reduce liver motion due to respiration. The usual method of abdominal compression is using a stereotactic body frame with a rigid frame and a customized vacuum pillow which can be altered to increase the abdominal pressure by a screw mechanism. The position of the diaphragm can be assessed daily by fluoroscopy to ensure daily reproducibility and setup can be verified by cone-beam CT. The use of abdominal compression reduces the motion of the diaphragm to a tune of 7 mm in liver tumors [16].

Gating and tracking are often confused entities. Respiratory gating involves the delivery of radiation during a particular phase of the patient's respiratory cycle. The specific coordinates of a gate for a particular patient are determined by an external respiratory signal or internal fiducial markers. The most commonly available external gating systems are the Real-time Position Management (RPM) system and linear accelerator gating interface with an Anzai belt. The external gating systems are placed on the patient's abdomen between the xiphoid process and the umbilicus and the in-room camera detects the markers in the gating system when a 4D scan is performed [17]. Tumor tracking involves dynamic repositioning of the radiation beam based on the relative changing motion of the tumor. Tumor tracking usually involves the placement of gold fiducials in the vicinity of the tumor. The major components of tumor tracking involve real-time identification of spatial coordinates of the tumor, anticipate the time lag between relative tumor motion and beam, and repositioning

the beam [18]. Liver tumors are easily accessible for ultrasound-guided placement of gold fiducials for tumor tracking with a very high success rate and low chances of fiducial migration [19].

6.3.3 Tumor Surrogates and Setup Verification

To ensure reproducibility of the initial CT simulation and day-to-day radiation treatment delivery, setup verification is a core component of the radiation delivery process. The daily setup reproducibility of liver tumors can be ensured by kv-based imaging, MV cone-beam CT (CBCT), or visualization of tumor surrogates like implanted fiducials, surrogate breathing signals or non-radiographic tumor tracking with implantable powered radiofrequency (rf) coil, wireless rf seed-tracking system [20–24]. The most common methods of daily setup verification are kv imaging and CBCT. The kv imaging setup is based on the correlation of the bony anatomy and MV CBCT assesses the tumor similar to a non-4D CT scan. Both these methods do not account for interfraction variability of respiratory motion and tumor motion. Some studies have reported the use of IV contrast during CBCT for better identification of the liver tumors though practical applicability is limited by the need for repeated contrast injections [25, 26].

6.4   Conformal Avoidance

Higher doses of tumor-directed radiation can be given if adjacent normal tissues can be adequately spared. For liver tumors, the biggest consideration is the sparing of uninvolved "normal" liver. Potential differential radiosensitivities of the liver based on the cirrhotic, necrotic, and viable liver tissue make anatomic liver-based dose volume constraints less accurate in sparing the functionally active areas of the liver. Classification systems like the Child–Pugh (CP) score serve as surrogates for residual functional activity of the liver but do not provide information on which part of the liver is functional. The use of functional liver imaging techniques like [^{99m}Tc] sulfur colloid single-photon emission tomography (SPECT) may aid in the radiation planning process by facilitating conformal avoidance of functioning uninvolved liver. The sulfur colloid is taken up by the Kupffer cells in the liver which aids in quantitative molecular imaging, allowing assessment of spatial heterogeneity of liver function. Preliminary reports on Differential Hepatic Avoidance Radiation Therapy (DHART) or conformal avoidance RT suggest that this approach is technically feasible with functional liver metrics derived from SPECT being complementary to anatomic imaging and can permit dose painting of liver tumors while minimizing radiation-induced hepatotoxicity [27, 28].

6.5 Stereotactic Ablative Body Radiotherapy

The advent of advanced imaging modalities for target delineation like tri-phasic CT and MR imaging coupled with respiratory motion management strategies that allow gating as well as tracking of tumor allow highly ablative doses of radiation to be delivered in very few fractions. In a meta-analysis of 70 observational studies of studies comparing photon versus charged particle therapy (CPT) in HCC, it was found that the OS, PFS, and LC rates were similar in CPT and SBRT arms whereas the conventional radiotherapy had inferior tumor-specific outcomes as well as increased toxicity [29]. Yoon et al. reported a prospective trial that assessed 90 CP-A patients with liver-confined HCC and macrovascular invasion to sorafenib or TACE with hypofractionated RT. TACE with RT resulted in superior PFS, OS rates compared to sorafenib suggesting that SBRT may be used in synergy with other local therapies [30]. Sun et al. reported that biologically effective dose (BED) in excess of 100 Gy is an important factor in predicting the outcomes with SBRT in patients with HCC ($\leq$5 cm). There has been increased interest in the ability of ablative doses of radiation in releasing sequestered tumor-associated antigens and priming the circulating T and NK cells in augmenting tumor

control outcomes in HCC [31]. There has also been increasing interest in combining SBRT with immune checkpoint therapies to synergize the tumor antigen release (in situ autovaccination) with stimulation of immune cells in HCC.

6.6 MR Linac-Based Radiotherapy

The MRIdian Linac system (ViewRay, Oakwood Village, OH) is a breakthrough technology that allows real-time tumor tracking with the aid of MR imaging. This system is a composite of 0.345-T field strength and a 6-MV flattening filter-free linear accelerator and can be used to deliver radiation only when the region of interest is in the target position. The main advantages of this approach are the ability to have tighter target volumes with the ability to deliver increased dose per fraction and to account for day-to-day physiological changes in the normal organ position [32]. Preliminary reports of liver SBRT on the MR-linac have shown that it is safe and feasible with good tumor control outcomes [33, 34]. A similar platform with a 1.5-T field strength and a linear accelerator is being advanced by Elekta and Phillips.

6.7 Proton Beam Therapy

Proton beam therapy (PBT) has distinct dosimetric attributes compared to photon radiation treatment. In photon radiotherapy, the radiation energy is continuously deposited along the beam path both upstream (entrance dose) and downstream (exit dose) of the target volume, leading to unwanted radiation exposure in adjacent liver parenchyma and other critical normal structures. In contrast, protons are positively charged particles, with a rest mass of 1.67262×10^{-27} kg per atom. As high-energy protons traverse the tissue, the dose deposition is relatively small and constant per unit distance. At the end of beam path, however, the electromagnetic and nuclear interactions abruptly increase as the proton velocity decreases, resulting in a massive energy transfer over a short path length which is referred to as the "Bragg peak" [35]. This unique physical property of protons allows a finite range of dose deposition in tissue with a near-zero dose beyond the treatment target (near zero exit dose). Importantly, the liver parenchyma is inherently sensitive to radiation injury which could cause radiation-induced liver disease (RILD), especially in the setting of liver cirrhosis [36]. The elimination of exit doses by PBT enables safe delivery of ablative doses to liver tumors without augmenting the risk of posttreatment liver decompensation, thereby widening the therapeutic index of radiation treatment [37].

6.7.1 Passively Scattered Proton Therapy

Passive scattering delivery systems are the most commonly used PBT techniques in treating liver tumors, with planning concepts akin to 3D pho-

ton plans [38]. The pristine proton beam is spread out by physical scatterers to create a broad radiation field and conformed to the individual tumor shape with collimators (Fig. 6.1). In depth, a range modulator wheel is utilized to generate the spread-out Bragg peak (SOBP). The proton range is subsequently adjusted with a compensator to account for the distal edge conformity, target motion, daily setup variations, and the range uncertainty [39]. Passive scattered PBT provides dosimetric advantages of a large uniform proton field which can be exploited to encompass the potential positions of moving targets such as lung and liver tumors.

Recent studies have demonstrated that passively scattered PBT conferred durable LC and OS benefits to patients with locally advanced HCC. A phase II trial by Fukumitsu et al. included 51 patients with peripheral HCC (>2 cm away from the alimentary tract and porta hepatis) without tumor vascular thrombosis (TVT) who underwent hypofractionated PBT with 66 GyE in 10

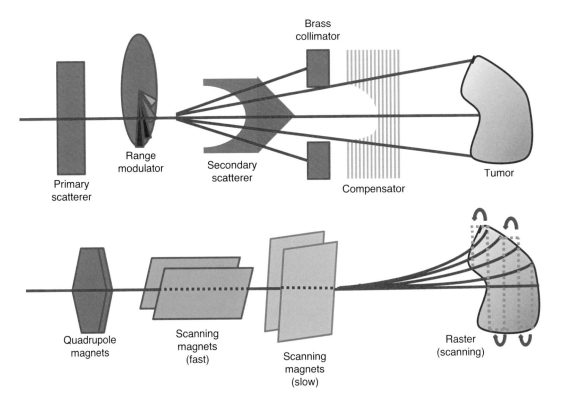

Fig. 6.1 Passive scattering and spot scanning proton delivery systems

fractions [40]. After a median follow-up of 34 months, their study documented outstanding 3- and 5-year LC rates of 94.5% and 87.8%, respectively. Strikingly, the 3- and 5-year OS rates were 49.2% and 38.7%, respectively, which were comparable to the favorable outcomes observed in hepatectomy series. Another phase II study by Bush et al. enrolled 76 HCC patients with larger tumor size (mean, 5.5 cm) and severe cirrhosis (CP-B, 47%; CP-C, 24%) treated with 63 GyE in 15 fractions [41]. The 5-year LC was 80%, with encouraging median OS of 34, 13, and 12 months for patients with CP-A, CP-B, and CP-C liver cirrhosis, respectively. These promising results were further confirmed in a multi-institutional phase II study of 44 patients with locally advanced HCC (median, 5.7 cm; TVT, 34%) undergoing hypofractionated PBT by Hong et al. [42]. The 2-year LC and OS rates were 94.8% and 63.2%, respectively, indicating that passively scattered PBT is highly effective in eradicating localized HCC with survival outcomes that compare favorably with resection for these poor prognostic populations.

In comparison to photon radiotherapy, passively scattered PBT allows safe delivery of ablative doses to liver cancers. Previous studies demonstrated that a higher biologically effective dose (BED) was associated with improved LC and OS outcomes for unresectable HCC [43–48]. Nonetheless, the liver represents a major dose-limiting organ. Even low-dose radiation could result in potentially lethal complications such as RILD [49–52]. In conventional photon radiotherapy, delivery of high-dose treatment for centrally located or large volume tumors unavoidably produces a "low-dose bath" to the liver due to the exit doses beyond the targets [53–55]. This low-dose exposure poses an elevated RILD risk which could in turn diminish the therapeutic benefits of ablative irradiation. In contrast, PBT eliminates the exit doses associated with photons and reduces the risks of treatment-related complications. A recent study by Sanford et al. retrospectively compared the outcomes in 133 patients with unresectable HCC treated with either passively scattered PBT ($N = 49$) or photon radiotherapy ($N = 84$) [56]. Although the same ablative

doses were delivered in both arms, patients who underwent PBT had a significantly lower V10 of liver compared with those treated with photons. After a median follow-up of 14 months, there was no significant difference in 2-year LC results (proton, 93% vs. photon, 90%) between the two modalities. However, patients undergoing PBT had a significantly lower incidence of non-classic RILD (odds ratio, 0.26) and prolonged median overall survival (31 vs. 14 months) compared with the photon arm, suggesting that elimination of low-dose exposure remarkably decreases the risk of severe hepatic complications. Another study by Hasan et al. retrospectively compared the outcomes of T1–2N0 HCC patients treated with either PBT ($N = 71$) or photon stereotactic ablation body radiotherapy (SABR) ($N = 918$) using the National Cancer Database [57]. Both arms received similar median BED (PBT, 98 Gy vs. photon, 100 Gy). However, patients who were treated with protons had significantly improved OS (HR =0.48, 95% CI: 0.29–0.78) compared with the photon SABR patients, corroborating the wider therapeutic index alluded to in the previous study.

For intrahepatic cholangiocarcinoma, long-term survival can be achieved using high-dose passively scattered PBT. A recent study by Tao et al. demonstrated that a BED higher than 80.5 Gy was associated with superior LC and OS results in patients with unresectable cholangiocarcinoma [58]. Due to the dosimetric advantages of protons, ablative irradiation is more likely achievable using PBT without exceeding the normal tissue constraints. The therapeutic efficacy of high-dose hypofractionated PBT for unresectable cholangiocarcinoma has been prospectively proven in a multicenter prospective phase II trial by Hong et al. [42]. Thirty-nine patients with intrahepatic cholangiocarcinoma (including two mixed HCC and cholangiocarcinoma) were treated with either 67.5 GyE in 15 fractions (>2 cm from the porta hepatis) or 58 GyE in 15 fractions (within 2 cm from the porta hepatis). A sustainable 2-year LC rate of 94.1% was achieved, with favorable median OS of 22.5 months. Retrospective series also reported similar results. A study of 30 cholangiocarcinoma patients treated with passively scattered PBT by Hung et al. demonstrated 1-year LC rate of 88%, with median OS of 19.3 months [59]. Another proton series including 28 cholangiocarcinoma patients by Makita et al. reported 1-year LC and OS rates of 67.7% and 49%, respectively [60]. In a cohort of 12 cholangiocarcinoma patients treated with curative PBT by Ohkawa et al., the 1-year LC was 88%, with median OS of 27.5 months [61]. Collectively, these studies suggest that PBT with ablative doses can lead to durable control of irradiated tumors with encouraging survival outcome for patients with locally advanced cholangiocarcinoma who were not amenable to curative resection.

Passively scattered PBT has recently emerged as an ablative treatment technique for metastatic liver cancers with improved ability to manage larger size tumors without severe adverse events. A phase II trial by Hong et al. prospectively evaluated the efficacy and toxicity of proton SABR with 50, 40, or 30 GyE in 5 fractions in 89 patients with one to four liver metastases from solid cancers (colorectal, $n = 34$; pancreatic, $n = 13$; esophagogastric, $n = 12$; other, $n = 30$) [62]. The median tumor size was 2.5 cm, and 24 tumors were larger than 6 cm in diameter. After a median follow-up of 30.1 months, a favorable median OS of 18.1 months was observed. No grade 3 to 5 toxicity was recorded. The 1- and 3-year LC rates were 71.9% and 61.2%, respectively, suggesting that proton SABR is a safe and efficacious liver-directed treatment modality for oligometastases. In photon radiotherapy, notably, a larger tumor volume is frequently associated with inferior LC outcome due to lower maximum tolerable tumor doses. In a phase I study of photon SABR for 68 patients with liver metastases by Lee et al., larger tumors (≥ 75.2 mL) and lower target doses significantly correlated with higher local failure rates [63]. In contrast, the dosimetric advantages of PBT enable safe deposition of ablative doses to large-volume tumors [53–55]. In the study by Hong et al., the 1-year LC rate for bulky metastatic tumors (≥ 6 cm) remained high at 73.9%, suggesting that PBT may derive greater therapeutic benefits for patients with larger metastatic tumors who were not amenable to ablative photon irradiation [62] (Table 6.1).

6.7.2 Intensity-Modulated Proton Therapy

Intensity-modulated proton therapy (IMPT), commonly referred to as "pencil beam" or "spot scanning," is a sophisticated proton delivery system that offers the promise of highly conformal target coverage and optimized dose distributions. IMPT utilizes an electromagnetic field to deflect the proton "pencil" beams to encompass the target volume in layers of spots and manipulates the proton doses and depths by altering the fluency and energy for individual spots. When multiple IMPT beams are used, all spots from all fields can be optimized simultaneously using the multifield optimization (MFO) technique that allows for greater degrees of freedom to produce highly modulated and steep dose gradients [68, 69]. In general, IMPT provides superior dose conformity to the proximal extent of the target with improved dose optimization compared with passive scattered PBT [70]. In addition, the requirement of patient-specific collimators and compensators are omitted using IMPT techniques, conferring potential operational advantages over passive scattering delivery systems. Nonetheless, IMPT is highly sensitive to target movement. The interplay effect between respiratory organ motion and the movement of the scanning beam can lead to extreme focal tumor under-dosage or critical normal structure overdosage, particularly in proton SABR with ≤ 5 fractions [71–73]. The challenges regarding the range uncertainties in complex heterogeneous structures, daily setup errors, and other aspects of treatment planning and quality assurance are also more pronounced in IMPT compared with passive scattering PBT or photon radiotherapy [71–73].

A propensity score-matched study by Yoo et al. retrospectively compared the outcomes in HCC patients treated with IMPT ($N = 33$) or passive scattering PBT ($N = 70$) [74]. The majority of patients on the IMPT arm received 10 or more

Table 6.1 Recent studies on the efficacy of proton beam therapy for liver cancers

Reference	Country, period	Type of study	Patient number	Dose regimen	Tumor size	Vascular invasion	Liver function	Local control	Overall survival
HCC									
Hong et al. [42]	USA, 2009–2015	Prosp	44	67.5 GyE/15 Fr (peripheral tumors) 58 GyE/15 Fr (central tumors)	Median = 5.7 cm	Yes = 15	CP-A = 32 CP-B = 9	2 − y = 94.8%	1 − y = 76.5% 2 − y = 63.2% Median = 49.9 mo
Bush et al. [41]	USA, 1998–2006	Prosp	76	63 Gy/15 Fr	Mean = 5.5 cm	PVTT = 4	CP-A = 22 CP-B = 36 CP-C = 18	5 − y = 80%	Median, CP-A = 34 mo CP-B = 13 mo CP-C = 12 mo
Fukumitsu et al. [40]	Japan, 2001–2004	Prosp	51	66 GyE/10 Fr	≤5 cm = 45 >5 cm = 6	Yes = 0	CP-A = 41 CP-B = 10	3 − y = 94.5% 5 − y = 87.8%	3 − y = 49.2% 5 − y = 38.7%
Sanford et al. [56]	USA, 2008–2017	Retro	49	Median = 67 Gy	Median GTV = 106 ml	Yes = 13	CP-A = 38 CP-B = 8	2 − y = 93%	2 − y = 59.1% Median = 31 mo
Chadha et al. [48]	USA, 2007–2016	Retro	46	Median = 67.5 GyE/15 Fr	Median = 6 cm	Yes = 13	CP-A = 38 CP-B = 8	1 − y = 95% 2 − y = 81%	1 − y = 73% 2 − y = 62% Median = 30.7 mo
Komatsu et al. [64]	Japan, 2001–2009	Retro	242	Median = 76 GyE/20 Fr	<5 cm = 196 5–10 cm = 65 >10 cm = 17	Yes = 73	CP-A = 184 CP-B = 55 CP-C = 3	5 − y = 90.2%	5 − y = 38%
Nakayama et al. [65]	Japan, 2001–2007	Retro	318	66 GyE/10 Fr (peripheral tumors) 72.6 GyE/22 Fr (≤2 cm from PH) 77 GyE/35 Fr (≤2 cm from GI tract)	T1 = 150 T2 = 107 T3 = 61	PVTT = 49 IVCTT = 5	CP-A = 234 CP-B = 77 CP-C = 7	5 − y = 83.3%	1 − y = 89.5% 3 − y = 64.7% 5 − y = 44.6%
Kawashima et al. [66]	Japan, 1999–2007	Retro	60	Median = 76 GyE/20 Fr	Median = 4.5 cm	Yes = 42	CP-A = 47 CP-B = 13	3 − y = 90% 5 − y = 86%	3 − y = 56% 5 − y = 25% Median = 41 mo
Cholangiocarcinoma									
Hong et al. [42]	USA, 2009–2015	Prosp	39	67.5 GyE/15 Fr (peripheral tumors) 58 GyE/15 Fr (central tumors)	Median = 6 cm	Yes = 11	CP-A = 34 CP-B = 4	2 − y = 94.1%	1 − y = 69.7% 2 − y = 46.5% Median = 22.5 mo

(continued)

Table 6.1 (continued)

Reference	Country, period	Type of study	Patient number	Dose regimen	Tumor size	Vascular invasion	Liver function	Local control	Overall survival
Hung et al. [59]	Taiwan, 2015–2017	Retro	30	Median = 72.6 GyE/22 Fr	Median = 7 cm	Yes = 7	No cirrhosis = 28 CP-A = 2	1 – y = 88%	1 – y = 83% Median = 19.3 mo
Makita et al. [60]	Japan, 2009–2011	Retro	28	Median = 68.2 GyE	Median = 5.2 cm	Yes = 10	Not reported	1 – y = 67.7%	1 – y = 49%
Ohkawa et al. [61]	Japan, 1995–2009	Retro	20 (curative group = 12)	Median = 72.6 GyE/22 Fr	Median = 5 cm	Yes = 3	CP-A = 14 CP-B = 6	Curative group: 1 – y = 88% 2 – y = 60% 3 – y = 60%	Curative group: 1 – y = 82% 3 – y = 38% Median = 27.5 mo
Liver metastasis									
Hong et al. [62]	USA, 2010–2015	Prosp	89	50 GyE/5 Fr = 31 40 GyE/5 Fr = 51 30 GyE/5 Fr = 7	Median = 2.5 cm	Not reported	No cirrhosis = 83 CP-A = 6	1 – y = 71.9% 3 – y = 61.2%	1 – y = 66.3% 2 – y = 35.9% 3 – y = 20.8% Median = 18.1 mo
Fukumitsu et al. [67]	Japan, 2002–2012	Retro	9 (gastric cancer)	Median = 72.6 GyE/22 Fr	Median = 3 cm	Not reported	Not reported	1 – y = 89% 3 – y = 71% 5 – y = 71%	1 – y = 100% 3 – y = 78% 5 – y = 56%

treatment fractions, with the radiation field encompassing whole respiratory amplitudes during regular breathing. After a median follow-up of 14 months, the 2-year OS and LC rates were 83.2% and 81.4% for the IMPT patients, respectively. No significant differences in OS, LC, and toxicity profiles were recorded between the two modalities. Another retrospective series by Dionisi et al. reported the outcomes of 18 patients (HCC, $N = 14$; intrahepatic cholangiocarcinoma, $N = 3$; mixed, $N = 1$) who were treated with IMPT using 15-fraction schedule (median, 58.05 GyE), with a median follow-up of 10 months [75]. The 1-year OS and LC rates were 63% and 90%, respectively. These data suggest that the use of higher fractionation numbers may mitigate the interplay effect. However, considering the small subject numbers, short median follow-up lengths, and obscure oncological benefits (as compared with passive scattering PBT) in these studies, the use of IMPT for liver cancer treatment should be approached with caution. Recent dosimetric analyses indicate that the dose perturbation caused by the interplay effect is relative to the speed of scanning beams and the directions of beam and target movements [76, 77]. Further studies optimizing the delivery system of scanning beams and eval-

uating the clinical utility of IMPT are urgently needed.

6.8   Carbon Ion Radiation Therapy

Carbon ion radiation therapy (CIRT) is similar to PBT in its use of a charged particle with characteristic Bragg peak-defined depth dose profiles to treat tumors. They interact similarly with tissues primarily by Coulomb interactions leading to the release of secondary electrons with very low energies, mostly in the keV range. The consequent short path lengths of these electrons result in very tight lateral penumbras for CIRT compared to PBT. As noted for PBT, the amount of energy deposited depends on the velocity of these particles, which is maximum at beam entry where there is sparse energy deposition and gradually, as the velocity declines while traversing tissues, more energy is deposited near the end of their track to form the Bragg peak region with a sharp distal fall off [78].(Fig. 6.2) The reduced velocity at the end of range of carbon ions also results in nuclear interactions and consequent fragmentation into low atomic number particles that create a characteristic fragmentation tail beyond the

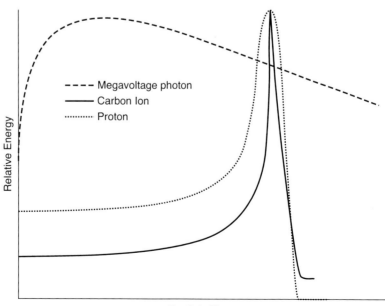

Fig. 6.2 Dose depth curves for 6 MV photons, protons, and carbon ions

Bragg peak. The biological effect of these fragments is small because of their low atomic number. Nonetheless, this creates some additional uncertainty regarding dose distal to the target volume. As with PBT, in clinical practice the narrow Bragg peak region is broadened using ridge filters that absorb variable amounts of energy to create the so-called spread-out Bragg peak or SOBP covering the target size. Alternatively, as with PBT, CIRT can also deliver intensity-modulated treatment using three-dimensional pencil beam raster scanning techniques where the modulation of beam energy allows for highly conformal targeting of tumors with pinpoint accuracy without the excess proximal dose seen with the passive method [79–82].

Compared to proton beams, carbon ions have a charge that is 6 times higher and a mass that is 12 times higher, which contributes to a mean energy deposited per unit path length of the beam (linear energy transfer, or LET) that is 36 times greater for a given velocity. These attributes of carbon ions, including their lower charge-to-mass ratio, contribute to their sharper penumbra and steeper lateral dose fall-off around the target volume than proton beams. On the other hand, no dose is deposited in the region beyond the distal end of the Bragg peak in proton therapy [82].

6.8.1 Biological Effects of CIRT

A distinct consequence of these physical characteristics of the carbon ion beam is that the higher LET results in greater density of ionizations along the beam track, and a greater likelihood of complex and clustered DNA damage (two or more closely spaced DNA lesions [single- or double-strand breaks, basic sites, or oxidized bases]) within one or two helical turns of the DNA. These clustered DNA lesions or multiply damaged sites are more difficult to repair, and therefore, CIRT has a higher RBE (in the range of 2–4) compared to PBT (with a nominal RBE of 1.1). Preclinical studies suggest that the RBE increases with increasing LET up to about 150 Kev/μm but decreases thereafter. The RBE also increases with decreasing fractional dose and the

repair capacity of the biological system. The lower the α/β value of a given tissue, the higher the RBE of CIT. Another biological factor that influences the RBE is oxygenation of tissue. Whereas low-LET radiation is more effective at eradicating normoxic tumor cells/tissues than hypoxic tumor cells/tissues, CIRT is less discriminating in its efficacy against hypoxic and normoxic tissues. Consequently, the ratio of doses required for equivalent tumor control for hypoxic and well-oxygenated tumors, the oxygen enhancement ratio (OER), is also greater for higher LETs of CIRT, approaching a value of 1 at LETs >500 KeV/μm [38, 83, 84].

6.8.2 Modeling, Prescribing, and Reporting CIRT

As a result of these radiobiological features of CIRT, dose prescriptions for CIRT are not merely defined by the traditional parameters of total physical (absorbed) dose in Gy, number of fractions, absorbed dose per fraction, and overall treatment time. The variable RBE along the beam path (by a factor of 2–4) introduces great complexity in benchmarking beam parameters and defining the biological effect of a given dose and LET of CIRT. Multiple efforts have been undertaken over the years to define ways of prescribing CIRT dose and indexing it to photon therapy, in a manner akin to the arbitrary use of a nominal RBE of 1.1 for protons, but considerably more challenging for CIRT due to its variable RBE. In the early days of CIRT in Japan, the only available data for modeling biological (and therefore clinical) effects of CIRT were preclinical data with human salivary gland cells treated with an SOBP carbon beam and clinical data of patients treated with fast neutron beams. Assuming that the salivary gland represented early responding tumor tissue, the relative RBE of each voxel was indexed to the preclinical in vitro data. This relative RBE was then converted to an absolute RBE by a scaling factor that equated the RBE at a dose-averaged LET of 80 keV/μm to a value of 3 which came from recognition of biological equivalence of this LET CIRT to a clinical fast neutron treatment of 0.9 Gy for 16 fractions. This was the classical mixed-effects model (or the Kanai model) which served well as a close computational approximation of true biological effect. With the advent of intensity-modulated CIRT, this model needed refining. Recognizing that the crucial determinant of RBE is the spatial deposition of dose at the microscopic scale or region of interest ("domain"), a model based on the theory of dual radiation action was developed in Japan, the Microdosimetric kinetic model (MKM). Yet again, the salivary gland in vitro data was used to generate a relative RBE value but here the conversion to absolute RBE was achieved by indexing to a previously defined clinical CIRT RBE at the center of a reference 6 cm SOBP generated by a carbon ion beam with an initial energy of 350 MeV/μ. In essence, this seeks to achieve the same biological effect for the pencil beam CIRT as the mixed-beam model would have achieved for the same dose prescription of a passively scattered CIRT beam before. Contemporaneously with these formulism being developed and implemented in Japan, German CIRT centers adopted a different approach to model and prescribe dose that also recognized that microscopic-scale spatial dose deposition dictated RBE. This model, the local effects model or LEM, derives RBE values of microscopic dose distributions by comparing the survival of cells treated in vitro with the same absorbed dose of photons or carbon ions. By benchmarking RBE of CIRT to that of late responding normal tissue (the central nervous system) with an α/β pegged at 2, this model aimed to be conservative with prediction of adverse events secondary to CIRT. Increasing complexity of input parameters in the LEM model (for example, accounting for isolated vs. clustered double-strand breaks within the topology of chromatin loops) have led to progressive refinements of the models in version I–IV of the LEM model. Given the differences in underlying assumptions of these models, there are differences in dose prescriptions between treatment regimens using these models; the RBE-weighted dose (expressed as GyRBE) being the product of the physical dose deposited by the carbon beam and the assumed RBE value.

Nonetheless, to date, all of the models have performed reasonably well at modeling a stochastic phenomenon of biological effects of dense ionization tracks along a carbon ion beam path with variable LET all along its course [82, 85–88].

6.8.3 Clinical Attributes of CIRT for HCC

6.8.3.1 Dose Conformality
One of the most striking advantages of CIRT for HCC is the homogeneity of dose distribution throughout the target and high dose conformality around the target tumor. This allows escalation of radiation dose to ablative levels inside the target lesion while sparing the healthy tissue inside and outside the liver, thereby broadening the therapeutic index with increased tumor control probability (TCP) and decreased normal tissue complication probability (NTCP). Striking this balance is especially difficult when the dose-limiting structure is the non-tumor-bearing liver that triggers RILD as a function of the low dose bath of radiation it receives. Previous photon studies have shown a positive correlation between radiotherapy dose to the tumor and local control rate; whereas the incidence of RILD negatively correlates with mean liver dose (MLD) seen by the non-tumor-bearing "normal" liver [89].

CIRT is administered in most centers using one or two beams with minimal or even no exit dose and minimal dose scattered to normal liver. This beam arrangement maximally spares normal liver tissue. Normal liver V5–V20 are considerably lower for CIRT than for SABR and IMRT [90, 91], possibly contributing to prolonged survival. In a comparative dosimetric study between CIRT and SABR in ten HCC patients, the prescribed total dose was 60 Gy in 4 fractions. Patients were simulated, and the planning images of the expiratory phase were used to generate contours that were then used in both plans. Respiratory motion was minimized by setting a gating window from 30% of the expiratory phase to 30% of the inspiratory phase. Using a planning directive of coverage of the planning target volume (PTV) by at least 90% of the prescribed dose, the PTV D90 was significantly higher in the CIRT group [59.6 ± 0.2 Gy(RBE)] than the SABR group [56.6 Gy] ($p < 0.05$). The homogeneity index [HI = maximum dose/minimum dose] in the target was lower for CIRT, indicating better homogeneity of dose distribution within the PTV, and the conformity index (CI; volume receiving the prescribed dose/target volume) was significantly higher for CIRT. This was achieved while maintaining a considerably lower MLD for CIRT. The treatment planning constraint of MLD <22 Gy was achieved in all ten CIRT plans but only 60% of SABR plans, especially when tumor size exceeded 4 cm. Although and gastrointestinal tract maximal dose (Dmax) was higher for SABR plans than CIRT plans (17.4 ± 7.1 Gy vs. 8.4 ± 4.3 GyRBE), this difference was not statistically significant [91].

In dosimetric comparison between 60 Gy(RBE) CIRT and 50 Gy or 60 Gy IMRT for locally advanced HCC with macroscopic vascular invasion noted that MLD was significantly lower in patients who received 60 Gy of CIRT than in those who received 50 or 60 Gy of IMRT. Only 10% of patients exceeded an MLD of 23 Gy in the CIRT 60 Gy(RBE) group compared to 30% of patients in the 50 and 60 Gy IMRT groups [90].

6.8.3.2 Hypofractionation

Accumulating evidence suggests that hypofractionated heavy particle radiotherapy is cost-effective compared to the conventional fractionated approaches, allowing more efficient use of clinical resources. It is even more convenient for the patient, as it greatly reduces the treatment course. Radiosurgery in HCC is no more exclusive to SABR. CIRT is proven to be effective and safe when administered over an extremely low number of fractions. While no data are available about the effectiveness of HCC PBT with less than 10 fractions of treatment, to the best of our knowledge; multiple CIRT studies have addressed the safety and effectiveness of hypofractionated therapy [92, 93].

In the first prospective study investigating CIRT for HCC in 1995, patients received 49.5–79.5 Gy in 15 fractions in 5 weeks. The estimated

3-year LC and OS rates were 81% and 50%, respectively. Subsequently, a series of studies were carried investigating progressive hypofractionation schedules. In a multicenter retrospective study of patients treated with a variety of hypofractionation schedules, patients receiving 48.0 Gy ($n = 46$) in two fractions, 52.8 Gy ($n = 108$) and 60.0 Gy ($n = 20$) in four fractions had LC and OS rates at 3 years of 81% and 73.3%, respectively. Only three patients (1.7%) experienced RILD. These data suggest that hypofractionated CIRT can yield excellent results, comparable to those of more protracted fractionation regimens [94].

Thereafter, increasing numbers of clinical studies adopted these hypofractionated regimens more routinely. The shortest CIRT schedule for HCC evaluated to date has been the two-fraction regimen. In one such study of 57 patients with localized HCC who received a CIRT dose of 45 Gy(RBE) in 2 fractions, with a median follow-up duration of 54 months (range, 7–103 months), the LC rate at 3 years was 91% after CIRT. Notably, CIRT achieved excellent control of all HCC lesions, including those that did not respond to the previous treatments. The 3-year OS rate was 67%. only two patients experienced grade 3 acute skin reactions, but no other grade 3 or higher toxicities were observed in any organ. No patient exhibited an increase in the Child–Pugh score of 2 or more points [89].

6.8.3.3 Dose Escalation

CIRT is an attractive option for radiation dose escalation in HCC, especially for large tumors that are not readily amenable to dose escalation with SABR. Clinical CIRT doses of 76 Gy(RBE) in 13 fractions and 60 Gy(RBE) in four fractions are equivalent to 125 Gy at 2 Gy per fraction. Despite these high BEDs, the CIRT treatments were well-tolerated with no increase in treatment-related toxicity. The feasibility of high-dose hypofractionated CIRT for patients with HCC was further investigated in 21 patients who received 60 Gy(RBE) in 4 fractions. No grade 3 or greater severe acute toxicity was observed in those patients. Grade 2 toxicities were observed in 4 patients (19.0%). Only 2 patients (9.5%) had

Table 6.2 Clinical outcomes after CIRT for HCC

Study	N	Study type	Fractionation	Child–Pugh score	Local control 1 years	3 years	5 years	Overall survival 1 years	3 years	5 years
Yasuda [89]	57	Retro	45 Gy/2 Fr	A or B	98%,	91%	91%	97%	67%	45%
Shibuya [95]	21	Retro	60 Gy/4 Fr	A or B	100%	92.3%	81.0%	90.5%		
Shibuya [96]	174	Retro	48 Gy/2 Fr 52.8 Gy/4 Fr 60 Gy/4 Fr		95.4%	82.5%	73.3%	94.6%	81.0%	
Imada [97]	64	Retro	52.8 Gy/4 Fr			95.8	92.4%		58.3%	29.2
Komatsu [64]	101	Retro	52.8 GyE/8 Fr 76 GyE/20 Fr 66 GyE/10 Fr 52.8 GyE/4 Fr	A, B, C			93%			36.3%
Kasuya	124	Retro	52.8 Gy/4 Fr	A or B	94.7%	91.4%	90.0%	90.3%	50.0%	25.0%
Kato [94]	24	Prosp	49.5–79.5 Gy/15 Fr	A, B	92%	81%	81%	92%	50%	25%

worsening of Child–Pugh score at 3 months. There was no significant difference in Child–Pugh score at 3 and 6 months after CIRT compared to that before treatment ($p = 0.846$). The 1- and 2-year LC rates were 100% and 92.3%, respectively [95] (Table 6.2).

6.9 Conclusions

Technological improvements in radiation therapy have dramatically increased the feasibility and widespread adoption of curative-intent radiation therapy for HCC. As noted in this chapter, these advances have spanned the range from improvement in target delineation, respiratory motion management, image-guided therapy with real-time verification, adaptive treatment modifications, RILD prediction algorithms, and sophisticated treatment delivery techniques including SABR, PBT, and CIRT. Collectively, these advances have increased the probability of tumor control and overall survival in patients with localized HCCs who are treated with radiotherapy, with results often rivaling those of surgery. However, more universal adoption of such ablative treatments will require randomized clinical trials conducted in increasingly homogeneous groups of patients with clearly defined inclusion and exclusion criteria. It may well be that there is no "one-size-fits-all" solution where advanced radiation techniques trump other liver-directed modalities in every instance but an increased awareness of the scenarios where such treatment may offer meaningful clinical value could guide the personalization of treatment. Patients with HCC can only stand to gain when more options are available to them and hepatobiliary tumor boards and oncology practices are aware of the full spectrum of available options for patients.

References

1. Bray F, Ferlay J, Soerjomataram I, Siegel RL, Torre LA, Jemal A. Global cancer statistics 2018: GLOBOCAN estimates of incidence and mortality worldwide for 36 cancers in 185 countries. CA Cancer J Clin. 2018;68(6):394–424.
2. Delis SG, Dervenis C. Selection criteria for liver resection in patients with hepatocellular carcinoma and chronic liver disease. World J Gastroenterol. 2008;14(22):3452–60.
3. Couto OF, Dvorchik I, Carr BI. Causes of death in patients with unresectable hepatocellular carcinoma. Dig Dis Sci. 2007;52(11):3285–9.
4. Lawrence TS, Robertson JM, Anscher MS, Jirtle RL, Ensminger WD, Fajardo LF. Hepatic toxicity resulting from cancer treatment. Int J Radiat Oncol Biol Phys. 1995;31(5):1237–48.

5. Ben-Josef E, Normolle D, Ensminger WD, Walker S, Tatro D, Haken RKT, et al. Phase II trial of high-dose conformal radiation therapy with concurrent hepatic artery floxuridine for unresectable intrahepatic malignancies. J Clin Oncol. 2005;23(34):8739–47.

6. Mornex F, Girard N, Beziat C, Kubas A, Khodri M, Trepo C, et al. Feasibility and efficacy of high-dose three-dimensional-conformal radiotherapy in cirrhotic patients with small-size hepatocellular carcinoma non-eligible for curative therapies—mature results of the French Phase II RTF-1 trial. Int J Radiat Oncol Biol Phys. 2006;66(4):1152–8.

7. Yoon HI, Lee IJ, Han KH, Seong J. Improved oncologic outcomes with image-guided intensity-modulated radiation therapy using helical tomotherapy in locally advanced hepatocellular carcinoma. J Cancer Res Clin Oncol. 2014;140(9):1595–605.

8. Hou JZ, Zeng ZC, Wang BL, Yang P, Zhang JY, Mo HF. High dose radiotherapy with image-guided hypo-IMRT for hepatocellular carcinoma with portal vein and/or inferior vena cava tumor thrombi is more feasible and efficacious than conventional 3D-CRT. Jpn J Clin Oncol. 2016;46(4):357–62.

9. Forner A, Vilana R, Ayuso C, Bianchi L, Solé M, Ayuso JR, et al. Diagnosis of hepatic nodules 20 mm or smaller in cirrhosis: prospective validation of the noninvasive diagnostic criteria for hepatocellular carcinoma. Hepatology (Baltimore, MD). 2008;47(1):97–104.

10. Voroney JP, Brock KK, Eccles C, Haider M, Dawson LA. Prospective comparison of computed tomography and magnetic resonance imaging for liver cancer delineation using deformable image registration. Int J Radiat Oncol Biol Phys. 2006;66(3):780–91.

11. Wang H, Krishnan S, Wang X, Beddar AS, Briere TM, Crane CH, et al. Improving soft-tissue contrast in four-dimensional computed tomography images of liver cancer patients using a deformable image registration method. Int J Radiat Oncol Biol Phys. 2008;72(1):201–9.

12. Keall PJ, Mageras GS, Balter JM, Emery RS, Forster KM, Jiang SB, et al. The management of respiratory motion in radiation oncology report of AAPM Task Group 76. Med Phys. 2006;33(10):3874–900.

13. Tsai YL, Wu CJ, Shaw S, Yu PC, Nien HH, Lui LT. Quantitative analysis of respiration-induced motion of each liver segment with helical computed tomography and 4-dimensional computed tomography. Radiat Oncol (London, Engl). 2018;13(1):59.

14. Oh SA, Yea JW, Kim SK, Park JW. Optimal gating window for respiratory-gated radiotherapy with real-time position management and respiration guiding system for liver cancer treatment. Sci Rep. 2019;9(1):4384.

15. Eccles C, Brock KK, Bissonnette JP, Hawkins M, Dawson LA. Reproducibility of liver position using active breathing coordinator for liver cancer radiotherapy. Int J Radiat Oncol Biol Phys. 2006;64(3):751–9.

16. Herfarth KK, Debus J, Lohr F, Bahner ML, Fritz P, Höss A, et al. Extracranial stereotactic radiation therapy: set-up accuracy of patients treated for liver metastases. Int J Radiat Oncol Biol Phys. 2000;46(2):329–35.

17. Wagman R, Yorke E, Ford E, Giraud P, Mageras G, Minsky B, et al. Respiratory gating for liver tumors: use in dose escalation. Int J Radiat Oncol Biol Phys. 2003;55(3):659–68.

18. Beddar AS, Kainz K, Briere TM, Tsunashima Y, Pan T, Prado K, et al. Correlation between internal fiducial tumor motion and external marker motion for liver tumors imaged with 4D-CT. Int J Radiat Oncol Biol Phys. 2007;67(2):630–8.

19. Park SH, Won HJ, Kim SY, Shin YM, Kim PN, Yoon SM, et al. Efficacy and safety of ultrasound-guided implantation of fiducial markers in the liver for stereotactic body radiation therapy. PLoS One. 2017;12(6):e0179676.

20. Hawkins MA, Brock KK, Eccles C, Moseley D, Jaffray D, Dawson LA. Assessment of residual error in liver position using kV cone-beam computed tomography for liver cancer high-precision radiation therapy. Int J Radiat Oncol Biol Phys. 2006;66(2):610–9.

21. Yang J, Cai J, Wang H, Chang Z, Czito BG, Bashir MR, et al. Is diaphragm motion a good surrogate for liver tumor motion? Int J Radiat Oncol Biol Phys. 2014;90(4):952–8.

22. Fahmi S, Simonis FFJ, Abayazid M. Respiratory motion estimation of the liver with abdominal motion as a surrogate. Int J Med Robot. 2018;14(6):e1940.

23. Seiler PG, Blattmann H, Kirsch S, Muench RK, Schilling C. A novel tracking technique for the continuous precise measurement of tumour positions in conformal radiotherapy. Phys Med Biol. 2000;45(9):N103–10.

24. Balter JM, Wright JN, Newell LJ, Friemel B, Dimmer S, Cheng Y, et al. Accuracy of a wireless localization system for radiotherapy. Int J Radiat Oncol Biol Phys. 2005;61(3):933–7.

25. Eccles CL, Tse RV, Hawkins MA, Lee MT, Moseley DJ, Dawson LA. Intravenous contrast-enhanced cone beam computed tomography (IVCBCT) of intrahepatic tumors and vessels. Adv Radiat Oncol. 2016;1(1):43–50.

26. Schernthaner RE, Haroun RR, Duran R, Lee H, Sahu S, Sohn JH, et al. Improved visibility of metastatic disease in the liver during intra-arterial therapy using delayed arterial phase cone-beam CT. Cardiovasc Intervent Radiol. 2016;39(10):1429–37.

27. Price RG, Apisarnthanarax S, Schaub SK, Nyflot MJ, Chapman TR, Matesan M, et al. Regional radiation dose-response modeling of functional liver in hepatocellular carcinoma patients with longitudinal sulfur colloid SPECT/CT: a proof of concept. Int J Radiat Oncol Biol Phys. 2018;102(4):1349–56.

28. Schaub SK, Apisarnthanarax S, Price RG, Nyflot MJ, Chapman TR, Matesan M, et al. Functional liver imaging and dosimetry to predict hepatotoxicity risk in cirrhotic patients with primary liver cancer. Int J Radiat Oncol Biol Phys. 2018;102(4):1339–48.

29. Qi WX, Fu S, Zhang Q, Guo XM. Charged particle therapy versus photon therapy for patients with hepatocellular carcinoma: a systematic review and meta-analysis. Radiother Oncol. 2015;114(3):289–95.

30. Yoon SM, Ryoo BY, Lee SJ, Kim JH, Shin JH, An JH, et al. Efficacy and safety of transarterial chemoembolization plus external beam radiotherapy vs sorafenib in hepatocellular carcinoma with macroscopic vascular invasion: a randomized clinical trial. JAMA Oncol. 2018;4(5):661–9.

31. Schaue D, Ratikan JA, Iwamoto KS, McBride WH. Maximizing tumor immunity with fractionated radiation. Int J Radiat Oncol Biol Phys. 2012;83(4):1306–10.

32. Wen N, Kim J, Doemer A, Glide-Hurst C, Chetty IJ, Liu C, et al. Evaluation of a magnetic resonance guided linear accelerator for stereotactic radiosurgery treatment. Radiother Oncol J Eur Soc Therap Radiol Oncol. 2018;127(3):460–6.

33. Fast M, van de Schoot A, van de Lindt T, Carbaat C, van der Heide U, Sonke JJ. Tumor trailing for liver SBRT on the MR-linac. Int J Radiat Oncol Biol Phys. 2019;103(2):468–78.

34. Feldman AM, Modh A, Glide-Hurst C, Chetty IJ, Movsas B. Real-time magnetic resonance-guided liver stereotactic body radiation therapy: an institutional report using a magnetic resonance-linac system. Cureus. 2019;11(9):e5774.

35. Newhauser WD, Zhang R. The physics of proton therapy. Phys Med Biol. 2015;60(8):R155–209.

36. Munoz-Schuffenegger P, Ng S, Dawson LA. Radiation-induced liver toxicity. Semin Radiat Oncol. 2017;27(4):350–7.

37. Dionisi F, Widesott L, Lorentini S, Amichetti M. Is there a role for proton therapy in the treatment of hepatocellular carcinoma? A systematic review. Radiother Oncol. 2014;111(1):1–10.

38. Skinner HD, Hong TS, Krishnan S. Charged-particle therapy for hepatocellular carcinoma. Semin Radiat Oncol. 2011;21(4):278–86.

39. Langen K, Zhu M. Concepts of PTV and robustness in passively scattered and pencil beam scanning proton therapy. Semin Radiat Oncol. 2018;28(3):248–55.

40. Fukumitsu N, Sugahara S, Nakayama H, Fukuda K, Mizumoto M, Abei M, et al. A prospective study of hypofractionated proton beam therapy for patients with hepatocellular carcinoma. Int J Radiat Oncol Biol Phys. 2009;74(3):831–6.

41. Bush DA, Kayali Z, Grove R, Slater JD. The safety and efficacy of high-dose proton beam radiotherapy for hepatocellular carcinoma: a phase 2 prospective trial. Cancer. 2011;117(13):3053–9.

42. Hong TS, Wo JY, Yeap BY, Ben-Josef E, McDonnell EI, Blaszkowsky LS, et al. Multi-institutional phase II study of high-dose hypofractionated proton beam therapy in patients with localized, unresectable hepatocellular carcinoma and intrahepatic cholangiocarcinoma. J Clin Oncol. 2016;34(5):460–8.

43. Robbins JR, Schmid RK, Hammad AY, Gamblin TC, Erickson BA. Stereotactic body radiation therapy for hepatocellular carcinoma: practice patterns, dose selection and factors impacting survival. Cancer Med. 2019;8(3):928–38.

44. Holliday EB, Tao R, Brownlee Z, Das P, Krishnan S, Taniguchi C, et al. Definitive radiation therapy for hepatocellular carcinoma with portal vein tumor thrombus. Clin Transl Radiat Oncol. 2017;4:39–45.

45. Lausch A, Sinclair K, Lock M, Fisher B, Jensen N, Gaede S, et al. Determination and comparison of radiotherapy dose responses for hepatocellular carcinoma and metastatic colorectal liver tumours. Br J Radiol. 2013;86(1027):20130147.

46. Jang WI, Kim M-S, Bae SH, Cho CK, Yoo HJ, Seo YS, et al. High-dose stereotactic body radiotherapy correlates increased local control and overall survival in patients with inoperable hepatocellular carcinoma. Radiat Oncol. 2013;8(1):250.

47. Scorsetti M, Comito T, Cozzi L, Clerici E, Tozzi A, Franzese C, et al. The challenge of inoperable hepatocellular carcinoma (HCC): results of a single-institutional experience on stereotactic body radiation therapy (SBRT). J Cancer Res Clin Oncol. 2015;141(7):1301–9.

48. Chadha AS, Gunther JR, Hsieh CE, Aliru M, Mahadevan LS, Venkatesulu BP, et al. Proton beam therapy outcomes for localized unresectable hepatocellular carcinoma. Radiother Oncol J Eur Soc Therap Radiol Oncol. 2019;133:54–61.

49. Pursley J, El Naqa I, Sanford NN, Noe B, Wo JY, Eyler CE, et al. Dosimetric analysis and normal tissue complication probability modeling of Child-Pugh score and Albumin-Bilirubin grade increase after hepatic irradiation. Int J Radiat Oncol Biol Phys. 2020;107(5):986–95.

50. Son SH, Kay CS, Song JH, Lee S-W, Choi BO, Kang YN, et al. Dosimetric parameter predicting the deterioration of hepatic function after helical tomotherapy in patients with unresectable locally advanced hepatocellular carcinoma. Radiat Oncol. 2013;8(1):11.

51. Pan CC, Kavanagh BD, Dawson LA, Li XA, Das SK, Miften M, et al. Radiation-associated liver injury. Int J Radiat Oncol Biol Phys. 2010;76(3 Suppl):S94–S100.

52. Hsieh C-E, Venkatesulu BP, Lee C-H, Hung S-P, Wong P-F, Aithala SP, et al. Predictors of radiation-induced liver disease in eastern and western patients with hepatocellular carcinoma undergoing proton beam therapy. Int J Radiat Oncol Biol Phys. 2019;105:73–86.

53. Gandhi SJ, Liang X, Ding X, Zhu TC, Ben-Josef E, Plastaras JP, et al. Clinical decision tool for optimal delivery of liver stereotactic body radiation therapy: Photons versus protons. Pract Radiat Oncol. 2015;5(4):209–18.

54. Toramatsu C, Katoh N, Shimizu S, Nihongi H, Matsuura T, Takao S, et al. What is the appropriate size criterion for proton radiotherapy for hepatocellular carcinoma? A dosimetric comparison of spot-scanning proton therapy versus intensity-modulated radiation therapy. Radiat Oncol (London, Engl). 2013;8:48.

55. Wang X, Krishnan S, Zhang X, Dong L, Briere T, Crane CH, et al. Proton radiotherapy for liver tumors: dosimetric advantages over photon plans. Med Dosim. 2008;33(4):259–67.

56. Sanford NN, Pursley J, Noe B, Yeap BY, Goyal L, Clark JW, et al. Protons versus photons for unresectable hepatocellular carcinoma: liver decompensation and overall survival. Int J Radiat Oncol Biol Phys. 2019;105(1):64–72.

57. Hasan S, Abel S, Verma V, Webster P, Arscott WT, Wegner RE, et al. Proton beam therapy versus stereotactic body radiotherapy for hepatocellular carcinoma: practice patterns, outcomes, and the effect of biologically effective dose escalation. J Gastrointest Oncol. 2019;10(5):999–1009.

58. Tao R, Krishnan S, Bhosale PR, Javle MM, Aloia TA, Shroff RT, et al. Ablative radiotherapy doses lead to a substantial prolongation of survival in patients with inoperable intrahepatic cholangiocarcinoma: a retrospective dose response analysis. J Clin Oncol Off J Am Soc Clin Oncol. 2016;34(3):219–26.

59. Hung S-P, Huang B-S, Hsieh C-E, Lee C-H, Tsang N-M, Chang JT-C, et al. Clinical outcomes of patients with unresectable cholangiocarcinoma treated with proton beam therapy. Am J Clin Oncol. 2020;43(3):180–6.

60. Makita C, Nakamura T, Takada A, Takayama K, Suzuki M, Ishikawa Y, et al. Clinical outcomes and toxicity of proton beam therapy for advanced cholangiocarcinoma. Radiat Oncol. 2014;9(1):26.

61. Ohkawa A, Mizumoto M, Ishikawa H, Abei M, Fukuda K, Hashimoto T, et al. Proton beam therapy for unresectable intrahepatic cholangiocarcinoma. J Gastroenterol Hepatol. 2015;30(5):957–63.

62. Hong TS, Wo JY, Borger DR, Yeap BY, McDonnell EI, Willers H, et al. Phase II study of proton-based stereotactic body radiation therapy for liver metastases: importance of tumor genotype. J Natl Cancer Inst, 2017. 109(9) https://doi.org/10.1093/jnci/djx031.

63. Lee MT, Kim JJ, Dinniwell R, Brierley J, Lockwood G, Wong R, et al. Phase I study of individualized stereotactic body radiotherapy of liver metastases. J Clin Oncol Off J Am Soc Clin Oncol. 2009;27(10):1585–91.

64. Komatsu S, Fukumoto T, Demizu Y, Miyawaki D, Terashima K, Sasaki R, et al. Clinical results and risk factors of proton and carbon ion therapy for hepatocellular carcinoma. Cancer. 2011;117(21):4890–904.

65. Nakayama H, Sugahara S, Tokita M, Fukuda K, Mizumoto M, Abei M, et al. Proton beam therapy for hepatocellular carcinoma: the University of Tsukuba experience. Cancer. 2009;115(23):5499–506.

66. Kawashima M, Kohno R, Nakachi K, Nishio T, Mitsunaga S, Ikeda M, et al. Dose-volume histogram analysis of the safety of proton beam therapy for unresectable hepatocellular carcinoma. Int J Radiat Oncol Biol Phys. 2011;79(5):1479–86.

67. Fukumitsu N, Okumura T, Takizawa D, Numajiri H, Ohnishi K, Mizumoto M, et al. Proton beam therapy for liver metastases from gastric cancer. J Radiat Res. 2017;58(3):357–62.

68. Moreno AC, Frank SJ, Garden AS, Rosenthal DI, Fuller CD, Gunn GB, et al. Intensity modulated proton therapy (IMPT) – The future of IMRT for head and neck cancer. Oral Oncol. 2019;88:66–74.

69. Pugh TJ, Amos RA, John Baptiste S, Choi S, Nhu Nguyen Q, Ronald Zhu X, et al. Multifield optimization intensity-modulated proton therapy (MFO-IMPT) for prostate cancer: robustness analysis through simulation of rotational and translational alignment errors. Med Dosim. 2013;38(3):344–50.

70. Park PC, Zhu XR, Lee AK, Sahoo N, Melancon AD, Zhang L, et al. A beam-specific planning target volume (PTV) design for proton therapy to account for setup and range uncertainties. Int J Radiat Oncol Biol Phys. 2012;82(2):e329–e36.

71. Grassberger C, Dowdell S, Lomax A, Sharp G, Shackleford J, Choi N, et al. Motion interplay as a function of patient parameters and spot size in spot scanning proton therapy for lung cancer. Int J Radiat Oncol Biol Phys. 2013;86(2):380–6.

72. Knopf A-C, Lomax AJ. In the context of radiosurgery – pros and cons of rescanning as a solution for treating moving targets with scanned particle beams. Phys Med. 2014;30(5):551–4.

73. Dolde K, Zhang Y, Chaudhri N, Dávid C, Kachelrieß M, Lomax AJ, et al. 4DMRI-based investigation on the interplay effect for pencil beam scanning proton therapy of pancreatic cancer patients. Radiat Oncol. 2019;14(1):30.

74. Yoo GS, Yu JI, Cho S, Jung SH, Han Y, Park S, et al. Comparison of clinical outcomes between passive scattering versus pencil-beam scanning proton beam therapy for hepatocellular carcinoma. Radiother Oncol. 2020;146:187–93.

75. Dionisi F, Brolese A, Siniscalchi B, Giacomelli I, Fracchiolla F, Righetto R, et al. Clinical results of active scanning proton therapy for primary liver tumors. Tumori J. 2020; https://doi.org/10.1177/0300891620937809.

76. Akino Y, Wu H, Oh R-J, Das IJ. An effective method to reduce the interplay effects between respiratory motion and a uniform scanning proton beam irradiation for liver tumors: a case study. J Appl Clin Med Phys. 2019;20(1):220–8.

77. Lambert J, Suchowerska N, McKenzie DR, Jackson M. Intrafractional motion during proton beam scanning. Phys Med Biol. 2005;50(20):4853–62.

78. Ray S, Cekanaviciute E, Lima IP, Sørensen BS, Costes SV. Comparing photon and charged particle therapy using DNA damage biomarkers. Int J Part Ther. 2018;5(1):15–24.

79. Ebner DK, Tsuji H, Yasuda S, Yamamoto N, Mori S, Kamada T. Respiration-gated fast-rescanning carbon-ion radiotherapy. Jpn J Clin Oncol. 2017;47(1):80–3.

80. Zeitlin C, La Tessa C. The role of nuclear fragmentation in particle therapy and space radiation protection. Front Oncol. 2016;6:65.

81. Tsujii H, Kamada T. A review of update clinical results of carbon ion radiotherapy. Jpn J Clin Oncol. 2012;42(8):670–85.

82. Karger CP, Peschke P. RBE and related modeling in carbon-ion therapy. Phys Med Biol. 2017;63(1):01TR02.

83. Choi J, Kang JO. Basics of particle therapy II: relative biological effectiveness. Radiat Oncol J. 2012;30(1):1–13.

84. Mohamad O, Makishima H, Kamada T. Evolution of carbon ion radiotherapy at the national institute of radiological sciences in Japan. Cancers (Basel). 2018;10(3):66.

85. Fossati P, Matsufuji N, Kamada T, Karger CP. Radiobiological issues in prospective carbon ion therapy trials. Med Phys. 2018;45(11):e1096–e110.

86. Fossati P, Molinelli S, Matsufuji N, Ciocca M, Mirandola A, Mairani A, et al. Dose prescription in carbon ion radiotherapy: a planning study to compare NIRS and LEM approaches with a clinically-oriented strategy. Phys Med Biol. 2012;57:7543–54.

87. Kagawa K, Murakami M, Hishikawa Y, Abe M, Akagi T, Yanou T, et al. Preclinical biological assessment of proton and carbon ion beams at Hyogo Ion Beam Medical Center. Int J Radiat Oncol Biol Phys. 2002;54:928–38.

88. Wang W, Huang Z, Sheng Y, Zhao J, Shahnazi K, Zhang Q, et al. RBE-weighted dose conversions for carbon ionradiotherapy between microdosimetric kinetic model and local effect model for the targets and organs at risk in prostate carcinoma. Radiother Oncol. 2020;144:30–6.

89. Yasuda S, Kato H, Imada H, Isozaki Y, Kasuya G, Makishima H, et al. Long-term results of high-dose 2-fraction carbon ion radiation therapy for hepatocellular carcinoma. Adv Radiat Oncol. 2020;5(2):196–203.

90. Shiba S, Shibuya K, Kawashima M, Okano N, Kaminuma T, Okamoto M, et al. Comparison of dose distributions when using carbon ion radiotherapy versus intensity-modulated radiotherapy for hepatocellular carcinoma with macroscopic vascular invasion: a retrospective analysis. Anticancer Res. 2020;40(1):459–64.

91. Abe T, Saitoh J-I, Kobayashi D, Shibuya K, Koyama Y, Shimada H, et al. Dosimetric comparison of carbon ion radiotherapy and stereotactic body radiotherapy with photon beams for the treatment of hepatocellular carcinoma. Radiat Oncol (London, Engl). 2015;10:187.

92. Hsu C-Y, Wang C-W, Cheng A-L, Kuo S-H. Hypofractionated particle beam therapy for hepatocellular carcinoma: a brief review of clinical effectiveness. World J Gastrointest Oncol. 2019;11(8):579–88.

93. Kasuya G, Kato H, Yasuda S, Tsuji H, Yamada S, Haruyama Y, et al. Progressive hypofractionated carbon-ion radiotherapy for hepatocellular carcinoma: combined analyses of 2 prospective trials. Cancer. 2017;123(20):3955–65.

94. Kato H, Tsujii H, Miyamoto T, Mizoe J-E, Kamada T, Tsuji H, et al. Results of the first prospective study of carbon ion radiotherapy for hepatocellular carcinoma with liver cirrhosis. Int J Radiat Oncol Biol Phys. 2004;59(5):1468–76.

95. Shibuya K, Ohno T, Katoh H, Okamoto M, Shiba S, Koyama Y, et al. A feasibility study of high-dose hypofractionated carbon ion radiation therapy using four fractions for localized hepatocellular carcinoma measuring 3 cm or larger. Radiother Oncol. 2019;132:230–5.

96. Shibuya K, Ohno T, Terashima K, Toyama S, Yasuda S, Tsuji H, et al. Short-course carbon-ion radiotherapy for hepatocellular carcinoma: a multi-institutional retrospective study. Liver Int. 2018;38(12):2239–47.

97. Imada H, Kato H, Yasuda S, Yamada S, Yanagi T, Kishimoto R, et al. Comparison of efficacy and toxicity of short-course carbon ion radiotherapy for hepatocellular carcinoma depending on their proximity to the porta hepatis. Radiother Oncol. 2010;96(2):231–5.

Basics of Ablative Radiotherapy: The Background Knowledge Necessary to Practicing Stereotactic Body Radiotherapy for Hepatocellular Carcinoma

7

Alejandra Méndez Romero, Steven Habraken, and Dave Sprengers

Abstract

While stereotactic body radiation therapy (SBRT) is a promising treatment option for patients with hepatocellular carcinoma (HCC), this fragile population is relatively unknown to radiation oncologists starting a liver SBRT program. This chapter summarizes information that will aid understanding of the population and of the benefits and limitations of SBRT.

This information is based on the international HCC management guidelines, the inclusion criteria and outcomes reported in prospective and retrospective cohort studies on SBRT, and the results of propensity-score analyses performed between SBRT and other local treatment options, such as radiofrequency ablation or transarterial chemoembolization. The chapter also reviews the toxicity related to SBRT and the role of underlying liver cirrhosis in decreasing the liver's tolerance of irradiation. Last but not least, it presents topics related to target delineation, treatment planning, and the requirements of medical physics relevant to starting an SBRT program for HCC.

Keywords

Practice · Knowledge · Stereotactic body radiation therapy (SBRT) · Hepatocellular carcinoma (HCC)

7.1 Introduction

Hepatocellular carcinoma (HCC) is a global health burden. Its pattern of occurrence shows a significant geographic imbalance, with the highest incidence in East Asia and Sub-Saharan Africa [1]. Most HCCs are associated with a known underlying etiology, most frequently chronic viral hepatitis (B and C), alcohol intake, and aflatoxin exposure. An important risk factor is liver cirrhosis, which is defined as a response to chronic liver injury that involves the histological development of regenerative nodules surrounded by fibrous bands that lead to portal hypertension and end-stage liver disease [2]. Cirrhosis can be caused by chronic viral hepatitis, alcohol intake, and aflatoxin exposure [1].

A. Méndez Romero (✉) · S. Habraken
Department of Radiotherapy, Erasmus MC Cancer Institute, Erasmus MC University Medical Center, Rotterdam, The Netherlands
e-mail: a.mendezromero@erasmusmc.nl; s.habraken@erasmusmc.nl

D. Sprengers
Department of Gastroenterology and Hepatology, Erasmus MC University Medical Center Rotterdam, Rotterdam, The Netherlands
e-mail: d.sprengers@erasmusmc.nl

Several clinical practice guidelines have been published on the management of HCC in different geographical areas, such as Europe, North American, and the Asia-Pacific region [1, 3, 4]. These guidelines provide excellent overviews for assisting physicians in the decision-making process.

Traditionally, radiation therapy (RT) has played only a limited role in the treatment of liver tumors. This was due to the evidence that conventional radiation could treat the whole liver safely with moderate doses of up to 30 Gy, and that such doses could lead only to the short-term palliation of symptoms [5, 6]. Technological developments in the 1990s then made it possible to deliver high doses of radiation to limited volumes of the liver with acceptable toxicity and promising outcomes regarding local control and toxicity [7, 8]. Over the subsequent decades, new advances contributed to the implementation of stereotactic body radiation therapy (SBRT)—including the possibility of imaging during the treatment to correct for inter- and intrafraction variations in the tumor position—and advances in treatment planning. More clinical information was collected on patient selection and outcomes, and on factors influencing liver toxicity, such as the presence of liver cirrhosis [9–11].

In recent years, more evidence has been collected on SBRT, mainly in retrospective studies, but also in prospective phase I–II studies [12–19]. However, as no large randomized control trials have compared RT with other treatments, RT has not been recommended in treatment guidelines, although it is considered to be a promising treatment option [1, 3, 4]. Although studies have been developed to provide the evidence required, definitive results are still pending (NCT 02470533, NCT 01730937, NCT 02323360, NCT 02182687). However, three recent studies showed positive results in favor of radiotherapy. Two large comparative studies (propensity-score analysis) on the results of radiofrequency ablation (RFA) and SBRT showed improved local recurrence rates [20, 21]. The first phase III randomized non-inferiority trial between RT in the form of proton therapy and RFA showed improved local progression-free survival [22].

SBRT for HCC involves a multidisciplinary team of gastroenterologists, surgeons, imaging and interventional radiologists, pathologists, medical oncologists and radiation oncologists. To discuss the best treatment option for their patients, specialized tumor boards are required. Within the radiotherapy department, close collaboration with physicists and technicians is also essential. Due to their underlying impaired liver function, these patients constitute a fragile and complex population. It should therefore be remembered that the aim of the treatment is not only to control the tumor but also to preserve the liver function in ways that avoid decompensations.

To further understanding this fragile patient population and of the benefits and limitations of SBRT, the following chapter summarizes information for radiation oncologists who are starting to treat HCC patients.

7.2   Materials and Methods

As the treatment of HCC is multidisciplinary, we have sought to outline the most important issues that radiation oncologists should bear in mind before starting to treat patients diagnosed with HCC. Each author has compiled the knowledge specific to his or her own discipline. In this way, (1) DS has focused on aspects of hepatology such as incidence, diagnosis, staging, treatment options (other than radiotherapy), and guidelines; (2) AMR has described aspects of SBRT, such as patient selection, outcomes regarding local control and toxicity, and the evidence generated by comparisons of SBRT with other recognized local treatment options; and (3) SH has summarized the aspects of medical physics considerations that are essential to an SBRT program for HCC. The last considerations may be used for quality assurance in clinical trials including SBRT. The authors also propose target definitions and the organs-at-risk (OAR) constraints currently used at their center.

To retrieve the most relevant and recent publications on RT studies with a particular focus on SBRT, we searched in PubMed using the terms hepatocellular carcinoma, SBRT, and stereotactic radiotherapy. In this chapter, an account was also taken of the authors' experience in treating patients in daily clinical practice and in developing trials involving HCC patients.

7.3 Results

7.3.1 Epidemiology, Risk Factors, Guidelines, and Treatment Options

Liver cancer is the sixth most common cancer in the world and the third cause of cancer-related mortality as estimated by the World Health Organization (globacan.iarc.fr; 2018 data). In 2018, the annual number of new cases was almost 850,000, over 600,000 of which occurred in Asia, the highest incidence rates being in East Asia (with over 50% of cases occurring in China) and sub-Saharan Africa. Hepatocellular carcinoma (HCC) represents about 90% of primary liver cancers. On a global scale, its incidence has been growing: between 1990 and 2015, the number of newly diagnosed HCC cases increased by 75%. Age-standardized incidence rates have increased in many high socio-demographic index countries, including the USA and most European countries. In contrast, some countries with high incidence rates, such as China and eastern Sub-Saharan Africa, have experienced decreases of more than 20% [23]. These data suggest that geographical heterogeneity is related primarily to differences in the exposure rate to risk factors.

Cirrhosis should be considered as a risk factor for HCC. Preexisting cirrhosis is found in more than 80% of people diagnosed with HCC [24]. The major causes of cirrhosis, and hence HCC, are the hepatitis B virus (HBV), the hepatitis C virus (HCV), alcohol, and nonalcoholic fatty liver disease (NAFLD). Less-prevalent causes of liver cirrhosis—such as hereditary hemochromatosis, primary biliary cholangitis (PBC), and Wilson's disease—have also been associated with HCC development. However, there is little significant data on HCC that occurs in a non-cirrhotic liver. NAFLD predisposes to HCC in non-cirrhotic patients, and as the obesity epi-

demic progresses, the number of patients who develop HCC against the background of NAFLD is expected to increase [25, 26]. Additionally, 15% of HBV-related HCC occur in non-cirrhotic patients—possibly due partly to exposure to aflatoxin B1, a major hepatocarcinogen that is more common in areas such as sub-Saharan Africa, South-East Asia, and China, where HBV is the dominant virus [27, 28].

As the prognosis of HCC depends largely on the stage at which the tumor is detected, detecting HCC early in its development is critical to improving the survival of affected patients. For this reason, clinical practice guidelines by the European Association for the Study of the Liver (EASL), the American Association for the Study of Liver Diseases (AASLD), and the Asian Pacific Association for the Study of the Liver (APASL) all promote a screening strategy for high-risk patients that involves biannual ultrasound with or without measurement of serum alpha-fetoprotein (AFP) [1, 3, 4]. In the context of liver cirrhosis, HCC can usually—depending on the characteristic imaging features these guidelines describe—be diagnosed using multiphasic CT, dynamic contrast-enhanced MRI, or contrast-enhanced ultrasound (CEUS). If these criteria are not present but HCC or other malignancy is considered probable, a liver biopsy should be considered for diagnosis. HCC cannot be diagnosed by imaging in patients without cirrhosis, in whom biopsy is therefore required.

Once the diagnosis has been established, cancer staging is intended to establish a prognosis and to allow the most appropriate treatment to be selected for the best candidates. The options for HCC depend on tumor burden, degree of liver dysfunction, and performance status. Although there is no single universally accepted staging system, the Barcelona Clinic for Liver Cancer (BCLC) system, which pairs these parameters with a recommended therapy, is advocated by EASL and AASLD, and is, therefore, the most widely used in Western countries [1, 4]. While the median overall survival associated with therapy based on the BCLC stage indicates the average anticipated life expectancy, there is scope for further refining the estimation of prognosis. In

Asia, several different staging systems are used, only one of which—the Hong Kong Liver Cancer (HKLC) staging system—takes account of prognostic factors—and also pairs each stage with a recommended therapy. Among subsets of patients, the HKLC also recommends more aggressive therapy than the BCLC—a system that will require prospective validation in Western patients [29].

Although regional differences in disease staging may lead to differences in treatment approaches, surgical resection is the curative treatment of choice worldwide for resectable HCC in patients without cirrhosis. As detailed in the EASL, AASLD, and APASL guidelines, it is also favored in patients with Child–Pugh class A without clinically significant portal hypertension (CSPH). Technically, there is no size cutoff for tumor diameter, and if there is sufficient functional liver remnant, large tumors can be resected safely. HCCs presenting with multiple nodules are not necessarily a contraindication for surgical intervention, provided patient performance status and co-morbidities allow surgical consideration, and provided liver function and remnant liver volume-preserving principles are met [30]. Liver transplantation (LT) is the treatment of choice for unresectable tumors, for patients with CSPH or hepatic decompensation with HCC within the Milan criteria (i.e., 1 tumor up to 5 cm, or two to three tumors, the largest being <3 cm, no vascular invasion). Sometimes, however, the Milan criteria are extended on the basis of regional considerations [1, 3, 4]. If successful locoregional therapies achieve downstaging to within the Milan criteria, patients who previously exceeded these criteria can be considered for LT. Additionally, as studies have shown that improved post-LT cancer recurrence rates are correlated with response to locoregional therapies for HCCs while waiting for LT, such treatment is recommended [1, 31].

Locoregional therapies for HCC include a broad spectrum of techniques, such as hyperthermic ablative approaches like RFA and microwave ablation (MWA), transarterial chemoembolization (TACE), selective internal radiation therapy (SIRT), and SBRT. The most widely used locoregional therapies are radiofrequency and microwave techniques that subject the tissue to cytotoxic temperatures, causing coagulation necrosis. As RFA yields the best results in HCCs smaller than 2 cm, it can be used as the first-line curative therapy in the patients concerned, even surgical patients [1, 3, 27]. Depending both on the location of the tumor and on hepatic and extrahepatic patient conditions, hyperthermic ablation is also an alternative to surgical resection in tumors 2–3 cm in size.

TACE—which relies on targeting the arterial hypervascularization of HCC—achieves tumor necrosis by embolization of the arterial blood supply, either with a suspension of lipiodol and a chemotherapeutic agent and gelatin sponge or with drug-eluting beads loaded with doxorubicin. It is intended for use in a palliative setting for incurable patients with large or multifocal but intrahepatic disease [1, 3, 27]. Its survival benefits relative to those of best supportive care were demonstrated in two randomized controlled trials [32, 33]. SIRT involves exposing the tumor to highly concentrated radiation while protecting the normal parenchyma by injecting implantable radioactive microspheres into tumor-feeding arteries. SIRT using Yttrium-90 (Y-90) might be recommended to patients who are not good candidates for TACE due to bulky tumor and/or portal vein invasion. Although the available studies that compared SIRT with TACE were retrospective and involved small numbers of patients, they suggested that SIRT significantly lengthens the time to progression, and also provides better tumor control, but not longer survival [34, 35]. As patients with advanced HCC (macrovascular invasion and extrahepatic disease) are ineligible for the therapies referred to above, the standard for them is treatment with systemic tyrosine kinase inhibitors such as Sorafenib and Lenvatinib or immunotherapies.

Although the use of radiotherapy is not included in the EASL, AASLD, and APASL guidelines, a growing body of evidence refers to radiotherapy as a potential tool for primary treatment or for bridging/downsizing purposes.

7.3.2 SBRT Patient Selection, Outcomes, and Comparative Studies

According to the European, American, and Asia-Pacific management guidelines for HCC, SBRT does not currently play a primary role in the treatment of HCC [1, 3, 4]. Over the years, experience has nonetheless been accumulated in retrospective and phase I–II studies, in which patients treated with SBRT were ineligible for resection and in many cases ineligible for thermic ablation or for TACE, or had an incomplete response after TACE [12, 13, 15, 19, 36–40]. Local control rates at 2 years were 78–97%, and the overall survival rate at 2 years was 47–84% (Table 7.1). SBRT has also been used as bridging or downstaging for transplantation where it provided 100% local control rates until transplantation (Table 7.2) [41–46].

Most patients treated with SBRT as the definitive treatment include patients with Barcelona Liver Cancer (BCLC) A, B, and C score, most of those with C score mainly due to the inclusion of patients with portal invasion. In the pretransplant setting, SBRT has been used with both intentions, i.e., to bridge and to down-stage the tumors until transplantation. Patients with BCLC score A, B, and D (due to Child–Pugh class C) have been treated. In one series, patients with segmental portal thrombosis were also eligible for transplant [44].

More experience with definitive SBRT has been gained in patients with Child–Pugh class A liver cirrhosis (Table 7.1). Those with Child–Pugh class B have been also treated with SBRT, but in much lower numbers (Table 7.1). A maximum of seven points has been proposed for using definitive SBRT [14, 15, 38, 47]. The reasons for Cullemborg et al. and Cardenes et al. to propose this limit lay in the finding that survival was more impaired and the risk of developing hepatic toxicity (RILD) was higher in the group with Child–Pugh > 7 points than in the group with ≤7 points [14, 47]. Similarly, Valakh et al. published the outcomes of SBRT for HCC in a group of patients with severe cirrhosis (Child–Pugh 8–11 points) who were ineligible for transplant due either to

being outside the Milan criteria or to medical contraindications [48]. The authors concluded that although SBRT—which had been delivered in a median of 35 Gy in 4–5 fractions—achieved local tumor control (91% at 6 months), progressive cirrhosis was a common cause of death. On the other hand, more experience has been accumulated by using SBRT to treat patients with more advanced cirrhosis in a pretransplant setting than in a definitive one, and thus with patients with Child–Pugh class B, or even C, liver cirrhosis.

Although there is no strict cutoff value regarding the maximum tumor size that can be treated with SBRT, a number of studies have considered which maximum diameter should apply in patient recruitment. The limits tended to range from 4 cm though 5 cm and 6 cm to <10 cm [14, 15, 19, 36, 38, 40, 47, 49–52]. Neither was there a fixed maximum number of tumors for SBRT. While patients with 1–3 tumors are often treated, many other options have been reported [14, 17, 51, 52]. One solitary tumor was requested by Takeda et al. in a phase II trial, while Kimura et al. included patients with <3 nodules, and Yeung et al., and Goodman et al. recruited patients with <5 nodules [19, 40, 49, 50]. The maximum diameter and the number of tumors that may be treated safely will in fact be limited by the volume of the normal liver, the impairment of the liver function, the target localization, and the treatment technique.

The dose–response relationship in SBRT for HCC has been investigated by the Liver Working Group of the American Association for Physics in Medicine (AAPM), and also by the Asian Liver Radiation Therapy Study Group [53, 54]. In data from 5 HCC studies (394 patients) collected by Ohri et al. on behalf of the AAPM group, local control was 93% at 1 year, 89% at 2 years, and 86% at 3 years. Within the range of schedules used in this pooled analysis (33–60 Gy, 3–5 fractions, BED 60–180 Gy_{10}), local control in these patients was not influenced by a biologically effective dose (BED) > or ≤ 100 Gy_{10}. It was not possible to analyze possible confounding factors (such as tumor size) that required patient-level data. The absence of a dose–response rela-

Table 7.1 SBRT as definitive therapy for HCC

Author/publication year	Design	Child–Pugh/BCLC	Number of patients	Dose-fractionation scheme	2 years local control %	2 years overall survival %
Andolino [12] No transplant 2011	Retrospective	A B/A–C	24 13	3 × 12–16 Gy 5 × 8 Gy	87	47
Kang [15] 2012	Phase II	A B/A–C	41 6	3 × 14–20 Gy	95	69
Bujold [13] 2013	Phase I–II	A A–C	102	6 × 4–9 Gy	87 (1 year)	34
Takeda [19] 2016	Phase II	A B/A–C	91 9	5 × 8 Gy 5 × 7 Gy	96.3	80
Gkika [37] 2017	Retrospective	A B/B–C	27 19	3–12 × 4–15 Gy	77 (1 year)	Not reported
Yeung [40] 2019	Retrospective	A B/A–C	28 3	3 × 15 Gy (65%) 5 × 9 Gy (24%)	94	74
Jang [38] 2020	Phase II	A B/A–C	64 1	3 × 15–20 Gy	97	84
Durand–Labrunie [36] 2020	Phase II	A B Unknown/A–C	88 12 1	3 × 15 Gy	95	70
Loi [39] 2020	Retrospective	A B/A–C	92 36	54 Gy[a] (30–75) in 6 (3–10) fractions	78	58

[a]Median dose

Table 7.2 SBRT as a pretransplant therapy

Author/ publication year	Design	Child–Pugh/ BCLC	Number of patients	Dose-fractionation scheme	Local control until transplant %	Median/5 years overall survival %
Facciuto [41] 2011	Retrospective	A, B/A	27	2 × 12–18 Gy 4 × 7 Gy	100 10 delisted	32 m 82 at 3 years
Katz [42] 2011	Retrospective	A B C Unknown/ A–B, D	3 8 4 3	10 × 5	100 (6 delisted)	Not reported
O'Connor [43] 2012	Retrospective	A B C/ A–B, D	7 2 1	3 × 11–18 Gy	100	Not reached 100
Mannina [44] 2017	Retrospective	A B (7)/A–C[a]	17 21	3 × 16 Gy (26%) 5 × 8 Gy (61%)	100	Not estimable 73
Sapisochin[b] [45] 2017	Retrospective	A B/A–B	36	Median 6 × 6 Gy (30–40 Gy)	100 (6 delisted)	Not reported 61
Nugent[c] 2017 (abstract)	Randomized Phase II SBRT vs. TACE	A B/A–B	SBRT 12 TACE 15	5 × 9 Gy	Equally effective	Not reported
Uemura [46] 2019	Retrospective	A B C/ A–B, D	11 9 2	Median 5 (4–6) fractions Median 45 Gy (36–50)	100 (2 delisted)	Not reported 81 at 3 years

[a]Segmental PVT
[b]Comparative study (intention-to-treat analysis) SBRT, RFA, TACE
[c]Only abstract format DOI: https://doi.org/10.1200/JCO.2017.35.4_suppl.223

tionship in this pooled analysis may be partly explained by tumor radiosensitivity and by a less viable tumor burden after other local or regional treatments. However, Kim et al. analyzed a multi-institutional retrospective cohort of 510 Asian patients diagnosed with HCC. Baseline characteristics were less favorable in the BED < 100 Gy_{10} group (Child–Pugh class B, advanced stage, median size 4 cm) than in the BED ≥ 100 Gy_{10} group. The respective rates of 2-year freedom from local progression (FFLP) were 89 vs. 69% ($p < 0.001$). After propensity-score matching, multivariate analysis identified a BED < 100 Gy as the only significant factor related to poor local control. The authors discussed that although BED ≥ 100 Gy may be favorable, underlying liver dysfunction and proximity to OAR might increase toxicity, subsequently requiring a dose reduction. In these situations, the best trade-off should be reached on the basis of a meticulous SBRT plan and rigorous quality assurance. The authors commented that institutional experience may have affected the results and that treatment selection may depend not only on clinical factors but also on demographic and socioeconomic factors, and even hospital type.

Various retrospective studies have compared SBRT and RFA outcomes. A Japanese group performed a propensity-score analysis between patients treated with RFA and with SBRT [20]. Overall survival at 3 years was comparable (69.1 vs. 70.4%), and the 3-year local recurrence rates were significantly lower for SBRT (6.4 vs. 20.2%). As for liver toxicity, the rates at which Child–Pugh scores of ≥2 deteriorated after RFA and SBRT were 10.2 and 8.2% within the 12-month period after treatment. However, regarding liver function according to liver failure death, SBRT had significantly worse outcomes (4 vs. 1 liver failure death). Regarding other grade ≥ 3 toxicities, one case of grade 5 peritonitis and one of grade 5 hemorrhagic gastric ulcers were observed in the RFA group. Other studies have also used propensity-score-weighted and propensity-score-matched analysis to evaluate the efficacy of the two treatments [55–57]. On the basis of data from the National Cancer Database regarding HCC stage I or II, Rajyaguru et al. found that 5-year overall survival was significantly better after RFA (29.8%) than after SBRT (19.3%) [56]. However, other groups published results similar to those described above. Kim et al. in a single institution study observed no significant differences in 2-year overall survival between SBRT (71.8%) and RFA (76.4%), and local control rates at 2 years that were superior for SBRT in tumors larger than 2 cm [55]. Recently, the same author published the results of a large multicenter Asian cooperation [21]. Similar to the previous study, the cumulative mortality rate at 2 years was not significantly different between SBRT and RFA while SBRT was associated with a significantly lower chance of local recurrence at 2 years (16.4 vs. 31.1%). Grade 3–4 toxicity did not differ between groups although a change in Child–Pugh score > 2 points at 3 months was more frequent in the SBRT group (11.2 vs. 4.7%; $p < 0.001$). Although overall toxicity did not differ significantly between treatment arms, 6.7% of the patients in the SBRT arm developed the radiation-induced liver disease (RILD). Wahl et al. also reported similar 2-year overall survival between groups (52.9 vs. 46.3%) and that RFA was followed by lower freedom from local progression in tumors ≥2 cm (Hazard Ratio 3.35) [57]. While Child–Pugh mean scores 12 months after treatment worsened by 0.3 after RFA and 1.2 after SBRT ($p = 0.005$), adjustment for patient and treatment factors showed that not treatment modality but an increasing number of previous treatments was associated with Child–Pugh deterioration.

In a retrospective study comparing SBRT with TACE outcomes, Sapir et al. conducted a propensity-score analysis to compare outcomes in a single-institution cohort with 1–2 tumors [58]. While 2-year local control favored SBRT (91 vs. 23%), overall survival at 2 years did not differ significantly (54.9 vs. 34.9%). Overall, more grade ≥ 3 toxicities occurred in patients after TACE than after SBRT.

Strategies combining SBRT and TACE have produced positive results. A phase II study using optional TACE followed by SBRT for solitary tumors ≤ 4 cm reported local control rates as high as 93% at 3 years and overall survival of 66.7% [19]. The Child–Pugh score worsened in 8.9% of the patients. A retrospective comparison of TACE followed by SBRT in a group of 30 patients found complete response rates that were significantly higher than those in a group of 335 patients who received TACE alone (96.3 vs. 3.3%) [59]. No patients developed liver-radiation-induced liver damage.

With regard to radiation-induced liver disease (RILD), the QUANTEC report differentiated between "classic" and "nonclassic" RILD [60]. Classic RILD involves anicteric hepatomegaly and ascites, which typically occur between 2 weeks and 3 months after therapy. It also involves an elevation of alkaline phosphatase more than twice the upper limit of normal or baseline value. Nonclassic RILD typically occurs between 1 week and 3 months after therapy, and either involves elevated liver transaminases of over 5 times the upper normal limit, or a decline in liver function (measured by a ≥2 point deterioration in the Child–Pugh score).

The development of hepatic toxicity after radiotherapy has been associated with various biological factors, such as the hepatitis virus B carrier virus and the presence and severity of liver cirrhosis [9, 61, 62]. Patients at risk for hepatitis virus B reactivation should have appropriate serum testing, and prophylactic antiretroviral therapy should be considered [63].

Radiation dose–volume effects for liver SBRT have been studied by Pan et al., and more recently by Miften et al. [60, 64]. In a study on the predictors of liver toxicity, Velec et al. observed that baseline Child–Pugh scores and higher liver doses, e.g., mean dose, dose delivered to 800 cc (D800), and effective volume (Veff), were strongly associated with an increase in Child–

Pugh score of ≥ 2 points 3 months after SBRT [65]. Mean liver dose appeared to be important to risk estimation—a finding consistent with the QUANTEC report, in which the suggested limit was <18 Gy for 6-fraction SBRT. Song et al. found that hepatic complication was predicted by a specific dose-volume parameter, i.e., liver volume receiving <18 Gy in three fractions [66]. When the total liver volume receiving 18 Gy was less than 800 cc, there was an abrupt increase in the probability that the Child–Pugh class (hepatic complication) would progress.

In the review series, common toxicity criteria (CTC) events ≥ 3 ranged approximately from 3.8 to 30% and from 6 to 27% [67, 68]. Special attention should be paid to the possible development of intestinal complications such as bowel ulceration. Some authors see this as indicating that the utmost importance of ensuring that treatment is delivered in experienced centers [68]. In approximately 10–30% of the patients treated with SBRT decline in liver function as indicated by a worsening of Child–Pugh score has been reported, and episodes of liver failure resulting in death have also been described [64, 67].

Account should be taken of the influence of liver toxicities on the prognosis of the HCC patients after SBRT. Over a 12-month period, Sanuki et al. observed a fatal hepatic failure rate of 4% [69]. Hepatic failure was significantly predicted by a Child–Pugh score of ≥ 8, grade ≥ 3 elevated transaminases, and grade ≥ 3 platelet count. Two-year overall survival rates for patients without and with hepatic toxicity (RILD) differed significantly (64.9 vs. 83.8%). Similarly, Lasley et al. observed grade 3 or 4 hepatic toxicity in 11% of Child–Pugh class A patients and 38% of Child–Pugh B class patients [70]. Overall, the risk of death was significantly higher (4.95%) in Child–Pugh class A patients with grade 3 or 4 liver toxicity than in patients without toxicity. No correlation was seen in Child–Pugh B patients, although 3 of these 8 patients underwent a liver transplant.

As an alternative to conventional bridging therapies, SBRT can be safely used as a bridge to a liver transplant [45]. Reported grade 3 toxicities range from 0 to 35% [68]. Even though the com-

parison of patients in the first 3 months after SBRT showed that their liver function was more impaired than that of patients treated with RFA or TACE, none of them had to be urgently transplanted due to further liver decompensation, and no patients in either group were delisted due to treatment toxicity [45]. Neither were their surgical complication rates higher, though in one study a modification of the initial surgical approach was needed [68].

7.3.3 SBRT Target Delineation, Treatment Planning, and Medical Physics Considerations

7.3.3.1 Target Definition and Delineation

Although the clinical target volume (CTV) in these patients often corresponds with the gross tumor volume (GTV), several groups have described the addition of a CTV margin of 3–10 mm [12, 13, 15, 17, 36, 52, 71]. Usually, the GTV (the contrast-enhanced tumor) is delineated on the hepatic arterial phase on the expiration breath-hold-planning contrast-enhanced (dual or multiphase) CT, although a contrast-enhanced 4D-CT can also be used [72, 73]. Whenever possible, target definition may be supported by additional magnetic resonance imaging (MRI) registered to the radiotherapy planning CT [74].

Abdominal OAR should be delineated. It is recommended that the delineation process is approached in a systematic fashion. Guidelines such as the Radiation Therapy Oncology Group (RTOG) guideline can be very helpful for radiation oncologists and technicians [75]. Parallel OARs in the vicinity of the target—such as the liver and kidneys, for which the mean dose (Dmean) constraints apply in treatment planning—must be delineated completely. But for serial OAR—such as the spinal cord, esophagus, duodenum and bowel, for which the maximum dose (Dmax) or the near-maximum (i.e., D2%) constraints apply in treatment planning—partial delineation near the high dose volume may suffice. The revision of the contours by a diagnostic abdominal radiologist may be both useful and educational.

7.3.3.2 Breathing Motion

During treatment planning and treatment delivery, breathing-motion management—i.e., voluntary breath-hold, active breath-hold, gating, or tracking—is highly recommended. If breathing-motion management is not feasible, an internal target volume (ITV) shall be defined as the union of GTV delineations on all breathing phases of a 4D-CT scan.

When defining expansion margins from the CTV (or ITV) to the planning target volume (PTV), full account must be taken of residual breathing-motion uncertainty and other treatment uncertainties, such as patient setup, deformations, and anatomical variation.

7.3.3.3 Treatment Planning

The use of intensity-modulated radiotherapy (IMRT) or equivalently an arc technique, and inverse optimization is highly recommended in treatment planning. Due to underlying disease (such as hepatitis or cirrhosis), functional healthy-liver tissue is a critical organ at risk in many HCC patients. Dose to the healthy liver (liver minus GTV) shall be evaluated in terms of a Dmean constraint and/or a volumetric constraint. Evaluation of the healthy-liver normal tissue complication probability (NTCP) on the basis of the model by Dawson et al. may be valuable [76]. For HCC with underlying Child–Pugh grade A liver cirrhosis treated in six fractions, our center accepts an NCTP value of $\leq$5% together with a Dmean liver constraint of <18 Gy and a volumetric constraint of D800 cc < 23.4 Gy (Table 7.3). Standard dosimetric constraints must be achieved for the abovementioned parallel and serial OARs. Different constraint parameters have been reported in the literature, each of which may represent a very valid choice [12–15, 18, 20, 36].

7.3.3.4 Treatment Unit

The periodic independent verification of machine output (cGy/monitor unit) by an independent standard laboratory is highly recommended, as is

Table 7.3 Planning organs at risk constraints

Organ at risk	Hard constraint
Healthy liver	NTCP liver-GTV $\leq$ 5% [76] >800 ml liver-GTV < 23.4 Gy [66] Mean liver-GTV dose < 18 Gy [60]
Stomach	Max point dose < 39 Gy and Volume receiving $\geq$ 30 Gy should be $\leq$5 cc [77]
Duodenum/Small and large bowel	Max point dose < 39 Gy [77]
Esophagus	Max point dose $\leq$ 36 Gy [78]
Spinal cord	Max point dose < 24 Gy [79]
Kidney	2/3 right kidney < 19.2 Gy [79]

Footnote: Constraints have been converted in six fractions using the EQD2 formula with $\alpha/\beta = 3$ for all organs except for the spinal cord ($\alpha/\beta = 2$)
Treatment delivered in six fractions of 8–9 Gy

periodic pretreatment dosimetric 2D or 3D verification of clinical treatment plans for individual patients.

7.4   Discussion

In this chapter, we have reviewed the most important considerations for a radiation oncologist to bear in mind when starting an HCC program. The information presented here is multidisciplinary, as only multidisciplinarity will make it possible to develop an SBRT program for this patient group. Due to their underlying liver cirrhosis, it is important to note that these patients constitute a fragile population who need special care, whatever the choice of treatment. Decisions on the most suitable treatment for an individual patient will be tailored on the basis not only of the tumor size, number, or extension but also of the liver function.

HCC management guidelines in Europe, North America, and Asia-Pacific allocate no official role to SBRT [1, 3, 4]. The reason for this lies mainly in the absence of any randomized trials comparing SBRT and other treatment techniques. However, phase I–II trials have reported high rates of local control with acceptable toxicity [12, 13, 15, 19, 36–40]. To limit toxicity, patient selection is important. Some groups proposed that treatment with SBRT as a definitive option should be limited to patients with Child–Pugh A and B7 points [14, 15, 38, 47]. After rigorous consideration of patient safety, it may be possible to extend these criteria in pretransplant settings or in trials. As SBRT has emerged favorably from propensity analyses comparing it with RFA and TACE [20, 21, 57, 58], randomized trials are now needed to compare SBRT with these treatment modalities. Their outcomes will help to define the role of SBRT in the management of HCC (NCT 02470533, NCT 01730937, NCT 02323360, NCT 02182687).

Due to the physical properties of protons, the dose delivered in the normal liver with protons may be reduced when compared with a treatment delivered with photons. To treat patients with large or multiple tumors and impaired liver function due to liver cirrhosis, proton therapy may be more favorable than photons [80, 81]. This technique may help to safely extend the indications of SBRT to patients with more and/or larger lesions. In a recent phase III randomized non-inferiority trial that compared proton therapy and RFA in patients with ≤ 2 tumors sized <3 cm, 2-year local progression-free survival in the intention-to-treat groups was 92.8% for proton therapy and 83.2% for RFA [22]. Such a difference of 9.6% points meets the criteria for statistical non-inferiority. No grade 4 toxicity or mortality were reported. The most common adverse events were radiation pneumonitis and a decrease leukocyte count for proton therapy and an increase of alanine aminotransferase levels and abdominal pain for RFA.

To start an SBRT program for HCC, one needs not only to choose a treatment protocol but also to consider the characteristics of the population in the region where the treatment will be given [53]. Ethnicity may play a role in the behavior of HCC and also in the development of toxicity [82, 83].

To deliver safe, high-quality treatment, the greatest possible importance should be attached to ensuring quality assurance in all the steps involved in SBRT.

SBRT consumes time and resources and requires inputs from a whole team of profession-als within and outside the radiotherapy department. However, it is also an extremely rewarding technique: definitive SBRT helps patients to achieve local tumor control safely, and bridging SBRT helps to bring them safely to the time of transplant.Conflict of InterestNo conflict of interests to declare. This statement applies to all the authors.

References

1. European Association for the Study of the Liver. EASL Clinical Practice Guidelines: management of hepatocellular carcinoma. J Hepatol. 2018;69(1):182–236.
2. Schuppan D, Afdhal NH. Liver cirrhosis. Lancet. 2008;371(9615):838–51.
3. Omata M, Cheng AL, Kokudo N, Kudo M, Lee JM, Jia J, et al. Asia-Pacific clinical practice guidelines on the management of hepatocellular carcinoma: a 2017 update. Hepatol Int. 2017;11(4):317–70.
4. Marrero JA, Kulik LM, Sirlin CB, Zhu AX, Finn RS, Abecassis MM, et al. Diagnosis, staging, and management of hepatocellular carcinoma: 2018 practice guidance by the American Association for the Study of Liver Diseases. Hepatology. 2018;68(2):723–50.
5. Borgelt BB, Gelber R, Brady LW, Griffin T, Hendrickson FR. The palliation of hepatic metastases: results of the Radiation Therapy Oncology Group pilot study. Int J Radiat Oncol Biol Phys. 1981;7(5):587–91.
6. Emami B, Lyman J, Brown A, Coia L, Goitein M, Munzenrider JE, et al. Tolerance of normal tissue to therapeutic irradiation. Int J Radiat Oncol Biol Phys. 1991;21(1):109–22.
7. Lax I, Blomgren H, Naslund I, Svanstrom R. Stereotactic radiotherapy of malignancies in the abdomen. Methodological aspects. Acta Oncol. 1994;33(6):677–83.
8. McGinn CJ, Ten Haken RK, Ensminger WD, Walker S, Wang S, Lawrence TS. Treatment of intrahepatic cancers with radiation doses based on a normal tissue complication probability model. J Clin Oncol. 1998;16(6):2246–52.
9. Dawson LA, Normolle D, Balter JM, McGinn CJ, Lawrence TS, Ten Haken RK. Analysis of radiation-induced liver disease using the Lyman NTCP model. Int J Radiat Oncol Biol Phys. 2002;53(4):810–21.
10. Herfarth KK, Debus J, Lohr F, Bahner ML, Rhein B, Fritz P, et al. Stereotactic single-dose radiation therapy of liver tumors: results of a phase I/II trial. J Clin Oncol. 2001;19(1):164–70.
11. Wulf J, Hadinger U, Oppitz U, Thiele W, Ness-Dourdoumas R, Flentje M. Stereotactic radiotherapy of targets in the lung and liver. Strahlenther Onkol. 2001;177(12):645–55.

12. Andolino DL, Johnson CS, Maluccio M, Kwo P, Tector AJ, Zook J, et al. Stereotactic body radiotherapy for primary hepatocellular carcinoma. Int J Radiat Oncol Biol Phys. 2011;81(4):e447–53.

13. Bujold A, Massey CA, Kim JJ, Brierley J, Cho C, Wong RK, et al. Sequential phase I and II trials of stereotactic body radiotherapy for locally advanced hepatocellular carcinoma. J Clin Oncol. 2013;31(13):1631–9.

14. Cardenes HR, Price TR, Perkins SM, Maluccio M, Kwo P, Breen TE, et al. Phase I feasibility trial of stereotactic body radiation therapy for primary hepatocellular carcinoma. Clin Transl Oncol. 2010;12(3):218–25.

15. Kang JK, Kim MS, Cho CK, Yang KM, Yoo HJ, Kim JH, et al. Stereotactic body radiation therapy for inoperable hepatocellular carcinoma as a local salvage treatment after incomplete transarterial chemoembolization. Cancer. 2012;118(21):5424–31.

16. Louis C, Dewas S, Mirabel X, Lacornerie T, Adenis A, Bonodeau F, et al. Stereotactic radiotherapy of hepatocellular carcinoma: preliminary results. Technol Cancer Res Treat. 2010;9(5):479–87.

17. Mendez Romero A, Wunderink W, Hussain SM, De Pooter JA, Heijmen BJ, Nowak PC, et al. Stereotactic body radiation therapy for primary and metastatic liver tumors: a single institution phase i-ii study. Acta Oncol. 2006;45(7):831–7.

18. Sanuki N, Takeda A, Oku Y, Mizuno T, Aoki Y, Eriguchi T, et al. Stereotactic body radiotherapy for small hepatocellular carcinoma: a retrospective outcome analysis in 185 patients. Acta Oncol. 2014;53(3):399–404.

19. Takeda A, Sanuki N, Tsurugai Y, Iwabuchi S, Matsunaga K, Ebinuma H, et al. Phase 2 study of stereotactic body radiotherapy and optional transarterial chemoembolization for solitary hepatocellular carcinoma not amenable to resection and radiofrequency ablation. Cancer. 2016;122(13):2041–9.

20. Hara K, Takeda A, Tsurugai Y, Saigusa Y, Sanuki N, Eriguchi T, et al. Radiotherapy for hepatocellular carcinoma results in comparable survival to radiofrequency ablation: a propensity score analysis. Hepatology. 2019;69(6):2533–45.

21. Kim N, Cheng J, Jung I, Liang J, Shih YL, Huang WY, et al. Stereotactic body radiation therapy vs. radiofrequency ablation in Asian patients with hepatocellular carcinoma. J Hepatol. 2020;73(1):121–9.

22. Kim TH, Koh YH, Kim BH, Kim MJ, Lee JH, Park B, et al. Proton beam radiotherapy vs. radiofrequency ablation for recurrent hepatocellular carcinoma: a randomized phase III trial. J Hepatol. 2020;74(3):603–12.

23. Global Burden of Disease Liver Cancer Collaboration, Akinyemiju T, Abera S, Ahmed M, Alam N, Alemayohu MA, et al. The burden of primary liver cancer and underlying etiologies from 1990 to 2015 at the global, regional, and national level: results from the global burden of disease study 2015. JAMA Oncol. 2017;3(12):1683–91.

24. Bruix J, Sherman M, American Association for the Study of Liver Diseases. Management of hepatocellular carcinoma: an update. Hepatology. 2011;53(3):1020–2.

25. Balakrishnan M, El-Serag HB. Editorial: NAFLD-related hepatocellular carcinoma—increasing or not? With or without cirrhosis? Aliment Pharmacol Ther. 2018;47(3):437–8.

26. White DL, Kanwal F, El-Serag HB. Association between nonalcoholic fatty liver disease and risk for hepatocellular cancer, based on systematic review. Clin Gastroenterol Hepatol. 2012;10(12):1342–59.e2.

27. Kulik L, El-Serag HB. Epidemiology and management of hepatocellular carcinoma. Gastroenterology. 2019;156(2):477–91.e1.

28. Ross RK, Yuan JM, Yu MC, Wogan GN, Qian GS, Tu JT, et al. Urinary aflatoxin biomarkers and risk of hepatocellular carcinoma. Lancet. 1992;339(8799):943–6.

29. Choo SP, Tan WL, Goh BKP, Tai WM, Zhu AX. Comparison of hepatocellular carcinoma in Eastern versus Western populations. Cancer. 2016;122(22):3430–46.

30. Lurje I, Czigany Z, Bednarsch J, Roderburg C, Isfort P, Neumann UP, et al. Treatment strategies for hepatocellular carcinoma (-) a multidisciplinary approach. Int J Mol Sci. 2019;20(6):1465.

31. Montalti R, Mimmo A, Rompianesi G, Di Gregorio C, Serra V, Cautero N, et al. Absence of viable HCC in the native liver is an independent protective factor of tumor recurrence after liver transplantation. Transplantation. 2014;97(2):220–6.

32. Llovet JM, Real MI, Montana X, Planas R, Coll S, Aponte J, et al. Arterial embolisation or chemoembolisation versus symptomatic treatment in patients with unresectable hepatocellular carcinoma: a randomised controlled trial. Lancet. 2002;359(9319):1734–9.

33. Lo CM, Ngan H, Tso WK, Liu CL, Lam CM, Poon RT, et al. Randomized controlled trial of transarterial lipiodol chemoembolization for unresectable hepatocellular carcinoma. Hepatology. 2002;35(5):1164–71.

34. Salem R, Gordon AC, Mouli S, Hickey R, Kallini J, Gabr A, et al. Y90 radioembolization significantly prolongs time to progression compared with chemoembolization in patients with hepatocellular carcinoma. Gastroenterology. 2016;151(6):1155–63.e2.

35. Salem R, Lewandowski RJ, Kulik L, Wang E, Riaz A, Ryu RK, et al. Radioembolization results in longer time-to-progression and reduced toxicity compared with chemoembolization in patients with hepatocellular carcinoma. Gastroenterology. 2011;140(2):497–507.e2.

36. Durand-Labrunie J, Baumann AS, Ayav A, Laurent V, Boleslawski E, Cattan S, et al. Curative irradiation treatment of hepatocellular carcinoma: a multicenter phase 2 trial. Int J Radiat Oncol Biol Phys. 2020;107(1):116–25.

37. Gkika E, Schultheiss M, Bettinger D, Maruschke L, Neeff HP, Schulenburg M, et al. Excellent local control and tolerance profile after stereotactic body radio-

therapy of advanced hepatocellular carcinoma. Radiat Oncol. 2017;12(1):116.

38. Jang WI, Bae SH, Kim MS, Han CJ, Park SC, Kim SB, et al. A phase 2 multicenter study of stereotactic body radiotherapy for hepatocellular carcinoma: safety and efficacy. Cancer. 2020;126(2):363–72.

39. Loi M, Comito T, Franzese C, Dominici L, Lo Faro L, Clerici E, et al. Stereotactic body radiotherapy in hepatocellular carcinoma: patient selection and predictors of outcome and toxicity. J Cancer Res Clin Oncol. 2020;147(3):927–36.

40. Yeung R, Beaton L, Rackley T, Weber B, Hamm J, Lee R, et al. Stereotactic body radiotherapy for small unresectable hepatocellular carcinomas. Clin Oncol (R Coll Radiol). 2019;31(6):365–73.

41. Facciuto ME, Singh MK, Rochon C, Sharma J, Gimenez C, Katta U, et al. Stereotactic body radiation therapy in hepatocellular carcinoma and cirrhosis: evaluation of radiological and pathological response. J Surg Oncol. 2012;105(7):692–8.

42. Katz AW, Chawla S, Qu Z, Kashyap R, Milano MT, Hezel AF. Stereotactic hypofractionated radiation therapy as a bridge to transplantation for hepatocellular carcinoma: clinical outcome and pathologic correlation. Int J Radiat Oncol Biol Phys. 2012;83(3):895–900.

43. O'Connor JK, Trotter J, Davis GL, Dempster J, Klintmalm GB, Goldstein RM. Long-term outcomes of stereotactic body radiation therapy in the treatment of hepatocellular cancer as a bridge to transplantation. Liver Transpl. 2012;18(8):949–54.

44. Mannina EM, Cardenes HR, Lasley FD, Goodman B, Zook J, Althouse S, et al. Role of stereotactic body radiation therapy before orthotopic liver transplantation: retrospective evaluation of pathologic response and outcomes. Int J Radiat Oncol Biol Phys. 2017;97(5):931–8.

45. Sapisochin G, Barry A, Doherty M, Fischer S, Goldaracena N, Rosales R, et al. Stereotactic body radiotherapy vs. TACE or RFA as a bridge to transplant in patients with hepatocellular carcinoma. An intention-to-treat analysis. J Hepatol. 2017;67(1):92–9.

46. Uemura T, Kirichenko A, Bunker M, Vincent M, Machado L, Thai N. Stereotactic body radiation therapy: a new strategy for loco-regional treatment for hepatocellular carcinoma while awaiting liver transplantation. World J Surg. 2019;43(3):886–93.

47. Culleton S, Jiang H, Haddad CR, Kim J, Brierley J, Brade A, et al. Outcomes following definitive stereotactic body radiotherapy for patients with Child-Pugh B or C hepatocellular carcinoma. Radiother Oncol. 2014;111(3):412–7.

48. Valakh V, Gresswell S, Kirichenko A. Outcomes of stereotactic body radiotherapy for hepatocellular carcinoma with severe cirrhosis and ineligibility for transplant. Anticancer Res. 2018;38(12):6815–20.

49. Goodman KA, Wiegner EA, Maturen KE, Zhang Z, Mo Q, Yang G, et al. Dose-escalation study of single-fraction stereotactic body radiotherapy for liver malignancies. Int J Radiat Oncol Biol Phys. 2010;78(2):486–93.

50. Kimura T, Aikata H, Takahashi S, Takahashi I, Nishibuchi I, Doi Y, et al. Stereotactic body radiotherapy for patients with small hepatocellular carcinoma ineligible for resection or ablation therapies. Hepatol Res. 2015;45(4):378–86.

51. Park JH, Yoon SM, Lim YS, Kim SY, Shim JH, Kim KM, et al. Two-week schedule of hypofractionated radiotherapy as a local salvage treatment for small hepatocellular carcinoma. J Gastroenterol Hepatol. 2013;28(10):1638–42.

52. Scorsetti M, Comito T, Cozzi L, Clerici E, Tozzi A, Franzese C, et al. The challenge of inoperable hepatocellular carcinoma (HCC): results of a single-institutional experience on stereotactic body radiation therapy (SBRT). J Cancer Res Clin Oncol. 2015;141(7):1301–9.

53. Kim N, Cheng J, Huang WY, Kimura T, Zeng ZC, Lee VHF, et al. Dose-response relationship in stereotactic body radiation therapy for hepatocellular carcinoma: a pooled analysis of an Asian liver radiation therapy group study. Int J Radiat Oncol Biol Phys. 2020;109(2):464–73.

54. Ohri N, Tome WA, Mendez Romero A, Miften M, Ten Haken RK, Dawson LA, et al. Local control after stereotactic body radiation therapy for liver tumors. Int J Radiat Oncol Biol Phys. 2018; https://doi.org/10.1016/j.ijrobp.2017.12.288.

55. Kim N, Kim HJ, Won JY, Kim DY, Han KH, Jung I, et al. Retrospective analysis of stereotactic body radiation therapy efficacy over radiofrequency ablation for hepatocellular carcinoma. Radiother Oncol. 2019;131:81–7.

56. Rajyaguru DJ, Borgert AJ, Smith AL, Thomes RM, Conway PD, Halfdanarson TR, et al. Radiofrequency ablation versus stereotactic body radiotherapy for localized hepatocellular carcinoma in nonsurgically managed patients: analysis of the national cancer database. J Clin Oncol. 2018;36(6):600–8.

57. Wahl DR, Stenmark MH, Tao Y, Pollom EL, Caoili EM, Lawrence TS, et al. Outcomes after stereotactic body radiotherapy or radiofrequency ablation for hepatocellular carcinoma. J Clin Oncol. 2016;34(5):452–9.

58. Sapir E, Tao Y, Schipper MJ, Bazzi L, Novelli PM, Devlin P, et al. Stereotactic body radiation therapy as an alternative to transarterial chemoembolization for hepatocellular carcinoma. Int J Radiat Oncol Biol Phys. 2018;100(1):122–30.

59. Honda Y, Kimura T, Aikata H, Kobayashi T, Fukuhara T, Masaki K, et al. Stereotactic body radiation therapy combined with transcatheter arterial chemoembolization for small hepatocellular carcinoma. J Gastroenterol Hepatol. 2013;28(3):530–6.

60. Pan CC, Kavanagh BD, Dawson LA, Li XA, Das SK, Miften M, et al. Radiation-associated liver injury. Int J Radiat Oncol Biol Phys. 2010;76(3 Suppl):S94–100.

61. Cheng JC, Wu JK, Lee PC, Liu HS, Jian JJ, Lin YM, et al. Biologic susceptibility of hepatocellular carci-

noma patients treated with radiotherapy to radiation-induced liver disease. Int J Radiat Oncol Biol Phys. 2004;60(5):1502–9.

62. Liang SX, Zhu XD, Xu ZY, Zhu J, Zhao JD, Lu HJ, et al. Radiation-induced liver disease in three-dimensional conformal radiation therapy for primary liver carcinoma: the risk factors and hepatic radiation tolerance. Int J Radiat Oncol Biol Phys. 2006;65(2):426–34.

63. Jang JW, Kwon JH, You CR, Kim JD, Woo HY, Bae SH, et al. Risk of HBV reactivation according to viral status and treatment intensity in patients with hepatocellular carcinoma. Antivir Ther. 2011;16(7):969–77.

64. Miften M, Vinogradskiy Y, Moiseenko V, Grimm J, Yorke E, Jackson A, et al. Radiation dose-volume effects for liver SBRT. Int J Radiat Oncol Biol Phys. 2018; https://doi.org/10.1016/j.ijrobp.2017.12.290.

65. Velec M, Haddad CR, Craig T, Wang L, Lindsay P, Brierley J, et al. Predictors of liver toxicity following stereotactic body radiation therapy for hepatocellular carcinoma. Int J Radiat Oncol Biol Phys. 2017;97(5):939–46.

66. Son SH, Choi BO, Ryu MR, Kang YN, Jang JS, Bae SH, et al. Stereotactic body radiotherapy for patients with unresectable primary hepatocellular carcinoma: dose-volumetric parameters predicting the hepatic complication. Int J Radiat Oncol Biol Phys. 2010;78(4):1073–80.

67. Mendez Romero A, de Man RA. Stereotactic body radiation therapy for primary and metastatic liver tumors: from technological evolution to improved patient care. Best Pract Res Clin Gastroenterol. 2016;30(4):603–16.

68. Xu MJ, Feng M. Radiation therapy in HCC: what data exist and what data do we need to incorporate into guidelines? Semin Liver Dis. 2019;39(1):43–52.

69. Sanuki N, Takeda A, Oku Y, Eriguchi T, Nishimura S, Aoki Y, et al. Influence of liver toxicities on prognosis after stereotactic body radiation therapy for hepatocellular carcinoma. Hepatol Res. 2015;45(5):540–7.

70. Lasley FD, Mannina EM, Johnson CS, Perkins SM, Althouse S, Maluccio M, et al. Treatment variables related to liver toxicity in patients with hepatocellular carcinoma, Child-Pugh class A and B enrolled in a phase 1-2 trial of stereotactic body radiation therapy. Pract Radiat Oncol. 2015;5(5):e443–e9.

71. Choi SH, Seong J. Stereotactic body radiotherapy: does it have a role in management of hepatocellular carcinoma? Yonsei Med J. 2018;59(8):912–22.

72. Beddar AS, Briere TM, Balter P, Pan T, Tolani N, Ng C, et al. 4D-CT imaging with synchronized intravenous contrast injection to improve delineation of liver tumors for treatment planning. Radiother Oncol. 2008;87(3):445–8.

73. Jensen NK, Mulder D, Lock M, Fisher B, Zener R, Beech B, et al. Dynamic contrast enhanced CT aiding gross tumor volume delineation of liver tumors: an interobserver variability study. Radiother Oncol. 2014;111(1):153–7.

74. Roberts LR, Sirlin CB, Zaiem F, Almasri J, Prokop LJ, Heimbach JK, et al. Imaging for the diagnosis of hepatocellular carcinoma: a systematic review and meta-analysis. Hepatology. 2018;67(1):401–21.

75. Jabbour SK, Hashem SA, Bosch W, Kim TK, Finkelstein SE, Anderson BM, et al. Upper abdominal normal organ contouring guidelines and atlas: a Radiation Therapy Oncology Group consensus. Pract Radiat Oncol. 2014;4(2):82–9.

76. Dawson LA, Eccles C, Craig T. Individualized image guided iso-NTCP based liver cancer SBRT. Acta Oncol. 2006;45(7):856–64.

77. Kavanagh BD, Pan CC, Dawson LA, Das SK, Li XA, Ten Haken RK, et al. Radiation dose-volume effects in the stomach and small bowel. Int J Radiat Oncol Biol Phys. 2010;76(3 Suppl):S101–7.

78. Kong FM, Ritter T, Quint DJ, Senan S, Gaspar LE, Komaki RU, et al. Consideration of dose limits for organs at risk of thoracic radiotherapy: atlas for lung, proximal bronchial tree, esophagus, spinal cord, ribs, and brachial plexus. Int J Radiat Oncol Biol Phys. 2011;81(5):1442–57.

79. Schefter TE, Kavanagh BD, Timmerman RD, Cardenes HR, Baron A, Gaspar LE. A phase I trial of stereotactic body radiation therapy (SBRT) for liver metastases. Int J Radiat Oncol Biol Phys. 2005;62(5):1371–8.

80. Hong TS, Wo JY, Yeap BY, Ben-Josef E, McDonnell EI, Blaszkowsky LS, et al. Multi-institutional phase II study of high-dose hypofractionated proton beam therapy in patients with localized, unresectable hepatocellular carcinoma and intrahepatic cholangiocarcinoma. J Clin Oncol. 2016;34(5):460–8.

81. Sanford NN, Pursley J, Noe B, Yeap BY, Goyal L, Clark JW, et al. Protons versus photons for unresectable hepatocellular carcinoma: liver decompensation and overall survival. Int J Radiat Oncol Biol Phys. 2019;105(1):64–72.

82. Chin PL, Chu DZ, Clarke KG, Odom-Maryon T, Yen Y, Wagman LD. Ethnic differences in the behavior of hepatocellular carcinoma. Cancer. 1999;85(9):1931–6.

83. Xu ZY, Liang SX, Zhu J, Zhu XD, Zhao JD, Lu HJ, et al. Prediction of radiation-induced liver disease by Lyman normal-tissue complication probability model in three-dimensional conformal radiation therapy for primary liver carcinoma. Int J Radiat Oncol Biol Phys. 2006;65(1):189–95.

Image-Guided Radiotherapy

8

Pablo Munoz-Schuffenegger, Teo Stanescu,
and Laura A. Dawson

Abstract

The role of radiation therapy (RT) in the treatment of liver malignancies has historically been low, in part due to challenges in delivering ablative doses of RT safely while respecting the radiation dose limits of numerous normal tissues in the upper abdomen, including the liver itself. Challenges to the routine use of RT to treat hepatic malignancies include the low whole liver tolerance to RT and the proximity of liver tumors to other organs at risk (OAR), such as the stomach and bowel. Since the liver moves with breathing and its mean position relative to the vertebral bodies changes daily, delivering highly conformal RT can be challenging.

Advances in imaging, RT planning, and delivery have made it possible for RT to be used to treat liver cancers effectively and safely. Image-guided radiation therapy (IGRT) at the time of RT delivery is a crucial component of the RT process. IGRT accounts for baseline shifts and reduces the impact of liver motion, improving precision and accuracy of RT delivery, reducing the risk of toxicity while improving the chance of tumor control. As IGRT technological solutions and image quality continue to improve, the opportunity for adapting to change that occurs at the treatment unit between fractions and during RT delivery becomes more feasible. MR-guided RT helps in this regard due to the improved ability to visualize liver tumors directly and an increased ability to identify and avoid irradiation to adjacent OAR.

Novel IGRT systems will continue to evolve, with next-generation IGRT solutions becoming more automated and efficient, potentially allowing higher throughput, more generalized utilization, new RT paradigms to be studied (such as dose accumulation and dose painting), and more liver cancer patients to be effectively and safely irradiated.

P. Munoz-Schuffenegger
Radiation Oncology Unit, Department of
Hematology – Oncology, Pontificia Universidad
Catolica de Chile, Santiago, Chile

T. Stanescu · L. A. Dawson (✉)
Radiation Medicine Program, Princess Margaret
Cancer Centre, University Health Network,
Toronto, ON, Canada

Department of Radiation Oncology, University of
Toronto, Toronto, ON, Canada
e-mail: Laura.Dawson@rmp.uhn.ca

Keywords

Image-guided radiation therapy · IGRT ·
Cone-beam CT · MR-guided radiation
therapy · Motion management ·
Hepatocellular carcinoma

8.1   Introduction

Primary liver cancer and liver metastases from other malignancies are responsible for a substantial proportion of cancer morbidity and mortality worldwide. Although advances in systemic therapy in the past decades have led to improved survival for many cancer patients, the benefits have been modest in patients with primary liver cancer such as hepatocellular carcinoma (HCC) or intrahepatic cholangiocarcinoma (IHC), and a multidisciplinary approach is likely to lead to larger benefit than with one modality of treatment. The role of radiation therapy (RT) in the treatment of primary liver malignancies has historically been low, in part due to challenges in delivering ablative doses of RT safely while respecting the radiation dose limits of numerous normal tissues in the upper abdomen, including the liver itself, which often has a reduced capacity due to underlying cirrhosis. There has been more rapid adoption of RT for the treatment of liver (and other oligo) metastases with the advent of stereotactic body radiation therapy (SBRT) with recent randomized phase II data demonstrating a benefit of SBRT for patients with one to three sites of metastases in progression-free survival and survival, compared to best supportive care alone [1, 2]. Although most randomized studies to date have been heterogeneous and/or small, larger phase III studies are ongoing and expected to confirm the promising outcomes described in earlier studies. As more patients with liver metastases are treated with SBRT, it is crucial to ensure that the risk of acute and long-term toxicity is kept to a minimum.

Challenges to the routine use of RT to treat hepatic malignancies include the low whole liver tolerance to RT and the proximity of liver tumors to other dose-limiting normal tissues including the stomach and bowel. RT needs to be delivered conformally around liver tumors, sparing enough liver volume and respecting the RT tolerance limits of all adjacent normal tissues. Also, as the liver moves with breathing and its mean position relative to the vertebral bodies changes on a day-to-day basis, delivering highly conformal RT can be challenging.

Despite these previously mentioned challenges, advances in imaging have been a backbone to advances in RT planning and delivery that have made it possible for RT to be used to treat liver cancers safely. Image-guided radiation therapy (IGRT) at the time of RT delivery can account for baseline shifts and motion in the liver, and improve precision and accuracy of RT delivery, reducing the risk of toxicity while improving the chance of tumor control. Nonetheless, the safe application of IGRT technology is not limited to the operation of the treatment unit; it extends back to the treatment planning process (including image acquisition) where the treatment plans are developed under the assumption that high IGRT performance will be present at the time of treatment, emphasizing the need for strong coordination between the planning process and the image guidance activities at the treatment unit [3].

The purpose of this chapter is to review the current status of IGRT options for the treatment of liver cancers and to highlight challenges and potential solutions for the future for this clinical scenario.

8.2   Imaging for Radiation Treatment Planning

As the imaging guidance strategy used at the time of RT delivery needs to consider liver motion due to breathing and the treatment planning strategy, imaging used for RT planning and breathing motion management will be described briefly in addition to the image guidance strategy used at the time of delivery (i.e., IGRT).

8.2.1   Simulation

The first step in the treatment planning process is to obtain high-quality computed tomography (CT) images of the patient in the treatment position. The planning CT image acquisition parameters, including image resolution and intravenous (IV) contrast, must be optimized to visualize the tumor and normal tissues of interest. The optimal phase of contrast for tumor enhancement depends on the tumor type (e.g., primary liver cancer or metastases). Multiphasic IV CT is particularly important in primary hepatic malignancies. Magnetic resonance imaging (MRI) is also useful in identifying and characterizing liver malignancies and may be done in addition to CT simulation to aid in gross tumor volume (GTV) delineation. Methods commonly employed to consider motion at the time of planning include obtaining the image during repeat breath holds (exhale or inhale) or obtaining respiration correlated CT (4DCT). Acquiring a full multiphasic CT using 4DCT is challenging. However, techniques for 4DCT simulation with synchronized contrast injection in liver SBRT patients have been previously described [4]. A practical solution is to obtain breath hold multiphasic imaging, then follow with a 4DCT that may acquire imaging during the lengthier delayed phase of imaging.

8.2.2 Defining Treatment Volumes

Once the simulation images have been obtained, treatment planning volumes must be defined, as well as delineation of organs at risk (OAR). The GTV is usually defined using IV contrast-enhanced CT imaging; the optimal phase for image acquisition post-IV depends on the disease type, with an arterial image (after 20–30 s) typically showing enhancement for HCC and a venous image (delayed, after 50–70 s) demonstrating liver metastases best. HCC demonstrates washout in venous and delayed phases of imaging. MRI (with and without IV contrast) is helpful for GTV definition, particularly in HCC patients [5]. Given the variability in imaging interpretation, radiation oncologists are encouraged to consult with a diagnostic hepatobiliary radiologist to aid in GTV definition, especially for rapidly changing tumors or to query new findings on the simulation scans relative to prior diagnostic imaging. In a study by Hong et al. [6], in a group of experts, excellent agreement was seen in contouring total GTV; however, there was important heterogeneity in the defini-

tion of portal vein thrombus that may impact treatment planning, especially if differential dosing is contemplated.

8.2.3 Quantification of Motion

The internal treatment volume (ITV) encompassing internal organ motion (e.g., breathing motion) and the setup uncertainty expected at treatment delivery need to be considered in the determination of fixed or patient-specific planning treatment volume (PTV) margins. There is a large interpatient variation in respiratory motion, in which the superior-inferior direction tends to exhibit the largest motion, ranging from 5 to 40 mm [7]. The ITV should be quantified by measuring the respiratory motion for patients treated while free breathing or with abdominal compression.

The motion of either the tumor itself, or a surrogate such as the liver, or inserted fiducial markers, can be measured using several methods:

- Fluoroscopy (from a simulation scan or at the treatment unit) provides real-time imaging of the diaphragm and lung interface, which can be used as a surrogate of liver tumor motion in the superior-inferior direction [8]; left-right (LR) and anterior-posterior (AP) motions, however, are not discernable.
- 4DCT provides multiphase 3D image sets which can be used to measure motion in all directions, as well as hysteresis. Using 4DCT for calculating tumor specific motion may be challenging because tumors in the liver are difficult to see without IV contrast. The feasibility of incorporating IV contrast to delineate the tumor edges for all CT phases has been described [4, 9]. This is the most common and reliable strategy to measure breathing motion. Note, a 4DCT is acquired in a short snapshot of time and may not represent changes in motion observed during the full course of RT especially if the patient setup is not achieved consistently (with/without immobilization devices).

- MRI imaging can provide tumor visualization even in the absence of contrast. Cine MRI imaging can be used to measure tumor-specific motion using 2D temporal images in multiple planes (e.g., coronal and sagittal) [10, 11]. Although the temporal resolution is better than 4DCT out of plane motion can compromise the assessment of the true tumor motion. More advanced 4D MRI techniques can also be used for the full target motion assessment; however, they are not widely available on the clinical MR scanners.

8.3   Motion Management

For patients with large breathing excursions, several options are available to manage motion and reduce the size of the planning treatment volume (PTV) margins, and hence, reduce the amount of irradiated normal tissue. The simplest strategy is to apply a patient-specific PTV margin according to each patient's breathing motion. Other methods include reducing or eliminating tumor motion, incorporating this motion directly into the treatment delivery process, or accounting for it at the time of treatment planning.

Motion Reduction Abdominal compression (AC) can be used to reduce respiratory liver motion in patients undergoing liver SBRT. Eccles et al. [12] compared liver motion with and without AC in 60 patients treated as part of a clinical trial; the mean tumor motion without AC was 11.7 mm (range 4.8–23.3 mm) in the craniocaudal (CC) direction and was reduced down to 9.4 mm (range 1.6–23.4 mm) with abdominal compression. Tumor motion was significantly reduced in both CC and AP directions in 52% of the patients and in a single direction (CC or AP) in 90% of the patients [12]. Another strategy to reduce motion is to use lorazepam [13].

Motion Elimination Assisted or voluntary breath hold enables the PTV to be substantially reduced in patients with large breathing excursions. Assisted breath hold at the exhale position has a short-term reproducibility that enables a reduction of PTV margins, with an average intrafraction CC reproducibility of diaphragm relative to vertebral bodies of 1.5 mm (range, 0.6–3.9 mm); however, even with breath hold, the interfraction CC reproducibility may be substantial due to baseline shifts (e.g., an average of 3.4 mm, range of 1.5–7.9 mm), and thus IGRT continues to be as important, even if breath hold motion management is used [14].

Motion Incorporation Many methods based on incorporating motion into the treatment process, including tumor gating, tracking, and trailing, are currently available. For tumor gating, the treatment beam is only turned on when the tumor or a surrogate is in a predefined region of interest. As baseline shifts in liver position relative to vertebral bodies occur day to day, imaging of any fiducial marker and correcting for the daily change in liver position is fundamental before initiating gating based on an external surrogate. Tumor trailing, by incorporating continuous motion monitoring, is a treatment delivery technique that continuously adjusts the beam aperture according to the last time-averaged position of the target [15]. Unlike tumor tracking, in the tumor trailing strategy, the treatment delivery does not track the target position exactly but follows the relatively slow ultracyclic trend—e.g., following the mean position that may shift over time.

8.4   Rationale for Image-Guided Radiation Therapy (IGRT)

Shifts in liver position relative to vertebral bodies occur despite all means of motion management, with the largest baseline shifts seen day to day (interfraction), and smaller but non-negligible residual changes observed over the duration of a treatment fraction (intrafraction). IGRT before each fraction corrects for mostly CC shifts. The risk of a larger intrafraction baseline shift increases as the treatment time lengthens. In a prior study by Case et al., there were negligible anatomical changes within a 20-min treatment window; however, the risk of drift or more substantial baseline shifts increased as the RT time further increased. Monitoring during RT delivery may be required/desired to measure residual intrafraction changes. Real-time IGRT may be needed, in conjunction with gating or tracking, to further reduce the PTV margins.

8.5 IGRT Technologies

8.5.1 Pre-IGRT Preparation

Although IGRT can help reduce the PTV and volume irradiated, it cannot "move" targets away from dose-limiting OARs. Thus, immobilization and positioning strategies should be considered to widen the "space" between the OARs and GTV. For example, abdominal compression may move the bowel closer to the liver and may not be desirable for anterior mid- or left-sided liver tumors. Inhale breath hold may move the liver away from the heart and maybe helpful for tumors adjacent to the heart. Finally, internal spacers may be used to move the adjacent bowel away from hepatic tumors [16].

Before bringing a patient to simulation, inserted fiducial markers are often used to aid in kilovoltage (kV) fluoroscopy or cone-beam computed tomography (CBCT) based IGRT. The fiducials placement procedure should be done at least a few days prior to simulation if fiducials are part of the IGRT process. Three fiducials are generally preferred to be inserted around the tumor with a non-coplanar distribution, rather than inside the tumor, to avoid the risk of tumor seeding [17]. Note that breath hold 3D-CBCT and 4D-CBCT facilitate IGRT to take place without the use of fiducials in certain programs [18].

Finally, patient education and coaching prior to the simulation and treatment delivery sessions may be useful for achieving a more reproducible treatment setup throughout the RT course. For example, nutrition/dietary guidelines such as maintaining a stomach empty for simulation may be beneficial for some patients. Also, avoiding a diet high in gas may reduce imaging artifact due to moving gas.

8.5.2 Orthogonal X-Ray Projection Imaging and Fluoroscopy

2D orthogonal imaging, using the megavoltage (MV) treatment beam and a portal imager, was the first type of in-room IGRT technique implemented in the clinic. This approach was the precursor of current widely available kV imaging, which relies on a dedicated X-ray source and detector panel system mounted on the LINAC treatment machine. Although the diaphragm might be discernible in breath hold with the MV portal imaging and might aid in correcting the dominant CC baseline shifts of the liver, residual positional uncertainties still existed. Large fiducials inserted around the tumor were required for MV-based IGRT to allow for substantial reductions of PTV margins [19]. On-board kV imaging, available at the treatment unit, allowed for smaller fiducials to support IGRT, and also facilitated fluoroscopic evaluation before and during treatment.

Shirato et al. described the first kV system where the tumor was tracked during RT delivery by means of floor and ceiling mounted pairs of kV tubes and imagers [20]. Liver tumors that moved due to breathing were exposed to radiation only when previously inserted fiducial markers, placed near the liver cancer, were within a predefined volume. The CyberKnife (Accuray, Sunnyvale, CA, USA) consists of a compact LINAC mounted on a robotic arm. This system uses the coupling of an orthogonal pair of X-ray cameras to dynamically manipulate the robot-mounted LINAC with six degrees of freedom (translations and rotations). Nowadays, most LINAC vendors can measure motion with fluoroscopy at the treatment unit, sometimes combining this functionality with CBCT-based IGRT such as in the VERO System (BrainLAB AG, Feldkirchen, Germany).

Fluoroscopic IGRT has the advantages of real-time motion assessment and real-time gating or tracking. The main disadvantages include: (a) the need for inserted fiducials which are associated with a small risk of infection or bleeding in the larger population and an increased risk in patients with cirrhosis and (b) higher dose to the patient, although this can be reduced with modifications of imaging frequency and technical specifications. An alternative to inserted fiducials is Lipiodol (an ethiodized oil, Guerbet, Villepinte, France), which may be used with prior transarterial chemoembolization (TACE) therapies for HCC patients and stay in-situ for many months. Lipiodol is radio-opaque and has been reported to be successfully used in place of inserted fiducials [21]. Note, volumetric information is not available if fluoroscopic IGRT is used on its own, and thus, potential setup issues related to organ deformations or rotations may not be detected. This is particularly important when neighboring dose-limiting OARs may transit into the high dose gradient regions.

8.5.3 MV Volumetric Image Guidance

Helical MVCT scans can be obtained using a tomotherapy system (TomoTherapy, Madison, WI, USA), which allows the MV treatment beam to rotate around the patient while the couch moves through the bore. Single slice or volumetric MV images of the irradiated region can be reconstructed. Although soft-tissue contrast is not as good as kV-based CT imaging, MVCT has been shown to be usable for image guidance in liver SBRT [22].

8.5.4 In-room CT

Strategies using a CT scan before each treatment fraction have been described. Wunderink et al. discussed a strategy relying on the use of a Stereotactic Body Frame device and daily CT imaging in which the frame and patient were transported via a trolley from CT to the treatment room and subsequently positioned on the LINAC's treatment table. Further, the position of the spine was verified with electronic portal images to confirm the correct treatment setup [23].

In the case of other devices, such as the EXaCT Targeting system (Varian Medical Systems Inc., Palo Alto, CA, USA) the same patient couch is used for both the CT imaging and LINAC-based treatment, meaning that imaging can be performed with the patient in the actual treatment position. As an added value, the CT images provide the anatomical and electron density information (Hounsfield units), which is required to calculate and reconstruct the planned dose to the patient in the treatment position. A disadvantage, however, is that a couch shift or "swing" is needed after imaging is acquired, introducing a potential source of positioning uncertainty [24].

8.5.5 Cone-Beam CT (CBCT)

CBCT refers to the tomographic reconstruction of volumetric anatomical information from a series of digital radiographs acquired at different angles as the gantry rotates around the patient [25]. Kilo-voltage CBCT systems integrate a kV tube and a flat panel detector mounted on a LINAC. The same rotation axis is shared between the kV imaging and MV treatments, and CBCT's central axis is oriented perpendicular to the treatment MV beam.

As breathing motion can be substantial, breath hold techniques such as active breathing control (ABC—Elekta, Stockholm, Sweden) can minimize organ motion considerably [26]. In patients treated with ABC breath hold, volumetric/3D CBCT imaging is acquired in a "stop-and-go" fashion, since patient breath holds are typically between 15 and 20 s long and the requirement for a 3D CBCT is in the order of 1 min. This means that over a partial or full 360° gantry rotation CBCT projections are collected over three to four sequences separated by breaks to allow the patient to breathe normally and reestablish a subsequent breath hold. In the majority of patients, intrafraction reproducibility of liver position is reliable. In 2006, Hawkins et al. discussed the advantages of stop-and-go breath hold CBCT over 2D orthogonal kV imaging in liver cancer patients [19]. The study showed that the volumetric image guidance improved accuracy over 2D orthogonal imaging and qualified CBCT to be a feasible, low-dose, image guidance strategy (Fig. 8.1).

Respiratory sorted 4D CBCT is beneficial for patients who are unable to be treated with breath hold CBCT [27]. The breathing amplitude of the liver can be automatically measured, and match-

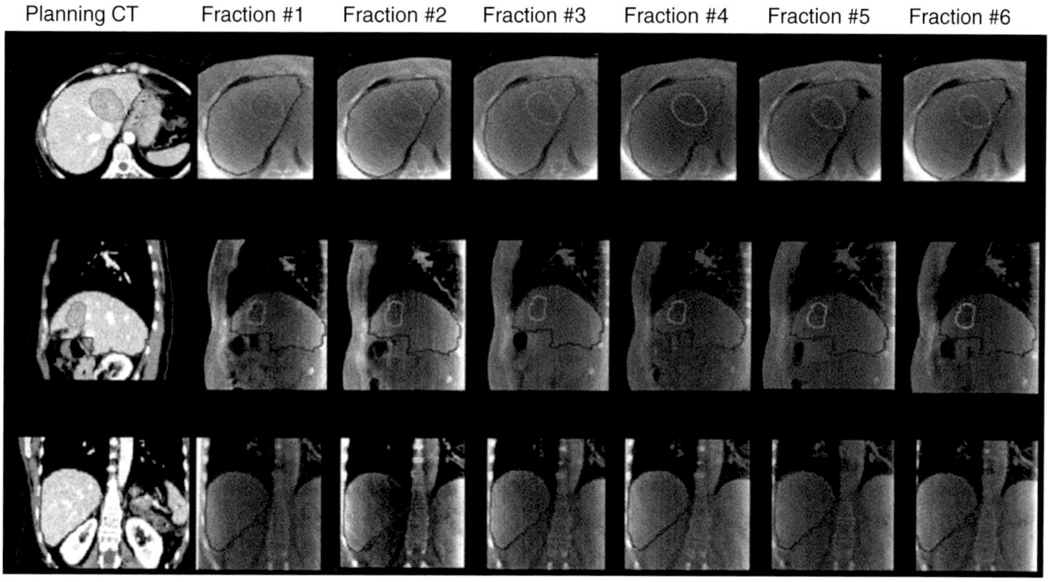

Fig. 8.1 Planning CT and kV stop-and-go CBCT images obtained in the treatment position prior to each fraction, with liver and GTV contours from the CT simulation overlaid on each CBCT, showing good alignment (with permission from Hawkins et al. [19])

ing to a phase (e.g., exhale) of the 4D CBCT or the time-weighted mean liver position, can improve the accuracy of the setup, and allow IGRT without fiducials, which are often helpful when using 3D CBCT.

At the treatment unit, image matching may be automated or manual, e.g., liver-to-liver, followed by minor adjustments in the region of the tumor. Alternatively, fiducial-to-fiducial matching can be used, for example, in the case when 3D CBCT is used. Following the liver matching process, care should be taken to review the adjacent OARs position to ensure there are no unexpected shifts in anatomy that could lead to excessive doses being delivered to these structures. Direct tumor visualization is uncommon although Lipiodol can be useful as a radio-opaque marker if the patient was previously treated with TACE [21].

8.5.6 MR-Guided Radiation Therapy (MRgRT)

MRgRT is the most recent advance in IGRT and refers to the use of an integrated MR scanner with a radiation treatment unit [1]. Two systems are currently in clinical practice for the treatment of liver cancers, i.e., Unity equipped with a 1.5 T on-board MR imaging device (Elekta, Stockholm, Sweden) [28] and MRIdian featuring a 0.35 T MR system (ViewRay, Oakwood Village, OH, USA) [28, 29]. Additionally, two other designs have been investigated by research groups and are at different stages of prototype development [30, 31].

Liver cancers are well suited for MRgRT applications for many reasons. Liver tumors may be visualized without the use of IV contrast as opposed to kV-based imaging (CT or CBCT), allowing direct targeting of the liver tumor for IGRT which is expected to allow for reduced treatment margins (Fig. 8.2). Also, some OARs such as the biliary tract and vessels are better visualized on MR than on CT.

The liver moves due to breathing and its continuous spatial and temporal displacement can be directly assessed using fast 2D-cine MR imaging acquired in any arbitrary plane (e.g., sagittal, coronal). Since 2D-cine is a standard imaging functionality of any modern MR scanner, both Unity and MRIdian systems are capable of acquiring good quality imaging relevant to liver RT. In particular, the MRIdian platform allows direct tumor monitoring and treatment gating based on MR

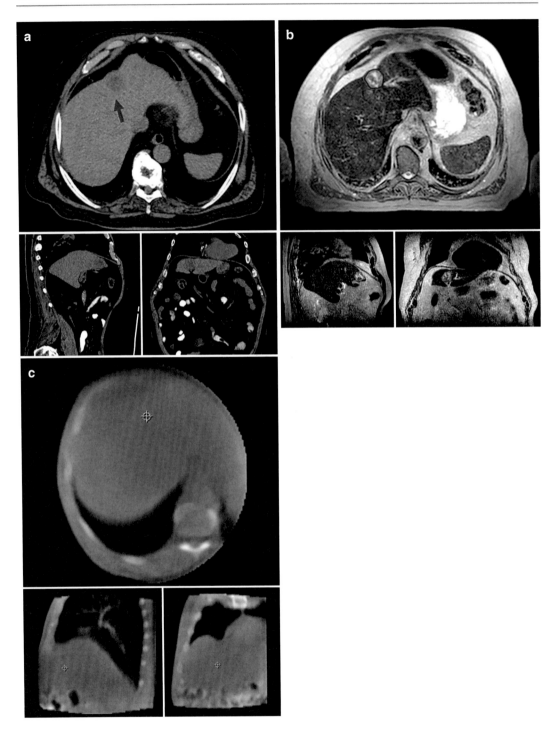

Fig. 8.2 Liver mixed cholangiocarcinoma/hepatocellular carcinoma imaged with (**a**) diagnostic CT, (**b**) MR acquired with a T2-weighted navigator triggered sequence on the Unity system—dataset can be used for both adaptive online planning and treatment verification and (**c**) CBCT reconstructed for IGRT

imaging; on the other hand, the Unity system allows for cine real-time monitoring, but gating is not yet clinically available [32]. Recently, 4D-MRI driven MR-guided online adaptive radiotherapy methods for abdominal SBRT have been implemented on the Unity platform [33, 34] (Fig. 8.3).

Many hepatic tumors are adjacent to luminal GI tissues which may limit the ability to escalate treatment dose. MRgRT provides a platform for online adaptive RT for these patients, with replanning occurring every day, and possible dose escalation, if luminal OARs move away from the tumor (Fig. 8.4). Also, frequent MR acquired during the course of RT provides a platform for biomarker discovery, such as diffusion-weighted imaging (DWI), which has shown promise as a biomarker for tumor response in early studies [35].

MRgRT requires the identification and contouring of the tumor and relevant OARs on the MR images acquired at the treatment unit. Thus, education and standardization of how target volumes and OARs should be contoured are paramount. At the time of MR simulation, imaging from the MRgRT treatment unit may be obtained to ensure that the image data is of adequate quality to identify the tumor well enough and achieve a feasible treatment plan. Lukovic et al. recently published an upper organs-at-risk (OAR) contouring atlas for MRgRT [36] (Fig. 8.5), which is consistent with the CT-based OAR consensus paper from Jabbour et al. [37].

Hepatocyte-specific contrast agents, such as gadoxetate disodium, can significantly enhance the visualization of liver lesions during MR and may be desired at the time of MR simulation. The agents have also been investigated at the time of MRgRT to further improve target identification and characterization. However, it is not practical to use IV contrast on a routine daily basis. On dynamic IV contrast MR imaging, tumors tend to enhance in a similar manner to what is seen with IV contrast CT. HCC appears hypervascular on arterial imaging, with washout in venous and delayed phases. IHC tends to be best seen in venous phase imaging, sometimes with some tumor necrosis and ring enhancement. Most metastases are well visualized on venous phase imaging [38]. For MR simulation, the acquisition of IV contrast imaging is useful.

In the case of MRgRT, non-contrast MR imaging is routinely used in the clinic, generally with little (or no) choice of sequences, outside a research platform. A default sequence with mixed T2- and T1-weighted contrast (vendor-specific) is used for both 0.35 T and 1.5 T clinical MRgRT units, with a variable degree of visibility for liver metastases and primary cancers. In general, liver metastases appear hypointense in T1-weighted imaging and mildly hyperintense in T2-weighted imaging. Hypervascularization is seen in dynamic phases of neuroendocrine tumors, and milder hypervascularization is seen in metastases from thyroid, melanoma, and renal cell carcinoma. On the 0.35 T system, liver metastases tend to appear hypoisointense in comparison with the adjacent liver when imaged with the TrueFISP imaging sequence, which is used for motion monitoring and image guidance.

An early multi-center study analyzed the clinical results of 26 patients treated with 0.35 T MRgRT SBRT [39]. In this study, two institutions performed gating with maximum inspiratory breath hold for each patient, and one institution used a modified shallow internal target volume or exhale-based setup for treatment. In cases where the liver tumor was not directly visible on commercially available cine MR imaging, real-time tracking was done using surrogate anatomy, such as the portal vein or the liver lobe. The local control of treated tumors was 80% at 21 months, with grade 3 gastrointestinal toxicity in two patients—one portal hypertension and one hilar stricture (7.7%). Others have not reported grade 3 or higher toxicity following MRgRT used for patients with primary or metastatic liver cancer [40]. In a prospective phase I study by Henke et al., stereotactic MR-guided adaptive radiation therapy (e.g., SMART approach) was used in six patients with liver oligometastases, and four patients with primary liver cancer. Early outcomes were promising with a 6-month local progression-free survival rate of 89% and 1-year survival rate of 75%, with no reported grade 3 or higher toxicity [41].

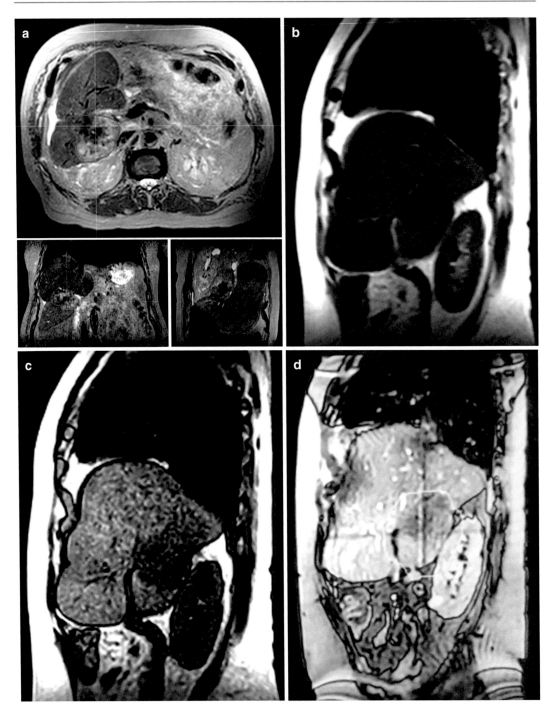

Fig. 8.3 Liver metastases imaged on the Unity platform: (**a**) 3D T2-weighted scan acquired in the exhale phase of the breathing cycle—sample images shown for the transverse, coronal, and sagittal planes; 2D-cine sagittal acquisitions with (**b**) T2-weighted contrast, (**c**) T1-weighted contrast, and (**d**) a balanced steady-state free precession sequence providing mixed T2/T1-weighted contrast; (**b**) and (**c**) were acquired on the MR console while (**d**) was acquired in the motion monitoring environment

Fraction 1   Fraction 2   Fraction 3   Fraction 4

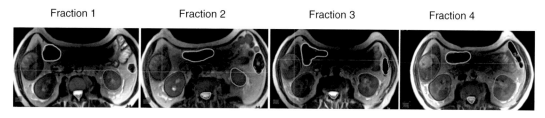

Fig. 8.4 Repeat MR images of a segment VI liver tumor in close proximity to the large bowel over a course of SBRT, showing the potential for adaption. On fraction 2 and 4, the large bowel moves away from the GTV, providing an opportunity for dose escalation. GTV: red. Large bowel: yellow. Liver: brown. Pink: duodenum

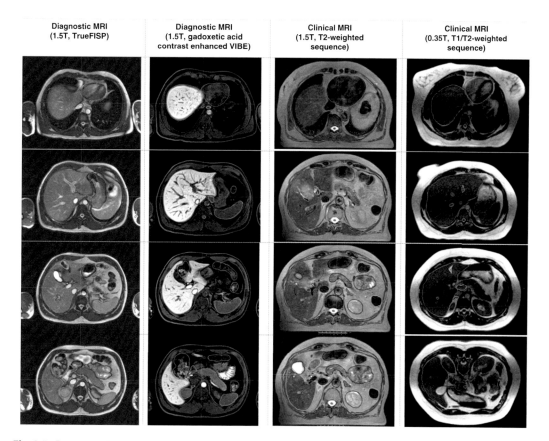

Fig. 8.5 Representative axial images acquired using various sequences from 1.5 T diagnostic MR scanner (TrueFISP and contrast-enhanced VIBE), 1.5 T MR Unity unit (Elekta, Stockholm), and 0.35 T MR ViewRay unit (Oakwood Village, OH, USA). DICOM/DICOM-RT images available at econtour.org (with permission from Lukovic et al. [36])

8.6   Conclusions

IGRT has greatly facilitated safe dose escalation and hypofractionation, including SBRT, for the treatment of liver cancers. As IGRT technological solutions and image quality continue to improve, the opportunity for adapting to change that occurs at the treatment unit between fractions and during RT delivery becomes more feasible for more patients. MRgRT helps in this regard due to the improved ability to visualize liver tumors directly and an increased ability to identify and avoid irradiation to adjacent OAR. We expect that the novel IGRT systems will continue to evolve, with next-generation IGRT solutions becoming more automated and efficient, potentially allowing higher throughout, more generalized utilization, new RT paradigms to be studies (such as dose accumulation and dose painting), and possibly more liver cancer patients to be effectively and safely irradiated.

Acknowledgments We thank Dr. Jelena Lukovic for her help with Figs. 8.2 and 8.5.

References

1. Palma DA, Olson R, Harrow S, Gaede S, Louie AV, Haasbeek C, et al. Stereotactic ablative radiotherapy versus standard of care palliative treatment in patients with oligometastatic cancers (SABR-COMET): a randomised, phase 2, open-label trial. Lancet. 2019;393(10185):2051–8.
2. Palma DA, Olson R, Harrow S, Gaede S, Louie AV, Haasbeek C, et al. Stereotactic ablative radiotherapy for the comprehensive treatment of oligometastatic cancers: long-term results of the SABR-COMET phase II randomized trial. J Clin Oncol. 2020;38(25):2830–8.
3. Jaffray DA, Langen KM, Mageras G, Dawson LA, Yan D, Ed DR, et al. Safety considerations for IGRT: executive summary. Pract Radiat Oncol. 2013;3(3):167–70.
4. Helou J, Karotki A, Milot L, Chu W, Erler D, Chung HT. 4DCT simulation with synchronized contrast injection in liver SBRT patients. Technol Cancer Res Treat. 2016;15(1):55–9.
5. Voroney JP, Brock KK, Eccles C, Haider M, Dawson LA. Prospective comparison of computed tomography and magnetic resonance imaging for liver cancer delineation using deformable image registration. Int J Radiat Oncol Biol Phys. 2006;66(3):780–91.
6. Hong TS, Bosch WR, Krishnan S, Kim TK, Mamon HJ, Shyn P, et al. Interobserver variability in target definition for hepatocellular carcinoma with and without portal vein thrombus: radiation therapy oncology group consensus guidelines. Int J Radiat Oncol Biol Phys. 2014;89(4):804–13.
7. Langen KM, Jones DT. Organ motion and its management. Int J Radiat Oncol Biol Phys. 2001;50(1):265–78.
8. Balter JM, Dawson LA, Kazanjian S, McGinn C, Brock KK, Lawrence T, et al. Determination of ventilatory liver movement via radiographic evaluation of diaphragm position. Int J Radiat Oncol Biol Phys. 2001;51(1):267–70.
9. Beddar AS, Briere TM, Balter P, Pan T, Tolani N, Ng C, et al. 4D-CT imaging with synchronized intravenous contrast injection to improve delineation of liver tumors for treatment planning. Radiother Oncol. 2008;87(3):445–8.
10. Kirilova A, Lockwood G, Choi P, Bana N, Haider MA, Brock KK, et al. Three-dimensional motion of liver tumors using cine-magnetic resonance imaging. Int J Radiat Oncol Biol Phys. 2008;71(4):1189–95.
11. Shimizu S, Shirato H, Xo B, Kagei K, Nishioka T, Hashimoto S, et al. Three-dimensional movement of a liver tumor detected by high-speed magnetic resonance imaging. Radiother Oncol. 1999;50(3):367–70.
12. Eccles CL, Patel R, Simeonov AK, Lockwood G, Haider M, Dawson LA. Comparison of liver tumor motion with and without abdominal compression using cine-magnetic resonance imaging. Int J Radiat Oncol Biol Phys. 2011;79(2):602–8.
13. Tsang DS, Voncken FE, Tse RV, Sykes J, Wong RK, Dinniwell RE, et al. A randomized controlled trial of lorazepam to reduce liver motion in patients receiving upper abdominal radiation therapy. Int J Radiat Oncol Biol Phys. 2013;87(5):881–7.
14. Eccles C, Brock KK, Bissonnette JP, Hawkins M, Dawson LA. Reproducibility of liver position using active breathing coordinator for liver cancer radiotherapy. Int J Radiat Oncol Biol Phys. 2006;64(3):751–9.
15. Fast M, van de Schoot A, van de Lindt T, Carbaat C, van der Heide U, Sonke JJ. Tumor trailing for liver SBRT on the MR-Linac. Int J Radiat Oncol Biol Phys. 2019;103(2):468–78.
16. Yoon SS, Aloia TA, Haynes AB, Kambadakone A, Kaur H, Vauthey JN, et al. Surgical placement of biologic mesh spacers to displace bowel away from unresectable liver tumors followed by delivery of dose-intense radiation therapy. Pract Radiat Oncol. 2014;4(3):167–73.
17. Llovet JM, Vilana R, Bru C, Bianchi L, Salmeron JM, Boix L, et al. Increased risk of tumor seeding after percutaneous radiofrequency ablation for single hepatocellular carcinoma. Hepatology. 2001;33(5):1124–9.
18. Dawson LA, Eccles C, Craig T. Individualized image guided iso-NTCP based liver cancer SBRT. Acta Oncol. 2006;45(7):856–64.
19. Hawkins MA, Brock KK, Eccles C, Moseley D, Jaffray D, Dawson LA. Assessment of residual error in liver position using kV cone-beam computed tomography for liver cancer high-precision radiation therapy. Int J Radiat Oncol Biol Phys. 2006;66(2):610–9.
20. Shirato H, Oita M, Fujita K, Shimizu S, Onimaru R, Uegaki S, et al. Three-dimensional conformal setup (3D-CSU) of patients using the coordinate system provided by three internal fiducial markers and two orthogonal diagnostic X-ray systems in the treatment room. Int J Radiat Oncol Biol Phys. 2004;60(2):607–12.
21. Yue J, Sun X, Cai J, Yin FF, Yin Y, Zhu J, et al. Lipiodol: a potential direct surrogate for cone-beam computed tomography image guidance in radiotherapy of liver tumor. Int J Radiat Oncol Biol Phys. 2012;82(2):834–41.
22. Engels B, Everaert H, Gevaert T, Duchateau M, Neyns B, Sermeus A, et al. Phase II study of helical tomotherapy for oligometastatic colorectal cancer. Ann Oncol. 2011;22(2):362–8.

23. Wunderink W, Mendez Romero A, Vasquez Osorio EM, de Boer HC, Brandwijk RP, Levendag PC, et al. Target coverage in image-guided stereotactic body radiotherapy of liver tumors. Int J Radiat Oncol Biol Phys. 2007;68(1):282–90.

24. Court L, Rosen I, Mohan R, Dong L. Evaluation of mechanical precision and alignment uncertainties for an integrated CT/LINAC system. Med Phys. 2003;30(6):1198–210.

25. Jaffray DA, Siewerdsen JH, Wong JW, Martinez AA. Flat-panel cone-beam computed tomography for image-guided radiation therapy. Int J Radiat Oncol Biol Phys. 2002;53(5):1337–49.

26. Wong JW, Sharpe MB, Jaffray DA, Kini VR, Robertson JM, Stromberg JS, et al. The use of active breathing control (ABC) to reduce margin for breathing motion. Int J Radiat Oncol Biol Phys. 1999;44(4):911–9.

27. Sonke JJ, Zijp L, Remeijer P, van Herk M. Respiratory correlated cone beam CT. Med Phys. 2005;32(4):1176–86.

28. Raaymakers BW, Jurgenliemk-Schulz IM, Bol GH, Glitzner M, Kotte A, van Asselen B, et al. First patients treated with a 1.5 T MRI-Linac: clinical proof of concept of a high-precision, high-field MRI guided radiotherapy treatment. Phys Med Biol. 2017;62(23):L41–50.

29. Kluter S. Technical design and concept of a 0.35 T MR-Linac. Clin Transl Radiat Oncol. 2019;18:98–101.

30. Keall PJ, Barton M, Crozier S. Australian Mri-Linac program icfIIICCCLHSUUoNQSWS, Wollongong. The Australian magnetic resonance imaging-linac program. Semin Radiat Oncol. 2014;24(3):203–6.

31. Fallone BG. The rotating biplanar linac-magnetic resonance imaging system. Semin Radiat Oncol. 2014;24(3):200–2.

32. Bertholet J, Knopf A, Eiben B, McClelland J, Grimwood A, Harris E, et al. Real-time intrafraction motion monitoring in external beam radiotherapy. Phys Med Biol. 2019;64(15):15TR01.

33. Paulson ES, Ahunbay E, Chen X, Mickevicius NJ, Chen GP, Schultz C, et al. 4D-MRI driven MR-guided online adaptive radiotherapy for abdominal stereotactic body radiation therapy on a high field MR-Linac: implementation and initial clinical experience. Clin Transl Radiat Oncol. 2020;23:72–9.

34. Stemkens B, Paulson ES, Tijssen RHN. Nuts and bolts of 4D-MRI for radiotherapy. Phys Med Biol. 2018;63(21):21TR01.

35. Eccles CL, Haider EA, Haider MA, Fung S, Lockwood G, Dawson LA. Change in diffusion weighted MRI during liver cancer radiotherapy: preliminary observations. Acta Oncol. 2009;48(7):1034–43.

36. Lukovic J, Henke L, Gani C, Kim TK, Stanescu T, Hosni A, et al. MRI-based upper abdominal organs-at-risk atlas for radiation oncology. Int J Radiat Oncol Biol Phys. 2020;106(4):743–53.

37. Jabbour SK, Hashem SA, Bosch W, Kim TK, Finkelstein SE, Anderson BM, et al. Upper abdominal normal organ contouring guidelines and atlas: a Radiation Therapy Oncology Group consensus. Pract Radiat Oncol. 2014;4(2):82–9.

38. Vilgrain V, Esvan M, Ronot M, Caumont-Prim A, Aube C, Chatellier G. A meta-analysis of diffusion-weighted and gadoxetic acid-enhanced MR imaging for the detection of liver metastases. Eur Radiol. 2016;26(12):4595–615.

39. Rosenberg SA, Henke LE, Shaverdian N, Mittauer K, Wojcieszynski AP, Hullett CR, et al. A multi-institutional experience of MR-guided liver stereotactic body radiation therapy. Adv Radiat Oncol. 2019;4(1):142–9.

40. Feldman AM, Modh A, Glide-Hurst C, Chetty IJ, Movsas B. Real-time magnetic resonance-guided liver stereotactic body radiation therapy: an institutional report using a magnetic resonance-Linac system. Cureus. 2019;11(9):e5774.

41. Henke L, Kashani R, Robinson C, Curcuru A, DeWees T, Bradley J, et al. Phase I trial of stereotactic MR-guided online adaptive radiation therapy (SMART) for the treatment of oligometastatic or unresectable primary malignancies of the abdomen. Radiother Oncol. 2018;126(3):519–26.

Particle Beam Radiotherapy

9

Masashi Mizumoto, Yoshito Oshiro,
and Hideyuki Sakurai

Abstract

Particle therapy has progressed over 40 years and there are now many results for outcomes for hepatocellular carcinoma (HCC). The local control rate of HCC by particle therapy is expected to be 85–90% at 3 years and 80–90% at 5 years. Overall survival rate is expected to be 55–65% at 2 years and 20–50% at 5 years. The prognostic factors for survival considered are hepatic function and number and size of tumors.

Adverse events due to particle therapy are considered acceptable. Acute adverse effects, such as dermatitis and hepatic dysfunction, occur in most cases. They are generally transient, easily managed, and acceptable. Late adverse effects, including bile duct damage, ulcer, dermatitis, and rib fracture, can also occur. Basically, these severe toxicities are quite rare and can be avoided using recent fractionation schedules. Hepatic dysfunction is not dependent on irradiation dose, and proton beam therapy (PBT) can reduce the risk of radiation induced liver disease (RILD) compared to photon radiotherapy.

In conclusion, particle therapy for HCC is effective and safe, even for cases with portal vein tumor thrombosis (PVTT) or inferior vena cava tumor thrombosis (IVCTT), poor liver function, and coexisting disease, and is a good alternative to other treatment.

Keywords

Particle therapy · Proton beam therapy Carbon ion therapy · Radiotherapy Radiation therapy · Liver · Hepatocellular carcinoma · HCC

9.1 Introduction

Charged particle radiotherapy is classified into proton beam therapy (PBT) and carbon ion therapy and has a unique dose distribution. In treatment of hepatocellular carcinoma (HCC), liver dysfunction and radiation induced liver disease (RILD) can be major problems, with RILD being one of the most important treatment-related complications in hepatic radiation therapy. Whole-liver radiation therapy is limited and unsatisfactory for patients with HCC, mainly due to poor hepatic tolerance to ionizing radiation. Emami et al. reported tolerance doses of 30, 35, and 50 Gy for the entire liver, two-thirds, and one-third of the liver, respectively [1]. The RTOG 84-05 trial found incidence of RILD caused by whole-liver irradiation at a single dose of 1.5 Gy twice a day of 0/122 and 5/51 (9.8%) at total doses of 27–30 Gy and 33 Gy, respectively, and it was not

M. Mizumoto · Y. Oshiro · H. Sakurai (✉)
Department of Radiation Oncology, University of Tsukuba Hospital, Tsukuba, Ibaraki, Japan
e-mail: hsakurai@pmrc.tsukuba.ac.jp

possible to control tumors for a sustained period of time at either of these doses.

The dose distribution of a proton beam offers advantages compared to photon radiotherapy, especially in treatment of HCC. The American Society for Radiation Oncology (ASTRO) issued the Model Policy on PBT in 2014 [2], and this therapy for HCC is now covered by medical insurance in the United States. In this chapter, we discuss PBT for HCC.

9.2 Physical Characteristics of Proton Beams

A photon beam is a kind of electromagnetic wave, whereas a proton beam is a charged particle beam that is similar to a carbon ion beam. When charged particle beams pass through tissue, they deposit most of their energy at the end of the path, which produces a sharp energy peak that is referred to as the Bragg peak. William Henry Bragg, a professor of mathematics and physics, first demonstrated this phenomenon in 1904. Charged particles (protons and light ions) have a facultative range. Thereafter, the dose rapidly decreases to almost zero within about 1 cm, and this sharp fall-off of dose beyond the peak is the main advantage of charged particle beams.

Proton beams are accelerated to therapeutic energies of 70–250 MeV with the cyclotron of a synchrotron and delivered to the treatment room. For clinical application, it is necessary to adjust the depth of the Bragg peak to the tumor depth and spread this peak to create a flat dose distribution to irradiate the target tumor homogenously. This is referred to as the spread-out Bragg Peak (SOBP) (Fig. 9.1). The lateral edge is also sharper than in photon beams due to less large-angle scattering. However, PBT does not have the build-up effect observed in photoradiotherapy; therefore, careful attention to skin reactions is required for a target tumor located just beneath the surface of the skin.

The proton range and sharpness of the Bragg peak is strongly affected by the energy and density of the tissues through which the beam passes in the body. The particle range is inversely proportional to tissue density [3]. The CT density of the liver is almost homogeneous with the CT value of around 60 HU; therefore, the beam end is relatively clear. However, the beam range is changed in the lung due to lower density and in the rib due to higher density, Therefore, beam angle selection and distant margin decisions are important in use of PBT.

9.3 Biological Characteristics

A proton beam is categorized as low linear energy transfer (LET) radiation, similar to photon radiotherapy, whereas a carbon ion beam is categorized as high LET. LET is a measure of energy transfer to matter from an ionizing particle travelling through the matter. It is closely related to energy per unit distance and provides an indication of ion-induced damages. Higher LET radiation is thought to be more effective for destroying cells. Differences in biological effects due to radiation quality are quantified as the relative biological effective (RBE) dose. The RBE is defined as the ratio of the photon dose to the proton dose required to give the same biological effect under identical irradiation conditions. The effect may use various endpoints, such as cell death, mutation, and transformation. Consensus has been reached that the RBE of proton beams is 1.1 in clinical applications [4, 5]. That is, the biological effects of protons are similar to those of photons; therefore, PBT is generally thought to be applicable for most uses of photon radiotherapy. However, there may be differences in the kinetics and extent of apoptosis induction between protons and photons [6, 7].

9.4 History of Particle Beam Therapy

Ernest Rutherford discovered that nuclei of oxygen and hydrogen atoms were produced when nitrogen gas was irradiated by α radiation from uranium in 1899 and demonstrated the presence of atoms (that were named protons) in 1919 [8, 9]. In the 1930s, Ernest Lawrence invented the cyclotron to accelerate protons, and thereafter, Robert R. Wilson of Harvard University [10] pro-

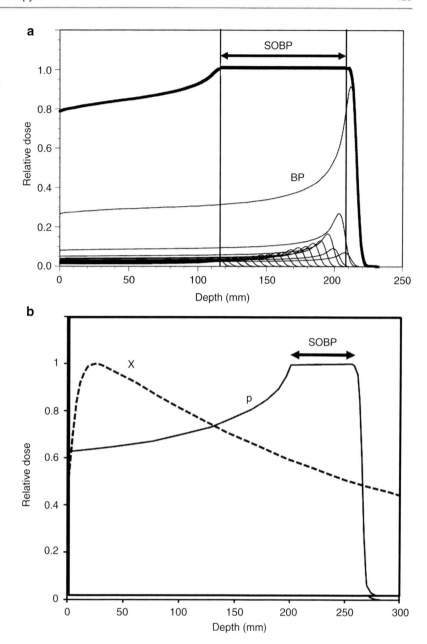

Fig. 9.1 Proton beam releases its maximum energy dose, called the "Bragg peak." In proton beam therapy, this Bragg peak is set to match the location and size of the tumor (**a**). Proton beam therapy is highly effective because it allows the energy dose released by an emitted beam to be more accurately concentrated on a tumor than is possible in traditional radiation therapy (**b**)

posed the first medical application in 1946. The acquisition of proton beams for medical applications became possible using an accelerator when research facilities for high-energy physics were constructed after World War II, and the first study of their medical use worldwide was performed at Berkeley in 1954, followed by Uppsala, Sweden, in 1957, and Harvard in 1961. At that time, PBT was used for benign diseases such as pituitary adenoma and intracranial arteriovenous malformation. One reason for this was uncertainty in the

dose calculation. In 1973, however, CT was developed and calculation of ion beam dose distributions became possible, leading to PBT being indicated for malignant tumors in the 1970s.

The initial target was limited to sarcoma at the skull base, and indications were gradually expanded thereafter. Among these subsequent indications, melanoma of the uvea was particularly notable [11], and >70% of PBT indications in the 1980s were melanoma of the uvea and skull base or upper cervical tumor. PBT was indicated for body trunk tumors only at the University of Tsukuba, after PBT for the liver was initiated in the 1980s at Tsukuba [12, 13]. A fluoroscopic device for positioning was designed to ensure accurate irradiation of deep targets that moved with respiration [13]. A technique to insert a fiducial marker in the liver to confirm positioning of the target [14] and a system to intermittently emit proton beams in synchronization with respiratory motion [15] were also developed. These are now used as basic treatment techniques for the liver. Currently, many particle beam facilities are available for treatment of the liver, and the clinical outcomes continue to accumulate.

9.5   Techniques in Proton Therapy

9.5.1   Passive Scattered Proton Therapy

Passive scattered proton therapy is the traditional method of PBT. A narrow proton beam is scattered in the gantry nozzle component over a larger area to cover the entire target volume. Lateral and longitudinal spreading is achieved by rotation modulation wheels and scatters. Distal spreading is achieved by spread-out Bragg Peak (SOBP) using a ridge filter rotating in the beam to obtain the required range of proton energies entering the patient. After spreading, the beam is shaped to fit the treatment field. The lateral and longitudinal shape is formed by using a collimator and the distal range is controlled by a bolus or range shifter to fit the target shape. In this method, SOBP is uniform over the treatment field; normal tissue at the proximal side of the treatment field may therefore be included within the SOBP when tumor thickness is heterogeneous and irradiated with an overdose.

9.5.2   Spot Scanning Therapy

Proton scanning beams have been in use for treatment at the Paul Scherrer Institute since 1996. In spot scanning therapy, a narrow beam is used without modification. The position where the beam stops is controlled by using a scanning electromagnet three-dimensionally in the domain of the tumor, and then beams are delivered in the shape of the tumor to paint it over in total. The depth of the proton beam is regulated by its energy from the synchrotron. For each scanned beam, the treatment beam is delivered in layers, depending on energy. In clinical practice, beams are delivered to the deepest layer from the body surface with maximum energy. For a moving target, respiratory movement and change of the beam range due to a change of beam path density is carefully take into consideration.

9.5.3   Intensity-Modulated Proton Therapy (IMPT)

IMPT is an application of spot scanning that improves on X-ray intensity modulated beams with dose modulation along the lateral and beam axis through in-field modulation. In IMPT, proton beams are delivered from multiple angles, modulating the intensity. The proton pencil beam allows dose modulation in the patient using the number of protons to control local dose deposition, energy to control local penetration, and magnetic deflection to control the off-axis position [16]. A high dose concentration can be reached even if the tumor shape is complicated or normal tissue is adjacent to the tumor. Figure 9.2 shows the image of passive scattered proton therapy, spot scanning therapy, and IMPT.

9.6   Proton Therapy for HCC

Utilizing the characteristics of the dose distribution of proton beams, i.e., the capacity to markedly reduce the dose for regions deeper than the target and produced an ideal dose distribution with a small number of ports, the dose for tumors can be set at a higher level in PBT. Non-exposed non-cancerous regions can be secured in a large volume, which may increase safety in patients with liver cirrhosis and low hepatic function. These properties have facilitated use

Fig. 9.2 The image of passive scattered proton therapy, spot scanning therapy, and IMPT. Passive scattered proton therapy is the traditional method of PBT. Compared to passive scattered proton therapy, spot scanning therapy and IMPT are expected better dose concentration for tumor. Dotted line indicates hepatocellular carcinoma and dark red is prescription dose area and light red is low dose are. IMPT minimized both prescription dose area and low dose area

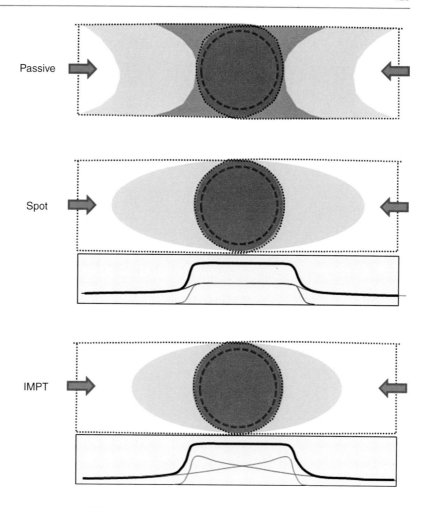

of high fractional and total doses in PBT compared with those in conventional fractionated X-ray radiotherapy.

PBT for primary liver cancer was first attempted at the University of Tsukuba, and results equivalent to radical surgery were obtained with high-dose irradiation (fractions of 3.0–4.0 Gy). These studies included patients with portal vein tumor thrombosis (PVTT), inferior vena cava tumor thrombosis (IVCTT), large tumors, and normal tissue adjacent to the tumor, and many patients for whom other treatment modalities were contraindicated or not feasible, such as elderly patients and cases with repeated treatment. The largest study was reported by Fukuda et al. in 2017. The study was retrospective, but included 129 patients who received PBT as initial treatment and a median follow-up period of 55 months. The treatment dose was 66.0–77.0 Gy(RBE) in 10–35 fractions. The five-year local control (LC) and overall survival (OS) rates

were 87% (95% CI:) and 66%, respectively, in all patients, and there were no grade 3 or more severe toxicities. In addition, 12% of the patients had a tumor thrombi in the first branch or main trunk of the portal vein (Vp3/4) or inferior vena cava, and these cases had 5-year LC and OS rates of 90% and 54% respectively. It was concluded that PBT can be an alternative treatment for localized HCC, especially when accompanied with tumor thrombi. Bush et al. conducted randomized clinical trial comparing PBT to transarterial chemoembolization (TACE) for HCC [17]. They suggested there was a trend toward improved two-year LC (88 vs. 45%, $p = 0.06$) and PFS (48 vs. 31%, $p = 0.06$) favoring the PBT group. Table 9.1 shows the treatment result of PBT for HCC.

Most studies of PBT for HCC are retrospective and small. However, these studies are important and may represent the true efficacy of PBT; therefore, they are included in this chapter. The results

Table 9.1 Treatment results of proton therapy for HCC

Authors (year)	Study	Number of patients	Proton therapy	Local control	Survival	Adverse effects
Bush et al. (2011) [18]	Phase 2	66	63 Gy(RBE)/15 fr	Local failure 20%	3y-PFS 60%	5 gastrointestinal adverse events (not need surgery)
Kawashima et al. (2005) [19]	Phase 2	30	76 Gy(RBE)/20 fr	2y-LC 96%	1/2/3y-OS 77/66/62%	No G2 or more gastrointestinal or pulmonary toxicity
Fukumitsu et al. (2009) [20]	Phase 2	51	66 Gy(RBE)/10 fr	3/5y-LC 94.5/87.8%	3/5y-OS 49.2/38.7%	Three G2 or more toxicity
Fukuda et al. (2017) [21]	Retrospective	129 (Previously untreated)	66-77 Gy(RBE)/10-35 fr	5y-LC 94/87/75% (Stage 0A/B/C)	5y-OS 69/66/25% (Stage 0A/B/C)	No G3 or more late toxicity
Mizumoto et al. (2011) [22]	Retrospective	266 (3 treatment protocol)	66 Gy(RBE)/10 fr 72.6 Gy(RBE)/22 fr 77 Gy(RBE)/35 fr	1/3/5y-LC 98/87/81 %	1/3/5y-OS 87/61/48%	12 patients had symptomatic toxicity (No G4 or more)
Kimura et al. (2017) [23]	Retrospective	24 (>5 cm)	72.6 Gy(RBE)/22 fr (60.8–85.8)	2y-LC 87.0%	2y-OS 52.4%	No G3 or more toxicity
Sugahara et al. (2010) [24]	Retrospective	22 (>10 cm)	72.6 Gy(RBE)/22 fr (47.3–89.1)	2y-LC 87.0%	2y-OS 36.0%	No G3 or more toxicity
Oshiro et al. (2017) [25]	Retrospective	83 (repeated)	Median 70.5 Gy(RBE)	N/A	2/5y-OS 87.5/49.4%	No radiation-induced liver dysfunction

fr fraction, *y-OS* year overall survival, *y-PFS* year progression free survival, *y-LC* year local control

for local control, survival, and adverse effects from previous studies are introduced separately.

9.6.1 Local Control

Bush et al. reported 34 cases of HCC in 2004 [18]. A dose of 63 Gy(RBE)/15 fr decreased alpha-fetoprotein (AFP) and achieved the lowest levels between three and six months after completion of treatment. One case with no AFP change had gross residual disease, and three cases showed local recurrence in the treated area. The two-year LC rate was 75%. In an update in 2011, the same group reported that 15 of 76 cases had local failure between two and 60 months after treatment [19]. Only 3 of 15 cases experienced local treatment failure without having new lesions develop in other parts of the liver. A total of 7 cases showed increased AFP levels, indicating LC failure.

Kawashima et al. reported 30 cases of HCC in 2005 [20]. A protocol of 72.6 Gy(RBE)/16 fr achieved complete disappearance of the primary tumor for 5–20 months in 24 cases. A residual tumor was present until death or at final follow-up in five cases, and one case with a single nodular tumor of 4.2 cm in diameter had local recurrence at five months after treatment. Of the 30 patients, 29 were free from local progression until death or at final follow-up. The two-year LC rate was 96%.

Chiba et al. retrospectively reviewed 162 cases of HCC in 2005 [21]. Based on various treatment schedules from 55 Gy(RBE)/10 fr to 92.4 Gy(RBE)/24 fr, 13 cases showed local recurrence between 7 and 43 months after treatment. The diameter of the tumors that recurred was 2.0–7.0 cm. However, since the tumor diameter did not show a significant relationship with the LC rate, it was suggested that PBT could be used to treat patients with relatively large tumors for which conventional local treatments, such as percutaneous ethanol injection, microwave coagulation therapy, and radiofrequency ablation, were not successful. The five-year LC rate was 86.9%.

Hata et al. retrospectively reviewed 19 cases of HCC with hepatic function of Child-Pugh class C [22]. Treatment schedules of 55–92.4 Gy(RBE)/10–24 fr gave an objective response rate (complete response (CR) or partial response (PR)) of 63%, and all but one of the irradiated tumors was controlled in a median follow-up period of 17 months.

Fukumitsu et al. reported 51 cases of HCC in which tumors were not adjacent to the porta hepatis or digestive organs in 2009 [23]. A dose of 66 Gy(RBE)/10 fr resulted in only three cases with local recurrence at 16, 18, and 41 months after treatment. The LC rate had no relationship with prior treatment, number of tumors, tumor diameter, and AFP level. The five-year LC rate was 87.8%.

Mizumoto et al. reported 53 cases of HCC in which the tumors were located adjacent to the porta hepatis in 2008 [24]. A protocol of 72.6 Gy(RBE)/22 fr resulted in three cases of HCC adjacent to the porta hepatis developing local recurrence at 7, 14, and 30 months after treatment and simultaneously developing new liver tumors outside the irradiated area. The three-year LC rate was 86%. The same group retrospectively reviewed 266 cases treated with three different treatment protocols (66 Gy(RBE)/10 fr, 72.6 Gy(RBE)/22 fr, and 77 Gy(RBE)/35 fr) in 2011 [25], and found LC rates of 98%, 87%, and 81% at 1, 3, and 5 years, respectively. It was concluded that there was no significant difference in LC rate among the three protocols, and no prognostic factor for the response rate was found in the review.

Hong et al. evaluated PBT for 11 patients with HCC and one with intrahepatic cholangiocarcinoma (ICC) in 2013. A median dose of 60 Gy(RBE)/15 fr (range: 45–75 Gy(RBE)) resulted in one case with marginal recurrence in a median follow-up time of 69 months for survivors [26]. Kim et al. conducted a dose-escalation study in HCC patients in 2015 [27], using three levels of 1: 60 Gy(RBE)/20 fr (equivalent to 2 Gy[EQD2] 65 Gy(RBE)$_{10}$); 2: 66 Gy(RBE)/22 fr (EQD2, 71.5 Gy(RBE)$_{10}$), and 3: 72 Gy(RBE) (EQD2, 78 Gy(RBE)$_{10}$)/24 fr. The complete response rates were 62.5%, 57.1% and 100% at dose levels 1, 2 and 3, respectively. There were no severe (>grade 3) acute toxicities. It was concluded that EQD2 > 78 Gy(RBE)$_{10}$ should be delivered to achieve LC.

In the randomized trial comparing PBT with TACE by Bush et al. [17], 36 patients were randomized to TACE and 33 to PBT with 70.2 Gy(RBE)/15fr. The two-year LC rate was 88% and 45% for PBT and TACE group, respectively.

Chadha et al. reported the results of PBT for 46 patients with HCC at a dose of 33.6–144 Gy (RBE)/15 fr in 2019 [28]. The two-year LC rate was 81% and the LC rates were 92% and 63% for cases that received BED ≥ 90 Gy(RBE) and <90 Gy(RBE), respectively. Sanford et al. conducted a comparison study of protons vs. photons for 133 patients with HCC in 2019[31]. In this study, 49 patients received PBT and 84 received photons. A dose of 45 Gy/15 fr or 30 Gy/5–6 fr was used, and the two-year LC rates were 93% and 90% for PBT and photons, respectively, with no difference in locoregional recurrence ($p = 0.93$).

Collectively, these reports show that the LC rate of HCC with single or multiple tumors that can be treated in a single irradiation field is about 85–90% at three years and 80–90% at five years. There are few differences among tumor lesion types and tumor shrinkage occurs after several months. The definition of LC was not exactly the same among the studies. Japanese groups use similar evaluation criteria, that is, "no sign of regrowth and no new tumors in the treated volume." In contrast, groups in the USA include, in addition to no new tumor growth, "AFP elevation without radiographic disease progression outside the primary treatment area," which is stricter than the Japanese definition. This stricter definition may largely explain the difference in LC rates between the US and Japanese studies.

9.6.2 Survival

Bush et al. reported a two-year OS rate of 55% in 34 cases [18] and Kawashima et al. found OS of 77%, 66%, and 62% at 1, 2 and 3 years in 30 cases [20]. The two-year OS rate of cases in which an indocyanine green (ICG) clearance test gave a retention rate at 15 min (ICG R15) ≤40% was significantly higher than that of cases with ICG R15 > 40% (80 vs. 30%) [20].

Chiba et al. reported a five-year OS rate of 23.5% in 162 cases in a retrospective study [21]. The five-year OS rate of cases with chronic hepatitis and Child-Pugh class A was significantly better than for those with Child-Pugh class B and C cirrhosis, with no significant difference between class B and C cases (class A: 35.1%, B: 10.3%, C: 0%). The OS rate of 80 cases with solitary lesions was significantly higher than that of 82 cases with multiple lesions. The causes of death were tumor progression (46.9%) and hepatic failure (37.9%).

Hata et al. found a two-year OS rate of 42% in HCC cases of Child-Pugh class C [22]. Even class C cases had better survival than the OS for patients treated only with supportive care. It was concluded that although most previous studies selected cases of Child-Pugh class A or B, PBT was also viable for treatment of cases with severe hepatic function. Fukumitsu et al. reported OS rates of 49.2% at three years and 38.7% at five years in 51 cases in which the tumor was not adjacent to the porta hepatis or digestive organ [23]. The causes of death were tumor progression (71%) and hepatic failure (10%).

Mizumoto et al. reported OS rates of 57% and 45% at two and three years in 53 cases in which the tumor was located adjacent to the porta hepatis [24]. The two-year OS rate of 63.6% in 46 cases in Child-Pugh class A was significantly higher than that in 7 cases in class B or C (14.3%). The two-year OS rate of 22 cases with a solitary lesion was 76.3%, which was significantly higher than that of 43.4% in 31 cases with multiple lesions. The three-year OS rate was 83.9% in 14 cases in Child-Pugh class A with a solitary HCC and AFP < 100 ng/ml, which was an excellent outcome. The causes of death were intrahepatic recurrence (69.2%), dis-

tant metastasis (7.7%), and hepatic failure (11.5%), which were similar to the data in Fukumitsu et al. [23]. In a retrospective review of 266 cases treated by three different treatment protocols in 2011, the same group found a five-year OS rate of 55.1% for 198 cases in Child-Pugh class A, which was significantly higher than that in 61 cases in class B or C (11.4%) [25]. The OS rates of all cases were 61% at three years and 48% at five years, and the OS rates of cases treated with the 66 Gy(RBE)/10 fr, 72.6 Gy(RBE)/22 fr, or 77 Gy(RBE)/35 fr protocol were quite similar to each other.

Komatsu et al. reported a five-year OS rate of 38% in 242 cases [29] in a study using various treatment schedules of 52.8 Gy(RBE)/4 fr to 84 Gy(RBE)/20 fr to investigate whether the dose affects the survival time. The five-year OS rate of 46.6% in 184 cases in Child-Pugh class A was significantly higher than those of 8.7% in 55 cases in class B (8.7%) and 0% in three cases in class C (0%). The prognostic factors were performance status (PS), Child-Pugh class, and vascular invasion.

Hong et al. found one-, two- and three-year OS rates of 53%, 40% and 33%, respectively, in 11 patients with HCC and 3 patients with ICC [22]. In a dose escalation study by Kim et al. [27], the three-year OS rate did not differ significantly among dose levels. However, the three-year OS rates were 25%, 66.7%, and 73.3% for dose levels 1, 2 and 3, respectively, and the OS rate was significantly higher for patients who achieved CR compared with those who did not (65.2 vs. 20%, p = 0.033). In Chadha et al., the OS rate was significantly better for patients who received BED > 90 Gy(RBE). The two-year OS rate was 62% for all patients, and the median survival times were 49.9 and 15.8 months for those who received ≥90 Gy(RBE) and <90 Gy(RBE), respectively [28].

A comparison study of PBT vs. photon therapy by Sanford et al. [30] suggested that the median Child Pugh score and ALBI before treatment can identify patients who should receive PBT (p = 0.08 and 0.03). The two-year OS rates were 59.1% and 28.6% for patients who received PBT and photon therapy, respectively (p = 0.03). The LC rate did not differ significantly between

PBT and photon therapy, but the incidence of RILD was significantly higher for photon therapy, and development of non-classical RILD at three months was significantly correlated with a worse OS.

In the randomized trial comparing PBT with TACE by Bush et al. [17], two-year OS for entire group was 59% and there was no significant difference between PBT and TACE group.

Collectively, these studies suggest an OS rate for HCC of about 55–65% at two years and 20–50% at five years. The causes of death are 50–70% due to tumor progression, followed by 10–40% due to hepatic dysfunction. The prognostic factors for survival are hepatic function, and number and size of tumors. The AFP level, PS, and vascular invasion are also included as prognostic factors. Dose escalation suggests that a higher dose is necessary for LC, and survival is better for patients who achieve LC.

9.6.3 Adverse Effects

Bush et al. observed acute adverse effects, such as fatigue, radiation dermatitis, and abdominal discomfort, in approximately 60% of patients [18], but none required hospitalization or interruption of treatment. A small decrease in serum albumin and a small elevation in total serum bilirubin were found after treatment. Serum albumin returned to baseline at six months, and no patient was clinically jaundiced. It was concluded that both acute and chronic adverse effects of PBT in HCC were mild. Severe adverse effects of more than Grade 3 were not present in acute and late-stage treatment in an updated report from the same group in 2011 [19].

Kawashima et al. found proton-induced hepatic insufficiency involving ascites and/or asterixis without a large elevation of serum bilirubin or transaminase at one–four months after treatment in 8 of 30 cases [20]. It was suggested that V30% in combination with ICG R15 might be a useful indicator for estimation of liver tolerance to PBT from a dose-volume histogram analysis.

Chiba et al. reported late adverse effects of Grade 2 or higher in 5 of 162 cases [21], including fibrotic stenosis of the common bile duct at 13 months, biloma at 29 and 36 months, and gastrointestinal tract bleeding at 4 and 6 months after treatment. There were no deaths due to the late adverse effects. Some acute adverse effects were noted, but they subsided quickly without causing any problems. The acute adverse effects included elevation of aspartate transaminase and alanine transaminases in 18 cases.

Fukumitsu et al. found that 4 of 51 cases had late adverse effects of more than Grade 3, including 3 cases with rib fracture at 3–27 months and one of pneumonitis at three months [23]. No patients died of these late adverse effects. It was concluded that cases in which the tumor is located close to the body surface should be monitored more carefully with regard to the dose distribution to the skin and ribs.

Mizumoto et al. examined 53 cases in which the tumor was adjacent to the porta hepatis [24]. In Chiba et al., cases with severe late adverse effects, such as fibrotic stenosis of the common bile duct or biloma, had been treated with 79.2 Gy(RBE)/16 fr or 91.3 Gy(RBE)/23 fr [21]. Thus, a protocol of 72.6 Gy(RBE) 22 fr was used as a lower dose fractionation schedule[26] and there was no difference in LC rate for tumors adjacent to the porta hepatis. Consequently, only five cases had Grade 2 acute adverse effects in the skin and gastrointestinal tract, and none of the 53 cases had acute or late adverse effects of more than Grade 3. In a retrospective review of 266 cases treated with three different treatment protocols in 2011, the adverse effects of more than Grade 3 were acute dermatitis ($n = 2$), late rib fracture ($n = 3$), dermatitis ($n = 1$), and perforation, bleeding, or inflammation of the digestive tract ($n = 3$) [25].

Komatsu et al. reported that all acute toxicities in 242 cases were transient, easily managed, and acceptable [29]. However, four cases had late adverse effects, including refractory skin ulcers, and one case required skin transplantation. Moreover, a salvage drainage operation was required for one case of biloma at 10 months after treatment. Eight cases showed late adverse effects on hepatic function of more than Grade 3, but all these cases with hematological disorders were asymptomatic and required no further treatment.

Hong et al. found Grade 2 bilirubinemia ($n = 2$), Grade 3 gastrointestinal bleeding ($n = 1$), and stomach perforation ($n = 1$) in 11 HCC and 3 ICC cases treated with a median dose of 60 Gy(RBE) in 15 fractions [26]. Chadha et al. found no Grade ≥ 3 hepatic toxicity regardless of the irradiation dose of BED ≥ 90 Gy(RBE) or <90 Gy(RBE), but Grade ≥ 3 acute toxicities of non-maligning ascites (9%), hyperbilirubinemia (4%), and diarrhea and upper gastrointestinal bleeding (2%) were found [28].

In a comparison of PBT vs. photon therapy, Sanford et al. [30] found no significant difference in LC rate. However, the risk of development of RILD was significantly worse for photon therapy ($p = 0.03$), and development of RILD at three months was associated with worse OS ($p < 0.01$). In 2020, Sumiya et al. examined changes in liver and biliary enzymes during PBT for 300 patients with HCC. The liver enzymes and bilirubin were almost stable during treatment, with only transient elevation observed [31].

Overall, these studies suggest that acute adverse effects, such as dermatitis and hepatic dysfunction, occur in most cases. They are, however, generally transient, easily managed, and acceptable. With regard to late adverse effects, bile duct damage, ulcer, dermatitis, and rib fracture can occur. However, these effects are quite rare and can be avoided using recent fractionation schedules. Hepatic dysfunction is not dependent on irradiation dose, and PBT can reduce the risk of RILD compared to photon radiotherapy. These data suggest that PBT at a high dose is safe and well tolerable when a fractionated dose is selected depending on the tumor location.

9.6.4   Efficacy of PBT for HCC

In conclusion, most studies have suggested that PBT at biologically effective doses of 75–100 Gy(RBE) ($\alpha/\beta = 10$) and 80–130 Gy(RBE) ($\alpha/\beta = 3$) used clinically results in an LC rate of about 85–90% at three years and 80–90% at five years. However, intrahepatic recurrence, which is common in HCC, occurs in many cases. Consequently, the OS rate is about 55–65% at two years and 20–50% at five years. Adverse effects are quite rare in the acute and late phases. Most reports suggest the superiority of PBT over photon therapy for treatment of HCC. Reports of use of PBT for HCC are summarized in Table 9.1.

9.7   Treatment Factors in Proton Therapy

9.7.1   Liver Function and Coexisting Disease

HCC often develops from a cirrhotic liver. Liver cirrhosis is a progressive disease and treatment modalities for HCC are strictly limited for these patients because of the potential risk of liver failure. Therefore, HCC patients with severe cirrhosis are usually treated with palliative care. The median survival time for these patients is three–nine months and all die within three years [32–34]. Radiotherapy is not an option because the risk of RILD increases for patients with poor liver function. Chang et al. reported the results of stereotactic body radiotherapy (SBRT) for 16 patients [35]. There was no treatment-related toxicity for Child-Pugh class A cases, but severe liver failure was observed for two class B cases. In a dose escalation study using SBRT, Cardenes et al. [36] planned to use 48 Gy/3 fr for Child-Pugh class A cases and 42 Gy/3 fr for class B cases. However, toxicity was observed in the class B cases; therefore, the dose was decreased to 40 Gy/5 fr, but RILD still occurred in three cases with a Child-Pugh score ≥ 7.

Liver function is a risk factor for RILD and an important determining factor for use of PBT. Mizumoto et al. found that a favorable Child-Pugh score was significantly associated with a good prognosis [25], and Kawashima et al. showed that ICG 15 is related to good overall survival [20]. In an evaluation of the relationship of ICG 15 with Child-Pugh score, Mizumoto et al. [37] found that ICG 15 was related to a good prognosis and that the survival period depended on the ICG 15 score, even in Child-Pugh class A cases.

PBT can be indicated for cases with poor liver function or coexisting disease. Hata et al. studied use of PBT in 19 patients with Child-Pugh C cirrhosis [22] at total doses of 50–84 Gy(RBE) in 3–5 Gy(RBE) fractions. The two-year OS rate was 42% with a 63% objective response rate (CR and PR), and neither Grade 3 nor more severe treatment toxicity was observed. There was also no deterioration in the Child-Pugh score, but instead this score improved in 14 patients. These results suggest that PBT is less toxic for normal liver, and that inhibition of tumor progression improves liver function.

PBT has also been examined in patients with limited treatment options due to old age, unfavorable conditions, and comorbidities [38, 39]. For patients >80 years old, 66 Gy(RBE)/10 fr, 72.6 Gy(RBE)/22 fr, and 77 Gy(RBE)/35 fr were delivered based on the tumor locations, as mentioned above. Severe toxicity was not observed and three-year cause-specific survival was 88%, even though OS at three years was 62%. These results are comparable with data from other patients but were all from retrospective and small studies. However, PBT seems to be applicable for a variety of patients with HCC who are not suitable for other treatments, but poor PS is related to a poor prognosis based on a report by Fukuda et al. [40].

9.7.2 Tumor Size

There are various treatment options for patients with HCC. Surgery may be the best choice for large HCC, but <20% of patients are candidates for surgical resection. Tumor size is an important factor determining the treatment modality. For example, percutaneous ethanol injection is indicated for tumors <3 cm [41]. Radiofrequency ablation is usually indicated for tumors <5 cm and is contraindicated for tumors adjacent to a large vessel, such as the portal vein or inferior vena cava [42–44].

Radical photon radiotherapy has recently been used for HCC. The radiation tolerance of the liver is an important factor and can be determined by the preserved functional capacity [45]. In photon radiotherapy, large tumors require a wide low dose area in normal liver, and the risk of RILD is

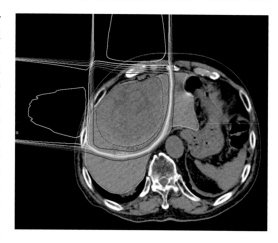

Fig. 9.3 Isodose curves of proton therapy for large HCC administered through the anterior and anterior right-lateral oblique ports represent 100–10% of the prescribed dose at 10% intervals. Proton therapy easily covers the HCC and avoids risk organs such as the digestive tract, normal liver, and spinal cord

increased. Even with intensity modulated radiotherapy (IMRT), the low dose area cannot be reduced, and may be increased. Therefore, for photon radiotherapy, only SBRT is usually indicated for small tumors of <5 cm, and large tumors are contraindicated for radical photon radiotherapy. In contrast, a proton beam can create give an appropriate dose distribution with a small number of ports (1–3 ports). Therefore, PBT can offer radical treatment for larger HCC beyond the ability of photon radiotherapy. Figure 9.3 shows the dose distribution in PBT for large HCC.

Kimura et al. reported that 24 patients with HCC > 5 cm received proton beam therapy with a median dose of 72.6 Gy(RBE)/22 fr [46]. The two-year LC and OS rates were 87.0% and 52.4%, respectively, and there were no severe acute or late toxicities. Sugahara et al. reported the results of 22 patients with large HCC of >10 cm in diameter [47] using a median dose of 72.6 Gy(RBE)/22 fr (range: 47.3–89.1 Gy(RBE)/10–35 fr). The two-year LC and OS rates were 87% (95% CI 65–100%) and 36% (15–56%), respectively, and there were no severe toxicities due to the treatment. Figure 9.3 shows isodose curves of proton beam therapy for large HCC. Proton therapy easily covere the HCC avoiding risk organ such as digestive tract, normal liver, and spinal cord. Nakamura et al. reported the results of PBT for nine patients with large HCC [48] with a cranio-caudal tumor size of 15.0–18.6 cm. In many centers, the treatment field is limited to ≤15 cm, and therefore a patch-field technique was used to irradiate these tumors. No local recurrence was observed, and the one- and two-year OS rates were 55 and 14%, respectively, with a median OS rate of 13.6%. A severe late effect of liver abscess was observed in one patient.

Experience with PBT for large HCC has not been extensive enough for this method to be accepted as a standard treatment modality. However, PBT seems to be worthy of evaluation when other treatment modalities are not effective due to tumor size.

9.7.3 Tumor Location and Protocol

Liver tumors occur in various locations, with some developing peripherally and some centrally in the liver parenchyma. Also, some tumors grow in the hepatic portal region and may invade the portal vein. Depending on the tumor location, different treatment protocols are used to protect surrounding tissues and organs. For a tumor in the hepatic portal region, bile duct stenosis is a severe problem after high dose radiotherapy. Chiba et al. reported that three of 162 patients had bile duct stenosis after PBT at doses of 79.2 Gy(RBE)/16 fr and 92.4 Gy(RBE)/24 fr [21]. Based on this finding, Mizumoto et al. conducted PBT in 55 patients with HCC adjacent to the porta hepatis at 72.6 Gy(RBE)/22 fr [24]. The three-year LC and OS rates were 86% and 50.0%, respectively, with no severe late toxicities, including bile duct stenosis.

HCC is also sometimes adjacent to the gastrointestinal tract, and in such cases hemorrhage, ulceration, and perforation of the gastrointestinal tract should be prevented. Nakayama et al. delivered doses of 72.6 Gy(RBE)/22 fr and 77 Gy(RBE)/35 fr in 47 patients with HCC located within 2 cm of the gastrointestinal tract [49]. The treatment margin was reduced to avoid excess radiation doses to the gastrointestinal tract at 33–39.6 Gy(RBE)/10–12 fr for a total dose of 72.6 Gy(RBE) or 50.6–55 Gy(RBE)/10–21 fr for a total dose of 77 Gy(RBE). The three-year local

progression-free survival (PFS) and OS were 88% and 50%, respectively, and gastrointestinal toxicity was observed in four patients: Grade 2 hemorrhage of the stomach ($n = 1$), Grade 2 and 3 colonic hemorrhage ($n = 2$), and Grade 2 hemorrhage in the hepatic flexure of the colon ($n = 1$). The irradiated volume of ≥50 Gy was 5.4, 5.1, and 25.8 ml for the patients with stomach, Grade 3 colonic, and Grade 2 hepatic flexure hemorrhages, respectively.

Dose escalation is possible for a peripherally located tumor. Fukumitsu et al. reported treatment results for HCC located >2 cm from the porta hepatis or gastrointestinal tract with PBT of 66 Gy(RBE)/10 fr [23]. The three- and five-year LC rates were 94.5% and 87.3%, respectively, and the three- and five-year OS rates were 49.2 and 38.7%, respectively. Three of the 51 patients developed rib fractures, but none had liver failure secondary to PBT. In this protocol, a V60 (60 Gy(RBE) dose at 2 Gy fractions [EQD2], when the alpha/beta ratio = 3) of the rib ≥ 4.48 cm^3 is a useful guide to predict rib fracture [50]. A comparison of three treatment protocols was performed by Mizumoto et al., but there were no significant differences in the results. The three- and five-year OS rates were 61% (95% CI: 53–68%) and 48% (38–57%), respectively, and the three- and five-year LC rates were 87% (81–97%) and 81% (68–94%), respectively [25].

Kawashima et al. and Bush et al. recently reported phase 2 studies for HCC treated with PBT[21,41]. The tumor location was not mentioned in these reports. Kawashima et al. used 76 Gy(RBE) in 3.8 Gy(RBE) once-daily fractions at four fractions in a week, and the two-year local PFS and OS were 96% (95% CI, 88–100%) and 66% (48–84%), respectively. Four of the 30 patients died of hepatic insufficiency without recurrence during the six–nine months after PBT. Bush et al. used 63 Gy(RBE) in 4.2-Gy daily fractions in 15 fractions over three weeks, the median survival time was 36 months (95% CI, 30–42 months), and local recurrence occurred in 15/76 patients (20%) with a mild treatment toxicity of Grade 2.

LC was excellent and OS was favorable in all these reports. Since the feasible treatment schedule varied, it is important that tumor location, especially for those near the gastrointestinal tract, is taken into consideration in selection of the treatment schedule.

9.7.4 Portal Vein Tumor Thrombosis (PVTT) and Inferior Vena Cava Tumor Thrombosis (IVCTT)

The prognosis of advanced HCC remains poor, especially in patients with PVTT or IVCTT. The incidence of PVTT and IVCTT is 44–84% and 31–50% in autopsy and clinical data, respectively [51–53]. The treatment options are strictly limited for these patients, and the prognosis for these patients remains extremely poor without treatment, with a median survival of only two–three months [54–57].

Standalone photon radiotherapy has been used for patients with tumor thrombosis, but the objective is often palliative care due to the low tolerance of the liver to radiation. Photon radiotherapy in combination with transarterial chemoembolization (TACE) has also been used [58–62]. In this treatment, radiotherapy was usually used to irradiate tumor thrombi only with a median total dose of 45–50 Gy delivered to the PVTT in fractions of 1.8–2.0 Gy, and TACE is used for intrahepatic tumors. The objective response rate was 50–79%, and OS at one and two years was 25–45% and 10–25%, respectively, with median survival ranging from 5.3 to 8.0 months. Severe treatment toxicities including gastrointestinal ulcers and bleeding were reported in 2–26% of cases.

There are also reports of use of PBT for PVTT and IVCTT therapy. The first use of PBT for PVTT was at the University of Tsukuba [63]. Twelve patients with a PVTT in the main trunk and the major branches of the portal vein were treated with a total dose of 50–72 Gy(RBE)/10–22 fr (RBE was calculated as 1.0 at the time). All treated tumor thrombi were controlled in a follow-up period of 0.3–7.3 years without ≥Grade 3 toxicities. Sugahara et al. [64] reported the results for 35 cases with PVTT treated by PBT of 72.6 Gy(RBE)/22 fr, of which 29 showed an objective response. The two- and five-year OS rates were 48% and 21%, respectively, and the median survival time was 22 months (range: 2–88 months). There were no severe toxicities.

In 2014, Lee et al. [65] reported the results of PBT for 27 patients with PVTT at a median dose of 50 Gy(RBE)/20–22 fr to the PVTT and primary tumor. PVTT showed an objective response and was stable in 56% and 37% of cases, respectively, and PBTT responders had significantly higher one-year OS (80 vs. 25%). No case had severe (>grade 3) toxicities. In 2017, Kim et al. used a simultaneous integrated boost (SIB) technique and treated tumor vascular thrombosis (TVT) to avoid overdoses to the gastrointestinal structure [66]. PTV2 was defined as ITV plus a 5–7 mm margin in all directions, and PTV1 as PTV2 minus the overlapping volume of PTV2 and a 10-mm expanded volume of the gastrointestinal tract. A dose of 50, 60 or 66 Gy/10 fr was delivered to PTV1 depending on the distance of the tumor from the gastrointestinal structure, and 30 Gy/10 fr was delivered to PTV2. The two-year LC rate was 88.1% and patients who received EQD2 ≥ 80 Gy(RBE)10 tended to show a better TVT response.

The first results for PBT for IVCTT were reported by Mizumoto et al. [67] PBT was performed for three patients, and the IVC was recanalized in all patients after treatment without severe toxicities. In 2011, Komatsu et al. reported results for 16 patients with IVCTT treated with particle radiotherapy [68], including 13 treated by PBT at 56–76 Gy(RBE)/8–38 fr. The other three patients were treated with carbon ions. The one- and three-year OS rates were 100% and 60%, respectively, in the curative treatment group, and all irradiated tumors showed complete shrinkage without severe toxicities. Sekino et al. used PBT for 21 patients with IVCTT in 2020 [69], and found no severe toxicities or local recurrence in the treatment region, including IVCTT, in a median follow-up period of 21 months. The OS rates were 62%, 33% and 19% at one, two, and three years, respectively.

The results of PBT for PVTT and IVCTT are positive and suggest that PBT may be effective and safe for patients who cannot receive other treatment modalities. However, these reports are all from retrospective studies from a single facility. Thus, additional larger and prospective studies are required to establish the efficacy of PBT for both PVTT and IVCTT.

9.7.5 Re-irradiation

HCC is generally a multicentric disease, especially when it is associated with HCV. Therefore, new tumors often develop sequentially, and repeated treatment is an unavoidable necessity. When the liver is irradiated widely at a high dose, RILD may occur. Emami et al. reported tolerance doses of 30, 35 and 50 Gy for the entire liver, two-thirds of the liver, and one-third of the liver, respectively [1]. Lawrence et al. suggested that the risk of radiation hepatitis increases with a mean dose to the whole liver >37 Gy [70]. Dawson et al. reported that the tolerance dose was >90 Gy when the irradiated volume was limited to one-third of the liver [71].

SBRT using photon beams is commonly used for small liver tumors (mainly liver metastases). In SBRT, multiple HCC can be treated at one time. Treatment beams can be selected without overlap for distant tumors, or adjacent small tumors can be treated as a single target. However, repeated radiotherapy for HCC is not common because it is difficult to avoid overlap of the beams and the tissue functional capacity is decreased. In contrast, PBT can be performed with minimal ports. Generally, 1–3 ports are used for one tumor; therefore, the low dose area is much smaller than with photon SBRT, and repeated PBT can be considered.

In a study of repeated PBT for 68 lesions in 27 patients [72], Hashimoto et al. found a LC rate of 87.8% and acute hepatic failure in only two patients in Child-Pugh classes B and C. It was concluded that repeated PBT for HCC was safe when the tumor was located in the peripheral region of the liver and liver function was Child-Pugh class A. Subsequently, Oshiro et al. reported a DVH analysis for 83 patients who received PBT two–four times for HCC, including cases with PVTT (19.2%) and IVCTT (9.6%) [73]. The maximal median cumulative dose to the liver was 131.2 Gy(RBE) (range: 66.7–248.1 Gy(RBE)), and the median mean liver dose was 21.7 Gy(RBE) (range: 5.4–66.5 Gy(RBE)) The two- and five-

year OS rates from the first PBT were 87.5% (95% CI: 80.2–94.8%) and 49.4% (95% CI: 37.6–61.2%), respectively. Eight patients (9.6%) died of hepatic failure and one had intestinal bleeding and underwent hemicolectomy eight months after the first PBT, but then received three further courses of PBT. Thus, repeated PBT for HCC seems to be safe and should be considered when other treatment modalities are not recommended.

9.8 Carbon Ion Radiotherapy

Carbon ion radiotherapy (CIRT) for HCC was first performed in Japan in 1995 at the National Institute of Radiological Science (NIRS) [74]. CIRT is also known to possess the Bragg peak and has biologically unique characteristics resulting in a higher cytocidal effect than PBT. Carbon ion radiotherapy has been used for HCC because of its excellent dose localization property. Most reports of CIRT for HCC were from NIRS and Gunma University.

Kato et al. showed the result of a phase I/II study by dose escalation with total dose of 49.5–79.5Gy(RBE) in 15 fractions [75]. No severe complications, no radiation induced liver disease, and no treatment death were observed even at the highest dose at 79.5 Gy(RBE). The cumulative three-year local control and survival were 81% and 50%, respectively. Kasuya et al. suggested treatment results for 124 patients with 133 HCCs treated with CIRT. In this study, 69.6 Gy(RBE)/12fr, 58.0 Gy(RBE)/8fr, and 52.8Gy(RBE)/4fr were used. The one-, three-, and five- year local control rate was 94.7% (95% CI: 89.9–97.6%), 91.4% (95% CI: 85.7–95.5%), and 90.0% (95% CI: 83.5–94.6%), and one-, three-, and five- year OS was 90.3% (95% CI: 83.6–94.4%), 50.0% (95% CI: 40.9–58.4%), and 25.0% (17.8–32.9%), respectively. They suggested that Child-Pugh class B and the presence of a tumor thrombus were significant factors for mortality [76].

CIRT with high dose and hypofractionation were progressed at NIRS. Shibuya et al. [77] reported treatment results with 48.0Gy(RBE)/2fr, 52.8 Gy(RBE)/4 fr and 60.0Gy(RBE)/4fr. The OS and LC at one, two, and three years were 95.4%,

82.5% and 73.3%; and 94.6%, 87.7% and 81.0%, respectively. Grade 3 or 4 toxicities and RILD were reported 5.7% and 1.7% of the patients, respectively. In this report, tumor size of <3 cm was one of the significant factors for better tumor control. After this report, they conducted another study of high dose hypo-fractionated CIRT for HCC of 3 cm or grater [78]. 60Gy(RBE)/4fr were delivered for 21 patients. The one- and two-year LC and OS were 100% and 92.3%; and 90.5% and 80.0%, respectively. Worsening Child- Pugh score at three and six months were reported in two of the 21 patients (15%). Yasuda et al. suggested long term results of CIRT with 45Gy(RBE)/2fr for 57 patients [79]. The one-, three-, and five-year tumor control rate was 98% (95% CI: 95–100%), 91% (95% CI: 87–95%) and 91% (95% CI: 87–95%), respectively, and the one-, three-, and five- year OS was 97% (95% CI: 95–100%), 67% (95% CI: 61–74%), and 45% (95% CI: 38–51%), respectively. No grade 3 or severer late toxicity was observed.

Shiba et al. [80] reported CIRT for 31 elder patients with HCC who are 80 years or older with the treatment dose of 52.8 Gy(RBE) or 60.0 Gy(RBE) in 4 fr, and they suggested there were no severe late toxicities and estimated two-year LC and OS were 89.2% and 82.3%, respectively. They also conducted comparison study of CIRT vs TACE for single HCC [81]. One hundred twenty-four patients received CIRT and 353 received TACE, and the treatment results were favored in the CIRT group. The three-year OS, LC, and PFS in CIRT vs. TACE were 88 vs. 58% ($p < 0.05$), 80 vs. 26% ($p < 0.01$), and 51 vs. 15% ($p < 0.05$), respectively.

9.9 Summary

PBT has progressed over 40 years and there are now many results for outcomes of PBT for HCC (Table 9.1). Proton beams are advantageous for liver tumors due to the energy peak. PBT for HCC is effective and safe, even for cases with PVTT or IVCTT, poor liver function, and coexisting disease, and is a good alternative to other treatment.

References

1. Emami B, Lyman J, Brown A, Coia L, Goitein M, Munzenrider JE, Shank B, Solin LJ, Wesson M. Tolerance of normal tissue to therapeutic irradiation. Int J Radiat Oncol Biol Phys. 1991;21:109–22.
2. The American Society for Radiation Oncology. Proton beam therpay model policy issued by ASTRO 2014.
3. Breuer H, Smit BJ. Proton therapy and radio-surgery. 1st ed. Berlin: Springer; 2000.
4. Paganetti H, Niemierko A, Ancukiewicz M, Gerweck LE, Goitein M, Loeffler JS, Suit HD. Relative biological effectiveness (RBE) values for proton beam therapy. Int J Radiat Oncol Biol Phys. 2002;53:407–21.
5. Wambersie A. RBE, reference RBE and clinical RBE: applications of these concepts in hadron therapy. Strahlenther Onkol. 1999;175(Suppl 2):39–43.
6. Di Pietro C, Piro S, Tabbi G, Ragusa M, Di Pietro V, Zimmitti V, Cuda F, Anello M, Consoli U, Salinaro ET, Caruso M, Vancheri C, Crimi N, Sabini MG, Cirrone GA, Raffaele L, Privitera G, Pulvirenti A, Giugno R, Ferro A, Cuttone G, Lo Nigro S, Purrello R, Purrello F, Purrello M. Cellular and molecular effects of protons: apoptosis induction and potential implications for cancer therapy. Apoptosis. 2006;11:57–66.
7. Gerelchuluun A, Hong Z, Sun L, Suzuki K, Terunuma T, Yasuoka K, Sakae T, Moritake T, Tsuboi K. Induction of in situ DNA double-strand breaks and apoptosis by 200 MeV protons and 10 MV X-rays in human tumour cell lines. Int J Radiat Biol. 2011;87:57–70.
8. Rutherford E. Collisions of alpha particles with light atoms. II. Nitrogen and oxygen atoms. The Philosophical Magazine. 1919;37:571–80.
9. Rutherford E. Collision of a particle with light atoms. IV. An anomalous effect in nitrogen (Reprint from philosophical Magazine Series 6, Vol 37, pg 581–587. 1919). Philos Mag. 2010;90:31–7.
10. Wilson RR. Radiological use of fast protons. Radiology. 1946;47:487–91.
11. Gragoudas ES, Goitein M, Koehler AM, Verhey L, Tepper J, Suit HD, Brockhurst R, Constable IJ. Proton irradiation of small choroidal malignant melanomas. Am J Ophthalmol. 1977;83:665–73.
12. Matsuzaki Y, Osuga T, Saito Y, Chuganji Y, Tanaka N, Shoda J, Tsuji H, Tsujii H. A new, effective, and safe therapeutic option using proton irradiation for hepatocellular carcinoma. Gastroenterology. 1994;106:1032–41.
13. Tsujii H, Inada T, Maruhashi A, Hayakawa Y, Tsuji H, Ohara K, Akisada M, Kitagawa T. [Field localization and verification system for proton beam radiotherapy in deep-seated tumors]. Nihon Igaku Hoshasen Gakkai Zasshi. 1989;49:622–29.
14. Arimoto T, Takase Y, Ishikawa N, Yoshii Y, Ishikawa S, Otani M, Kaneko M, Nishida M, Kitagawa T. [Investigation of marking procedure for markers in deep-seated organs by proton beam therapy]. Gan No Rinsho. 1988;34:395–403.

15. Ohara K, Okumura T, Akisada M, Inada T, Mori T, Yokota H, Calaguas MJB. Irradiation synchronized with respiration gate. Int J Radiat Oncol. 1989;17:853–7.

16. Kooy HM, Grassberger C. Intensity modulated proton therapy. Br J Radiol. 2015;88:20150195.

17. Bush DA, Smith JC, Slater JD, Volk ML, Reeves ME, Cheng J, Grove R, de Vera ME. Randomized clinical trial comparing proton beam radiation therapy with transarterial chemoembolization for hepatocellular carcinoma: results of an interim analysis. Int J Radiat Oncol Biol Phys. 2016;95:477–82.

18. Bush DA, Hillebrand DJ, Slater JM, Slater JD. High-dose proton beam radiotherapy of hepatocellular carcinoma: preliminary results of a phase II trial. Gastroenterology. 2004;127:S189–93.

19. Bush DA, Kayali Z, Grove R, Slater JD. The safety and efficacy of high-dose proton beam radiotherapy for hepatocellular carcinoma: a phase 2 prospective trial. Cancer. 2011;117:3053–9.

20. Kawashima M, Furuse J, Nishio T, Konishi M, Ishii H, Kinoshita T, Nagase M, Nihei K, Ogino T. Phase II study of radiotherapy employing proton beam for hepatocellular carcinoma. J Clin Oncol. 2005;23:1839–46.

21. Chiba T, Tokuuye K, Matsuzaki Y, Sugahara S, Chuganji Y, Kagei K, Shoda J, Hata M, Abei M, Igaki H, Tanaka N, Akine Y. Proton beam therapy for hepatocellular carcinoma: a retrospective review of 162 patients. Clin Cancer Res. 2005;11:3799–805.

22. Hata M, Tokuuye K, Sugahara S, Fukumitsu N, Hashimoto T, Ohnishi K, Nemoto K, Ohara K, Matsuzaki Y, Akine Y. Proton beam therapy for hepatocellular carcinoma patients with severe cirrhosis. Strahlenther Onkol. 2006;182:713–20.

23. Fukumitsu N, Sugahara S, Nakayama H, Fukuda K, Mizumoto M, Abei M, Shoda J, Thono E, Tsuboi K, Tokuuye K. A prospective study of hypofractionated proton beam therapy for patients with hepatocellular carcinoma. Int J Radiat Oncol Biol Phys. 2009;74:831–6.

24. Mizumoto M, Tokuuye K, Sugahara S, Nakayama H, Fukumitsu N, Ohara K, Abei M, Shoda J, Tohno E, Minami M. Proton beam therapy for hepatocellular carcinoma adjacent to the porta hepatis. Int J Radiat Oncol Biol Phys. 2008;71:462–7.

25. Mizumoto M, Okumura T, Hashimoto T, Fukuda K, Oshiro Y, Fukumitsu N, Abei M, Kawaguchi A, Hayashi Y, Ookawa A, Hashii H, Kanemoto A, Moritake T, Tohno E, Tsuboi K, Sakae T, Sakurai H. Proton beam therapy for hepatocellular carcinoma: a comparison of three treatment protocols. Int J Radiat Oncol Biol Phys. 2011;81:1039–45.

26. Hong TS, DeLaney TF, Mamon HJ, Willett CG, Yeap BY, Niemierko A, Wolfgang JA, Lu HM, Adams J, Weyman EA, Arellano RS, Blaszkowsky LS, Allen JN, Tanabe KK, Ryan DP, Zhu AX. A prospective feasibility study of respiratory-gated proton beam therapy for liver tumors. Pract Radiat Oncol. 2014;4:316–22.

27. Kim TH, Park JW, Kim YJ, Kim BH, Woo SM, Moon SH, Kim SS, Koh YH, Lee WJ, Park SJ, Kim JY, Kim DY, Kim CM. Phase I dose-escalation study of proton beam therapy for inoperable hepatocellular carcinoma. Cancer Res Treat. 2015;47:34–45.

28. Chadha AS, Gunther JR, Hsieh CE, Aliru M, Mahadevan LS, Venkatesulu BP, Crane CH, Das P, Herman JM, Koay EJ, Taniguchi C, Holliday EB, Minsky BD, Suh Y, Park P, Sawakuchi G, Beddar S, Odisio BC, Gupta S, Loyer E, Kaur H, Raghav K, Javle MM, Kaseb AO, Krishnan S. Proton beam therapy outcomes for localized unresectable hepatocellular carcinoma. Radiother Oncol. 2019;133:54–61.

29. Komatsu S, Fukumoto T, Demizu Y, Miyawaki D, Terashima K, Sasaki R, Hori Y, Hishikawa Y, Ku Y, Murakami M. Clinical results and risk factors of proton and carbon ion therapy for hepatocellular carcinoma. Cancer. 2011;117:4890–904.

30. Sanford NN, Pursley J, Noe B, Yeap BY, Goyal L, Clark JW, Allen JN, Blaszkowsky LS, Ryan DP, Ferrone CR, Tanabe KK, Qadan M, Crane CH, Koay EJ, Eyler C, DeLaney TF, Zhu AX, Wo JY, Grassberger C, Hong TS. Protons versus photons for unresectable hepatocellular carcinoma: liver decompensation and overall survival. Int J Radiat Oncol Biol Phys. 2019;105:64–72.

31. Sumiya T, Mizumoto M, Oshiro Y, Baba K, Murakami M, Shimizu S, Nakamura M, Hiroshima Y, Ishida T, Iizumi T, Saito T, Numajiri H, Nakai K, Okumura T, Sakurai H. Transitions of liver and biliary enzymes during proton beam therapy for hepatocellular carcinoma. Cancers (Basel). 2020;12:1840.

32. Blum HE. Treatment of hepatocellular carcinoma. Best Pract Res Clin Gastroenterol. 2005;19:129–45.

33. Llovet JM, Bustamante J, Castells A, Vilana R, Ayuso Mdel C, Sala M, Bru C, Rodes J, Bruix J. Natural history of untreated nonsurgical hepatocellular carcinoma: rationale for the design and evaluation of therapeutic trials. Hepatology. 1999;29:62–7.

34. Markovic S, Gadzijev E, Stabuc B, Croce LS, Masutti F, Surlan M, Berden P, Brencic E, Visnar-Perovic A, Sasso F, Ferlan-Marolt V, Mucelli FP, Cesar R, Sponza M, Tiribelli C. Treatment options in Western hepatocellular carcinoma: a prospective study of 224 patients. J Hepatol. 1998;29:650–9.

35. Chan LC, Chiu SK, Chan SL. Stereotactic radiotherapy for hepatocellular carcinoma: report of a local single-centre experience. Hong Kong Med J. 2011;17:112–8.

36. Cardenes HR, Price TR, Perkins SM, Maluccio M, Kwo P, Breen TE, Henderson MA, Schefter TE, Tudor K, Deluca J, Johnstone PA. Phase I feasibility trial of stereotactic body radiation therapy for primary hepatocellular carcinoma. Clin Transl Oncol. 2010;12:218–25.

37. Mizumoto M, Oshiro Y, Okumura T, Fukuda K, Fukumitsu N, Abei M, Ishikawa H, Ohnishi K, Numajiri H, Tsuboi K, Sakurai H. Association between pretreatment retention rate of indocyanine green 15 min after administration and life prognosis in patients with HCC treated by proton beam therapy. Radiother Oncol. 2014;113:54–9.

38. Hata M, Tokuuye K, Sugahara S, Fukumitsu N, Hashimoto T, Ohnishi K, Nemoto K, Ohara K, Matsuzaki Y, Akine Y. Proton beam therapy for hepatocellular carcinoma with limited treatment options. Cancer. 2006;107:591–8.

39. Hata M, Tokuuye K, Sugahara S, Tohno E, Nakayama H, Fukumitsu N, Mizumoto M, Abei M, Shoda J, Minami M, Akine Y. Proton beam therapy for aged patients with hepatocellular carcinoma. Int J Radiat Oncol Biol Phys. 2007;69:805–12.

40. Fukuda K, Okumura T, Abei M, Fukumitsu N, Ishige K, Mizumoto M, Hasegawa N, Numajiri H, Ohnishi K, Ishikawa H, Tsuboi K, Sakurai H, Hyodo I. Long-term outcomes of proton beam therapy in patients with previously untreated hepatocellular carcinoma. Cancer Sci. 2017;108:497–503.

41. Sitruk V, Seror O, Grando-Lemaire V, Mohand D, N'Kontchou G, Ganne-Carrie N, Beaugrand M, Sellier N, Trinchet JC. [Percutaneous ablation of hepatocellular carcinoma]. Gastroenterol Clin Biol. 2003;27:381–90.

42. Lencioni RA, Allgaier HP, Cioni D, Olschewski M, Deibert P, Crocetti L, Frings H, Laubenberger J, Zuber I, Blum HE, Bartolozzi C. Small hepatocellular carcinoma in cirrhosis: randomized comparison of radio-frequency thermal ablation versus percutaneous ethanol injection. Radiology. 2003;228:235–40.

43. Lin SM, Lin CJ, Lin CC, Hsu CW, Chen YC. Radiofrequency ablation improves prognosis compared with ethanol injection for hepatocellular carcinoma < or =4 cm. Gastroenterology. 2004;127:1714–23.

44. Shiina S, Teratani T, Obi S, Sato S, Tateishi R, Fujishima T, Ishikawa T, Koike Y, Yoshida H, Kawabe T, Omata M. A randomized controlled trial of radiofrequency ablation with ethanol injection for small hepatocellular carcinoma. Gastroenterology. 2005;129:122–30.

45. Ohara K, Okumura T, Tsuji H, Chiba T, Min M, Tatsuzaki H, Tsujii H, Akine Y, Itai Y. Radiation tolerance of cirrhotic livers in relation to the preserved functional capacity: analysis of patients with hepatocellular carcinoma treated by focused proton beam radiotherapy. Int J Radiat Oncol Biol Phys. 1997;38:367–72.

46. Kimura K, Nakamura T, Ono T, Azami Y, Suzuki M, Wada H, Takayama K, Endo H, Takeyama T, Hirose K, Takai Y, Kikuchi Y. Clinical results of proton beam therapy for hepatocellular carcinoma over 5 cm. Hepatol Res. 2017;47:1368–74.

47. Sugahara S, Oshiro Y, Nakayama H, Fukuda K, Mizumoto M, Abei M, Shoda J, Matsuzaki Y, Thono E, Tokita M, Tsuboi K, Tokuuye K. Proton beam therapy for large hepatocellular carcinoma. Int J Radiat Oncol Biol Phys. 2010;76:460–6.

48. Nakamura M, Fukumitsu N, Kamizawa S, Numajiri H, Nemoto Murofushi K, Ohnishi K, Aihara T, Ishikawa H, Okumura T, Tsuboi K, Sakurai H. A validated proton beam therapy patch-field protocol for effective treatment of large hepatocellular carcinoma. J Radiat Res. 2018;59:632–8.

49. Nakayama H, Sugahara S, Fukuda K, Abei M, Shoda J, Sakurai H, Tsuboi K, Matsuzaki Y, Tokuuye K. Proton beam therapy for hepatocellular carcinoma located adjacent to the alimentary tract. Int J Radiat Oncol Biol Phys. 2011;80:992–5.

50. Kanemoto A, Mizumoto M, Okumura T, Takahashi H, Hashimoto T, Oshiro Y, Fukumitsu N, Moritake T, Tsuboi K, Sakae T, Sakurai H. Dose-volume histogram analysis for risk factors of radiation-induced rib fracture after hypofractionated proton beam therapy for hepatocellular carcinoma. Acta Oncol. 2013;52:538–44.

51. Pirisi M, Avellini C, Fabris C, Scott C, Bardus P, Soardo G, Beltrami CA, Bartoli E. Portal vein thrombosis in hepatocellular carcinoma: age and sex distribution in an autopsy study. J Cancer Res Clin Oncol. 1998;124:397–400.

52. Fong Y, Sun RL, Jarnagin W, Blumgart LH. An analysis of 412 cases of hepatocellular carcinoma at a Western center. Ann Surg. 1999;229:790–9. discussion 799-800

53. Stuart KE, Anand AJ, Jenkins RL. Hepatocellular carcinoma in the United States. Prognostic features, treatment outcome, and survival. Cancer. 1996;77:2217–22.

54. Lee HS, Kim JS, Choi IJ, Chung JW, Park JH, Kim CY. The safety and efficacy of transcatheter arterial chemoembolization in the treatment of patients with hepatocellular carcinoma and main portal vein obstruction. A prospective controlled study. Cancer. 1997;79:2087–94.

55. Okuda K, Ohtsuki T, Obata H, Tomimatsu M, Okazaki N, Hasegawa H, Nakajima Y, Ohnishi K. Natural history of hepatocellular carcinoma and prognosis in relation to treatment. Study of 850 patients. Cancer. 1985;56:918–28.

56. Pawarode A, Voravud N, Sriuranpong V, Kullavanijaya P, Patt YZ. Natural history of untreated primary hepatocellular carcinoma: a retrospective study of 157 patients. Am J Clin Oncol. 1998;21:386–91.

57. Nagasue N, Yukaya H, Hamada T, Hirose S, Kanashima R, Inokuchi K. The natural history of hepatocellular carcinoma. A study of 100 untreated cases. Cancer. 1984;54:1461–5.

58. Ishikura S, Ogino T, Furuse J, Satake M, Baba S, Kawashima M, Nihei K, Ito Y, Maru Y, Ikeda H. Radiotherapy after transcatheter arterial chemoembolization for patients with hepatocellular carcinoma and portal vein tumor thrombus. Am J Clin Oncol. 2002;25:189–93.

59. Obi S, Yoshida H, Toune R, Unuma T, Kanda M, Sato S, Tateishi R, Teratani T, Shiina S, Omata M. Combination therapy of intraarterial 5-fluorouracil and systemic interferon-alpha for advanced hepatocellular carcinoma with portal venous invasion. Cancer. 2006;106:1990–7.

60. Hsu WC, Chan SC, Ting LL, Chung NN, Wang PM, Ying KS, Shin JS, Chao CJ, Lin GD. Results of three-dimensional conformal radiotherapy and thalidomide for advanced hepatocellular carcinoma. Jpn J Clin Oncol. 2006;36:93–9.

61. Nakagawa K, Yamashita H, Shiraishi K, Nakamura N, Tago M, Igaki H, Hosoi Y, Shiina S, Omata M, Makuuchi M, Ohtomo K. Radiation therapy for portal venous invasion by hepatocellular carcinoma. World J Gastroenterol. 2005;11:7237–41.

62. Ota H, Nagano H, Sakon M, Eguchi H, Kondo M, Yamamoto T, Nakamura M, Damdinsuren B, Wada H, Marubashi S, Miyamoto A, Dono K, Umeshita K, Nakamori S, Wakasa K, Monden M. Treatment of hepatocellular carcinoma with major portal vein thrombosis by combined therapy with subcutaneous interferon-alpha and intra-arterial 5-fluorouracil; role of type 1 interferon receptor expression. Br J Cancer. 2005;93:557–64.

63. Hata M, Tokuuye K, Sugahara S, Kagei K, Igaki H, Hashimoto T, Ohara K, Matsuzaki Y, Tanaka N, Akine Y. Proton beam therapy for hepatocellular carcinoma with portal vein tumor thrombus. Cancer. 2005;104:794–801.

64. Sugahara S, Nakayama H, Fukuda K, Mizumoto M, Tokita M, Abei M, Shoda J, Matsuzaki Y, Thono E, Tsuboi K, Tokuuye K. Proton-beam therapy for hepatocellular carcinoma associated with portal vein tumor thrombosis. Strahlenther Onkol. 2009;185:782–8.

65. Lee SU, Park JW, Kim TH, Kim YJ, Woo SM, Koh YH, Lee WJ, Park SJ, Kim DY, Kim CM. Effectiveness and safety of proton beam therapy for advanced hepatocellular carcinoma with portal vein tumor thrombosis. Strahlenther Onkol. 2014;190:806–14.

66. Kim TH, Park JW, Kim BH, Kim DY, Moon SH, Kim SS, Lee JH, Woo SM, Koh YH, Lee WJ, Kim CM. Optimal time of tumour response evaluation and effectiveness of hypofractionated proton beam therapy for inoperable or recurrent hepatocellular carcinoma. Oncotarget. 2018;9:4034–43.

67. Mizumoto M, Tokuuye K, Sugahara S, Hata M, Fukumitsu N, Hashimoto T, Ohnishi K, Nemoto K, Ohara K, Matsuzaki Y, Tohno E, Akine Y. Proton beam therapy for hepatocellular carcinoma with inferior vena cava tumor thrombus: report of three cases. Jpn J Clin Oncol. 2007;37:459–62.

68. Komatsu S, Fukumoto T, Demizu Y, Miyawaki D, Terashima K, Niwa Y, Mima M, Fujii O, Sasaki R, Yamada I, Hori Y, Hishikawa Y, Abe M, Ku Y, Murakami M. The effectiveness of particle radiotherapy for hepatocellular carcinoma associated with inferior vena cava tumor thrombus. J Gastroenterol. 2011;46:913–20.

69. Sekino Y, Okumura T, Fukumitsu N, Iizumi T, Numajiri H, Mizumoto M, Nakai K, Nonaka T, Ishikawa H, Sakurai H. Proton beam therapy for hepatocellular carcinoma associated with inferior vena cava tumor thrombus. J Cancer Res Clin Oncol. 2020;146:711–20.

70. Lawrence TS, Ten Haken RK, Kessler ML, Robertson JM, Lyman JT, Lavigne ML, Brown MB, DuRoss DJ, Andrews JC, Ensminger WD, et al. The use of 3-D dose volume analysis to predict radiation hepatitis. Int J Radiat Oncol Biol Phys. 1992;23:781–8.

71. Dawson LA, Ten Haken RK, Lawrence TS. Partial irradiation of the liver. Semin Radiat Oncol. 2001;11:240–6.

72. Hashimoto T, Tokuuye K, Fukumitsu N, Igaki H, Hata M, Kagei K, Sugahara S, Ohara K, Matsuzaki Y, Akine Y. Repeated proton beam therapy for hepatocellular carcinoma. Int J Radiat Oncol Biol Phys. 2006;65:196–202.

73. Oshiro Y, Mizumoto M, Okumura T, Fukuda K, Fukumitsu N, Abei M, Ishikawa H, Takizawa D, Sakurai H. Analysis of repeated proton beam therapy for patients with hepatocellular carcinoma. Radiother Oncol. 2017;123:240–5.

74. Tsujii H, Mizoe J, Kamada T, Baba M, Tsuji H, Kato H, Kato S, Yamada S, Yasuda S, Ohno T, Yanagi T, Imai R, Kagei K, Kato H, Hara R, Hasegawa A, Nakajima M, Sugane N, Tamaki N, Takagi R, Kandatsu S, Yoshikawa K, Kishimoto R, Miyamoto T. Clinical results of carbon ion radiotherapy at NIRS. J Radiat Res. 2007;48(Suppl A):A1–A13.

75. Kato H, Tsujii H, Miyamoto T, Mizoe JE, Kamada T, Tsuji H, Yamada S, Kandatsu S, Yoshikawa K, Obata T, Ezawa H, Morita S, Tomizawa M, Morimoto N, Fujita J, Ohto M. Results of the first prospective study of carbon ion radiotherapy for hepatocellular carcinoma with liver cirrhosis. Int J Radiat Oncol Biol Phys. 2004;59:1468–76.

76. Kasuya G, Kato H, Yasuda S, Tsuji H, Yamada S, Haruyama Y, Kobashi G, Ebner DK, Okada NN, Makishima H, Miyazaki M, Kamada T, Tsujii H, Liver Cancer Working Group. Progressive hypofractionated carbon-ion radiotherapy for hepatocellular carcinoma: combined analyses of 2 prospective trials. Cancer. 2017;123:3955–65.

77. Shibuya K, Ohno T, Terashima K, Toyama S, Yasuda S, Tsuji H, Okimoto T, Shioyama Y, Nemoto K, Kamada T, Nakano T, Japan Carbon Ion Radiotherapy Study Group. Short-course carbon-ion radiotherapy for hepatocellular carcinoma: a multi-institutional retrospective study. Liver Int. 2018;38:2239–47.

78. Shibuya K, Ohno T, Katoh H, Okamoto M, Shiba S, Koyama Y, Kakizaki S, Shirabe K, Nakano T. A feasibility study of high-dose hypofractionated carbon ion radiation therapy using four fractions for localized hepatocellular carcinoma measuring 3cm or larger. Radiother Oncol. 2019;132:230–5.

79. Yasuda S, Kato H, Imada H, Isozaki Y, Kasuya G, Makishima H, Tsuji H, Ebner DK, Yamada S, Kamada T, Tsujii H, Kato N, Miyazaki M, Working Group for Liver Tumor. Long-term results of high-dose 2-fraction carbon ion radiation therapy for hepatocellular carcinoma. Adv Radiat Oncol. 2020;5:196–203.

80. Shiba S, Abe T, Shibuya K, Katoh H, Koyama Y, Shimada H, Kakizaki S, Shirabe K, Kuwano H, Ohno T, Nakano T. Carbon ion radiotherapy for 80 years or older patients with hepatocellular carcinoma. BMC Cancer. 2017;17:721.

81. Shiba S, Shibuya K, Katoh H, Kaminuma T, Miyazaki M, Kakizaki S, Shirabe K, Ohno T, Nakano T. A comparison of carbon ion radiotherapy and transarterial chemoembolization treatment outcomes for single hepatocellular carcinoma: a propensity score matching study. Radiat Oncol. 2019;14:137.

Internal Radiotherapy Using Radionuclides

10

Aaron Kian-Ti Tong, David Chee-Eng Ng, and Pierce Kah-Hoe Chow

Abstract

Selective internal radiation therapy (SIRT) is a form of locoregional treatment using radiation from radiolabelled particles or ligands for liver cancer. This modality has seen significant advancements in recent times with robust scientific evidence backing the expanding therapeutic applications. The common indications for SIRT are reviewed based on current evidence, including the results of major clinical trials. Technological advances in hybrid imaging and interventional radiology have contributed to the use of planning dosimetry for dose activity prescriptions. There is emerging data to show that this leads to better patient outcomes. The recent phase III trials have also highlighted a good safety profile and better tolerance of SIRT compared to the current standard of care systemic treatment. There is potential for combining external beam radiotherapy with SIRT under certain clinical circumstances and new data will be eagerly expected in this area.

Keywords

Yttrium-90 · Selective internal radiation therapy · Radioembolisation · Hepatocellular carcinoma · Liver tumours · Personalised dosimetry · MAA SPECT/CT · 90Y PET/CT

A. K.-T. Tong (✉) · D. C.-E. Ng
Department of Nuclear Medicine and Molecular Imaging, Singapore General Hospital, Singapore, Singapore

Radiological Sciences Academic Clinical Programme, DUKE-NUS Medical School, Singapore, Singapore
e-mail: aaron.tong.k.t@singhealth.com.sg; david.ng.c.e@singhealth.com.sg

P. K.-H. Chow
Surgery and Surgical Oncology, Singapore General Hospital and National Cancer Center Singapore, Singapore, Singapore

Surgery Academic Clinical Programme, DUKE-NUS Medical School, Singapore, Singapore
e-mail: pierce.chow.k.h@nccs.com.sg

10.1 Introduction

Liver cancer is one of the leading causes of cancer death worldwide. In the recent two decades, there have been significant advances in therapy for both primary and secondary liver tumours, including selective internal radiation therapy (SIRT). This chapter will provide an overview of liver cancer treatment in the form of selective internal administration of therapeutic radionuclides to the liver. A small section will address the combined roles of SIRT with external beam radiotherapy (EBRT).

To understand how SIRT is performed, one must first understand the anatomy and pathological changes in the diseased tumoural liver. Unlike most organs, a dual blood supply exists in the liver: the hepatic arterial supply and portal venous supply. Hepatocellular carcinoma (HCC) nodules have a reduced portal venous supply and a normal hepatic arterial supply while intranodular arterial supply through new abnormal arteries increases gradually. Liver metastases larger than 3 mm also derive most of their blood supply from arterial circulation instead of the portal vein. These pathological changes provide the basis for which radionuclides can be administered intraarterially to achieve a therapeutic effect.

A surgeon from New York was an early pioneer in SIRT using Yttrium-90 (Y-90) microspheres for therapy of hepatic metastases from colorectal carcinoma. This was performed in animal experiments and followed by a few human volunteers [1]. Subsequently, the use of Y-90 oxide was then described to treat hepatocellular carcinoma (HCC) in humans.

SIRT is commonly performed using the radioisotope Y-90 where microspheres containing Y-90 are injected into hepatic arteries that supply the hepatic tumour. The practice in many centres is to perform a planning angiogram to interrogate the liver vasculature a week or two before Y-90 microspheres treatment. A radiation simulation study is performed by injecting Technetium-99 m labelled macroaggregrated albumin (Tc-99m MAA) particles, which are similar in size to the Y-90 microspheres, at the time of the planning angiogram. Theranostics concepts are applied to SIRT by using the pre-treatment Tc-99m MAA scintigram, together with post-treatment scanning. The personalised dosimetric calculations from the imaging allow for radiation dose planning to the hepatic tumours and are strongly advocated.

10.2 Therapeutic Radionuclides: Iodine-131, Yttrium-90, Holmium-166, Rhenium-188

There are a few radionuclides identified to have suitable properties for SIRT of hepatic tumours by harnessing the beta radiation emitted.

I-131 is a beta-/gamma-emitting radionuclide with a physical half-life of 8.04 days. The maximum and mean beta particle energies are 0.61 MeV and 0.192 MeV, respectively. I-131 emits a principal gamma photon of 364 keV (81% abundance). It can be chemically bound to lipiodol which is a naturally iodinated fatty acid ethyl ester of poppy seed oil. I-131 lipiodol has been used since the 1990s for palliation in HCC. Another similar study using Rhenium-188 lipoidal has also been published.

Yttrium-90 is the most described radionuclide used for SIRT and is a stronger beta emitter than I-131 with a mean energy of 0.9367 MeV and a physical half-life of 64.1 h (2.67 days). Y-90 microspheres entrapped within the liver parenchyma have a mean tissue penetration of 2.5 mm and a maximum range of 11 mm in tissues. Greater than 90% of the Y-90 microspheres radiation dose is delivered during the first 11 days post treatment. According to the Medical Internal Radiation Dose (MIRD) principle, one gigabecquerel (GBq) of Y-90 distributed homogenously throughout 1 kg of tissue provides an absorbed dose of approximately 50 Gy [2]. It also has minimal internal pair production (32 ppm) which allows for diagnostic PET imaging. Currently, there are two types of Y-90 microspheres available: resin microspheres and glass microspheres. The average size of resin microspheres is about 30% larger than glass microspheres while glass microspheres have a higher specific activity than the resin microspheres. Glass microspheres contain 2500 Bq per microsphere and about 1–2 million microspheres are infused for a typical patient. Resin microspheres contain about 50 Bq per microsphere and a typical treatment contains 40–60 million microspheres.

Holmium-166 (Ho-166) microspheres are newly developed recently becoming available commercially in Europe for SIRT in unresectable hepatic tumours. These Ho-166 microspheres emit both gamma (81 keV) and beta radiation as compared to Y-90 microspheres, and hence this new modality has unique imaging as well as dosing possibilities. Additionally, Ho-166 microspheres can be used as a planning dose instead of infusing Tc-99m MAA, and in theory, this should have superior performance for a radiation simulation scan. In addition, there is some possibility of imaging holmium-166 using MRI. There are two known phase I and phase II studies done using Ho-166 SIRT for liver metastases from mixed origins showing safety and tumour response [3]. There is also a completed phase II study that recruited 30 patients with metastatic neuroendocrine tumour pretreated with four cycles of Lu-177 Peptide Receptor Radionuclide Therapy (PRRT) and subsequently treated with Ho-166 SIRT which demonstrated safety and efficacious results [4]. It is anticipated that this new modality may change the way SIRT is practised.

10.3 Patient Selection and Evidence for Y-90 SIRT in Hepatic Malignancies

Hepatocellular carcinoma (HCC) is the most common form of primary liver tumour. In early HCC, treatment with curative intent can be performed with surgical resection, liver transplantation, or local ablative therapy, e.g., cryo-, radiofrequency or microwave in a select clinical setting. However, locally advanced or metastatic HCC is the usual presentation in a large majority of patients while many patients are also poor surgical candidates for resection. In most cases, HCC is diagnosed in the intermediate-advanced stage (stage B and C according to the Barcelona Clinic Liver Cancer (BCLC) staging categories), when radical therapy is not feasible. The median survival of untreated inoperable HCC is usually several months and this calls for effective use of locoregional treatments as alternatives. Y-90 SIRT has been shown in many studies to be an effective treatment that is well tolerated in these patients.

The liver is the most frequent site of metastasis for patients with colorectal cancer. Historical data has shown that the median survival of patients without treatment ranges from 3 to 12 months, with overall median survival of 7 months [5]. Although surgical resection provides the most favourable outcomes, rates of hepatic resection for metastases at the point of diagnosis are generally low and only a minority of patients benefit from surgery. The use of cytoreduction can improve functionality as well as prolong survival and SIRT is one such modality that can encompass the entire liver as compared to other locoregional therapies such as percutaneous cryoablation or microwave ablation.

The current guidelines on patient selection for SIRT are largely in tandem, all requiring adequate liver function, good vascular access, and minimal hepatopulmonary shunting to prevent complications [6]. There are five main clinical scenarios for which SIRT can be employed:

1. The first situation is radiation segmentectomy with curative intent in which a small solitary tumour is detected in the liver, but the patient is unsuitable for or has declined surgery and are not amenable to other curative locoregional treatments. Radiation segmentectomy is a methodology that gives a high radiation dose activity administered to the tumour containing perfused hepatic segment essentially killing the tumour and its adjacent normal hepatic parenchyma. Details on radiation dose activity prescription and absorbed dose thresholds will be discussed in the personalised dosimetry section in the later part of this book chapter.

2. The second clinical scenario frequently referred to for SIRT would be downstaging to surgical resection. Such patients usually are found with a solitary large left or right hepatic tumour that is inoperable but holds potential for downstaging to curative surgery by shrinking the tumour via SIRT. Selected patients may also benefit from contralateral lobe hypertrophy of the normal liver if a unilobar SIRT treatment was performed, especially if the future remnant liver volume was a limiting factor for surgical resection initially. A recent systemic review has shown that the administration of unilobar SIRT results in significant hypertrophy of the contralateral liver lobe comparable to that of portal vein embolisation and helps explain why SIRT is of valuable interest to liver surgeons [7].

3. A third clinical scenario is to bridge to liver transplantation. There may be a prolonged waiting time experienced by patients while awaiting orthotopic liver transplantation and SIRT is beneficial to halt tumour progression in such patients and prevent dropout on the

waiting list while awaiting definitive treatment. Although uncommon, there have also been patients who did not fulfil Milan Criteria for liver transplantation initially but were successfully downstaged to meet criteria later after treatment with Y-90 SIRT [8].

4. The fourth situation in which SIRT plays a dominant role is when a patient is referred to with a hepatic tumour in the presence of portal vein tumour thrombosis. Patients with PVTT tend to have a poor prognosis and this tumour thrombosis affecting the portal veins can occur in about 10–40% of HCC cases. The median survival of such patients that have PVTT is about 2–4 months in contrast to those without PVTT (10–24 months) [9]. The presence of PVTT generally makes curative surgery, transplantation, or TACE unsuitable as management options. SIRT however can be safely performed in such a clinical scenario due to its negligible embolic effect as well as a demonstration of efficacy [10]. Several studies of Y-90 SIRT in HCC patients with PVTT have shown good outcomes.

5. Finally, SIRT can be used as salvage therapy with largely palliative intent. Studies have clearly shown the palliative role of SIRT by inducing tumour necrosis and delaying progression with a relatively wide safety margin.

While both are transarterial therapies, TACE deposits small embolic particles coated with chemotherapeutic drugs rather than radiation that is in SIRT. A large randomised controlled phase II trial has evaluated SIRT against TACE in HCC patients with BCLC stages A or B showing that the patients receiving SIRT had significantly longer median time-to-progression (>26 months) compared to the group that received TACE (6.8 months; $P = 0.0012$). The authors concluded that Y-90 SIRT gave superior tumour control and may reduce transplant waitlist dropout [11]. Y-90 SIRT also outperforms TACE in downstaging HCC from United Network for Organ Sharing (UNOS) T3 to T2 [12]. In general, published studies show that SIRT has comparable outcomes as TACE and in a few studies, SIRT may be superior to TACE especially for large or numerous tumours.

There are a few concluded phase III trials on SIRT using Y-90 microspheres which have recently been published. A multicentre randomised phase III trial performed in France, SARAH [13], compared Y-90 resin microspheres SIRT with sorafenib 800 mg/day in patients who had locally advanced HCC in a trial designed for superiority. The trial did not meet its primary endpoint as median OS was 8.0 months in the SIRT group vs. 9.9 months in the sorafenib group (hazard ratio, 1.15;95% CI: 0.94–1.41; $P = 0.18$). Another phase III trial performed in Asia Pacific, SIRveNIB [14], compared Y-90 resin microspheres SIRT with sorafenib 800 mg/day in patients who had locally advanced HCC in a two-tailed study designed for superiority. The primary endpoint measured was overall survival and the study did not meet its primary endpoint as median OS was 8.8 and 10.0 months with SIRT and sorafenib, respectively (hazard ratio, 1.1;95% CI, 0.9–1.4; $P = 0.36$). There was significantly fewer grade 3 or greater adverse effects in the SIRT group of patients than the sorafenib group. The study concluded that OS did not differ significantly between SIRT and sorafenib in patients with locally advanced HCC, but there was a better toxicity profile of SIRT over sorafenib which may inform treatment choice in a select group of patients. Critical analysis of the non-superiority results of SIRT in these two randomised controlled trials noted some of the participating centres having varying levels of experience in administrating SIRT, use of body surface area methodology without consideration for dosimetric calculations for the planning of Y-90 dose activity as well as up to 3 weeks of time discrepancy in receiving treatment between the two arms [15]. There is another randomised trial, SORAMIC, which recruited 424 patients into two separate arms of SIRT followed by sorafenib versus sorafenib monotherapy and the results showed no difference in OS between the two groups of patients [16]. In this study, the median OS was 12.1 months (95% CI: 10.6, 14.6) in the SIRT followed by the sorafenib arm whilst the sorafenib monotherapy arm had a median OS of

11.5 months (95% CI: 9.8, 13.9) (HR:1.01;95% CI: 0.82, 1.25; P = 0.93). Subgroup analysis in the study did however show a survival benefit in younger patients, those with a non-alcoholic aetiology of liver cirrhosis and those who had no liver cirrhosis.

The recent NEMESIS meta-analysis identified 33 papers and congress abstracts of which the above three trials (SARAH, SIRveNIB, and SORAMIC) fulfilled eligibility criteria and were included in the meta-analysis. The three data sets had a total involvement of 1243 patients comparing SIRT as monotherapy, or followed by sorafenib, to sorafenib monotherapy among patients with advanced HCC [17]. Median OS with SIRT, whether or not followed by sorafenib, was non-inferior to sorafenib (10.2 and 9.2 months, [HR 0.91, 95% CI 0.78–1.05]). Treatment-related severe adverse events were reported in 149/515 patients (28.9%) who received SIRT and 249/575 (43.3%) who received sorafenib only ($P < 0.01$). The authors concluded that SIRT as initial therapy for advanced HCC was non-inferior to sorafenib in terms of OS and had a better safety profile.

Importantly in the field of predictive dosimetry, a first-ever recent multi-centred randomised study of glass microspheres compared using personalised dosimetry against standard dosimetry (DOSISPHERE-01) and demonstrated dramatically improved results [18]. The authors noted that the SARAH and SIRveNIB trials may have had negative results due to a lack of accurate personalised dosing. The concepts of personalised dosimetry and the DOSISPHERE-01 trial results will be discussed further in this chapter.

10.4 Hepatic Angiography: Interventional Radiology Techniques and Procedure

The hepatic angiography conducted by the interventional radiologists is of importance in SIRT. Herein the process is described briefly. During the exploratory hepatic angiography with Tc-99m MAA administration, the hepatic vascular anatomy is delineated, and the tumoural blood supply is carefully interrogated. In conventional hepatic anatomy, cannulation of the celiac artery followed by a digital subtraction angiogram (DSA) is performed. Selection of the appropriate hepatic artery is done and DSA performed to search for contrast enhancement of the tumour and detect extrahepatic supply. Where possible, a catheter-directed intraarterial CT (IACT) or hybrid angiosuite CT or cone-beam CT is performed from the microcatheter position that Y-90 SIRT is planned for administration. This helps ensure that the tumour is adequately covered and is also useful to detect extrahepatic supply that may have been missed on DSA, thus improving patient safety. From the perspective of dosimetry planning, IACT also aids the delineation of targeted vascular territory when drawing regions of interests and guides the Tc-99m MAA SPECT/CT for predictive dosimetry [19]. When the hepatic angiography is deemed satisfactory, Tc-99m MAA is administered and the patient will then undergo a Tc-99m MAA SPECT/CT scan. Upon confirming that the patient is suitable for treatment, SIRT can be performed on the same day or up to the next week depending on logistics of supply. During the hepatic angiography for planning simulation study or before the infusion of Y90 microspheres, prophylactic coil embolisations that are necessary can be performed and IACT is done after to confirm the absence of extrahepatic enhancement. The Y-90 microspheres are slowly administered with caution to the theoretical risk flow stasis occurrence especially when using resin Y-90 microspheres or performing radiation segmentectomy due to a larger number of microspheres infused although one retrospective study showed that the median remnant prescribed activity after SIRT is relatively low [20].

10.5 Radiation Simulation Study: MAA Scintigraphy

The pre-treatment scintigram using Tc-99m MAA is historically performed for evaluation of the hepatopulmonary shunt and to detect any extrahepatic tracer uptake especially in particular within the gastrointestinal tract. This helps assess the patient's suitability for SIRT. Studies have validated the usefulness of Tc-99m MAA scintigraphy as a useful predictor of hepatopulmonary shunt by way of comparison to post-treatment scans. Hence, doing a pre-treatment Tc-99m MAA scan is routine and part of multiple practice guidelines. A typical example of a planar Tc-99m MAA scintigram and how the shunt fraction is derived is seen in Figs. 10.1 and 10.2, respectively.

Currently, many experienced institutions use the Tc-99m MAA scintigraphy as a radiation simulation scan with calculations of Y-90 dose activity performed by partition modelling and personalised predictive dosimetry. The Tc-99m

MAA scintigram was found useful in a retrospective study of predictive dosimetry for estimating absorbed doses in tumour and non-tumoural tissues as calculated from post-treatment Y-90 PET/CT [21]. Another study evaluated 62 HCC patients who had Y-90 SIRT using glass microspheres and concluded that post-treatment PET/CT could give dosimetry accurately for the SIRT [22]. More importantly, this study found that pre-treatment tumour to non-tumour count ratio using the Tc-99m MAA scintigraphy (T/NT$_{MAA}$) predicts post-treatment tumour to non-tumour count ratio from Y-90 PET (T/NT$_{Y90}$) which supports the usage of the Tc-99m MAA scintigram as a radiation simulation scan for predictive dosimetry and therapy. Additionally, an early study

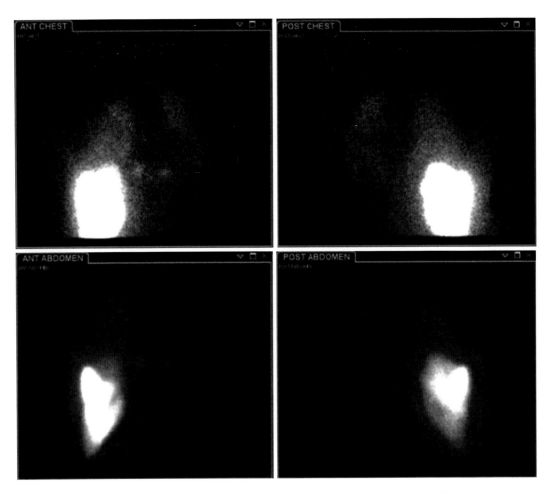

Fig. 10.1 Planar images of a Tc-99m MAA liver–lung shunt scintigram depicting tracer activity in the liver with some tracer activity seen in the lungs bilaterally due to hepatopulmonary shunting

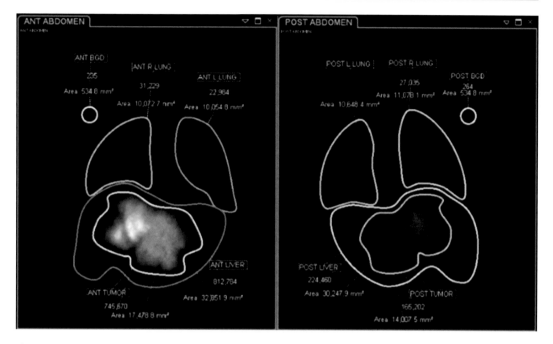

Fig. 10.2 Processed images of a liver–lung shunt scintigram with the region of interest (ROI) drawn in the liver, tumour and both lobes of the lungs. Numerical values of the radiotracer counts are calculated from the various ROIs

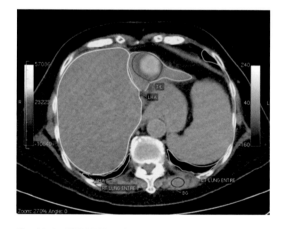

Fig. 10.3 SPECT/CT of Tc-99m MAA study. Contouring of the ROI is done for the lungs (blue outline), right hepatic lobe (white outline), left hepatic lobe (green outline) and tumour (red outline)

in excellent impact clinically with a median OS of 20.2 months for a good PVT candidate with Y-90 SIRT [24]. The role of a pre-treatment radiation simulation study in the form of a Tc-99m MAA SPECT/CT is expected to continue being validated in light of increasing predictive dosimetry use, although a Ho-166 microspheres scout scan may hold greater potential for this purpose. Figure 10.3 shows an example of how a Tc-99m MAA SPECT/CT can be analysed by drawing regions of interest for partition modelling and generating parameters to aid predictive dosimetry.

10.6   Dose Activity Prescription and Predictive Dosimetry

showed that usage of a Tc-99m MAA SPECT/CT quantitatively could predict response, PFS and OS in HCC patients with Y-90 SIRT [23] while another study done more recently by the same group led by Garin et al. evaluated HCC patients with PVT using dosimetry based on Tc-99m MAA scintigram and the PVT targeting resulted

For resin microspheres, the manufacturer provides an online calculator based on a body surface area (BSA) methodology to calculate the desired dose activity. The BSA methodology of a dose activity calculation is semi-empirical, used commonly for its simplicity and has been well-validated over the years. It is suitable for multifocal HCCs or metastases, usually when there are just too many lesions to feasibly perform dosimetry on. It is also useful in cases where the infiltrative disease is present and partition modelling is challenging as contouring the regions of interest is difficult due to a lack of clear tumour margins. For glass microspheres, an online MIRD-based dosimetry tool is provided by the manufacturer where the desired absorbed dose is assumed homogeneously distributed over the entire targeted arterial territory and the recommended dose is 120–150 Gy.

Another method uses partition modelling for personalised predictive dosimetry based on the absorbed doses in each region of interest drawn. Assuming the conditions during both planning and treatment angiography are similar, the Tc-99m MAA SPECT/CT scan is regarded as a radiation simulation study, this has been conceptually shown for both glass [25] and resin [19] microspheres. There are three dosimetric compartments in the partition model—tumour, normal hepatic parenchyma, and pulmonary parenchyma. Usage of radiotracer count ratios from the Tc-99m MAA hybrid SPECT/CT and parameters like the liver–lung shunt fraction and tumour-to-normal liver ratio allows for predictive dosimetry on a personalised patient basis. Modern angiographic techniques can target hepatic tumour selectively via two or more vessels. The use of hybrid angiosuite CT and SPECT/CT allows greater precision in sectoral tumour, hepatic vascular territory, and pulmonary volumes and hence better predictive vascular territory multi-partition dosimetry application with good effect [19]. Recently, there has been a greater push by many advocates towards using personalised predictive dosimetry against relying on older semi-empirical methodologies of dose calculations for SIRT [6]. A retrospective study of 58 patients with unresectable and chemorefractory intrahepatic cholangiocarcinoma that had Y-90 resin microspheres SIRT found that the median OS was shorter in patients treated with the BSA method (5.5 months) compared to partition modelling (14.9 months) (HR = 2.52, 95% CI: 1.23–5.16, $P < 0.001$) [26]. Just recently, Garin et al. conducted a multicentre randomised

phase II study in patients with unresectable HCC and compared outcomes of Y-90 glass microspheres using standard dosimetry (goal of 120 ± 20 Gy to treated volume) against personalised predictive dosimetry (goal of at least 205 Gy to index lesion). This study, DOSIPHERE-01, had a primary endpoint measuring response rate which was significantly increased in the personalised dosimetry arm versus the standard dosimetry arm in the intention-to-treat population (64.5 vs. 31% respectively, $P = 0.0095$). The median OS was significantly increased in the personalised dosimetry arm versus the standard dosimetry arm in the intention to treat the population (26.7 vs. 10.6 months, CI 95%:6–16.8, $P = 0.0096$) [18]. Evidence is in favour of personalised dose activity prescription using dosimetry instead of semi-empirical dosing for best outcomes. Softwares developed to estimating partition model dosimetry (for example, DAVYR—Dosimetry and Activity Visualizer for Yttrium-90 Radioembolization) help aid the use of personalised predictive dosimetry for patients undergoing SIRT and aim to increase feasibility for institutions with high caseloads.

An expert panel recommends that the mean absorbed dose thresholds for Y-90 resin microspheres used in HCC to be more than 120 Gy for tumour response, less than 50 Gy to normal liver and less than 20 Gy to the lung [27]. For Y-90 glass microspheres, the threshold for HCC was determined to be more than 205 Gy for tumour response, less than 120 Gy to normal liver and less than 30 Gy to the lung [25]. For Y-90 resin microspheres SIRT to colorectal metastasis in the liver, responders received a mean tumour absorbed dose of 82.7 ± 23.9 Gy [28]. There is limited literature to guide clinicians regarding repeated SIRT in a territory that has already been treated. There is a study that showed an increased risk of REILD after SIRT was re-performed especially after initial whole liver treatment [29]. A separate study showed acceptable toxicity when an average of 3 lobar treatments was performed, with 4–6 weeks between sequential lobar treatments; when a bilirubin cutoff of 1.75 mg/dL was used for both initial and repeated treatments; and when repeated radioembolisation was performed only for patients who initially demonstrated a response to radioembolisation (6 weeks after treatment) but then later showed disease progression [30].

Radiation segmentectomy has seen increasing interest due to its perceived curative intent. The concept is to deliver high doses of radiation to the tumour that involves 1 or 2 hepatic segments and essentially killing the tumour and its adjacent normal hepatic parenchyma much like surgical segmentectomy. This technique can be used in patients who refuse surgery; are ineligible for surgery due to poor liver function and inadequate future liver remnant or are not suitable for thermal ablation due to the tumour being in an unsafe location. The guidance of administered radiation dose has not been fully answered and one of the earliest studies had a median treatment dose of over 1200 Gy delivered [31]. A large multicentre study recruiting 102 patients used pathological correlation on Y-90 glass microsphere SIRT radiation segmentectomy and found more complete necrosis was observed when irradiation dose exceeded 190 Gy, suggestive of a threshold dose [32]. No major complications developed and this "super-selective" SIRT was deemed a safe and efficacious alternative if resection or thermal ablation is not feasible. Based on growing evidence, it is believed that with careful planning and meticulous dosimetry, the results of radiation segmentectomy can be excellent.

10.7   Post-treatment Imaging: Bremsstrahlung SPECT/CT and Y-90 PET/CT Imaging

PET/CT imaging after Y-90 SIRT has garnered much attention over the years. The use of Bremsstrahlung hybrid SPECT/CT is already a marked improvement from the past when only planar scintigraphy was available, and yet a problem of poor spatial resolution is still present. The technical advantages of Y-90 PET over Bremsstrahlung imaging are that it has better resolution than bremsstrahlung and potential for quantification for actual absorbed dose calculation. The disadvantages are that the small amount of positron emission (32 positrons per million

decays) results in a poor counts rate and poor signal-to-noise ratio and hence a long acquisition time (typically 20 min per bed position for an average treatment activity of Y-90). In clinical practise, Y-90 PET imaging allows for accurate localisation o the microspheres to determine if the targeting was appropriate and to predict tumour treatment response. Y-90 PET/CT imaging can be utilised for post-treatment dosimetry and identify tumour heterogeneity as well as provide intra-tumoural dose-histograms [33]. The findings may then have implications on further management especially with regards to the use of adjunctive external beam radiotherapy and how much radiation to give.

10.8   Side Effects of SIRT

There are known minor effects of SIRT due to the post-embolisation syndrome that may be considered treatment effects rather than complications and increased numbers of Y-90 microspheres injected is associated with this. Close to half of the patients may experience post-embolisation syndromes which include abdominal pain, fever, or lethargy and nausea, all of which are mild and can last up to 1 week after the procedure. Supportive management and low-dose steroid therapy may mitigate these effects and the vast majority of patients rarely require hospitalisation.

The more worrying complications typically arise from non-target deposition of the Y-90 microspheres into the lungs, gastrointestinal tract (such as the stomach, duodenum, or biliary tract) and the normal liver parenchyma. The overall complications rates are low especially with a good planning radiation simulation study but if it occurs it can result in significant morbidity or even fatality. Radiation pneumonitis is rare and reported in less than 1% of cases [34] but it can be fatal and is related to a high hepatopulmonary shunt greater than 20 Gy or in older literature 20%. Prevention can be by excluding those cases with a high hepatopulmonary shunt or limiting Y-90 treatment dose activities such that the lung should be safe. Administration of corticosteroids and pentoxifylline may help in the management of this condition. The deposition of Y-90 microspheres into the gastrointestinal tract, either from reflux or undetected collateral vessels, may result in stomach or duodenal ulcerations and a detailed review of previous scans and on-table IACT will be useful to exclude these small collateral vessels and reduce the risk of gastrointestinal ulceration. Excessive hepatic radiation of the normal liver parenchyma may result in Radioembolisation-Induced Liver Disease (REILD), a form of cholangiopathy/veno-occlusive disease which typically present 4–8 weeks following the procedure and can be exacerbated by pre-existing liver disease or previous radiation-related treatments to the liver. REILD is characterised by elevated bilirubin and alkaline phosphatase as well as ascites in the absence of tumour progression. Whole liver treatment with SIRT in a single setting increases the risk of hepatotoxicity as compared to sequential staged treatment of the right and left hepatic lobes with an interval of 6 weeks in between [35].

The best available datasets of Y-90 SIRT related adverse events are from the SARAH and SIRveNIB trials. From the SARAH trial, the most frequent grade 3 or worse treatment-related adverse events following SIRT were fatigue (20 [9%]), liver dysfunction (25 [11%]), increased laboratory liver values (20 [9%]), haematological abnormalities (23 [10%]), diarrhoea (3 [1%]), abdominal pain (6 [3%]), increased creatinine (4 [2%]), and hand–foot skin reaction (1 [<1%]) [13]. The grade 3 or worse treatment-related adverse events from performing SIRT in the SIRveNIB trial were abdominal pain (3 [2.3%]), ascites (5 [3.8%]), nausea (1 [0.8%]), hypoalbuminemia (1 [0.8%]), gastric ulcer (1 [0.8%]), upper GI haemorrhage (1 [0.8%]), jaundice (1 [0.8%]) and radiation hepatitis (2 [1.5%]) [14].

10.9 Miscellaneous Radionuclide Treatment of Liver Cancer: Peptide Receptor Radionuclide Therapy (PRRT)

Endoradiotherapy using peripheral intravascular radionuclide injection as a whole-body systemic treatment has been exemplified by PRRT which has seen a long history of usage in Europe for decades. However, the recent pivotal phase III trial, NETTER-1, is a phase III trial that showed the efficacy of treating neuroendocrine tumours using PRRT with a PFS at month 20 of 65.2% in the Lu-177 DOTATATE group and 10.8% in the control group. Response rates were 18% in the Lu-177 DOTATATE group versus 3% in the control group. The final findings of overall survival analysis are eagerly awaited as an interim analysis has already yielded positive preliminary results [36]. Moving beyond peripheral intravenous injections of PRRT, a small pilot study of patients with neuroendocrine hepatic metastases had SIRT performed with Y-90 DOTATOC and lead to good radiological and biochemical response [37]. More studies are currently ongoing with regards to the use of PRRT given in the form of SIRT.

10.10 Use of Adjunct External Beam Radiotherapy with SIRT

Scarce data exists with regards to usage of combined external beam radiotherapy and SIRT. The prognoses of patients with portal vein thrombosis, extrahepatic metastases, or residual tumours remain poor when treated with SIRT alone and this group of patients potentially may benefit from adjunctive EBRT especially in sites that had poor radionuclide uptake. The concern is that radiation toxicity to the liver is cumulative with risk of radiation-induced liver damage (a clinical syndrome of hepatomegaly, non-icteric ascites and elevated liver enzymes occurring 2 weeks to 6 months after external beam radiation exposure) or REILD.

There exist guidelines that call for vigilance in planning SIRT for patients with prior hepatic radiotherapy [38]. To the best of the authors' knowledge, there is only one report by Lam et al. who analysed 31 patients that received SIRT in the background of previous exposure of the liver to external beam radiation therapy [39]. They concluded that prior exposure of the liver to EBRT may lead to increased liver toxicity after

SIRT, depending on fractional liver exposure and dose level. The fraction of liver exposed to at least 30 Gy (V30) was the strongest predictor of toxicity with a threshold for hepatotoxicity at a volume of 13% and a threshold of REILD at a volume of 30%. It is noted that 84% of Lam's cohort were treated with whole liver SIRT, which may be associated with higher liver toxicity. SIRT appears to be safe for the treatment of hepatic malignancies only in patients who had limited hepatic exposure to prior EBRT, and there should be vigilance during evaluation whether a patient pre-treated with EBRT should continue with SIRT.

To the best of our knowledge, only one study by Wang et al. studied 22 patients who underwent EBRT after SIRT. The post-Y-90 SIRT Bremsstrahlung study was transferred to dose distribution and a patient-specific three-dimensional biological effective dose distribution of combined SIRT and EBRT was generated. The study team concluded that combining SIRT with EBRT was feasible and may provide survival benefit for selected patients especially those with portal vein thrombosis. They found that combined BED distribution was valuable for predicting toxicity outcome and the most relevant dosimetric parameters were V100Gy to V140Gy. Most of their patients (86%) were treated with selective segmental SIRT [40]. There were some concerns from the wider medical community that five patients in the study developed grade 5 liver toxicities, but from this initial data, radiation oncologists can get a dose level in which to avoid if doing EBRT after SIRT. The hope is that greater use of Y-90 PET imaging post SIRT treatment will lead to increased accuracy in preventing such radiation dose toxicities. With regards to the timing of adjunctive radiotherapy post SIRT, there is no existing data on this; hence, the timing has not been established although additional radiotherapy may not require any significant delay so long as acute side effects of SIRT does not interfere with the patient's ability to undergo SBRT simulation and treatment.

There is no known published data available of planned concurrent radiotherapy and Y-90 SIRT for hepatocellular carcinoma or other liver tumours. It is uncertain if there will be advantages in radiobiology using such an approach, but the total absorbed dose can be improved to all parts of the tumour. This in turn is expected to have a favourable outcome on the tumour treatment.

10.11 Conclusion

Current evidence demonstrates that selective internal radiation therapy using radionuclides for liver tumours is widely utilised with selected cases befitting from intention for cure either through radiation segmentectomy or as a bridge to definitive surgery. There is growing evidence from robust literature that SIRT using Y-90 microspheres to advanced hepatocellular carcinoma performs similarly as the current standard first-line systemic treatment with oral sorafenib and has a better safety profile. More precise personalised dosimetry for dose calculations will also play a pivotal role to determine better outcomes for patients undergoing SIRT as compared to using semi-empirical calculations of dose activity. We foresee a greater upcoming role in the combined use of external beam radiotherapy with SIRT either sequentially or concurrently.

References

1. Ariel IM. Radioactive isotopes for adjuvant cancer therapy; animal experimentation and preliminary results in human application. Arch Surg. 1964;89:244–9.
2. Kennedy A, Nag S, Salem R, Murthy R, McEwan AJ, Nutting CW, et al. Recommendations for radioembolization of hepatic malignancies using yttrium-90 microsphere brachytherapy: a consensus panel report from the radioembolization brachytherapy oncology consortium. Int J Radiat Oncol Biol Phys. 2007;68:13–23.
3. Reinders MTM, Smits MLJ, van Roekel C, Braat AJAT. Holmium-166 microsphere radioembolization of hepatic malignancies. Semin Nucl Med. 2019;49(3):237–43.
4. Braat AJAT, Bruijnen RCG, van Rooij R, et al. Additional holmium-166 radioembolisation after lutetium-177-dotatate in patients with neuroendocrine tumour liver metastases (HEPAR PLuS): a single-

centre, single-arm, open-label, phase 2 study. Lancet Oncol. 2020;21(4):561–70.

5. Gray BN. Colorectal cancer: the natural history of disseminated disease—a review. Aust N Z J Surg. 1980;50:643–6.

6. Tong AKT, Kao YH, Too CW, Chin KFW, Ng DCE, Chow PKH. Yttrium-90 hepatic radioembolization: clinical review and current techniques in interventional radiology and personalized dosimetry. Br J Radiol. 2016;89(1062):20150943.

7. Teo JY, Allen JC Jr, Ng DC, et al. A systematic review of contralateral liver lobe hypertrophy after unilobar selective internal radiation therapy with Y90. HPB (Oxford). 2016;18(1):7–12.

8. Tohme S, Sukato D, Chen HW, et al. Yttrium-90 radioembolization as a bridge to liver transplantation: a single-institution experience. J Vasc Interv Radiol. 2013;24(11):1632–8.

9. Llovet JM, Bustamante J, Castells A, Vilana R, Ayuso Mdel C, Sala M, et al. Natural history of untreated nonsurgical hepatocellular carcinoma: rationale for the design and evaluation of therapeutic trials. Hepatology. 1999;29:62–7.

10. Sangro B, Carpanese L, Cianni R, Golfieri R, Gasparini D, Ezziddin S, et al. Survival after yttrium-90 resin microsphere radioembolization of hepatocellular carcinoma across Barcelona clinic liver cancer stages: a European evaluation. Hepatology. 2011;54:868–78.

11. Salem R, Gordon AC, Mouli S, et al. Y90 Radioembolization significantly prolongs time to progression compared with chemoembolization in patients with hepatocellular carcinoma. Gastroenterology. 2016;151(6):1155–63.

12. Lewandowski RJ, Kulik LM, Riaz A, et al. A comparative analysis of transarterial downstaging for hepatocellular carcinoma: chemoembolization versus radioembolization. Am J Transplant. 2009;9(8):1920–8.

13. Vilgrain V, Pereira H, Assenat E, et al. Efficacy and safety of selective internal radiotherapy with yttrium-90 resin microspheres compared with sorafenib in locally advanced and inoperable hepatoccular carcinoma (SARAH): an open-label randomised controlled phase 3 trial. Lancet Oncol. 2017;18(12):1624–36.

14. Chow PKH, Gandhi M, Tan SB, et al. SIRveNIB: selective internal radiation therapy versus sorafenib in Asia-Pacific patients with hepatocellular carcinoma. J Clin Oncol. 2018;36(19):1913–21.

15. Sposito C, Mazzaferro V. The SIRveNIB and SARAH trials, radioembolization vs. sorafenib in advanced HCC patients: reasons for a failure, and perspectives for the future. Hepatobiliary Surg Nutr. 2018;7(6):487–9.

16. Ricke J, Klumpen HJ, Amthauer H, et al. Impact of combined selective internal radiation therapy and sorafenib on survival in advanced hepatocellular carcinoma. J Hepatol. 2019;71:1164–74.

17. Venerito M, Pech M, Canbay A, et al. NEMESIS: non-inferiority, individual patient meta-analysis of selective internal radiation therapy with yttrium-90 resin microspheres versus sorafenib in advanced hepatocellular carcinoma. J Nucl Med. 2020;61(12):1736–42. https://doi.org/10.2967/jnumed.120.242933.

18. Garin E, Tzelikas L, Guiu B, et al. Major impact of personalized dosimetry using 90Y loaded glass microspheres SIRT in HCC: final overall survival analysis of a multicentre randomized phase II study (DOSISPHERE-01). J Clin Oncol. 2020;38(4_suppl):516.

19. Kao YH, Hock Tan AE, Burgmans MC, Irani FG, Khoo LS, Gong Lo RH, et al. Image-guided personalized predictive dosimetry by artery-specific SPECT/CT partition modeling for safe and effective 90Y radioembolization. J Nucl Med. 2012;53:559–66.

20. Rodriguez LS, Thang SP, Li H, et al. A descriptive analysis of remnant activity during (90)Y resin microspheres radioembolization of hepatic tumors: technical factors and dosimetric implications. Ann Nucl Med. 2016;30(3):255–61.

21. Gnesin S, Canetti L, Adib S, et al. Partition model-based ^{99m}Tc-MAA SPECT/CT predictive dosimetry compared with ^{90Y} TOF PET/CT posttreatment dosimetry in radioembolization of hepatocellular carcinoma: a quantitative agreement comparison. J Nucl Med. 2016;57(11):1672–8.

22. Ho CL, Chen S, Cheung SK, et al. Radioembolization with Y-90 glass microspheres for hepatocellular carcinoma: significance of pretreatment C-11 acetate and FDG PET/CT and posttreatment Y-90 PET/CT in individualized dose prescription. Eur J Nucl Med Mol Imaging. 2018;45(12):2110–21.

23. Garin E, Lenoir L, Rolland Y, et al. Dosimetry based on ^{99m}Tc-macroaggregated albumin SPECT/CT accurately predicts tumor response and survival in hepatocellular carcinoma patients treated with ^{90}Y-loaded glass microspheres: preliminary results. J Nucl Med. 2012;53(2):255–63.

24. Garin E, Rolland Y, Edeline J. 90Y-loaded microsphere SIRT of HCC patients with portal vein thrombosis: high clinical impact of 99mTc-MAA SPECT/CT-based dosimetry. Semin Nucl Med. 2019;49(3):218–26.

25. Garin E, Lenoir L, Edeline J, et al. Boosted selective internal radiation therapy with 90Y-loaded glass microspheres (B-SIRT) for hepatocellular carcinoma patients: a new personalized promising concept. Eur J Nucl Med Mol Imaging. 2013;40:1057–68.

26. Levillain H, Duran Derijckere I, Ameye L, et al. Personalizsed radioembolization improves outcomes in refractory intrahepatic cholangiocarcinoma: a multicentre study. Eur J Nucl Med Mol Imag. 2019;46(11):2270–9.

27. Lau WY, Kennedy AS, Kim YH, et al. Patient selection and activity planning guide for selective internal radiotherapy with yttrium-90 resin microspheres. Int J Radiat Oncol Biol Phys. 2012;82:401–7.

28. Lam MG, Goris ML, Iagaru AH, et al. Prognostic utility of 90Y radioembolization dosimetry based on fusion

99mTc-macroaggregated albumin-99mTc-sulfur colloid SPECT. J Nucl Med. 2013;54(12):2055–61.

29. Lam MG, Louie JD, Iagaru AH, et al. Safety of repeated yttrium-90 radioembolization. Cardiovasc Intervent Radiol. 2013;36:1320–8.

30. Zarva A, Mohnike K, Damm R, et al. Safety of repeated radioembolizations in patients with advanced primary and secondary liver tumors and progressive disease after first selective internal radiotherapy. J Nucl Med. 2014;55:360–6.

31. Riaz A, Gates VL, Atassi B, et al. Radiation segmentectomy: a novel approach to increase safety and efficacy of radioembolization. Int J Radiat Oncol Biol Phys. 2011;79:163–71.

32. Vouche M, Habib A, Ward TJ, et al. Unresectable solitary hepatocellular carcinoma not amenable to radiofrequency ablation: multicentre radiology-pathology correlation and survival of radiation segmentectomy. Hepatology. 2014;60(1):192–201.

33. Kao YH, Steinberg JD, Tay YS, Lim GK, Yan J, Townsend DW, et al. Post-radioembolization yttrium-90 PET/CT—part 2: dose-response and tumor predictive dosimetry for resin microspheres. EJNMMI Res. 2013;3:57.

34. Leung TW, et al. Radiation pneumonitis after selective internal radiation treatment with intraarterial 90yttrium-microspheres for inoperable hepatic tumors. Int J Radiat Oncol Biol Phys. 1995;33(4):919–24.

35. Gil-Alzugaray B, Chopitea A, Inarrairaegui M, et al. Prognostic factors and prevention of radioembolization-induced liver disease. Hepatology. 2013;57:1078–87.

36. Strosberg J, El-Haddad G, Wolin E, et al. Phase 3 trial of Lu-177 Dotatate for midgut neuroendocrine tumours. N Engl J Med. 2017;376:125–35.

37. Kratochwil C, Lopez-Benitez R, Mier W, et al. Hepatic arterial infusion enhances DOTATOC radiopeptide therapy in patients with neuroendocrine liver metastases. Endocr Relat Cancer. 2011;18(5):595–602.

38. Murthy R, Kamat P, Nuñez R, Salem R. Radioembolization of yttrium-90 microspheres for hepatic malignancy. Semin Intervent Radiol. 2008;25(1):48–57.

39. Lam MG, Abdelmaksoud MH, Chang DT, et al. Safety of 90Y radioembolization in patients who have undergone previous external beam radiation therapy. Int J Radiat Oncol Biol Phys. 2013;87(2):323–9.

40. Wang TH, Huang PI, Hu YW, et al. Combined yttrium-90 microsphere selective internal radiation therapy and external beam radiotherapy in patients with hepatocellular carcinoma: from clinical aspects to dosimetry. PLoS One. 2018;13(1):e0190098.

Part III

Radiotherapeutic Strategies in Liver Cancer

Therapeutic Guidelines for Patients with Liver Cancer from the Perspective of Radiation Oncologists

11

Chai Hong Rim and Jinsil Seong

Abstract

Liver cancer has significant heterogeneities regarding its incidence, as well as disease etiology and characteristics among regions. Various staging systems have been developed, and the types of treatment available or commonly used for liver cancer are also different by region. Currently, there are more than 30 clinical guidelines for liver cancer treatment. In the past, external beam radiotherapy (EBRT) was used only for the purpose of palliation. Currently, EBRT is used for a variety of indications that range from curative approaches for early cases using techniques such as stereotactic body radiotherapy to bridging therapies for liver transplantation. EBRT is useful in locally advanced tumors by converting to curative surgery in selected cases and has also long been used for palliation. Nevertheless, data from radiotherapy studies are not yet sufficient and are often criticized for their low grades of evidence. This chapter reviews the current guidelines for the treatment of liver cancer from the perspective of radiation oncology and discusses how to apply them in clinical practice.

Keywords

Liver neoplasm · Hepatocellular carcinoma · External beam radiotherapy · Clinical guidelines

11.1 Introduction

Liver cancer is the fourth leading cause of cancer-related mortality worldwide; its mortality rate is similar to those of colorectal and gastric cancers (which are the second- and third-leading causes of cancer-related deaths, with mortality rates of 9.2% and 8.2%, respectively). Globally, East Asia has the highest incidence of liver cancer, with an age-standardized rate of 27 per 100,000 among men. The incidence of liver cancer is relatively low in western and northern Europe and in the United States, although the age-standardized rates in southern European countries are moderately high (exceeding 10 per 100,000 among men) [1]. Among all primary liver cancers, hepatocellular carcinoma (HCC) comprises the vast majority (up to 85%).

Cirrhosis is found to be the cause of HCC in ~80% of cases, and which is complicated by persistent viral hepatitis [2]. In East Asia, the most common cause of HCC is chronic inflammation due to hepatitis B infection. These patients are

C. H. Rim
Korea University Medical College, Seoul, South Korea

J. Seong (✉)
Department of Radiation Oncology, Yonsei Cancer Center, Yonsei University College of Medicine, Seoul, South Korea
e-mail: jsseong@yuhs.ac

J. Seong (ed.), *Radiotherapy of Liver Cancer*, https://doi.org/10.1007/978-981-16-1815-4_11

generally younger and are more often found to have locally advanced disease, but with relatively preserved liver function, than patients having other etiologies [3, 4]. Approximately one-third of patients with HCC are diagnosed with Barcelona Clinic of Liver Cancer (BCLC) stage C (advanced) disease, whereas 20–30% of patients are diagnosed with BCLC A (early) disease [5, 6]. Early HCC at diagnosis is rarer in China, of which <10% is diagnosed with BCLC A disease [6]. In contrast, HCC in the United States and Europe is mainly caused by alcohol use or chronic hepatitis due to hepatitis C virus. Those patients commonly have deteriorated liver function at the time of diagnosis [3]. Approximately 10–30% of HCC patients in these areas are diagnosed with BCLC A disease. In Japan, unlike in other East Asian countries, hepatitis C virus is the leading cause of HCC. With the comprehensive national screening by ultrasound and three tumor markers measurements, more than 60% of liver cancers are detected in their early stages. Median survival of HCC patients ranged from 14.8 to 25.5 months globally, whereas survival was as high as 79.6 months in Japan [7].

Treatment of HCC in the past depended largely on surgical approaches. However, accompanying cirrhosis or hepatic decompensation often hinders safe surgical attempt, and transplantation has been rarely performed due to shortage of donors in Asian countries [8, 9]. In recent decades, various locoregional modalities such as radiofrequency ablation (RFA) and transarterial chemotherapy (TACE) have shown their efficacy [10, 11]. External beam radiotherapy (EBRT) has also been increasingly applied, with availability to irradiate tumors selectively while sparing normal liver, based on CT-planning system [12]. Sorafenib became the first systemic agent that showed a survival benefit [13], and second-line agents such as regorafenib and cabozantinib have also recently shown significant efficacy [14, 15]. Given the diversity of treatment options and disease characteristics, various staging systems were developed to estimate patients' prognosis and optimize treatment. Major staging systems, including BCLC, Cancer of the Liver

Italian Program (CLIP), and Okuda were developed to measure combined contributions of cancer and hepatic dysfunction to overall prognosis [16]. Serum alpha-fetoprotein has been established as a negative prognostic factor from retrospective data, and included in subsets of staging systems including those of CLIP and Chinese University Prognostic Index (CUPI) [17]. In addition, the degree of socioeconomic support became another consideration, because modern HCC treatment requires multidisciplinary approaches involving well-equipped facilities, experts from multiple specialties, and up-to-date medicines.

Considering the diverse disease characteristics, evaluation methods, and available options according to region, various liver cancer associations have developed clinical practice guidelines to optimize treatment strategy according to regional circumstances.

11.2 Landmark Guidelines from International Associations

According to a recent systematic review by the Chinese Cochrane group, more than 30 treatment guidelines for HCC have been published [18]. Among them, the most well-known that are used internationally include those of the European Association for the Study of the Liver (EASL), National Comprehensive Cancer Network (NCCN) from the United States, and Asia-Pacific Association for the Study of the Liver (APASL).

The EASL is a community of European hepatologists that publishes guidelines not only for the treatment of cancer but for treating benign liver diseases such as chronic inflammation resulting from drug or alcohol use [19]. The board that devised the EASL guidelines included the developers of the BCLC classification system, which is the most commonly used staging and treatment recommendation system [20]. The BCLC system has its merits as a systematic staging system that takes into account widely validated liver function and disease characteristic parameters and also recommends a single standard treatment modality for each stage. The EASL focuses more on evidence-based medicine than on the practical aspects of cancer treatment, asserting that "the benefits of treatments should be assessed through randomized controlled trials in oncology"; as such, EBRT is not highly recommended. In 2012 version of the EASL, only a few sentences referred to EBRT, mentioning that no scientific evidence exists for using this type of radiotherapy and that its efficacy is outweighed by liver toxicity, except for a few palliative indications such as bone metastases [21]. However, in the EASL's updated 2018 version, indications for combination treatment with EBRT and TACE, palliation of portal vein thrombosis, and ablative treatment using stereotactic body radiotherapy (SBRT) were introduced across five paragraphs [20]. The recommendation level increased from the lowest category in the previous version to between the negative and weak categories, which is the same level as that of internal radiotherapy using yttrium.

The NCCN is a coalition formed by 28 major cancer centers in the United States. The NCCN panel comprises oncologists from various fields, and radiation oncologists were included on the board that developed treatment guidelines for liver cancer [22]. The guidelines are known for their comprehensive and applicable flow-chart form and are updated at least once a year according to NCCN policy. Throughout the development process of oncology treatment recommendations, the NCCN considers that: ". . . much of the evidence available for clinicians is based on data from indirect comparison among randomized trials, phase II or non-randomized trials, or clinical observations. . . In the field of oncology, it is crucial to include the experience and expertise of cancer specialists and other experts" [23]. The NCCN also uses its own evidence recommendation system, which is mostly based on panel discussions [24]. In contrast to those of the EASL, the NCCN guidelines are more concerned with oncological utility as well as the levels of evidence of relevant subjects. The NCCN guidelines for HCC use the Child-Pugh classification and United Network for Organ Sharing system to evaluate liver function

and operability, but do not use BCLC staging. Among the internationally used guidelines, those of the NCCN have acknowledged the benefits of EBRT. Since early 2018, radiation therapy has been recommended as a local modality for unresectable HCC at the same level as arterial-directed therapies and RFA (category 2A; there is uniform consensus that the intervention is appropriate based on lower-level evidence) [21]. The advantage of EBRT is its ability to treat tumors regardless of their locations, and the latest modalities for this type of treatment, such as intensity-modulated radiotherapy (IMRT) and proton therapy, are described in the guidelines, as is the ablative role of SBRT as an alternative to RFA or embolization [22].

Physicians from several countries in the Asia-Pacific regions participated in the development of the APASL Guidelines [25]. While most other guidelines are from developed countries, the APASL guidelines also included a number of doctors from developing countries such as India, Pakistan, the Philippines, and Indonesia. The socioeconomic status of developing countries in this region should, of course, be considered essential when determining optimal treatments. The guidelines allotted a substantial part of their contents to the disease etiology and epidemiology in each country. The official recommendation for EBRT is in the same vein as those in previous versions of the EASL and AASLD guidelines [21, 26]; in other words, the EBRT has not demonstrated a clear improvement in outcomes but can be used for palliation of bony metastases (C2: low quality of evidence with a weaker recommendation). However, the authors also stated that the latest therapeutic techniques, such as SBRT and proton therapy, could be advantageous for unresectable tumors and expressed a neutral stance by stating: "Even though strong evidence is lacking, RT may be one of the promising treatment options for HCC."

In summary, the above internationally used guidelines have generally been updated to view EBRT more positively. They all described the latest ablative modalities, such as SBRT or charged particle therapy, as supportive therapies.

11.3 Guidelines from National Associations

The AASLD is the society for hepatologists in the United States; it publishes guidelines not only for HCC but also for several inflammatory or benign liver diseases (available at: https://www.aasld.org/publications/practice-guidelines) and endorses the BCLC staging system for HCC treatment guidelines. In its previous version, no content was provided regarding EBRT [26]. In its 2018 update, however, EBRT was introduced as a locoregional modality along with TACE and internal radiotherapy. They recommend the use of locoregional therapy for patients who are not candidates for resection or transplantation. For those with advanced disease (i.e., macrovascular invasion and/or extrahepatic metastases), locoregional therapy can be considered, but its specific type (as well as the application of systemic therapy) should take into consideration the diversity of clinical situations [27]. The guidelines cited a meta-analysis that showed a survival benefit from combining TACE and EBRT compared to TACE alone [28], as well as a propensity-matched analysis that demonstrated the benefit of TACE and EBRT for patients with portal vein thrombosis [29].

Liver cancer associations in East Asian countries including China, Japan, Taiwan, Singapore, Hong Kong, and Korea have also published clinical guidelines [30–35]. Among them, the guidelines of the Japanese Society of Hepatology [30], which achieved excellent recommendations based on previous literature review studies, do not mention EBRT [36, 37]. Reasons for this include the fact that more than 60% of patients with HCC are diagnosed in their early stages and treated accordingly owing to excellent surveillance programs, disease etiologies, and a strong reliance on RFA and TACE in Japan [6].

In contrast, hepatitis B virus infection is the underlying cause of liver cancer in most patients in China, Singapore, Hong Kong, Taiwan, and Korea [25]. Hence, all guidelines from these countries include EBRT indications for patients with locally advanced disease (e.g., those with portal vein invasion) as well as early disease. The guideline development committee in China

encompasses many experts in various fields, including several radiation oncologists. These guidelines describe almost all known indications for which EBRT is feasible, which include major vessel invasion, bridging therapy to liver transplantation, extrahepatic metastases, and postoperative adjuvant settings. In addition, the guidelines have an additional benefit in that they describe substantial methodologic contents such as target volume setting, necessary hepatic reserve, and dose of irradiation [32]. The guidelines of the National Cancer Center of Singapore describe EBRT as an alternative option to RFA or transplantation for early HCCs (recommendation level 1b) and as a locoregional modality for patients with vascular invasion (recommendation level 2a); these guidelines fairly well recommended use of EBRT by the Oxford system [31].

The guidelines of the Taiwan Liver Cancer Association are authored in part by the radiotherapy group and adopt the BCLC staging system. These guidelines broadly describe the indication of EBRT for patients with HCC of BCLC stages A to D. They recommend this modality as an alternative local treatment for early HCCs (BCLC A), as a combined treatment with TACE for BCLC B disease, as a palliative option for portal vein thrombosis or cases refractory to TACE (BCLC C), and as palliation for metastatic disease (BCLC D) [34]. The levels of evidence for these recommendations were all 2B according to the GRADE system [38]. The guidelines by the Hong Kong Liver Cancer Association focused their indication of EBRT on the application of SBRT, which can be used for unresectable HCC, tumors close to biliary duct vessels, and bridging therapy for liver transplantation (recommendation level 4–5 in the Oxford system) [35]. The guidelines from the Korean Liver Cancer Study Group (KLCSG) also include several radiation oncologists as authors. The evidence and recommendation levels (using the GRADE system [38]) are B1 for the palliation of symptoms and metastases and B2 for treating patients who did not completely respond to TACE and those with portal vein invasion. Practical contents such as necessary liver remnants and dose-volume constraints are well described [33].

Liver cancer is not uncommon in developing countries [39]. As mentioned above, modern HCC treatment requires a multidisciplinary approach, including up-to-date medicines as well as interventions that require experts and facilities able to administer TACE, RFA, and EBRT [4]. Therefore, special consideration regarding socioeconomic status is necessary for developing countries. The guidelines of the Indian National Association for Study of the Liver mention that recommendations from the United States, Europe, and developed Asian countries mostly fail to apply to India owing to economic reasons [39]. The Indian guidelines had positive comments about EBRT; they noted the dose-response relationship and feasibility using 3-dimensional planning. They stated that EBRT is a promising tool for the management of some unresectable HCCs (evidence level 2B, Oxford system) but also mentioned that EBRT cannot be recommended outside of a clinical trial setting (evidence level 5).

The Latin American Association for the Study of the Liver included panelists from Mexico, Argentina, Brazil, Chile, Columbia, and Venezuela who were mostly hepatologists or hepatic surgeons. Their guidelines mention EBRT briefly in the context of its use for the palliation of mass effect or of pain without formal evidence grading or recommendations [40]. Meanwhile, the Egyptian Society of Liver Cancer guidelines are the only recommendations from Africa [41]; the authors cite socioeconomic status, the lack of a national insurance program, and the unavailability of cadaveric liver transplantation as reasons for developing their own guidelines. Content related to EBRT is limited to its application for bone metastases combined with sorafenib administration.

In summary, the indications of EBRT as a locoregional modality for unresectable or locally advanced HCC, bridging therapy for liver transplantation, and refractory disease after treatment with local modalities were suggested in many guidelines originating from a range of regions, from the United States to East Asian Countries. Practical contents that can help implement EBRT were also noted in guidelines from China and the KLCSG. Guidelines from developing countries tend to emphasize socioeconomic circumstances and suggest a limited role for EBRT as a palliative or exploratory option. A summary of information from the above-selected guidelines is shown in Table 11.1.

11.4 Appraisal of Guidelines

As noted above, the disease characteristics of liver cancer exhibit significant differences regionally, whereas socioeconomic circumstances also influence treatment decisions. Guidelines therefore exist from different associations reflecting this diversity. Even for the same or similar clinical situations, these guidelines may evaluate disease and suggest clinical strategies differently (Table 11.2). Thus, it is necessary to select guidelines that are relevant in the clinical and social situations of each region.

The primary consideration when selecting clinical guidelines may be whether they have been developed through the appropriate processes and whether they contain quality recommendations that are derived from the accumulation and interpretation of systematic evidence. The Appraisal of Guidelines for Research and Evaluation (AGREE) is a tool for the quantitative evaluation of clinical guidelines that has been validated internationally and endorsed by the World Health Organization advisory board [44]. The tool includes 23 question-items in six domains: "Scope and purpose," "Stakeholder involvement," "Rigor of development," "Clarity and presentation," and "Applicability." Previously, hepatic surgeons [36] and interventional radiologists [45] evaluated various HCC clinical guidelines using the AGREE tool based on their clinical perspectives. The Chinese Cochrane group also evaluated 30 guidelines and consensus recommendations [18]. Among those reviews, internationally known guidelines such as those from the EASL and AASLD were mostly well recommended. Of note, the guidelines from the KLCSG were also highly recommended when reviewed from the perspective of surgeons and interventional radiologists [36, 45].

Table 11.1 Summary and radiotherapy information of selected guidelines

Association	Country	Year of publication	Staging system	RO panel	Evaluation	RT recommendation	Practical consideration
AASLD	US	2018	AJCC system, Milan criteria	No	GRADE	Locoregional modality for unresectable HCCs (C1)	None
NCCN	US	Updated in 3–6 months	Child-Pugh score, UNOS system	Yes	Own system	Locoregional modality for unresectable HCCs (2A)	SBRT dosing (30–50 Gy in 3–5 fractions) Child-Pugh class A is recommended for SBRT, safety profile with B or poorer is limited. Availability of EBRT irrespective of location
EASL	Multinations in Europe	2018	BCLC system	No	GRADE	Targeting PVT, palliation of bone metastases, SBRT for bridging LT (no formal grading)	None
ESLC	Egypt	2011	BCLC, CLIP	No	None	Palliation of bone metastases (no formal grading)	None
KLCSG	Korea	2019	Modified UICC system	Yes	GRADE	Complementing TACE, palliation for PVT (B2) Metastases palliation (B1)	Child A or B7 is recommended for EBRT Safety liver volume: volume irradiated with ≤30 Gy must be ≥40% of total liver; for hypofraction, volume with <15 Gy must be ≥700 cc
APASL	Multinations in Asia-Pacific	2015	Child-Pugh score, own system considering the field practice of Asia-Pacific region	No	GRADE	Palliation of bone metastases (C2) No formal recommendation for EBRT to HCC	None
HKLC	Hong Kong	2018	Own system using Child-Pugh score, performance and anatomical tumor status	Yes	Oxford	SBRT for unresectable HCCs or bridging LT (4) and for tumors close to the MV or bile duct (5)	Indication of SBRT: Acceptable up to five lesions; up to Child-Pugh B8; alternative to tumors close to vessels or biliary ducts; bridging LT; uninvolved liver volume might be ≥700 cc

				GRADE		
TLCA	Taiwan	2018	BCLC	Yes	Cases not amenable to PEI/RFA or surgery, bridging LT, complementing TACE, palliating PVT and metastases (2B)	None
NCCS	Singapore	2016	Own system using Milan criteria, Child-Pugh score, and anatomical tumor status	Yes	Oxford	Alternative for cases not amenable to LT or RFA (1B), for vascular invasion cases (2B)	None
INASL	India	2014	BCLC	No	Oxford	Promising tool for some unresectable HCCs (2B) Definite use is not recommended outside of clinical trial (5)	None
Chinese	China	2017	Own system using Child-Pugh score, AFP level, anatomical tumor status	Yes	Oxford	Cases with major vessel invasion, palliation for symptoms or metastases, tumor downstaging, bridging LT, postoperative adjuvant setting (3)	SBRT: <45 Gy/3F with normal liver >700 cc; <54 Gy/3F with normal liver >800 cc for Child-Pugh A Conventional dose: 40–70 Gy CTV not necessarily include lymphatic drainage without metastasis Introduction of techniques including respiratory gating, breath control, abdominal compression

Abbreviations: *AASLD* American Association for the Study of Liver Disease, *AJCC* American Joint Committee on Cancer, *HCC* hepatocellular carcinoma, *EASL* European Association for the Study of the Liver, *RO* radiation oncology, *pRO* practical radiation oncology, *KLCSG* Korea Liver Cancer Study Group, *mUICC* modified Union for International Cancer Control, *TACE* transarterial chemoembolization, *PVT* portal vein thrombosis, *NCCN* national cancer comprehensive network, *CPS* Child-Pugh Score, *UNOS* United Network for Organ Sharing, *ESLC* Egyptian Study of Liver Cancer, *BCLC* Barcelona Clinic of Liver Cancer, *CLIP* Cancer of Liver Italian Program, *INASL* Indian National Association for the Study of the Liver, *APASL* Asia-Pacific Association for the Study of the Liver, *HKLC* Hong Kong Liver Cancer study group, *SBRT* stereotactic body radiotherapy, *LT* liver transplantation, *NCCS* National Cancer Center Singapore, *RFA* radiofrequency ablation, *PEI* percutaneous ethanol injection, *TLCA* Taiwan Liver Cancer Association

Table 11.2 Clinical example of treatment applications according to selected guidelines for HCC

Guidelines	EASL (BCLC)	NCCN	APASL	KLSCG-NCC
Classification	Early (A)	Resectable or transplantable	Own system (no extrahepatic metastases; Child-Pugh A/B; resectable)	mUICC II
Primary option	LT, resection or ablation	Resection or LT	Resection	Resection, LT (≤5 cm), RFA (≤3 cm)
Alternative option	(−)	Locoregional treatment (ablation, arterial directed therapy, EBRT)	Local ablation	TACE, TARE, other LRT (<3 cm, e.g., PEI) EBRT
Classification	Advanced (C)	Unresectable	Own system (no extrahepatic metastases; Child-Pugh A/B; macrovascular invasion)	mUICC II
Primary option	Systemic therapy	Locoregional treatment (ablation, arterial directed therapies, EBRT)	Systemic therapy (resection if resectable)	TACE, EBRT, Sorafenib, Lenvatinib
Alternative option	(−)	Systemic therapy, supportive care	TACE	Resection

Single, >2 cm, without VI

Single, ≤2 cm, with VI

Classification	Advanced (C)	Unresectable	Own system (no extrahepatic metastases; Child-Pugh A/B; macrovascular invasion)	mUICC III
Primary option	Systemic therapy	Locoregional treatment (ablation, arterial directed therapies, EBRT)	Systemic therapy (resection if resectable)	TACE + EBRT, TACE, Sorafenib, Lenvatinib (tumor occupation < 50%, Vp1–3)
Alternative option	(−)	Systemic treatment, supportive care	TACE	Resection EBRT

Single, >2 cm, with VI

Abbreviations: *BCLC* Barcelona Clinic Liver Cancer, *NCCN* National Comprehensive Cancer Network, *APASL* Asia-Pacific Association for the Study of the Liver, *KLSCG-NCC* Korean Liver Cancer Study Group and National Cancer Centre, *mUICC* modified Union for International Cancer Control, *LT* liver transplantation, *RFA* radiofrequency ablation, *PEI* percutaneous ethanol injection, *RT* radiotherapy, *TACE* trans-arterial chemoembolization, *EBRT* external beam radiotherapy, *VI* vascular invasion
Referenced from Rim et al. [43]

Recently, radiation oncologists from Japan, China, Hong Kong, Taiwan, and Korea who specialize in treating HCC collaborated to conduct an evaluation study of the HCC guidelines using the AGREE tool (Fig. 11.1) [42]. The evaluation was performed with an additional domain, "Radiotherapy contents," added to the original AGREE domains. The domain that most significantly affected the overall result was "Rigor of Development," which encompassed eight items evaluating the systemic method of evaluation and interpreting evidence and recommendations. Among the 18 guidelines that cited radiotherapy, four—from the NCCN, EASL, AASLD, and KLCSG—were assessed as "applicable without modification" considering both their overall scoring and individual recommendation. The NCCN guidelines were the only ones that received the highest recommendation from all the appraisers; these guidelines scored highly across all domains and had the highest score (84.7%) for the domain

of "Radiotherapy contents." The KLCSG guidelines achieved the highest recommendation from four of six appraisers and had the second-highest score (77.8%) for the "Radiotherapy contents" domain. The EASL and AASLD guidelines achieved the highest recommendation from three of six appraisers and scored well among all domains except "Radiotherapy contents," which scored as low as 44.4% and 26.4% respectively. The absence of radiation oncologists among developers, lack of practical content regarding EBRT, and a somewhat overly critical view regarding evidence and recommendations are thought to have resulted in these low domain scores. The main results from the appraisal studies of the HCC guidelines using the AGREE tool are shown in Table 11.3.

For physicians who devote themselves more to clinical practice than to academic endeavors, practical contents as well as the overall quality of the guidelines may be of greater concern. In other

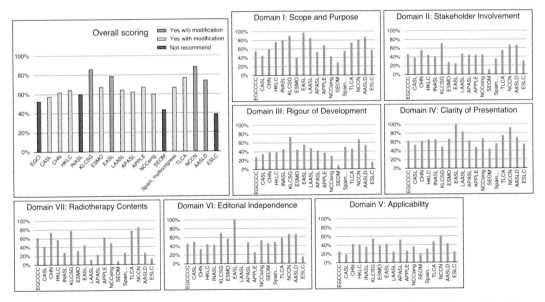

Fig. 11.1 Appraisal of hepatocellular carcinoma clinical guidelines by radiation oncologists, using AGREE II method (Referenced from Rim et al. [42]). Abbreviations: *ECGCCC* Eastern Canadian Gastrointestinal Cancer Consensus Conference, *HKLC* Hong Kong Liver Cancer association, *INASL* Indian National Association for Study of the Liver, *KLCSG* Korean Liver Cancer Study Group, *ESMO* European Society of Medical Oncology, *EASL* European Association for the Study of the Liver, *LAASL*

Latin America Association for the Study of the Liver, *APASL* Asia-Pacific Association for the Study of the Liver, *APPLE* Asia-Pacific Primary Liver Cancer Expert meeting, *NCC* National Cancer Center, *SEOM* Sociedad Española de Oncología Médica, *TLCA* Taiwan Liver Cancer Association, *NCCN* National Cancer Comprehensive Network, *AASLD* American Association for the Study of the Liver Disease, *ESLC* Egyptian Society of Liver Cancer

Table 11.3 Results of appraisals of clinical practice guidelines for HCC using the AGREE tool

Authors	Affiliation	Year, publication	Authors' disciplines	Strongly recommended guidelines
Schmidt et al. [46]	Hannover Medical School, US	2011, J Gastroenterol Hepatol	Hepatology	AASLD (2005), CCO (2006, 2008), SNLG (2009)
Wang et al. [18]	Chinese Cochrane Center	2014, PloS One	Medical administration, preventive medicine, safety evaluation of drugs	JMH (2008), AASLD (2011), EASL-EORTC (2012)
Gavriilidis et al. [36]	Surgical centers from France, UK, and Taipei	2017, J Hepatol	Surgery	Canadian consensus (2011), JSH (2010), KLSCG (2014)
Holvoet et al. [45]	Ghent University, Belgium	2015, Dig Liv Dis	Intervention (transarterial chemoembolization)	(EASL-EORTC (2012), AASLD (2011), Canadian consensus (2011)
Rim et al. [42]	Radiation oncology centers from China, Japan, Korea, Taiwan, and Hong Kong	2020, Radiother Oncol	Radiation oncology	NCCN, KLCSG (2019), EASL (2018), AASLD (2018)

Abbreviations: *AASLD* American Association for the Study of Liver Disease, *CCO* Cancer Care Ontario, *SNLG* Sisterna Nazionalle Linnee Guida, *JMH* Japanese Ministry of Health, *EASL-EORTC* European Association for the Study of the Liver-European Organization for Research and Treatment of Cancer, *JSH* Japan Society of Hepatology, *KLCSG* Korean Liver Cancer Study Group, *NCCN* National Comprehensive Cancer Network

words, no matter how well the literature reviews and recommendations are, it is more important to study the guidelines and obtain any necessary assistance to design the actual implementation of EBRT. The guidelines from the KLCSG, based on Union of International Cancer Control staging, graphically describe which EBRT indications can be considered in detail (Table 11.4) [33]. Hepatic reserve to retain the feasibility of EBRT is also addressed (e.g., adequate liver function is necessary [Child-Pugh class A or B7] and the volume receiving ≤30 Gy must be ≥40% of the total liver volume; in hypofractionated settings of ≤10 fractions, volumes receiving <15 Gy must be ≥700 mL) (Table 11.1). The NCCN guidelines state that EBRT can be applied irrespective of tumor location using modern modalities including 3D conformal radiotherapy, IMRT, and SBRT. They also suggest common doses and indications for SBRT (30–50 Gy in 3–5 fractions for 1–3 tumors without extrahepatic disease) and describe the necessity of strict dose constraints for patients with Child-Pugh B cirrhosis [47].

The guidelines by the Chinese National Health and Family Planning Commission described the practical aspects of EBRT in detail [32]. They

introduced basic principles to derive the gross tumor volume and clinical target volume, which are specialized terms in radiation oncology. The necessity of 4D CT, which considers the respiratory motion of the organs as well as a 5–15 mm margin for this movement, was also described. Conventional treatment was suggested using 40–70 Gy in 2 Gy per fraction. Regarding SBRT, a dose of <45 Gy in three fractions for normal liver volumes of >700 mL and of <54 Gy in three fractions for normal liver volumes of <800 mL were suggested as safe doses for Child-Pugh A patients, and a dose of ≥30–60 Gy in 3–6 fractions was suggested as the usual recommended dose (Table 11.1). In the evaluation study by international radiation oncologists using the AGREE tool, the domain score of "Radiotherapy contents" was fairly high at 73.6%.

Referencing internationally known guidelines such as those of the EASL, NCCN, and AASLD helps to understand the trends in standard treatment and establish an overall intervention strategy. The practical aspects of the KLCSG and Chinese guidelines can be helpful for actual EBRT applications, especially when dealing with hepatitis B virus-related liver cancer or locally

Table 11.4 Best and alternative options according to UICC system in guidelines of Korean Liver Cancer Study Group

mUICC stage		Best option	Alternative option
I	Single/≤2 cm/VI−	Resection RFA	TACE Other LRT EBRT
II	Single/>2 cm/VI−	Resection LT(tumor size ≤ 5 cm) RFA (tumor size ≤ 3 cm)	TACE, TARE Other LRT (tumor size ≤ 3 cm) EBRT
	Multiple/≤2cm/VI−	LT (within Milan criteria) TACE RFA (tumor number ≤ 3)	Resection (tumor number ≤ 2) Other LRT (tumor number ≤ 3) EBRT (tumor number ≤ 3)
	Single/≤2 cm/VI+	TACE EBRT Sorafenib Lenvatinib	Resection
III	Multiple/>2 cm/VI−	TACE LT (within Milan criteria) RFA (tumor number ≤ 3 and size ≤3 cm)	Resection (tumor number ≤ 2) TACE EBRT (tumor number ≤ 3 and size ≤ 3 cm) Other LRT (tumor number ≤ 3 and size ≤ 3 cm)
	Single/>2 cm/VI+	TACE + EBRT TACE Sorafenib Lenvatinib (tumor occupation < 50%, Vp1–3)	Resection EBRT
	Multiple/≤2 cm/VI+	TACE + EBRT TACE Sorafenib, Lenvatinib	
IVa	Multiple/>2 cm/VI+	Sorafenib Lenvatinib (tumor occupation < 50%, Vp1–3) TACE + EBRT	TACE
	Node+/no metastasis	Sorafenib Lenvatinib (tumor occupation < 50%, Vp1–3)	TACE EBRT
IVb	Metastasis+	Sorafenib Lenvatinib (tumor occupation < 50%, Vp1–3)	TACE EBRT

Abbreviations: *ECOG* Eastern Cooperative Oncolog Group, *mUICC* modified Union for International Cancer Control, *VI* vascular or bile duct invasion, *RFA* radiofrequency ablation, *TACE* transarterial chemoembolization, *LRT* locoregional therapy; other LRT includes percutaneous ethanol injection, microwave ablation, and cryoablation; *EBRT* external beam radiation therapy, *LT* liver transplantation, *TARE* transarterial embolization, *Vp* portal vein invasion
Referenced from [33]

advanced disease, which are common in Asia. Domestic guidelines that take into account the epidemiologic or socioeconomic circumstances in relevant countries should also be referenced.

11.5 Summary and Conclusions

The etiologies and disease characteristics of liver cancer vary significantly among regions. Socioeconomic support is essential for multidis-ciplinary approaches including up-to-date modalities and medications. Radiation oncologists should identify trends in standard therapy through referencing major guidelines that are internationally used, such as those from the EASL or NCCN, and determine treatment applications by referring to guidelines with practical and specific considerations that best apply to each region. Although the updated versions of the guidelines have more favorable views of EBRT, there remains a critical need for high-level evidence, including that from randomized controlled studies.

References

1. Bray F, Ferlay J, Soerjomataram I, Siegel RL, Torre LA, Jemal A. Global cancer statistics 2018: GLOBOCAN estimates of incidence and mortality worldwide for 36 cancers in 185 countries. CA Cancer J Clin. 2018;68(6):394–424.
2. El-Serag HB. Epidemiology of viral hepatitis and hepatocellular carcinoma. Gastroenterology. 2012;142(6):1264–73.e1.
3. Choo SP, Tan WL, Goh BK, Tai WM, Zhu AX. Comparison of hepatocellular carcinoma in Eastern versus Western populations. Cancer. 2016;122(22):3430–46.
4. Sinn DH, Choi G-S, Park HC, Kim JM, Kim H, Song KD, et al. Multidisciplinary approach is associated with improved survival of hepatocellular carcinoma patients. PLoS One. 2019;14(1):e0210730.
5. Rim CH, Kim CY, Yang DS, Yoon WS. The role of external beam radiotherapy for hepatocellular carcinoma patients with lymph node metastasis: a meta-analysis of observational studies. Cancer Manag Res. 2018;10:3305–15.
6. Kudo M. Management of hepatocellular carcinoma in Japan as a world-leading model. Liver Cancer. 2018;7(2):134–47.
7. Kudo M. Surveillance, diagnosis, treatment, and outcome of liver cancer in Japan. Liver Cancer. 2015;4(1):39–50.
8. KLCSG, NCCK. 2014 Korean Liver Cancer Study Group-National Cancer Center. Korea practice guideline for the management of hepatocellular carcinoma. Korean J Radiol. 2015;16(3):465–522.
9. Park S, Yoon WS, Rim CH. Indications of external radiotherapy for hepatocellular carcinoma from updated clinical guidelines: diverse global viewpoints. World J Gastroenterol. 2020;26(4):393–403.
10. Jia J, Zhang D, Ludwig J, Kim H. Radiofrequency ablation versus resection for hepatocellular carcinoma in patients with Child–Pugh A liver cirrhosis: a meta-analysis. Clin Radiol. 2017;72(12):1066–75.
11. Park JW, Chen M, Colombo M, Roberts LR, Schwartz M, Chen PJ, et al. Global patterns of hepatocellular carcinoma management from diagnosis to death: the BRIDGE Study. Liver Int. 2015;35(9):2155–66.
12. Rim CH, Yim HJ, Park S, Seong J. Recent clinical applications of external beam radiotherapy for hepatocellular carcinoma according to guidelines, major trials and meta-analyses. J Med Imaging Radiat Oncol. 2019;63(6):812–21. https://doi.org/10.1111/1754-9485.12948.
13. Llovet JM, Ricci S, Mazzaferro V, Hilgard P, Gane E, Blanc JF, et al. Sorafenib in advanced hepatocellular carcinoma. N Engl J Med. 2008;359(4):378–90.
14. Bruix J, Qin S, Merle P, Granito A, Huang YH, Bodoky G, et al. Regorafenib for patients with hepatocellular carcinoma who progressed on sorafenib treatment (RESORCE): a randomised, double-blind, placebo-controlled, phase 3 trial. Lancet. 2017;389(10064):56–66.
15. Abou-Alfa GK, Meyer T, Cheng AL, El-Khoueiry AB, Rimassa L, Ryoo BY, Cicin I, Merle P, Chen Y, Park JW, Blanc JF. Cabozantinib in patients with advanced and progressing hepatocellular carcinoma. N Engl J Med. 2018;379(1):54–63.
16. Levy I, Sherman M. Staging of hepatocellular carcinoma: assessment of the CLIP, Okuda, and Child-Pugh staging systems in a cohort of 257 patients in Toronto. Gut. 2002;50(6):881–5.
17. Subramaniam S, Kelley RK, Venook AP. A review of hepatocellular carcinoma (HCC) staging systems. Chin Clin Oncol. 2013;2(4):33.
18. Wang Y, Luo Q, Li Y, Wang H, Deng S, Wei S, et al. Quality assessment of clinical practice guidelines on the treatment of hepatocellular carcinoma or metastatic liver cancer. PLoS One. 2014;9(8):e103939.
19. European Association fot the Study of the Liver. EASL Clnical practice guideilnes. https://easl.eu/publications/clinical-practice-guidelines/. Assessed 15 Dec 2019.
20. Galle PR, Forner A, Llovet JM, Mazzaferro V, Piscaglia F, Raoul J-L, et al. EASL clinical practice guidelines: management of hepatocellular carcinoma. J Hepatol. 2018;69(1):182–236.
21. European Association for the Study of the Liver, European Organisation for Research and Treatment of Cancer. EASL-EORTC clinical practice guidelines: management of hepatocellular carcinoma. J Hepatol. 2012;56(4):908–43.
22. Pan CC, Kavanagh BD, Dawson LA, Li XA, Das SK, Miften M, et al. Radiation-associated liver injury. Int J Radiat Oncol Biol Phys. 2010;76(3):S94–S100.
23. Foerster F, Galle PR. Comparison of the current international guidelines on the management of HCC. JHEP Rep. 2019;1(2):114–9.
24. Chen S, Peng Z, Wei M, Liu W, Dai Z, Wang H, et al. Sorafenib versus transarterial chemoembolization for advanced-stage hepatocellular carcinoma: a cost-effectiveness analysis. BMC Cancer. 2018;18(1):392.
25. Omata M, Cheng A-L, Kokudo N, Kudo M, Lee JM, Jia J, et al. Asia–Pacific clinical practice guidelines on the management of hepatocellular carcinoma: a 2017 update. Hepatol Int. 2017;11(4):317–70.
26. Bruix J, Sherman M. Management of hepatocellular carcinoma: an update. Hepatology. 2011;53(3):1020–2.
27. Heimbach JK, Kulik LM, Finn RS, Sirlin CB, Abecassis MM, Roberts LR, et al. AASLD guidelines for the treatment of hepatocellular carcinoma. Hepatology. 2018;67(1):358–80.
28. Huo YR, Eslick GD. Transcatheter arterial chemoembolization plus radiotherapy compared with chemoembolization alone for hepatocellular carcinoma: a

systematic review and meta-analysis. JAMA Oncol. 2015;1(6):756–65.

29. Nakazawa T, Hidaka H, Shibuya A, Okuwaki Y, Tanaka Y, Takada J, et al. Overall survival in response to sorafenib versus radiotherapy in unresectable hepatocellular carcinoma with major portal vein tumor thrombosis: propensity score analysis. BMC Gastroenterol. 2014;14(1):84.

30. Kokudo N, Hasegawa K, Akahane M, Igaki H, Izumi N, Ichida T, et al. Evidence-based C linical P ractice G uidelines for H epatocellular C arcinoma: the J apan S ociety of H epatology 2013 update (3rd JSH-HCC G uidelines). Hepatol Res. 2015;45(2) https://doi.org/10.1111/hepr.12464.

31. Chow PK, Choo SP, Ng DC, Lo RH, Wang ML, Toh HC, et al. National cancer centre Singapore consensus guidelines for hepatocellular carcinoma. Liver Cancer. 2016;5(2):97–106.

32. Zhou J, Sun H-C, Wang Z, Cong W-M, Wang J-H, Zeng M-S, et al. Guidelines for diagnosis and treatment of primary liver cancer in China (2017 edition). Liver Cancer. 2018;7(3):235–60.

33. Korean Liver Cancer Association. 2018 Korean Liver Cancer Association–National Cancer Center. Korea practice guidelines for the management of hepatocellular carcinoma. Gut Liver. 2019;13(3):227–99.

34. Lu S-N, Wang J-H, Su C-W, Wang T-E, Dai C-Y, Chen C-H, et al. Management consensus guideline for hepatocellular carcinoma: 2016 updated by the Taiwan Liver Cancer Association and the Gastroenterological Society of Taiwan. J Formos Med Assoc. 2018;117(5):381–403.

35. Cheung TT-T, Kwok PC-H, Chan S, Cheung C-C, Lee A-S, Lee V, et al. Hong Kong consensus statements for the management of unresectable hepatocellular carcinoma. Liver Cancer. 2018;7(1):40–54.

36. Gavriilidis P, Roberts KJ, Askari A, Sutcliffe RP, Liu P-H, Hidalgo E, et al. Evaluation of the current guidelines for resection of hepatocellular carcinoma using the Appraisal of Guidelines for Research and Evaluation II instrument. J Hepatol. 2017;67(5):991–8.

37. Yoon SM, Ryoo B-Y, Lee SJ, Kim JH, Shin JH, An JH, et al. Efficacy and safety of transarterial chemoembolization plus external beam radiotherapy vs sorafenib in hepatocellular carcinoma with macroscopic vascular invasion: a randomized clinical trial. JAMA Oncol. 2018;4(5):661–9.

38. Guyatt G, Oxman A, Vist G, GRADE Working Group. An emerging consensus on rating quality of evidence and strength of recommendations. Br Med J. 2007;336(7650):924–6.

39. Kumar A, Acharya SK, Singh SP, Saraswat VA, Arora A, Duseja A, et al. The Indian National Association for Study of the Liver (INASL) consensus on prevention, diagnosis and management of hepatocellular carcinoma in India: the Puri recommendations. J Clin Exp Hepatol. 2014;4:S3–S26.

40. Méndez-Sánchez N, Ridruejo E, de Mattos AA, Chávez-Tapia NC, Zapata R, Paraná R, et al. Latin American Association for the Study of the Liver (LAASL) clinical practice guidelines: management of hepatocellular carcinoma. Ann Hepatol. 2014;13:S4–S40.

41. Wehrenberg-Klee E, Goyal L, Dugan M, Zhu AX, Ganguli S. Y-90 radioembolization combined with a PD-1 inhibitor for advanced hepatocellular carcinoma. Cardiovasc Intervent Radiol. 2018;41(11):1799–802.

42. Rim CH, Cheng J, Huang W-Y, Kimura T, Lee V, Zeng Z-C, et al. An evaluation of hepatocellular carcinoma practice guidelines from a radiation oncology perspective. Radiother Oncol. 2020;2020(148):73–81.

43. Rim CH, Seong J. Application of radiotherapy for hepatocellular carcinoma in current clinical practice guidelines. Radiat Oncol J. 2016;34(3):160–7.

44. Brouwers MC, Kho ME, Browman GP, Burgers JS, Cluzeau F, Feder G, et al. AGREE II: advancing guideline development, reporting and evaluation in health care. CMAJ. 2010;182(18):E839–E42.

45. Holvoet T, Raevens S, Vandewynckel Y-P, Van Biesen W, Geboes K, Van Vlierberghe H. Systematic review of guidelines for management of intermediate hepatocellular carcinoma using the Appraisal of Guidelines Research and Evaluation II instrument. Dig Liver Dis. 2015;47(10):877–83.

46. Schmidt S, Follmann M, Malek N, Manns MP, Greten TF. Critical appraisal of clinical practice guidelines for diagnosis and treatment of hepatocellular carcinoma. J Gastroenterol Hepatol. 2011;26(12):1779–86.

47. National Cancer Comprehensive Network. Principle of locoregional therapy. NCCN guidelines version 3.2019, Hepatobiliary cancers. https://www.nccn.org/professionals/physician_gls/pdf/hepatobiliary.pdf. Assessed 1 Dec 2019.

Ablative Radiation Therapy for Early Hepatocellular Carcinoma

12

Naoko Sanuki, Atsuya Takeda, and Yuichiro Tsurugai

Abstract

Ablative radiation therapy, also known as stereotactic body radiation therapy (SBRT) or stereotactic ablative body radiotherapy (SABR), has an evolving role in the treatment of hepatocellular carcinoma (HCC), owing to recent advances in technology. SBRT is primarily used when other local therapies are not feasible. Although evidence is limited, SBRT has been demonstrated to be an effective treatment with excellent local control. In this chapter, we discuss the role of SBRT as a curative local therapy for patients with early HCC.

Keywords

Stereotactic body radiation therapy (SBRT)
Stereotactic ablative radiation therapy
(SABR) · Hepatocellular carcinoma
Liver cancer · Hypofractionation
Radiofrequency ablation

N. Sanuki (✉)
Department of Radiology, Yokkaichi Municipal Hospital, Yokkaichi, Mie, Japan

Department of Radiation Oncology, Ofuna Chuo Hospital, Kamakura, Kanagawa, Japan
e-mail: naokosanuki@icloud.com

A. Takeda · Y. Tsurugai
Department of Radiation Oncology, Ofuna Chuo Hospital, Kamakura, Kanagawa, Japan
e-mail: takeda@1994.jukuin.keio.ac.jp

12.1 Treatment of Early HCC

12.1.1 The Significance of Surveillance in Early HCC Detection

Major risk factors for HCC include viral hepatitis, alcohol consumption, morbid obesity, and metabolic syndrome. Advances in imaging techniques and surveillance programs for patients at increased risk for HCC have led to the detection of small hepatic nodules in patients with chronic liver disease, resulting in increased delivery of curative treatment [1]. In a Japanese cohort including 1432 patients, careful ultrasonography surveillance resulted in the average size of detected tumors being smaller than 2 cm, with <2% of tumors exceeding 3 cm [2].

Early detection of HCC has been suggested to have contributed to prolonged survival as a consequence of more HCC patients receiving curative therapy. In Japan, where a complete nationwide surveillance program covered by national health care has been established, as many as 66% of all cases are curatively treatable at initial diagnosis either by resection or percutaneous ablation [3]. In contrast, in other parts of Asia and in western countries, rates of early HCC diagnosis do not exceed 30% [4]. In addition, only 6% of Japanese patients have advanced HCC (Barcelona Clinic Liver Cancer [BCLC] stage C or D) at initial diagnosis, while 50% of

© Springer Nature Singapore Pte Ltd. 2021
J. Seong (ed.), *Radiotherapy of Liver Cancer*, https://doi.org/10.1007/978-981-16-1815-4_12

cases are advanced at diagnosis in western countries. Differences in patient and tumor characteristics and treatment availability are closely linked to the treatment approaches used in each county.

It has been suggested that overall, the prevalence of hepatitis infection is being reduced by vaccination and/or anti-viral drugs, so the percentage of HCC due to noninfectious causes, such as alcohol consumption or metabolic syndrome, is increasing. These factors are expected to continue to influence future trends in HCC occurrence. Regardless, the proportion of early HCC cases is expected to increase due to surveillance of patients at high risk. According to the BCLC staging and treatment strategy, resection, transplantation, and percutaneous ablation are recommended as first-line treatments for early-stage HCC [5]. However, due to issues such as underlying cirrhosis or the presence of multifocal tumors arising from viral infection, only about 38% of patients who are initially diagnosed with HCC are eligible for resection [3, 6]. As more HCCs are detected at an early stage, the number of patients who are deemed ineligible for currently available curative local therapies will increase. Although radiation therapy is not listed as a treatment option in the European Association for the Study of the Liver (EASL) treatment algorithm [5], its role in HCC is gradually gaining acceptance, and it is increasingly being viewed as a curative treatment rather than a palliative treatment. Therefore, increasing attention should be focused on possible indications of radiation therapy in patients with early HCC.

12.1.2 Early HCC that Should Be Treated

Clinically, very early HCC (BCLC stage 0) is defined as the presence of a single tumor <2 cm, while early HCC (BCLC stage A) is characterized by a single tumor >2 cm or up to three nodules <3 cm in patients with good health status and well-preserved liver function (Child-Pugh class A) [5]. Although histopathological diagnosis is the gold standard for defining HCC, it is not always feasible in all patients, due to comorbidities, technical difficulty, and/or false negative results. In fact, unlike most solid cancers, a diag-

nosis of HCC with typical radiologic findings can be established based on imaging without biopsy confirmation [7, 8]. The characteristic appearance of classic HCC on dynamic imaging is a hypervascular lesion that shows washout in the portal venous phase.

Histopathological diagnosis of early HCC refers to a spectrum of disease, beginning from a premalignant state. A sequence of events has been proposed to occur in hepatic nodules preceding emergence of HCC; these lesions are recognized as precursors, such as adenomatous hyperplasia or dysplastic nodules [5, 8, 9]. Thereafter, early HCC lesions progress from low-grade to high-grade dysplastic nodules via multistep carcinogenesis. Owing to the advancement of diagnostic imaging techniques such as dynamic magnetic resonance imaging (MRI) using gadoxetate disodium, hypovascular dysplastic nodules (and some early HCCs) are increasingly being detected.

Survival benefits associated with treatment of early HCC may be affected by lead time bias and might not be attributable to early treatment. Midorikawa et al. compared two series of patients undergoing resection versus observation for early and overt HCC to estimate lead time and survival benefit [10]. These researchers observed that surgery did not beneficially alter the natural history of early HCC lesions <20 mm. In contrast, Kumada et al. reported that it took as long as 12 months after diagnosis before hypovascular nodules <15 mm became vascularized [11]. The American Association for the Study of Liver Disease recommends that biopsy should be performed for nodules <2 cm if their radiologic findings are not characteristic of HCC [8]. With the increase of early HCC detection, patients with small tumors who are ineligible for biopsy may be referred for radiation therapy for management of possibly premalignant nodules. Radiation oncologists need to be aware that for small HCCs with atypical imaging findings and unknown etiology, careful discussion with hepatologists and patients is required.

In general, tumors <1 cm should not be treated [5]. However, even a lesion of nearly 1 cm in size detected by MRI may be a dysplasia that will progress over time. Figure 12.1 describes a

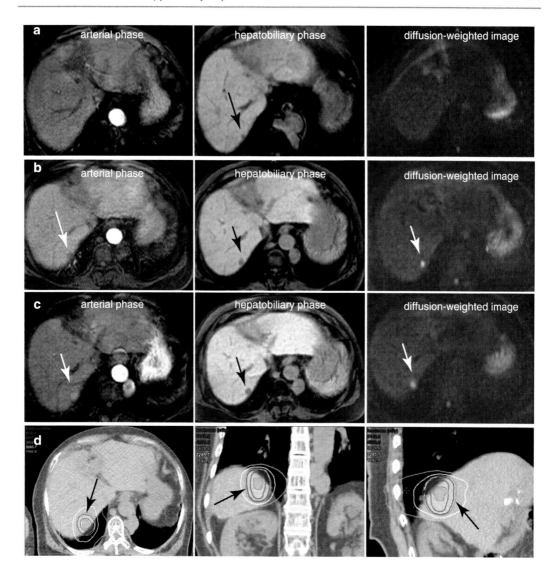

Fig. 12.1 A very early HCC that had been observed for about 30 months prior to SBRT. A 71-year-old female with HCC with repeated intrahepatic recurrences within a cirrhotic liver due to Budd-Chiali syndrome. Since 2006, she has developed three HCC lesions that sequentially occurred and were treated, with each showing durable local control. Approximately eight years after the onset of the initial HCC, a low signal nodule in the hepatobiliary phase of gadoxetic acid disodium-enhanced magnetic resonance imaging (EOB-MRI) appeared in segment 7 (S7), without early enhancement or decreased diffusion, which led to close monitoring without treatment (**a**). Twenty-eight months later, a signal reduction at the S7 lesion appeared in a diffusion-weighted image (**b**), and another two months passed before observation of early enhancement in a lesion 1.3 cm in diameter, for which the lesion was judged to be treatable (**c**). SBRT (40 Gy, 5 fractions) was administered to the S7 tumor (**d**). The dark-gray lines indicated by arrows coincide with the 40-Gy dose. Overall, it took about 30 months after the identification of the precancerous lesion to be indicated for local treatment. Two and a half years after SBRT, the patient died due to HCC progression without local recurrence of the irradiated lesion

patient with very early HCC treated with SBRT in segment 7. The patient had chronic liver disease accompanied by a 1.3-cm tumor detected by MRI. It took about 30 months for the tumor to be indicated for SBRT.

12.2 The Role of SBRT as a Curative Local Therapy

12.2.1 SBRT as an Ablative Therapy

The term *ablative* refers to the removal of a body part or tissue, and includes surgical resection, percutaneous "ablation" therapy, and stereotactic "ablative" body radiotherapy (SABR), each representing a different mode of attack. Liver transplantation is also a standard definitive treatment for nonmetastatic HCC. However, a very limited number of patients are ultimately candidates for transplantation, due to frequent comorbidities and graft shortage. According to the EASL treatment algorithm for HCC, a single tumor <2 cm in the preserved liver should be treated with liver transplantation, or if that is not possible, either resection or percutaneous ablation. Both of these ablative modalities are associated with local control rates >90% [6, 12, 13]. SBRT has also yielded an excellent local control rate >90% at two years, although its utility is not addressed in the EASL guidelines [14–17]. Nevertheless, ablative SBRT

could be a good option for patients unfit for resection and percutaneous ablation.

12.2.2 Local Control of SBRT and Other Local Therapies

In the absence of data from randomized trials comparing SBRT and other local therapies, the results of retrospective comparisons utilizing propensity score matching have been reported [18–22]. Local control is addressed in percutaneous ablation and SBRT studies (Table 12.1) but is not necessarily reported in surgical studies. However, local recurrence rates cannot simply be compared among studies, because the extent of resection and extent of irradiation often differ. Nevertheless, SBRT appears to result in equivalent or superior local control compared with radiofrequency ablation (RFA), especially for larger tumors and tumors in locations not amenable to RFA. Factors that cannot be matched by propensity score analysis, such as salvage intention and proximal vascularity, are some of the reasons why randomized trials are difficult to complete; however, these are the very areas where SBRT is expected to have great significance in clinical practice (Table 12.2). In other words, RFA and SBRT should be considered as complementary therapies, not equivalent therapies to be compared.

Table 12.1 Propensity score analysis comparing outcomes following RFA and SBRT

Author (year)	N (RFA/SBRT)	Follow-up duration (months)	Local control (RFA/SBRT)	Overall survival (RFA/SBRT)
Wahl [18] (2015)	332 (249/83)	20/13	80/84% @2 years	53/46% @2 years
Rajyaguru [19] (2018)	3980 (3684/296)	25	Not reported	30/19% @5 years ($p < 0.01$)
Hara[a] [20] (2019)	695 (474/221)	34/32	87/95% @3 years ($p < 0.01$)	69/70% @3 years ($p = 0.86$)
Kim [21] (2019)	850 (736/114)	22	65/75% @2 years ($p = 0.243$)	(−)
Kim [22] (2020)	2064 (1568/496)	28	72/79% @3 years ($p < 0.001$)	71/78% @2 years ($p = 0.308$)

Abbreviations: *RFA* radiofrequency ablation, *SBRT* stereotactic body radiation therapy
[a]SBRT and hypofractionated RT

Table 12.2 List of SBRT-preferable tumors and RFA-unpreferable tumors

Location
Directly below the diaphragm
Near the surface of the liver
Abutting a vessel
Near the luminal gastrointestinal tract
Hilar region near the biliary system
Large tumor (maximum diameter > 3 cm)
Residual tumor after TACE or RFA
Invisible on ultrasound
Obesity or fatty liver
Patients not suitable for holding breath
Bleeding tendency
Low platelet count (<50,000/mm³)
Current anticoagulant agents
Patients requiring dialysis
Fear of needles
Patient's refusal to RFA

Abbreviations: *SBRT* stereotactic body radiation therapy, *RFA* radiofrequency ablation, *TACE* transarterial chemoembolization
Modified from Hara et al. [20]

12.2.3 Survival after SBRT and Other Local Therapies

To evaluate survival after resection and SBRT, Su et al. compared clinical outcomes of patients who underwent resection and SBRT for one or two HCCs ≤5 cm. The five-year overall survival (OS) rates were comparable after propensity score matching: 69% in the resection group versus 74% in the SBRT group ($p = 0.405$) [23]. In contrast, Nakano et al. noted a very different result in patients who underwent resection (254 patients) and SBRT (27 patients) for one to three HCCs ≤3 cm. The five-year OS rate after propensity score matching was 75% for patients who underwent resection versus 48% for those who received SBRT ($p = 0.0149$) [24].

Among comparisons of RFA and SBRT, four published studies have utilized propensity score matching with partially conflicting results, possibly due to a variation in matching quality depending on which HCC prognostic factors were used (Table 12.1) [19–22]. Notably, liver function was not considered sufficient in some reports; therefore, serious selection bias could not be ruled out.

Nonetheless, three of the four studies reported comparable OS between patients treated with RFA and SBRT [20–22].

12.2.4 SBRT as a Definitive Treatment for Small HCC

As there are no available data from randomized trials, what data are required for SBRT to be accepted as a treatment option for small HCCs? Results reported from prospective trials and large databases have indicated that patients with newly diagnosed HCC who undergo surgery and RFA are likely to achieve OS rates >70% at three years [6, 25–28]. However, previous data from prospective trials of small HCCs indicate that the three-year OS rate after SBRT is unlikely to reach 70%, while more recently, three-year OS rates have been increasing (Table 12.3). Of note, most of the reports include a wide range of cases with local or intrahepatic recurrence, numerous previous treatments, and/or older age, which are disadvantageous factors with respect to SBRT when comparing OS rates with surgery or RFA.

Opportunities to perform SBRT as initial treatment for HCC remain limited. According to a retrospective study that investigated outcomes of up-front SBRT (with or without transarterial chemoembolization [TACE]) in 63 patients with previously untreated HCC, the three-year local control and OS rates were 92% and 73%, respectively [33]. The three-year OS rate of >70% is excellent, despite the fact that the median age of the study cohort was 74 years.

Two prospective phase II trials that evaluated SBRT for the treatment of newly diagnosed, solitary HCCs deemed unsuitable for standard locoregional therapies have been performed [30, 32]. These studies, conducted in France ($n = 43$; time period, 2009–2014; SBRT dose, 45 Gy/3 fractions) and Japan ($n = 36$; time period, 2014–2018; SBRT dose, 40 Gy/5 fractions), are similar in many ways. The median age (72 and 74 years in the French and Japanese studies, respectively) and tumor size (28 and 23 mm, respectively) were similar, as was baseline liver function (Child-Turcotte-Pugh [CTP]-A in 86% and 91%

Table 12.3 Prospective phase 1–2 studies of SBRT for patients with relatively small (≤6 cm) HCC lesions

Author (year)	N	Design and indication	Median follow-up (months)	Size (range)	Dose	Local control	Overall survival
Lasley [15] (2015)	59	Phase 1–2 ≤3 lesions ≤6 cm	33	33.6 ml (2.0–107.3)	CP-A 48 Gy/3 fr CP-B 40 Gy/5 fr	CP-A 91% CP-B 82% @3 years	CP-A 61% @3 years CP-B 26% @3 years
Takeda [14] (2016)	90	Phase 2 Solitary lesion ≤4 cm	42	2.3 cm (1.0–4.0)	35–40 Gy/5 fr	96% @3 years	67% @3 years
Kim [29] (2018)	32	Phase 1–2 ≤3 lesions, cumulative diameter ≤ 6 cm	23	2.1 cm (1.0–4.5)	36–60 Gy/4 fr	81% @2 years	81% @2 years
Kimura [30] (2019)	36	Phase 2 Newly diagnosed, solitary	21	2.3 cm (1.0–5.0)	40 Gy/5 fr	90% @3 years	78% @3 years
Jang [31] (2020)	74	Phase 2 Unresectable HCC	41	2.4 cm (1.0–9.9)	45–60 Gy/3 fr	95% @3 years	76% @3 years
Durand-Labrunie [32] (2020)	43	Phase 2 Newly diagnosed, solitary	48	2.8 cm (1.0–6.0)	45 Gy/3 fr	94% @2 years	69% @2 years

Abbreviations: *CP* Child-Pugh, *fr* fractions, *HCC* hepatocellular carcinoma, *SBRT* stereotactic body radiation therapy of cases, respectively). The local control and OS rates in both studies were also good: the 18-month local control and OS rates in the French study were 98% and 72%, respectively, while the three-year local control rates and OS rates in the Japanese study were 90% and 78%, respectively. Toxicities were mild and acceptable in both studies.

According to the EASL guidelines, five-year OS rates of 40–70% are expected following curative treatment of very early to early stage HCC tumors [34]. Although high-quality evidence based on randomized trials is not always available, the outcomes of SBRT based on existing evidence appear to meet the expected values of curative treatment. Because SBRT is essentially an alternative therapy in practice, many patients are elderly or have comorbidities for which the standard of care is not applicable. Nonetheless, the excellent OS might be attributed to the good local control, noninvasiveness, and mild toxicities associated with SBRT. The currently available data discussed above suggest a potential role of SBRT, particularly for small HCCs unfit for other local therapies. Further studies will be important to investigate which patients are most suitable for each local treatment.

12.2.5 Ongoing Trials Involving SBRT for HCC

There is one notable ongoing phase III trial being conducted in China (NCT03898921) [35]. Initiated in 2019, this study aims to compare RFA and SBRT for previously untreated small HCC (solitary tumor ≤5.0 cm without vascular invasion), expecting to accrue 270 participants with a primary endpoint of three-year OS rate. If the study is successfully completed, the results may contribute important evidence for consideration in clinical guidelines for HCC.

Additional approaches comparing SBRT and other treatments are also being evaluated, indicating this as an area of active investigation. For comparison with RFA, a randomized study of RFA alone versus RFA and SBRT is being conducted for postoperative recurrent HCC

(NCT04202523) [36]. For comparison with TACE, three head-to-head comparison trials (NCT03338647 [37], NCT02470533 [38], and NCT02762266 [39]) are ongoing in patients with unresectable or recurrent HCC. The addition of SBRT to systemic therapy (sorafenib) is also being compared to sorafenib alone in patients with unresectable or recurrent HCC (NCT01730937 [40], Radiation Therapy Oncology Group [RTOG] 1112). It should be noted that large tumors (e.g., up to 10 cm) are allowed in this study, with semi-radical intention, so the results may not be applicable for small HCCs that are otherwise eligible for resection or percutaneous ablation.

12.3 Optimal Prescribed Doses

12.3.1 Dose-Response in HCC

In patients treated with conventionally fractionated radiation therapy, a radiation dose-response has been observed in unresectable HCC [41]. Some models have suggested that dose escalation may improve local control, particularly in larger tumors, while others have observed that dose escalation is not effective, possibly due to the radiosensitive nature of HCC [42, 43] and liver tissue.

In contrast, for SBRT performed using hypofractionated regimens, the data regarding radiation dose response for HCC are inconsistent, although some data suggest improved local control with dose escalation, particularly for large tumors [42–44]. Various prescribed doses of SBRT are presently employed by different groups; the most common SBRT fractionation schemes for HCC are heterogeneous, ranging from 23 to 75 Gy in 3–6 fractions [45]. In a study aimed to establish tumor control probabilities (TCP) for liver tumors, the EQD2 (dose equivalent to treatment with 2 Gy per fraction) for a six-month local control rate of 90% in HCC was estimated to be 84 Gy [43]. Accordingly, a meta-analysis evaluating the efficacy of SBRT for HCC revealed a median EQD2 estimate of the prescribed dose of 83 Gy (range, 48–115 Gy) in the 32 studies evaluated [46]. Interpretation of these results should be done with caution, because the optimal dose may not be determined by the stated value of the prescribed dose but also by the dose prescription method. In addition, such doses reported in the literature may be larger than the optimal dose for small HCCs, because those studies included large tumors (>10 cm) [17, 47, 48]. In a retrospective investigation of the outcomes of relatively small HCCs (up to 5 cm; median tumor size, <3 cm) treated with SBRT, tumors were uniformly treated at two dose levels (35 and 40 Gy) in 5 fractions according to baseline liver function and normal liver dose. No significant differences in outcomes were observed between dose levels: the three-year local control rates in the 35-Gy and 40-Gy groups were 91% and 89% (log-rank $p = 0.99$), respectively, and the three-year OS rates were 66% and 72% ($p = 0.54$), respectively (EQD2 of 50 and 60 Gy, respectively) [49]. For the treatment of liver cancer, it is important to note that the radiosensitivity of both HCC and liver tissue is high [41] and liver reserve has a significant impact on survival; therefore, unnecessarily increasing doses can be detrimental and worsen prognosis. It is therefore important to preserve the normal liver at the lowest radiation dose that provides tumor control, particularly for small HCCs.

12.3.2 Dose Prescription in Consideration of Liver Preservation

Patients with HCC are prone to liver toxicity after radiation therapy due to underlying liver disease and comorbidities [50]. Therefore, in addition to local control, preservation of hepatic function is of great importance to the success of radiation therapy for HCC. In general, two types of approaches are used to determine the dose given to a tumor. One approach involves fixed doses that are employed for relatively small tumors with a median diameter of approximately 3 cm. In contrast, the other approach involves variable doses that are indicated for larger tumors, based on normal liver tolerance. Both fixed-dose and variable-dose prescription approaches have their own rationale, and it is important to understand the differences in treatment intention (curative or semi-radical), priority (local control or liver function preservation), and objectives (early or advanced) when referring to the literature. The fixed-dose approach provides the necessary minimum dose with sufficient efficacy for local control (i.e., as low as reasonably achievable). This concept may be reasonable for small HCCs to preserve liver function until possible retreatment; intrahepatic recurrences frequently occur after treatment (68% in five years) [51], and patients could possibly be repeatedly treated while underlying cirrhosis progressively develops over time.

12.4 SBRT in Special Situations and Future Directions

For patients with inoperable HCC, the indication for SBRT is broad and flexible, allowing for treatment of large tumors, multifocal disease, presence of tumor vascular invasion, and local recurrence after curative therapy. SBRT can also be applied to residual post-TACE tumors, portal vein tumor thrombi, and inferior vena cava tumor thrombi. In addition, the indication for SBRT can be further extended with technical advancement and accumulation of clinical evidence. Although the main subject of this chapter is early HCC, there are some special situations in which SBRT plays a significant role for various "small" lesions.

First, no strategy is listed in the EASL algorithm for patients with tumors >3 cm or for those with small tumors with relatively less decompensated livers. Although such tumors may actually be "beyond early" or "suboptimal early," respectively, they could be effectively and safely treated by SBRT with the intention to cure. As already mentioned in this chapter, SBRT has a durable role in patients with tumors that are too large (>3 cm) to be treated with percutaneous ablation (relatively unfeasible for ablation). SBRT should be recognized as a curative treatment option for patients with such tumors in the absence of results from randomized trials.

Second, for early and medially inoperable HCCs that are located close to luminal organs, such as the stomach and bowels, neither percutaneous ablation nor SBRT can be applied with full intensity. In these situations, a mild hypofractionated regimen will be applied to preserve bowel function, combined with novel systemic therapies (Fig. 12.2). Thus far, few reports of HCCs in the vicinity of the gastrointestinal tract treated with moderate oligo-fractionated irradiation have

been published, and the three-year local control rate appears to be compromised at 80%, even for small tumors [52, 53]. It would be unreasonable for small tumors to receive compromised treatment with reduced treatment intensity simply due to proximity to the intestinal tract. Regardless of whether the technique would still be called SBRT, it would be ideal to safely expand the indication for radiation therapy using the experience cultivated in SBRT.

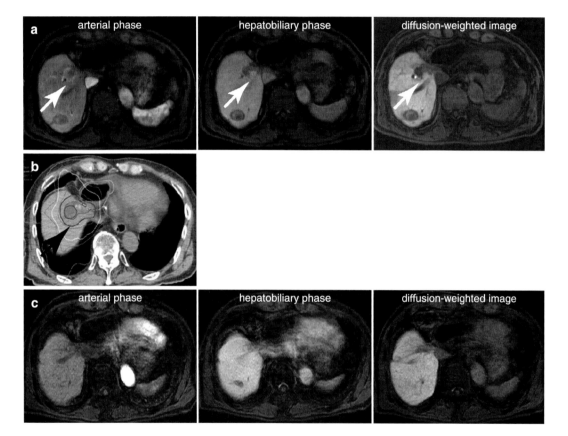

Fig. 12.2 Hypofractionated RT for HCC close to the stomach. A 79-year-old male with Child-Pugh class A cirrhosis. At the time of development of initial HCC, he underwent left liver lobectomy, then received multiple sequential local treatments for serial intrahepatic recurrences. Approximately four years after disease onset, intrahepatic recurrences were observed in S1 and S8 in the hepatobiliary phase of gadoxetic acid disodium-enhanced magnetic resonance imaging (EOB-MRI) (**a**). Local treatments such as RFA and TACE were not indicated due to proximity to the stomach. The patient agreed to undergo hypofractionated radiation therapy after a thorough explanation of the procedure, including the risks and benefits. A volumetric modulated therapy was performed at 42 Gy/14

fractions at a 70% isodose line (**b**). The dark-gray lines noted by arrows coincide with the 42-Gy dose. The volume 3 mm around the stomach received a flat dose distribution in the tumor-stomach overlapping regions and a steep dose distribution in the non-overlapping regions. The maximum dose was 44.2 Gy to the stomach and 45.0 Gy to the region 3 mm around the stomach, while the liver volume receiving >20 Gy (V20) was 19.7%. Intake of lansoprazole 15 mg and levamipide 300 mg/day was initiated at the start of treatment and was continued for six months. Although post-treatment malaise was noted, no gastrointestinal adverse events and no relapse had occurred at 32 months post-treatment (**c**)

Third, a treatment algorithm is supposed to be applied in the first-line setting. However, the algorithm is often used practically for salvage treatments for residual tumors or local progression after local treatment, or for focal intrahepatic recurrence. Such lesions can be repeatedly treated with local therapy, sometimes along with systemic therapy; however, curative treatment is not always feasible for medical and technical reasons. Noninvasive SBRT can serve as an effective salvage treatment in such patients, with the intention to cure. Given that much of the evidence for SBRT has focused on residual and recurrent cases, ample data already are available regarding the efficacy of SBRT in this patient population. The availability of multiple effective treatment options improves the overall outcomes of patients with this disease. Further investigations are warranted to define how and when patients with localized HCC are best treated.

References

1. Kanwal F, Singal AG. Surveillance for hepatocellular carcinoma: current best practice and future direction. Gastroenterology. 2019;157(1):54–64.
2. Sato T, Tateishi R, Yoshida H, Ohki T, Masuzaki R, Imamura J, et al. Ultrasound surveillance for early detection of hepatocellular carcinoma among patients with chronic hepatitis C. Hepatol Int. 2009;3(4):544–50.
3. Kudo M. Management of hepatocellular carcinoma in Japan: current trends. Liver Cancer. 2020;9(1):1–5.
4. Kudo M. Management of hepatocellular carcinoma in Japan as a world-leading model. Liver Cancer. 2018;7(2):134–47.
5. European Association for the Study of the Liver. EASL clinical practice guidelines: management of hepatocellular carcinoma. J Hepatol. 2018;69(1):182–236.
6. Kudo M, Izumi N, Kubo S, Kokudo N, Sakamoto M, Shiina S, et al. Report of the 20th Nationwide follow-up survey of primary liver cancer in Japan. Hepatol Res. 2020;50(1):15–46.
7. Marrero JA, Kulik LM, Sirlin CB, Zhu AX, Finn RS, Abecassis MM, et al. Diagnosis, staging, and management of hepatocellular carcinoma: 2018 practice guidance by the American Association for the Study of Liver Diseases. Hepatology. 2018;68(2):723–50.
8. Bruix J, Sherman M, American Association for the Study of Liver Diseases. Management of hepatocellular carcinoma: an update. Hepatology. 2011;53(3):1020–2.
9. International Consensus Group for Hepatocellular neoplasiathe International Consensus Group for Hepatocellular Neoplasia. Pathologic diagnosis of early hepatocellular carcinoma: a report of the international consensus group for hepatocellular neoplasia. Hepatology. 2009;49(2):658–64.
10. Midorikawa Y, Takayama T, Shimada K, Nakayama H, Higaki T, Moriguchi M, et al. Marginal survival benefit in the treatment of early hepatocellular carcinoma. J Hepatol. 2013;58(2):306–11.
11. Kumada T, Toyoda H, Tada T, Sone Y, Fujimori M, Ogawa S, et al. Evolution of hypointense hepatocellular nodules observed only in the hepatobiliary phase of gadoxetate disodium-enhanced MRI. AJR. 2011;197(1):58–63.
12. Regimbeau JM, Kianmanesh R, Farges O, Dondero F, Sauvanet A, Belghiti J. Extent of liver resection influences the outcome in patients with cirrhosis and small hepatocellular carcinoma. Surgery. 2002;131(3):311–7.
13. Lencioni R, Llovet JM. Modified RECIST (mRECIST) assessment for hepatocellular carcinoma. Semin Liver Dis. 2010;30(1):52–60.
14. Takeda A, Sanuki N, Tsurugai Y, Iwabuchi S, Matsunaga K, Ebinuma H, et al. Phase 2 study of stereotactic body radiotherapy and optional transarterial chemoembolization for solitary hepatocellular carcinoma not amenable to resection and radiofrequency ablation. Cancer. 2016;122(13):2041–9.
15. Lasley FD, Mannina EM, Johnson CS, Perkins SM, Althouse S, Maluccio M, et al. Treatment variables related to liver toxicity in patients with hepatocellular carcinoma, Child-Pugh class A and B enrolled in a phase 1-2 trial of stereotactic body radiation therapy. Pract Radiat Oncol. 2015;5(5):e443-e9.
16. Kang JK, Kim MS, Cho CK, Yang KM, Yoo HJ, Kim JH, et al. Stereotactic body radiation therapy for inoperable hepatocellular carcinoma as a local salvage treatment after incomplete transarterial chemoembolization. Cancer. 2012;118(21):5424–31.
17. Feng M, Suresh K, Schipper MJ, Bazzi L, Ben-Josef E, Matuszak MM, et al. Individualized adaptive stereotactic body radiotherapy for liver tumors in patients at high risk for liver damage: a phase 2 clinical trial. JAMA Oncol. 2018;4(1):40–7.
18. Wahl DR, Stenmark MH, Tao Y, Pollom EL, Caoili EM, Lawrence TS, et al. Outcomes after stereotactic body radiotherapy or radiofrequency ablation for hepatocellular carcinoma. J Clin Oncol. 2016;34(5):452–9.
19. Rajyaguru DJ, Borgert AJ, Smith AL, Thomes RM, Conway PD, Halfdanarson TR, et al. Radiofrequency ablation versus stereotactic body radiotherapy for localized hepatocellular carcinoma in nonsurgically managed patients: analysis of the national cancer database. J Clin Oncol. 2018;36(6):600–8.
20. Hara K, Takeda A, Tsurugai Y, Saigusa Y, Sanuki N, Eriguchi T, et al. Radiotherapy for hepatocellular carcinoma results in comparable survival to

radiofrequency ablation: a propensity score analysis. Hepatology. 2019;69(6):2533–45.

21. Kim N, Kim HJ, Won JY, Kim DY, Han KH, Jung I, et al. Retrospective analysis of stereotactic body radiation therapy efficacy over radiofrequency ablation for hepatocellular carcinoma. Radiother Oncol. 2019;131:81–7.

22. Kim N, Cheng J, Jung I, Liang J, Shih YL, Huang WY, et al. Stereotactic body radiation therapy vs. radiofrequency ablation in Asian patients with hepatocellular carcinoma. J Hepatol. 2020;73(1):121–9.

23. Su TS, Liang P, Liang J, Lu HZ, Jiang HY, Cheng T, et al. Long-term survival analysis of stereotactic ablative radiotherapy versus liver resection for small hepatocellular carcinoma. Int J Radiat Oncol Biol Phys. 2017;98(3):639–46.

24. Nakano R, Ohira M, Kobayashi T, Ide K, Tahara H, Kuroda S, et al. Hepatectomy versus stereotactic body radiotherapy for primary early hepatocellular carcinoma: a propensity-matched analysis in a single institution. Surgery. 2018;164(2):219–26.

25. Izumi N, Hasegawa K, Nishioka N, editors. A multicenter randomized controlled trial to evaluate the efficacy of surgery vs. radiofrequency ablation for small hepatocellular carcinoma (SURF trial). ASCO 2019 annual meeting; 2019.

26. Kim YS, Lim HK, Rhim H, Lee MW, Choi D, Lee WJ, et al. Ten-year outcomes of percutaneous radiofrequency ablation as first-line therapy of early hepatocellular carcinoma: analysis of prognostic factors. J Hepatol. 2013;58(1):89–97.

27. Feng K, Yan J, Li X, Xia F, Ma K, Wang S, et al. A randomized controlled trial of radiofrequency ablation and surgical resection in the treatment of small hepatocellular carcinoma. J Hepatol. 2012;57(4):794–802.

28. Huang J, Yan L, Cheng Z, Wu H, Du L, Wang J, et al. A randomized trial comparing radiofrequency ablation and surgical resection for HCC conforming to the Milan criteria. Ann Surg. 2010;252(6):903–12.

29. Kim JW, Kim DY, Han KH, Seong J. Phase I/II trial of helical IMRT-based stereotactic body radiotherapy for hepatocellular carcinoma. Dig Liver Dis. 2019;51(3):445–51.

30. Kimura T, Takeda A, Ishikura S, Ariyoshi K, Yamaguchi T, Imagumbai T, et al., editors. Multicenter prospective study of stereotactic body radiotherapy for untreated solitary primary hepatocellular carcinoma: the STRSPH Study. The Amercian Society for Radiation Oncology 61st Annual Meeting; 2019.

31. Jang WI, Bae SH, Kim MS, Han CJ, Park SC, Kim SB, et al. A phase 2 multicenter study of stereotactic body radiotherapy for hepatocellular carcinoma: safety and efficacy. Cancer. 2020;126(2):363–72.

32. Durand-Labrunie J, Baumann AS, Ayav A, Laurent V, Boleslawski E, Cattan S, et al. Curative irradiation treatment of hepatocellular carcinoma: a multicenter phase 2 trial. Int J Radiat Oncol Biol Phys. 2020;107(1):116–25.

33. Takeda A, Sanuki N, Eriguchi T, Kobayashi T, Iwabutchi S, Matsunaga K, et al. Stereotactic ablative body radiotherapy for previously untreated solitary hepatocellular carcinoma. J Gastroenterol Hepatol. 2014;29(2):372–9.

34. European Association for the Study of the Liver, European Organisation for Research and Treatment of Cancer. EASL-EORTC clinical practice guidelines: management of hepatocellular carcinoma. J Hepatol. 2012;56(4):908–43.

35. https://clinicaltrials.gov/ct2/show/NCT03898921?cond=NCT03898921&draw=2&rank=1 [Internet].

36. NCT04202523. https://clinicaltrials.gov/ct2/show/NCT04202523?cond=NCT04202523&draw=2&rank=1

37. NCT03338647. https://clinicaltrials.gov/ct2/show/NCT03338647?cond=NCT03338647&draw=2&rank=1

38. NCT02470533. https://clinicaltrials.gov/ct2/show/NCT02470533?cond=NCT02470533&draw=2&rank=1

39. NCT02762266. https://clinicaltrials.gov/ct2/show/NCT02762266?cond=NCT02762266&draw=2&rank=1

40. NCT01730937. https://clinicaltrials.gov/ct2/show/NCT01730937?cond=NCT01730937&draw=1&rank=1

41. Park HC, Seong J, Han KH, Chon CY, Moon YM, Suh CO. Dose-response relationship in local radiotherapy for hepatocellular carcinoma. Int J Radiat Oncol Biol Phys. 2002;54(1):150–5.

42. Jang WI, Kim MS, Bae SH, Cho CK, Yoo HJ, Seo YS, et al. High-dose stereotactic body radiotherapy correlates increased local control and overall survival in patients with inoperable hepatocellular carcinoma. Radiat Oncol. 2013;8:250.

43. Lausch A, Sinclair K, Lock M, Fisher B, Jensen N, Gaede S, et al. Determination and comparison of radiotherapy dose responses for hepatocellular carcinoma and metastatic colorectal liver tumours. Br J Radiol. 2013;86(1027):20130147.

44. Ohri N, Tome WA, Mendez Romero A, Miften M, Ten Haken RK, Dawson LA, et al. Local control after stereotactic body radiation therapy for liver tumors. Int J Rad Oncol Biol Phy. 2018; https://doi.org/10.1016/j.ijrobp.2017.12.288.

45. Bang A, Dawson LA. Radiotherapy for HCC: ready for prime time? JHEP Rep. 2019;1(2):131–7.

46. Rim CH, Kim HJ, Seong J. Clinical feasibility and efficacy of stereotactic body radiotherapy for hepatocellular carcinoma: a systematic review and meta-analysis of observational studies. Radiother Oncol. 2019;131:135–44.

47. Bujold A, Massey CA, Kim JJ, Brierley J, Cho C, Wong RK, et al. Sequential phase I and II trials of stereotactic body radiotherapy for locally advanced hepatocellular carcinoma. J Clin Oncol. 2013;31(13):1631–9.

48. Scorsetti M, Comito T, Cozzi L, Clerici E, Tozzi A, Franzese C, et al. The challenge of inoperable hepatocellular carcinoma (HCC): results of a single-institutional experience on stereotactic body

radiation therapy (SBRT). J Cancer Res Clin Oncol. 2015;141(7):1301–9.

49. Sanuki N, Takeda A, Oku Y, Mizuno T, Aoki Y, Eriguchi T, et al. Stereotactic body radiotherapy for small hepatocellular carcinoma: a retrospective outcome analysis in 185 patients. Acta oncologica (Stockholm, Sweden). 2014;53(3):399–404.

50. Bae SH, Kim MS, Jang WI, Cho CK, Yoo HJ, Kim KB, et al. Low hepatic toxicity in primary and metastatic liver cancers after stereotactic ablative radiotherapy using 3 fractions. J Korean Med Sci. 2015;30(8):1055–61.

51. Okuwaki Y, Nakazawa T, Shibuya A, Ono K, Hidaka H, Watanabe M, et al. Intrahepatic distant recurrence after radiofrequency ablation for a single small hepatocellular carcinoma: risk factors and patterns. J Gastroenterol. 2008;43(1):71–8.

52. Park JH, Yoon SM, Lim YS, Kim SY, Shim JH, Kim KM, et al. Two-week schedule of hypofractionated radiotherapy as a local salvage treatment for small hepatocellular carcinoma. J Gastroenterol Hepatol. 2013;28(10):1638–42.

53. Park J, Jung J, Kim D, Jung IH, Park JH, Kim JH, et al. Long-term outcomes of the 2-week schedule of hypofractionated radiotherapy for recurrent hepatocellular carcinoma. BMC Cancer. 2018;18(1):1040.

Transarterial Chemoembolization Plus External Beam Radiotherapy

13

Woong Sub Koom and Hwa Kyung Byun

Abstract

Transarterial chemoembolization (TACE) is the most commonly performed therapy for inoperable hepatocellular carcinoma (HCC). However, after initial success with TACE, treated tumors can be revascularized and retreated. When repeated many times, TACE often loses its efficacy and patients enter the state of TACE failure/refractoriness. Radiotherapy (RT) has been investigated as a component of combined treatment to compensate for the limitations of TACE. Recently, advancements in RT have enabled high-dose RT to be directed to the tumor while sparing the non-tumor-bearing surrounding liver parenchyma from these high doses. With the advancements in RT, considerable evidence indicates that there is a significant therapeutic benefit of TACE plus RT for unresectable HCC compared with TACE alone. Moreover, TACE plus RT has been used in various clinical situations such as tumors with portal vein tumor thrombosis. Optimal radiation technique, radiation dose, and optimal interval between TACE and RT needs to be clarified through further studies.

Keywords

Transarterial chemoembolization
Radiotherapy · Hepatocellular carcinoma
Tumor control · Combined modality therapy

13.1 Transarteral Chemoembolization

Transarterial chemoembolization (TACE) involves intraarterial infusion of a cytotoxic agent, followed immediately by embolization of the vessels that feed the tumor. The mixture of chemotherapeutic agents, such as doxorubicin, cisplatin, and mitomycin, with iodized oil injected into the feeding artery as an emulsion. Selective tumor ischemia is induced by embolization of the same feeding artery using gelatin sponge particles, polyvinyl alcohol particles, or microspheres. Adjacent nontumoral liver parenchyme is generally protected from TACE because, unlike the tumor, its blood supply comes mainly from the portal vein. To maximize the antitumor effect and minimize liver toxicity when performing TACE, it is important to superselect the feeding arteries of tumors as distally as possible [1]. Superselective chemoembolization of feeding arteries can significantly increase tumor necrosis and the local control rate [2]. In addition, cone-beam CT during chemoembolization helps detect tumors and tumor-feeding arteries more precisely, thus resulting in a better therapeutic outcome [3].

W. S. Koom (✉) · H. K. Byun
Department of Radiation Oncology, Yonsei Cancer Center, Yonsei University College of Medicine, Seoul, South Korea
e-mail: MDGOLD@yuhs.ac

The survival benefits of TACE as compared with the best supportive care was shown in randomized controlled trials and a meta-analysis [4]. In a systematic review of TACE including 101 studies and 12,372 patients, an objective response of 52.5% was shown [5]. Median survival with TACE ranges from 26 to 40 months, depending on patient selection [6, 7]. Adequate patient selection is needed because most treatment-related deaths were associated with liver failure, although the mortality associated with TACE was less than 1% [5]. Patients with decompensated cirrhosis is contraindicated for TACE. There is evidence that TACE using drug-eluting beads has antitumoral activity similar to that of conventional TACE, with fewer side effects [7]. Combining TACE with the systemic drug sorafenib (an inhibitor of the serine–threonine kinases Raf-1 and B-Raf and the receptor tyrosine kinase activity of vascular endothelial growth factor receptors [VEGFRs] and platelet-derived growth factor receptor β [PDGFR-β]) or brivanib (an inhibitor of VEGFR and fibroblast growth factor receptor) does not improve overall survival [6, 8]. TACE is the recommended treatment modality for Barcelona Clinic Liver Cancer (BCLC) B stage hepatocellular carcinoma (HCC). This stage is characterized by asymptomatic, large or multifocal HCC without macrovascular invasion or extrahepatic metastasis [9]. However, TACE is frequently used not only for BCLC-B stage but also for BCLC-C and D stage in real-life management, as shown in a multiregional cohort study [10].

13.2 The Weakness of TACE

TACE may become a double-edged sword independent from the presence of objective radiologic response if deterioration of liver function is caused by the intervention, which may obviate any type of further treatment and trigger liver-related death. For this reason, the best treatment strategy involves simultaneously achieving objective response and preserving liver function. This principle applies to every TACE treatment especially in the context of repeated, multiple TACE sessions, which may be necessary due to a

lack of adequate radiologic response after the previous intervention. After initial success with TACE, treated tumors can be revascularized and retreated. However, in the long term, the capacity to keep the cancer under control may be lost. Thus, retreatment decisions should be taken based on target lesion response or presence or absence of overall disease progression as well as on changes in liver function after TACE.

When repeated many times, TACE loses its efficacy at some point and patients enter the so-called state of TACE failure/refractoriness [11]. The concept of TACE refractoriness was first proposed in the clinical practice guidelines proposed by the Japan Society of Hepatology (JSH) [12] and then appeared in criteria published in Korea [13], in criteria established by the European Association for the Study of the Liver (EASL) [11], and in the Assessment for Retreatment (ART) score system [14]. The JSH defines TACE refractoriness as failure to control target lesions or the appearance of new lesions even after two or more consecutive TACE sessions. Table 13.1 shows the JSH criteria for TACE failure/refractoriness updated at the 50th LCSGJ Congress in 2014.

When TACE refractoriness/failure occurs, multifocal nodules scattered in both lobes or as a

Table 13.1 Definition of TACE failure/refractoriness

1	Intrahepatic lesion	
	i	Two or more consecutive insufficient responses of the treated tumor (viable lesion >50%) even after changing the chemotherapeutic agents and/or reanalysis of the feeding artery seen on response evaluation CT/MRI at 1–3 months after having adequately performed selective TACE
	ii	Two or more consecutive progressions in the liver (tumor number increases as compared to tumor number before the previous TACE procedure) even after having changed the chemotherapeutic agents and/or reanalysis of the feeding artery seen on response evaluation CT/MRI at 1–3 months after having adequately performed selective TACE
2	Continuous elevation of tumor markers immediately after TACE even though slight transient decrease is observed	
3	Appearance of vascular invasion	
4	Appearance of extrahepatic spread	

huge HCC mass are commonly seen, and the noncancerous liver tissue will have deteriorated because of the damage caused by TACE, which may result in a reduced survival time. Accordingly, it has become apparent in recent years that the treatment modality should be switched before patients enter this state.

Furthermore, tumor cells at the periphery of HCC are supplied by both arterial and portal blood, so they may remain viable. Thus, complete tumor necrosis may not be induced in large HCCs. Ischemic injury by TACE stimulates vascular endothelial growth factor production by residual tumor cells, which may induce neoangiogenesis, and thus, potentially cause disease recurrence [15]. For these reasons, multimodality treatment options combining with TACE can be considered to enhance treatment outcome and reduce treatment-related toxicity.

13.3 The Benefit of Combining TACE and RT

Radiotherapy (RT) has been well-investigated as a component of combined treatment to compensate for the limitations of TACE. Several studies, including meta-analyses and prospective trials, have reported significant therapeutic benefits of combination treatment using RT as a combination treatment with TACE [16, 17]. Huo et al. [17] suggested the rationales of combining TACE and RT as follows. First, residual cancer cells after TACE can be eradicated by RT, especially those at the tumor periphery which remain viable through the blood supply from the collateral circulation or recanalization of the embolized artery by the portal vein [18]; second, large numbers of cancer cells can be more radiosensitive, because TACE promotes the residual cells from a nonproliferative phase into cell proliferation [19]; third, tumor volume is decreased by TACE, which in turn reduces the radiation field and adverse events [20]; fourth, retention of chemotherapeutic agents from embolization in liver tumor cells has a radiosensitizing effect and accelerates tumornecrosis, which in turn results in a similar effect to concurrent chemoradiotherapy [21]; fifth, RT can enhance poor tumor response by TACE because

of little blood supply and poor filling of lipiodol emulsion; and sixth, RT performed after TACE extends the tumor retention of lipiodol and anticancer agents, which prevents the need for repeated TACE [22].

13.4 Approaches for Combining RT and TACE

In terms of combination strategies, TACE procedure followed by RT and RT sandwiched between TACE procedures are the most common. There are several approaches for combining RT with TACE. The first approach involves using RT to treat portal vein and inferior vena cava tumor thrombus to assist TACE. The rationale for this approach is that TACE is less effective in patients with portal vein tumor thrombus, and RT may make TACE more effective if portal vein disease can be decreased. The second approach is to administer RT as a "consolidation" planned procedure to target residual hepatic tumor after TACE. The rationale for this approach is that RT targets cancer cells at the tumor's periphery that may remain viable through blood supply from collateral circulation or recanalization of the embolized artery. The third approach is to administer RT as a "salvage" procedure for an unresponsive tumor after incomplete TACE [23]. In the fourth approach, tumor shrinkage after TACE allows the use of smaller irradiation fields, which enables the use of higher tumor doses and improves the normal liver tolerance [24].

13.5 Clinical Evidences of Combining RT with TACE

In many prospective or retrospective papers, unresectable HCCs were well treated with TACE followed by external beam RT, objective response rates (complete + partial response) were achieved in 63–76%, and a one-year survival rate was achieved in 72–82%, which is significantly higher compared to patients without RT (Table 13.2). Choi et al. [23] conducted a prospective phase II multicenter study to investigate the efficacy and toxicity of RT following incomplete TACE in

Table 13.2 Clinical outcome of TACE+RT for HCC

References	Design	Patient number	Patient	RT dose	Response rate	Survival
Prospective studies						
Li et al. [25]	Phase II, TACE+RT	45	All stage III, KPS ≥ 70, CP A, B	45 Gy/25 fx—>boost 5.4 Gy/3 fx	CR 6, PR 35, SD 4, PD 0	1-year 69%, 2-year 48%, 3-year 23%, median 23.5 months
Oh et al. [26]	Phase II, TACE+RT	40	HCC which failed after 1–2 courses of TACE	Median 54 Gy in 3 Gy/fx	ORR: 63% (CR 9, PR 18), 9 progressions within the irradiated field	1-year 72%, 2-year 46%
Koo et al. [27]	Phase II, TACE+RT (vs. historical control TACE alone)	42 vs. 29	All with IVCT, CP A, B	Median 45 Gy in 2.5–5 Gy/fx (determined by the extent of thrombosis)	ORR: 43 vs. 14%	Median 12 vs. 5 months, 1-year 48 vs. 17%
Choi et al. [23]	Phase II, TACE+RT	31	HCC which failed after 1–3 courses of TACE, CP A, B	Median 54 Gy in 1.8–2 Gy/fx	In-field CR 24%, PR 59% at 12 weeks Overall CR 10%, PR 52% at 12 weeks	2-year 61%
Yoon et al. [16]	Phase III, TACE+RT vs. sorafenib	90	liver confined, macroscopic vascular invasion, CP A	45 Gy in 2.5–3 Gy/fx	ORR at 12 weeks: Sorafenib 4.4% vs. TACE+RT 28.9%	
Retrospective studies						
Cheng et al. [28]	TACE+RT or RT alone	16, 6	Stage II–IV, CP A, B, median 10 cm	46.9 ± 5.9 Gy in 1.8–2 Gy/fx	Only 3 local progression (area treated with RT)	1-year 54%, 2-year 41%, median 19.2 months
Guo et al. [24]	TACE+RT vs. TACE	76 vs. 89	Stage I–III, KPS ≥ 70, CP A, B	1.8–2.0 Gy/fx * 15–28 fx	ORR: 47 vs. 28%	1-year 64 vs. 40%
Zeng et al. [29]	TACE+RT vs. TACE	54 vs. 203	Size > 10 cm: overall 31%, CP A, B	2 Gy/fx * 18–30 fx	ORR: 76 vs. 31%	1-year 72 vs. 60%, 3-year 24 vs. 11%
Chen et al. [22]	TACE+RT vs. TACE	78 vs. 80			ORR: 72 vs. 54%	1-year 78 vs. 59%, 3-year 26 vs. 16%
Shim et al. [30]	TACE+RT vs. TACE	38 vs. 35	Stage III, IV, size ≥ 5 cm, CP A, B	1.8 Gy/fx, 17–33 fx	TACE+RT: CR 0, PR 25	2-year 37 vs. 14% (higher benefit with large tumors)
Byun et al. [31]	TACE+RT	323	Liver confined, CP A, B	GTV: 50–75 Gy/20–25 fx PTV: 45–60 Gy/20–25 fx		Median 14.2 months

KPS Karnofsky performance status, *CP* child-pugh, *CR* complete response, *PR* partial response, *SD* stable disease, *PD* progressive disease, *ORR* objective response rate, *HCC* hepatocellular carcinoma, *PVT* portal vein thrombosis, *IVCT* inferior vena cava thrombosis, *TACE* transcatheter arterial chemoembolization, *RT* radiotherapy, *PTV* planning target volume

ORR was defined as CR+PR

unresectable HCCs. Patients with unresectable HCC who had a viable tumor after TACE of no more than three courses were included, and median 54 Gy of 3D-CRT was delivered. Best objective infield response rate was achieved in 84% of patients, with 23% of complete response rates and 61% of partial response rates within 12 weeks post-RT. The two-year in-field progression-free survival, overall progression-free survival, and overall survival rates were 45%, 29%, and 61%, respectively. These findings demonstrate that early application of 3D-CRT can be a promising option in multimodal approaches for patients with incomplete necrosis after TACE.

Meng et al. [32] performed meta-analysis from five randomized controlled trials and 12 non-randomized controlled clinical trials, which compared TACE+RT group and TACE alone group. As a result, TACE+RT significantly improved survival rates and complete response rates (OR, 2.58; 95% CI 1.64–4.06; $P = 0.0001$). Rates of adverse events were not significantly different, except for elevation of total bilirubin level.

Huo et al. [17] conducted a systemic review comparing TACE+RT and TACE alone in 25 trials including 11 randomized controlled trials. Patients receiving TACE plus RT showed significantly better one-year survival (HR, 1.36; 95% CI, 1.19–1.54) and complete response (clearance of the lesion after treatment) (HR, 2.73; 95% CI, 1.95–3.81) compared with TACE alone. There was an increased incidence of gastroduodenal ulcers and elevated levels of alanine transaminase and total bilirubin in patients receiving TACE+RT compared with those receiving TACE alone. Subgroup analyses showed nonsignificant trends in which survival was greater for TACE+RT in patients with portal vein tumor thrombus (PVTT) compared with those without PVTT.

13.6 Special Consideration

13.6.1 Portal-Vein Tumor Thrombosis

Despite recent progress in surveillance programs and imaging techniques for high-risk populations, PVTT is often observed in patients with advanced HCC. PVTT often causes extensive intrahepatic dissemination of the tumor through the portal tract, which can decrease blood supply to the normal liver, and finally causes portal hypertension resulting in the rupture of collateral vessels, ascites, hepatic encephalopathy, and deteriorating liver function.

Whether TACE plus RT is effective for patients with unresectable HCC with PVTT is an important issue for three reasons: first, there is currently no standard treatment for PVTT. Second, PVTT is an extremely poor prognostic condition in which the median survival time without treatment is approximately two months [33], and third, PVTT occurs in 20–70% of patients with intermediate HCC [34, 35]. Previously, numerous reports [28, 36] demonstrated the benefit of RT alone for PVTT. However, in contrast, TACE was associated with a theoretical risk that it could result in ischemic damage to normal liver parenchyma [37]. Because PVTT is a major obstacle to performing TACE, focal field RT targeting the PVTT, before or immediately after TACE for the tumor, may be a good treatment option. Whether the addition of TACE to RT doing more harm than good by reducing the benefit of RT alone is a remaining question. A comparative study has also shown that TACE plus RT compared with RT alone significantly improves survival for patients with UHCC with PVTT [28].

Huo et al. [17] showed in a meta-analysis that TACE plus RT compared with TACE alone was associated with significantly better one-, two-, and three-year survival rates in patients with PVTT. In addition, subgroup analysis showed that there was a nonsignificant trend in which TACE plus RT was more effective than TACE alone in patients with PVTT than in those without PVTT. Yoon et al. [16] conducted a randomized clinical trial to evaluate the efficacy and safety of TACE plus RT compared with sorafenib for patients with HCC and macroscopic vascular invasion. At week 12, the progression-free survival rate was significantly higher in the TACE+RT group than the sorafenib group (86.7 vs. 34.3%; $P < 0.001$). The TACE+RT group showed a significantly higher radiologic response rate than the sorafenib group at 24 weeks (15

[33.3%] vs. 1 [2.2%]; $P < 0.001$), a significantly longer median time to progression (31.0 vs. 11.7 weeks; $P < 0.001$), and significantly longer overall survival (55.0 vs. 43.0 weeks; $P = 0.04$). Curative surgical resection was conducted for five patients (11.1%) in the TACE-RT group owing to downstaging.

13.6.2 Optimal Timing of RT After TACE

Early administration of RT may enhance tumor control by eradicating residual tumor cells early. However, its application is limited because diffuse lipiodol retention around the tumor immediately after TACE may obscure the tumor margin, thereby hindering delineation of the RT target volume [38]. Furthermore, the post-TACE acute inflammatory status of the liver with elevated liver function parameters may prevent the early initiation of RT [39]. Consequently, RT is usually delayed for at least a few weeks. Therefore, it is of clinical importance to identify the optimal timing of RT initiation after TACE.

In a meta-analysis by Huo et al. [17], in patients who had received RT less than 28 days or 28 days or more after completion of TACE, for both studies, TACE plus RT was significantly more effective than TACE alone for one-year survival, but was not significant for two-year survival. TACE performed less than 28 days before RT was associated with significantly less no response (NR) than TACE alone, while TACE performed 28 days or more before RT was not significantly associated with better NR than TACE alone.

Seong et al. retrospectively investigated the optimal timing for initiating radiotherapy after incomplete TACE in patients with BCLC-B HCC. The optimal cut-off time interval appeared to be five weeks; using this cut-off, 65 and 39 patients were classified into the early and late radiotherapy groups. The one-year local failure-free rate was significantly higher in the early than in the late radiotherapy group (94.6 vs. 70.8%;

$P = 0.005$). On multivariate analysis, RT after TACE with time interval less than five weeks was identified as an independent predictor of favorable local failure-free survival (hazard ratio: 3.82, 95% confidence interval: 1.64–8.88, $P = 0.002$) [unpublished data].

13.6.3 Optimal Dose of RT After TACE

The RT dose–response relationship for HCC was reported by several investigators. Park et al. [40] has previously reported that RT dose was significantly associated with objective response in 158 patients with HCC (29% with <40 Gy vs. 69% with 40–50 Gy vs. 77% with >50 Gy [physical dose]). Toya et al. [41] reported that biologically effective dose (BED) ≥ 58 Gy was a significant factor for tumor response (22% with BED < 58 Gy vs. 80% with BED ≥ 58 Gy) of 38 patients with HCC showing portal vein invasion. The same principle may be applicable in TACE+RT scenario. Furthermore, recent developments in RT technology allowed application of higher RT doses to the tumor while sparing healthy liver tissue. Byun et al. [31] showed that radiation dose with BED ≥ 72 Gy improved local control and progression-free rate without increasing toxicity. Simultaneous integrated boost-intensity modulated radiation therapy was used significantly more frequently in the patients who received BED ≥ 72 Gy (64.5 vs. 12.9%; $P < 0.001$; Fig. 13.1).

13.7 Treatment-Associated Complications

Huo et al. showed in a meta-analysis that compared with TACE alone, TACE plus RT was associated with a greater incidence of gastroduodenal ulcers and elevation of alpha-lipoic acid and total bilirubin levels while having similar frequencies of nausea and/or vomiting, thrombocytopenia, and fever compared with TACE alone. Generally, these adverse effects were easily managed and treated.

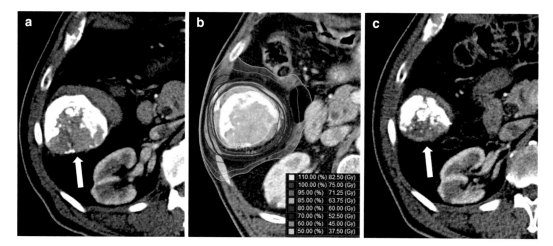

Fig. 13.1 Example of a simultaneous integrated boost-intensity-modulated radiation therapy (SIB-IMRT) plan. (**a**) Pretreatment computed tomography (CT) scan showing viable area in a post-TACE lesion (arrow). (**b**) The patient underwent SIB-IMRT with physical doses of 75 and 60 Gy in 25 fractions to the internal target volume (red contour) and planning target volume (blue contour), respectively. (**c**) CT scan at 4 months after SIB-IMRT showing the tumor shrinkage (arrow)

References

1. Matsui O, Kadoya M, Yoshikawa J, Gabata T, Arai K, Demachi H, et al. Small hepatocellular carcinoma: treatment with subsegmental transcatheter arterial embolization. Radiology. 1993;188(1):79–83.
2. Golfieri R, Cappelli A, Cucchetti A, Piscaglia F, Carpenzano M, Peri E, et al. Efficacy of selective transarterial chemoembolization in inducing tumor necrosis in small (<5 cm) hepatocellular carcinomas. Hepatology. 2011;53(5):1580–9.
3. Iwazawa J, Ohue S, Hashimoto N, Muramoto O, Mitani T. Survival after C-arm CT-assisted chemoembolization of unresectable hepatocellular carcinoma. Eur J Radiol. 2012;81(12):3985–92.
4. Llovet JM, Bruix J. Systematic review of randomized trials for unresectable hepatocellular carcinoma: chemoembolization improves survival. Hepatology. 2003;37(2):429–42.
5. Lencioni R, de Baere T, Soulen MC, Rilling WS, Geschwind JF. Lipiodol transarterial chemoembolization for hepatocellular carcinoma: a systematic review of efficacy and safety data. Hepatology. 2016;64(1):106–16.
6. Kudo M, Han G, Finn RS, Poon RT, Blanc JF, Yan L, et al. Brivanib as adjuvant therapy to transarterial chemoembolization in patients with hepatocellular carcinoma: a randomized phase III trial. Hepatology. 2014;60(5):1697–707.
7. Burrel M, Reig M, Forner A, Barrufet M, de Lope CR, Tremosini S, et al. Survival of patients with hepatocellular carcinoma treated by transarterial chemoembolisation (TACE) using Drug Eluting Beads.

Implications for clinical practice and trial design. J Hepatol. 2012;56(6):1330–5.
8. Meyer T, Fox R, Ma YT, Ross PJ, James MW, Sturgess R, et al. Sorafenib in combination with transarterial chemoembolisation in patients with unresectable hepatocellular carcinoma (TACE 2): a randomised placebo-controlled, double-blind, phase 3 trial. Lancet Gastroenterol Hepatol. 2017;2(8):565–75.
9. Bruix J, Sherman M. Management of hepatocellular carcinoma: an update. Hepatology. 2011;53(3):1020–2.
10. Park JW, Chen M, Colombo M, Roberts LR, Schwartz M, Chen PJ, et al. Global patterns of hepatocellular carcinoma management from diagnosis to death: the BRIDGE Study. Liver Int. 2015;35(9):2155–66.
11. Raoul JL, Gilabert M, Piana G. How to define transarterial chemoembolization failure or refractoriness: a European perspective. Liver Cancer. 2014;3(2):119–24.
12. Kudo M, Izumi N, Kokudo N, Matsui O, Sakamoto M, Nakashima O, et al. Management of hepatocellular carcinoma in Japan: Consensus-Based Clinical Practice Guidelines proposed by the Japan Society of Hepatology (JSH) 2010 updated version. Dig Dis. 2011;29(3):339–64.
13. Park JW, Amarapurkar D, Chao Y, Chen PJ, Geschwind JF, Goh KL, et al. Consensus recommendations and review by an International Expert Panel on Interventions in Hepatocellular Carcinoma (EPOIHCC). Liver Int. 2013;33(3):327–37.
14. Sieghart W, Hucke F, Pinter M, Graziadei I, Vogel W, Müller C, et al. The ART of decision making: retreatment with transarterial chemoembolization in

patients with hepatocellular carcinoma. Hepatology. 2013;57(6):2261–73.

15. Wang B, Xu H, Gao ZQ, Ning HF, Sun YQ, Cao GW. Increased expression of vascular endothelial growth factor in hepatocellular carcinoma after transcatheter arterial chemoembolization. Acta Radiol. 2008;49(5):523–9.

16. Yoon SM, Ryoo BY, Lee SJ, Kim JH, Shin JH, An JH, et al. Efficacy and safety of transarterial chemoembolization plus external beam radiotherapy vs sorafenib in hepatocellular carcinoma with macroscopic vascular invasion: a randomized clinical trial. JAMA Oncol. 2018;4(5):661–9.

17. Huo YR, Eslick GD. Transcatheter arterial chemoembolization plus radiotherapy compared with chemoembolization alone for hepatocellular carcinoma: a systematic review and meta-analysis. JAMA Oncol. 2015;1(6):756–65.

18. Hawkins MA, Dawson LA. Radiation therapy for hepatocellular carcinoma: from palliation to cure. Cancer. 2006;106(8):1653–63.

19. Aguirre-Ghiso JA. Models, mechanisms and clinical evidence for cancer dormancy. Nat Rev Cancer. 2007;7(11):834–46.

20. Steel GG, Peckham MJ. Exploitable mechanisms in combined radiotherapy-chemotherapy: the concept of additivity. Int J Radiat Oncol Biol Phys. 1979;5(1):85–91.

21. Seong J, Kim SH, Suh CO. Enhancement of tumor radioresponse by combined chemotherapy in murine hepatocarcinoma. J Gastroenterol Hepatol. 2001;16(8):883–9.

22. Chen WJ, Yuan SF, Zhu LJ, Sun XN, Zheng W. Three-dimensional conformal radiotherapy in combination with transcatheter arterial chemoembolization in the treatment of hepatocellular carcinoma. Journal of BUON. 2014;19(3):692–7.

23. Choi C, Koom WS, Kim TH, Yoon SM, Kim JH, Lee HS, et al. A prospective phase 2 multicenter study for the efficacy of radiation therapy following incomplete transarterial chemoembolization in unresectable hepatocellular carcinoma. Int J Radiat Oncol Biol Phys. 2014;90(5):1051–60.

24. Guo WJ, Yu EX, Liu LM, Li J, Chen Z, Lin JH, et al. Comparison between chemoembolization combined with radiotherapy and chemoembolization alone for large hepatocellular carcinoma. World J Gastroenterol. 2003;9(8):1697–701.

25. Li B, Yu J, Wang L, Li C, Zhou T, Zhai L, et al. Study of local three-dimensional conformal radiotherapy combined with transcatheter arterial chemoembolization for patients with stage III hepatocellular carcinoma. Am J Clin Oncol. 2003;26(4):e92–9.

26. Oh D, Lim DH, Park HC, Paik SW, Koh KC, Lee JH, et al. Early three-dimensional conformal radiotherapy for patients with unresectable hepatocellular carcinoma after incomplete transcatheter arterial chemoembolization: a prospective evalu-

ation of efficacy and toxicity. Am J Clin Oncol. 2010;33(4):370–5.

27. Koo JE, Kim JH, Lim YS, Park SJ, Won HJ, Sung KB, et al. Combination of transarterial chemoembolization and three-dimensional conformal radiotherapy for hepatocellular carcinoma with inferior vena cava tumor thrombus. Int J Radiat Oncol Biol Phys. 2010;78(1):180–7.

28. Cheng JC, Chuang VP, Cheng SH, Huang AT, Lin YM, Cheng TI, et al. Local radiotherapy with or without transcatheter arterial chemoembolization for patients with unresectable hepatocellular carcinoma. Int J Radiat Oncol Biol Phys. 2000;47(2):435–42.

29. Zeng ZC, Tang ZY, Fan J, Zhou J, Qin LX, Ye SL, et al. A comparison of chemoembolization combination with and without radiotherapy for unresectable hepatocellular carcinoma. Cancer J. 2004;10(5):307–16.

30. Shim SJ, Seong J, Han KH, Chon CY, Suh CO, Lee JT. Local radiotherapy as a complement to incomplete transcatheter arterial chemoembolization in locally advanced hepatocellular carcinoma. Liver Int. 2005;25(6):1189–96.

31. Byun HK, Kim HJ, Im YR, Kim DY, Han KH, Seong J. Dose escalation in radiotherapy for incomplete transarterial chemoembolization of hepatocellular carcinoma. Strahlenther Onkol. 2020;196(2): 132–41.

32. Meng MB, Cui YL, Lu Y, She B, Chen Y, Guan YS, et al. Transcatheter arterial chemoembolization in combination with radiotherapy for unresectable hepatocellular carcinoma: a systematic review and meta-analysis. Radiother Oncol. 2009;92(2):184–94.

33. Fujii T, Takayasu K, Muramatsu Y, Moriyama N, Wakao F, Kosuge T, et al. Hepatocellular carcinoma with portal tumor thrombus: analysis of factors determining prognosis. Jpn J Clin Oncol. 1993;23(2):105–9.

34. Albacete RA, Matthews MJ, Saini N. Portal vein thromboses in malignant hepatoma. Ann Intern Med. 1967;67(2):337–48.

35. Price J, Chan M, Hamilton-Wood C, Chronos NA, Mok SD, Metreweli C. Sonographic diagnosis of portal vein invasion in patients with hepatocellular carcinoma: comparison with arterial portography. Clin Radiol. 1990;41(1):9–12.

36. Tazawa J, Maeda M, Sakai Y, Yamane M, Ohbayashi H, Kakinuma S, et al. Radiation therapy in combination with transcatheter arterial chemoembolization for hepatocellular carcinoma with extensive portal vein involvement. J Gastroenterol Hepatol. 2001;16(6):660–5.

37. Yamada R, Sato M, Kawabata M, Nakatsuka H, Nakamura K, Takashima S. Hepatic artery embolization in 120 patients with unresectable hepatoma. Radiology. 1983;148(2):397–401.

38. Lim HS, Jeong YY, Kang HK, Kim JK, Park JG. Imaging features of hepatocellular carcinoma

after transcatheter arterial chemoembolization and radiofrequency ablation. AJR Am J Roentgenol. 2006;187(4):W341–9.

39. Chan AO, Yuen MF, Hui CK, Tso WK, Lai CL. A prospective study regarding the complications of transcatheter intraarterial lipiodol chemoembolization in patients with hepatocellular carcinoma. Cancer. 2002;94(6):1747–52.

40. Park HC, Seong J, Han KH, Chon CY, Moon YM, Suh CO. Dose-response relationship in local radiotherapy for hepatocellular carcinoma. Int J Radiat Oncol Biol Phys. 2002;54(1):150–5.

41. Toya R, Murakami R, Baba Y, Nishimura R, Morishita S, Ikeda O, et al. Conformal radiation therapy for portal vein tumor thrombosis of hepatocellular carcinoma. Radiother Oncol. 2007;84(3):266–71.

Definitive Radiotherapy for Locally Advanced Hepatocellular Carcinoma

14

Sang Min Yoon

Abstract

Locally advanced hepatocellular carcinoma (HCC) with macroscopic vascular invasion (MVI) showed a very poor prognosis owing to the early progression of HCC through the vasculature, decreased portal blood flow to the uninvolved liver, deterioration of hepatic function, and sometimes increased sudden death risk. Although systemic therapies are the current standard treatment in this advanced HCC, radiotherapy with or without combined locoregional treatments has increasingly been used to reverse the situation. Even in patients with HCC having MVI, the reported response rates held promise with regard to reducing the size of vascular invasion and improving the patients' outcomes after radiotherapy. Here, we summarize previous studies and recent updates of radiotherapy for HCC having MVI.

Keywords

Heaptocellular carcinoma · Thrombosis · Portal vein · Hepatic vein · Inferior vena cava · Radiotherapy

14.1 Introduction

Even though several staging systems in patients with hepatocellular carcinoma (HCC) have been proposed, there is no global consensus in predicting prognosis and selection of optimal therapy [1]. The most relevant and evaluated staging is the Barcelona Clinic Liver Cancer (BCLC) staging system, in which the BCLC C stage, termed *advanced stage*, includes the one or more of the following features: HCC was accompanied with vascular invasion, HCCs that have spread beyond the liver, and HCC-related symptoms of the Eastern Cooperative Oncology Group performance status of 1–2 [2]. Locally advanced HCC is not uncommonly used to categorize the prognosis of the patients and suggestion of the optimal treatments; however, the definition is not clear yet. According to a previous consensus workshop, locally advanced HCC is a subgroup of nonresectable HCC, and is categorized as nodular, massive with intrahepatic metastases, diffuse, and with vascular invasion [3]. This means locally advanced HCC is very heterogeneous including both the BCLC B and C stages of HCC. Among them, we want to focus on the role of radiotherapy in the management of HCC with macroscopic vascular invasion (MVI) in this chapter.

S. M. Yoon (✉)
Department of Radiation Oncology, Asan Liver Center, Asan Medical Center, University of Ulsan College of Medicine, Seoul, Republic of Korea
e-mail: drsmyoon@amc.seoul.kr

© Springer Nature Singapore Pte Ltd. 2021
J. Seong (ed.), *Radiotherapy of Liver Cancer*, https://doi.org/10.1007/978-981-16-1815-4_14

14.2 Macroscopic Vascular Invasion

HCC usually invades directly hepatic parenchyma as well as hepatic vasculature. MVI of the portal vein, hepatic vein, or inferior vena cava is common in patients with locally advanced HCC and is associated with a poor prognosis with an expected median survival time of 2–4 months without any treatment [4, 5]. The Liver Cancer Study Group of Japan suggested a macroscopic classification of HCC with portal vein tumor thrombus (PVTT) into four grades according to the extent of the thrombus: Vp1, presence of a tumor thrombus distal to, but not in, the second-order branches of the portal vein; Vp2, presence of a tumor thrombus in the second-order branches

of the portal vein; Vp3, presence of a tumor thrombus in the first-order branches of the portal vein; and Vp4, presence of a tumor thrombus in the main trunk of the portal vein or a portal vein branch contralateral to the primarily involved lobe (Fig. 14.1) [6]. In addition to the extent of PVTT impacts the patients' prognosis, PVTT causes extensive intrahepatic or extrahepatic dissemination of the tumor through the portal vasculature, decreased blood supply to the uninvolved healthy liver, and finally makes portal hypertension resulting in ascites, variceal bleeding, hepatic encephalopathy, and deterioration of hepatic function [7, 8]. Hepatic vein tumor thrombus usually spreads to inferior vena cava and/or right atrium (Fig. 14.2); lung metastasis, secondary Budd-Chiari syndrome, and heart fail-

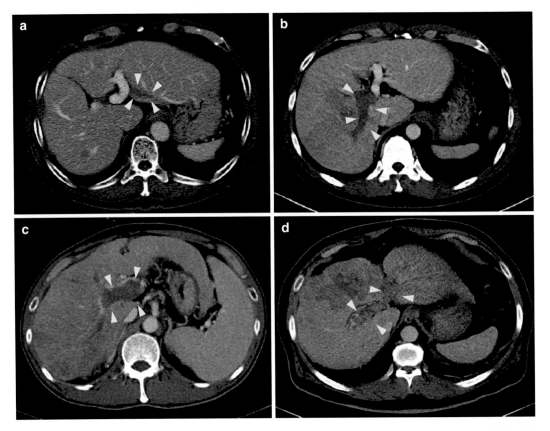

Fig. 14.1 Examples of hepatocellular carcinoma with portal vein tumor thrombus (yellow triangles) on portal phase of liver dynamic computed tomography. (**a**) Vp2, presence of a tumor thrombus in the second-order branches of the portal vein. (**b**) Vp3, presence of a tumor thrombus in the first-order branches of the portal vein. (**c**) Vp4, presence of a tumor thrombus in the main trunk of the portal vein. (**d**) Vp4, a portal vein branch contralateral to the primarily involved lobe (by the Liver Cancer Study Group of Japan)

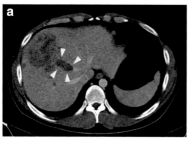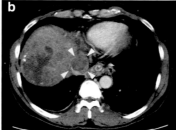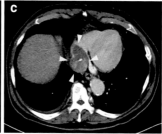

Fig. 14.2 Examples of hepatocellular carcinoma with macroscopic vascular invasion (yellow triangles) on portal phase of liver dynamic computed tomography. (**a**) Presence of a tumor thrombus in the middle hepatic vein. (**b**) Presence of a tumor thrombus in the inferior vena cava via hepatic vein invasion. (**c**) Presence of a tumor thrombus in right atrium through hepatic vein and inferior vena cava invasion

ure can occur if tumor thrombus was not controlled appropriately [9]. Moreover, this is associated with an increased risk of sudden death due to pulmonary thromboembolism [9].

14.3 Rationale of External Beam Radiotherapy for Macroscopic Vascular Invasion

The current guidelines recommend systemic therapies as the evidence-based treatment option for patients with advanced HCC including MVI [10, 11]. During the last 10-year period, sorafenib has been regarded as the only first-line systemic therapy based on the results of the phase III randomized trials that demonstrated overall survival benefit compared with placebo [12, 13]. Unfortunately, however, the efficacy of this treatment was not as good as expected with a low response rate (<5%) and modest survival gain of 2–3 months. Furthermore, the median overall survival of the patients with MVI was significantly lower than those without MVI after sorafenib treatment (184 vs. 386 days) according to a pooled analysis of the two randomized trials [4]. In the subgroup of patients with MVI, sorafenib prolonged the median survival time by only 47 days compared with placebo (184 vs. 137 days) [4]. Lenvatinib was acknowledged as another first-line systemic therapy in untreated advanced HCC according to the phase III, multicenter, non-inferiority clinical trial [14]. Although

the objective response and progression-free survival rates were superior in the lenvatinib arm compared with in the sorafenib arm, the median overall survival time was still lower in patients with MVI and extrahepatic metastases (11.5 months) even after lenvatinib treatment [14]. Recently, atezolizumab combined with bevacizumab resulted in better overall and progression-free survival outcomes than sorafenib in patients with unresectable HCC [15]; further analysis regarding the efficacy of this combination treatment in patients with HCC showing MVI will be necessary.

The role of external beam radiotherapy for HCC has been evaluated over several decades, and its usage has been increased recently owing to the evolution of radiotherapy techniques in the management of HCC. Because HCC is a radiation sensitive tumor, radiotherapy can lead to improved tumor control rates with the precision of modern radiotherapy [16]. Even in patients with HCC showing MVI, the reported response rates ranged from 30 to 70% after radiotherapy with or without combined locoregional therapies, which were higher than after standard systemic therapies [8, 9, 17–23]. This higher response rate is a prerequisite for the initial treatment of MVI because the objective response rate is a critical endpoint in the treatment of MVI due to the following reasons: (1) MVI is a well-known prognostic factor in patients with HCC, and early improvement of MVI extent can delay intravascular tumor growth in both intrahepatic and extrahepatic disease spreads [24]. (2) The decrease in the extent of

MVI can delay the deterioration of liver function by preserving portal flow [24]. (3) The decrease of MVI extent can also facilitate the subsequent treatment of primary tumor. A study reported that the mean number of repeated transarterial chemoembolization (TACE) sessions was significantly higher in patients treated with radiotherapy, suggesting that radiotherapy focused on vascular invasion could facilitate more aggressive TACE [25]. Therefore, the use of radiotherapy as an initial treatment can be a good treatment strategy to improve the oncologic outcomes in patients with advanced HCC having MVI.

14.4 Clinical Outcomes of Radiotherapy for HCC with Macroscopic Vascular Invasion

Treatment of advanced HCC with MVI is very complicated; it is not cured with a single session treatment, often requires subsequent repeated treatments, and/or it is necessary to change treatment policies from locoregional to systemic therapies or vice versa. Therefore, the multidisciplinary team approach is required during all courses of disease status to provide an optimal level of patient care [26]. Although various previous and/or subsequent treatments might be applied during the clinical courses, here we shall mainly summarize the results of radiotherapy for HCC with MVI according to the description of the articles. In addition, the prognosis of patients with HCC showing MVI varies widely [27, 28]; the survival outcomes should be compared cautiously considering baseline characteristics of the patients among the studies.

14.4.1 Pilot Study in the Initial Stage

The first study to evaluate the effect of radiotherapy in the control of PVTT in HCC was reported by Chen et al. in Taiwan [29]. They treated 10 HCC patients using a combined TACE for main tumors and radiotherapy with a dose of 30–50 Gy and reported complete response (CR) of the

PVTT in five patients and partial shrinkage in the other five patients by serial ultrasound examinations. Although survival outcomes were not evaluated, a promising result about size reduction of PVTT after combined TACE and radiotherapy was reported in this case series [29]. Yamada et al. also reported case series of local radiotherapy for PVTT in patients with unresectable HCC. After combined TACE and radiotherapy (dose range, 46–60 Gy) in eight patients, partial response (PR) was achieved in three patients (37.5%), with a median overall survival time of 5.7 months [30].

14.4.2 The Results of External Beam Radiotherapy Alone

As mentioned above, various treatments before or after radiotherapy were used in each study; many researchers have reported the role of radiotherapy without combined treatment for patients with MVI (Table 14.1). Kim et al. reported the impact of radiotherapy for PVTT of HCC in 59 patients with a total dose range of 30–54 Gy in 2–3 Gy daily dose [23]. They reported the objective response rate of 45.8% (CR: 6.8%, PR: 39%) and the responders to radiotherapy had a significantly longer overall survival rate than the nonresponders (median survival duration: 10.7 vs. 5.3 months; $p = 0.050$) [23]. Other researchers also reported similar response rates ranged from 33.3 to 44.7% after radiotherapy for both PVTT and inferior vena cava tumor thrombus (IVCTT) in relatively small patient cohorts [20, 31, 32]. Huang et al. published the response, survival, and prognostic factors for HCC with PVTT after radiotherapy in a large patient cohort of 326 patients [33]. The reported response rate was 25% (CR: 5.8%, PR: 12.2%, vascular transformation: 7%) in all patients (155 patients [47.5%], did not undergo imaging after radiotherapy and were classified as 'missing') and the median survival times were significantly higher among responder groups (CR: 13.3 months, PR: 11.6 months vs. no response: 4.5 months, missing: 2.1 months) [33]. Yu et al. reported that the objective response was observed in 151 patients

Table 14.1 Summary of treatment outcomes of external beam radiotherapy for hepatocellular carcinoma with macroscopic vascular invasion

Authors	Year	Study design	No. of patients	Combined Tx	MVI	RT	RT dose	Response rate	Survival outcomes	Toxicity (liver)	Toxicity (others)
Hata et al.	2005	R	12	None	PVT	PBT	50–72 GyE	CR: 16.7%, PR: 83.3%	2-Y: 88%, 5-Y: 58%	No change of C-P class	No Gr 3 toxicity
Kim et al.	2005	R	59	None	PVT	3D-CRT	30–54 Gy	CR: 6.8%, PR: 39%	Responder: median 10.7 mo., Non-responder: median 5.3 mo.	Classic RILD: 12 (20.3%)	Gr 2 GI toxicity: 10.2%
Lin et al.	2006	R	43	None	PVT	SRT: 22, 3D-CRT: 21	SRT: 45 Gy/15fx, 3D-CRT: 45 Gy/25fx	SRT - CR: 0%, PR: 75%, 3D-CRT - CR: 17%, PR: 67%	SRT: median 6 mo., 3D-CRT: median 6.7 mo.	None	No Gr 3 toxicity
Toya et al.	2007	R	38	None	PVT	3D-CRT	17.5–50.4 Gy	CR: 15.8%, PR: 28.9%	Median: 9.6 mo., 1-Y: 39.4%	No RILD	No Gr 3 toxicity
Igaki et al.	2008	R	18	None	IVCT	3D-CRT	30–60 Gy	RR: 33.3%	Median: 5.6 mo., 1-Y: 33.3%	N/E	N/E
Nakazawa et al.	2008	R	32	None	PVT, IVCT	3D-CRT	30–56 Gy	CR: 12.5%, PR: 31.3%	Responder: median 13.8 mo., Non-responder: median 7.0 mo.	No RILD	No Gr 3 toxicity
Huang et al.	2009	R	326	None	PVT	3D-CRT	60 Gy (goal)	CR: 5.8%, PR: 12.2%	Median: 3.8 mo., 1-Y: 16.7%, 2-Y: 5.5%, CR: median 13.3 mo., PR: median 11.6 mo.	N/E	N/E
Yu et al.	2011	R	281	None	PVT	3D-CRT	30–54 Gy	CR: 3.6%, PR: 50.2%	Median: 11.6 mo., 1-Y: 48.1%, 2-Y: 26.9%, Responder: 22.0 mo., Non-responder: 5.0 mo.	Gr 2,3 hepatic dysfunction: 5.3%	Gr 3 nausea: 10.4%, Gr 2,3 GI: 3.2%
Xi et al.	2013	R	41	Sorafenib (34.1%)	PVT, IVCT	SBRT	30–48 Gy/6fx	CR: 36.6%, PR: 39.0%	Median: 13 mo., 1-Y: 50.3%, Responder: 18 mo., Non-responder: 6 mo.	Gr 3 bilirubin: 2.4%	No Gr 3 toxicity
Lee et al.	2014	R	27	None	PVT	PBT	50–66 GyE	CR: 0%, PR: 55.6% (PVT)	Median: 13.2 mo.	None	Gr 2 GI toxicity: 7.4%

Abbreviations: *R* retrospective; *Tx* treatment, *MVI* macroscopic vascular invasion, *PVT* portal vein thrombus, *IVCT* inferior vena cava thrombus, *RT* radiotherapy, *PBT* proton beam therapy, *3D-CRT* 3-dimensional conformal radiotherapy, *SRT* stereotactic radiotherapy, *SBRT* stereotactic body radiotherapy, *GyE* gray equivalent, *Gy* gray, *fx* fraction, *CR* complete response, *PR* partial response, *RR* response rate, *Y* year, *mo* months, *C-P* Child-Pugh, *RILD* radiation-induced liver disease, *N/E* not evaluable, *Gr* grade, *GI* gastrointestinal

(53.8%) and the median survival rate was 11.6 months (range, 1–103.2) in 281 patients with HCC with PVTT after radiotherapy [17]. They proposed a predictive index for PVTT of the HCC (PITH) scores to stratify the patients' prognosis using seven clinical parameters including performance status, Child-Pugh classification, tumor size, multiplicity, the extent of PVTT, the status of occlusion of portal flow, and lymph node metastasis [17].

The most commonly used radiotherapy modality was 3-dimensional conformal radiotherapy (3D-CRT) for treatment of HCC with MVI. A couple of studies, however, reported the clinical outcomes of MVI after stereotactic body radiation therapy (SBRT) or proton beam therapy (PBT) [21, 34–37]. Lin et al. retrospectively compared the efficacy of SBRT to 3D-CRT in 43 patients [21]. The patients were assigned to receive either SBRT ($n = 22$, 45 Gy/15 fractions, using the Stereotactic Body Frame system) or 3D-CRT ($n = 21$, 45 Gy/25 fractions) arbitrarily. The response rates of evaluable patients were not statistically significant (SBRT group: 75%, 3D-CRT group: 84%; $p = 0.75$), and a similar median survival time was also observed between the two groups (SBRT group: 6 months, 3D-CRT group: 6.7 months; $p = 0.911$) [21]. Xi et al. studied the effectiveness of SBRT for HCC with PVTT and/or IVCTT using a hypofractionation regimen (30–48 Gy in 6 fractions) and reported a high response rate of 75.6% with the median survival time for all patients of 13 months (95% confidence interval [CI], 7.1–18.8 months) [35]. Two retrospective studies from Korea and Japan regarding the role of PBT in the management of HCC with PVTT also showed very promising response rates (75.6–100%) and survival outcomes with a relatively higher prescribed doses (range, 50–72 GyE) [34, 37].

14.4.3 Emergence of the Combined Radiotherapy with Transarterial Treatments

Advanced HCC with MVI is often accompanied with large, multiple, bilateral involvement, and/or infiltrative types of HCCs [28, 38, 39].

According to a recent radiologic review, PVTT is a common finding in patients with infiltrative HCC, often affecting both extra- and intra-hepatic branches, with a frequency ranging from 68 to 100% [40]. Therefore, the combined radiotherapy and locoregional treatment has been applied in treating the patients with advanced HCC showing MVI (Table 14.2). The most commonly used locoregional treatment in combination with radiotherapy was TACE to manage both intrahepatic HCC and MVI in these clinical settings.

In the early 2000s, two retrospective studies from Japan evaluated the feasibility and efficacy of radiotherapy in combination with TACE for HCC with PVTT [41, 42]. Although the number of enrolled patients was small, this combination treatment showed promising response rates (50%), minimal treatment-related toxicities, and was considered as a feasible and useful modality to improve the portal flow immediately in patients with HCC and PVTT [41, 42]. In 2003, the results of the first prospective trial of combined therapy of TACE and 3D-CRT for unresectable HCC with PVTT was published [43]. They enrolled the patients having unresectable HCC with PVTT in the first branch of the portal vein (no complete obstruction of the main portal trunk), without extrahepatic metastasis. The combination of TACE for the feeding arteries of each intrahepatic tumor and radiotherapy for targeting to PVTT (dose: 46–60 Gy with a daily dose of 2 Gy) yielded 57.9% of objective responses (CR: 0/19, PR: 11/19) with the median survival time of 7.0 months (a one-year survival rate of 40.6% and two-year survival rate of 10.2%), and low incidence of treatment-related toxicity in the liver and gastrointestinal tract [43]. Another study evaluated 136 patients with HCC having PVTT or IVCTT who received RT (90 patients received combined TACE) and reported a high response rate of 56.6% (CR: 41 [30.1%], PR: 36 [26.5%]) [18]. Yoon et al. reported the clinical outcomes of patients after TACE and 3D-CRT in a large registry database of 412 patients with HCC having PVTT [8]. They reported a 39.6% response rate for PVTT (CR: 6.6%, PR: 33%) and this response was the most powerful prognostic factor influencing overall mortality on multivariate analysis

Table 14.2   Summary of treatment outcomes of combined locoregional therapy and radiotherapy for hepatocellular carcinoma with macroscopic vascular invasion

Authors	Year	Study design	No. of patients	Combined Tx	MVI	RT	RT dose rate	Response rate	Survival outcomes	Toxicity (liver)	Toxicity (others)
Chen et al.	1994	C	10	TACE	PVT	2D	30–50 Gy	CR: 50%, PR: 50%		None	None
Yamada et al.	2001	C	8	TACE	PVT	3D-CRT	46–60 Gy	PR: 37.5%, SD: 62.5%	Median: 5.7 mo.	C-P ≥ 2: 37.5%	Gr 2 GI toxicity: 25%
Ishikura et al.	2002	R	20	TACE	PVT	3D-CRT	50 Gy	PR: 50%	Median: 5.3 mo., 1-Y: 25%	N/E	N/E
Tazawa et al.	2001	R	24	TACE	PVT	3D-CRT	50 Gy	CR: 16.7%, PR: 33.3%	Responder: median 9.7 mo., Non-responder: median 3.8 mo.	AST/ALT: 13%	Gr 3 nausea: 8.3%, Gr 3 diarrhea: 4.2%
Yamada et al.	2003	P	19	TACE	PVT	3D-CRT	46–60 Gy	PR: 57.9%	Median: 7 mo., 1-Y: 40.6%, 2-Y: 10.2%	Gr 2: 15.8%, Gr3: 10.5%	Gr 3 GI toxicity: 10.5%
Zeng et al.	2008	R	136	TACE (90)	PVT, IVCT	2D, 3D-CRT	30–60 Gy	CR: 30.1%, PR: 26.5%	Median: PV branch-10.1 mo.,PV trunk-7.4 mo., IVC-18.4 mo., PVT+IVCT-7.5 mo.	Gr 3 AST: 4.4%	Gr 3 nausea: 1.5%, Gr 3 anorexia: 2.2%, Gr 3 ulcer: 0.7%
Han et al.	2008	P	40	HAIC	PVT	3D-CRT	45 Gy	PR: 45%	Median: 13.1 mo. 1-Y: 57.6%, 2-Y: 32.2%	Grade 3-4 AST/ ALT: 62.5%, Gr 5: 2.5%	Gr 3-4 GI toxicity: 10%
Yoon et al.	2012	R	412	TACE	PVT	3D-CRT	21–60 Gy	CR: 6.6%, PR: 33%	Median: 10.6 mo., 1-Y: 42.5%, 2-Y: 22.8%, Responder: 19.4 mo., Non-responder: 7 mo.	Gr 3,4 AST/ALT: 8.5%, Gr 3,4 bilirubin: 4.2%	Gr 3 fatigue: 0.2%, Gr 2,3 GI toxicity: 3.6%
Kim et al.	2019	R	639	TACE	PVT, IVCT	3D-CRT	24–50 Gy		Median: 10.7 mo., 1-Y: 46.5%, 2-Y: 23.9%	N/E	N/E

Abbreviations: *C*, case series, *R* retrospective, *Tx* treatment, *TACE* transarterial chemoembolization, *HAIC* hepatic arterial infusion chemotherapy, *MVI* macroscopic vascular invasion, *PVT* portal vein thrombus, *IVCT* inferior vena cava thrombus, *RT* radiotherapy, *2D* 2-dimensional, *3D-CRT* 3-dimensional conformal radiotherapy, *Gy* gray, *CR* complete response, *PR* partial response, *SD* stable disease, *Y* year, *mo* months; *C-P* Child-Pugh, *N/E* not evaluable, *AST* aspartate transaminase, *ALT* alanine transaminase, *Gr* grade, *GI* gastrointestinal (median survival time of responders: 19.4 months vs. median survival of non-responders: 7.0 months) [8]. This combination regimen was complementary to each other; focal field radiotherapy targeting the PVTT maintained portal blood flow, allowing the maintenance of liver function and thereby allowing additional TACE; this therefore became the basis for the prospective clinical trial that would be discussed later [38]. Recently, Kim et al. reported the outcomes of combined TACE plus radiotherapy in a large cohort (639 patients) of treatment-naïve BCLC stage C HCC patients with MVI and proposed the subclassification model using the pretreatment patient and tumor characteristics (Child-Pugh class, status of extrahepatic metastasis, the extent of MVI, tumor size, and tumor type on imaging study) [28]. Regarding the optimal interval between TACE and radiotherapy, Yu et al. showed a two-week interval between TACE and radiotherapy was safe and efficient from their retrospective analysis [44].

Another combination therapy for advanced HCC is radiotherapy combined with hepatic arterial infusion chemotherapy (HAIC). Han et al. performed a prospective trial regarding the therapeutic effect of localized chemoradiation therapy followed by HAIC in patients with locally advanced HCC with PVTT [19]. The objective response was observed in 45% (18/40 patients) and the actuarial three-year overall survival rate was 24.1%, with the median survival time of 13.1 months. They suggested the high response rate encouraged the use of this approach in patients with locally advanced HCC to reduce tumor burden [19]. Recently, Kim et al. published the results of chemoradiation with HAIC (+/− TACE) followed by sequential sorafenib in patients with advanced HCC. They reported that the median overall survival was 24.6 months for the entire cohort and 13.0 months for the subgroup with tumor invasion into the main portal trunk or its first branch [45]. A nationwide, multicenter study investigated treatment outcomes as well as the optimal radiotherapeutic strategy in 985 patients with HCC and PVTT in Korea [46]. Treatment to PVTT was either radiotherapy alone (*n* = 328, 33.3%) or combined treatment (*n* = 657,

66.7%) with locoregional therapy (TACE: 527 patients, HAIC: 102 patients, TACE+HAIC: 28 patients). After propensity score matching, the median overall survival of the combined treatment was significantly better than that of no combined treatment group (10.4 vs. 8.7 months, *p* = 0.023) [46]. Although this result is not derived from a prospective controlled trial, the combined radiotherapy and other locoregional treatments is a recommended treatment option for patients with HCC and MVI.

14.4.4 Comparison Studies on the Management of HCC with Macroscopic Vascular Invasion

There have been several studies to compare the treatment modalities for HCC with MVI during the past 15 years (Table 14.3). The main study design was a retrospective comparison with/without statistical adjustment between the treatment groups; however, two prospective randomized studies were also published regarding the role of radiotherapy in the management of HCC with MVI compared with other modalities [38, 47].

14.4.4.1 Treatment Combinations with and Without Radiotherapy

Zeng et al. performed a retrospective comparison study between the patients who received radiotherapy (EBRT group) and the patients treated without radiotherapy (non-EBRT group) in HCC with PVTT and/or IVCTT [22]. Thirty-four patients in the EBRT group received various combined locoregional therapies (surgery: 9, TACE: 25) and 10 patients received radiotherapy only. Among the non-EBRT group, 18 patients underwent surgery, 73 received TACE, and 23 received no treatment. Despite the heterogeneity in treatments, the survival outcomes were significantly better in the EBRT group (median survival: eight months, one-year survival rate: 34%) compared with the non-EBRT group (median survival: four months, one-year survival rate: 11.4%) [22].

Table 14.3 Comparisons studies with or without radiotherapy on the management of hepatocellular carcinoma with macroscopic vascular invasion

Authors	Year	Study design	Comparison	No. of patients	Tx modality	MVI	RT	RT dose	Response rate	DFS/PFS/TTP	p-value	Overall survival	p-value
Zeng et al.	2005	R	Standard	44	RT	PVT, IVCT	3D-CRT	36–60 Gy	CR: 34.1%, PR: 11.4%			Median: 8 mo, 1-Y: 34.8%	<0.001
				114	None	PVT, IVCT						Median: 4 mo, 1-Y: 11.4%	
Koo et al.	2010	R	Standard	42	TACE+RT	IVCT	3D-CRT	28–50 Gy	CR: 14.3%, PR: 28.6%			Median: 11.7 mo, 1-Y: 47.7%	<0.01
				29	TACE	IVCT			CR: 0%, PR: 13.8%			Median: 4.7 mo, 1-Y: 17.2%	
Cho et al.	2014	R	PS	67 (PS: 27)	TACE+RT	MVI (95.5%)	3D-CRT	30–45 Gy				Median (PS): 8.9 mo	<0.001
				35 (PS: 27)	Sorafenib	MVI (100%)						Median (PS): 3.1 mo	
Onishi et al.	2015	R	Standard	33	CCRT	PVT	3D-CRT	50 Gy (82%)	CR: 3%, PR: 42% (PVT)			Median: 12.4 mo	0.14
				34	HAIC alone	PVT			CR: 6%, PR: 12% (PVT)			Median: 5.7 mo	
Fujino et al.	2015	R	Standard	41	CCRT	PVT	3D-CRT	30–45 Gy	CR: 15%, PR: 41% (PVT)			Median: 12.1 mo	0.308
				42	HAIC alone	PVT			CR: 12%, PR: 21% (PVT)			Median: 7.2 mo	
Lu et al.	2015	R	Standard	30	TACE+RT	PVT	3D-CRT	40–52.5 Gy	CR: 16.7%, PR: 53.3%			Median: 13.0 mo, 1-Y: 62.4%	NS

(continued)

Table 14.3 (continued)

Authors	Year	Study design	Comparison	No. of patients	Tx modality	MVI	RT	RT dose	Response rate	DFS/PFS/TTP	p-value	Overall survival	p-value
Kim et al.	2015	R	PS, IPTW	33	TACE	PVT			CR: 15.2%, PR: 30.3%			Median: 9 mo, 1-Y: 56.5%	
				196 (PS: 30)	TACE+RT	PVT	3D-CRT	21–60 Gy		Median TTP (PS): 3.4 mo	<0.001	Median (PS): 8.2 mo	<0.001
				66 (PS: 30)	Sorafenib	PVT				Median TTP (PS): 1.8 mo		Median (PS): 3.2 mo	
Lee et al.	2018	R	Matched cohort	43	TACE+RT	PVT	3D-CRT			Median PFS: 4.0 mo	>0.05	Median: 14.2 mo, 1-Y: 51%	0.04
				43	Resection	PVT				Median PFS: 5.6 mo		Median: 26.9 mo, 1-Y: 70%	
Chu et al.	2020	R	PS	203 (PS: 87)	TACE+RT	PVT	3D-CRT		CR: 24.1%, PR: 34.5%	Median PFS (PS): 5.9 mo	0.258	Median (PS): 13.2 mo	0.299
				104 (PS: 87)	TACE+Sorafenib	PVT			CR: 17.3%, PR: 24%	Median PFS (PS): 4.8 mo		Median (PS): 12 mo	
Yoon et al.	2018	P	Randomized	45	TACE+RT	MVI	3D-CRT	30–45 Gy	CR: 0%, PR: 33.3%	Median PFS: 30 wk	<0.001	Median: 55 wk	0.04
				45	Sorafenib	MVI			CR: 0%, PR: 2.2%	Median PFS: 11.3 wk		Median: 43 wk	
Wei et al.	2019	P	Randomized	82	Neoadjuvant. RT+Surgery	PVT	3D-CRT	18 Gy/6fx	CR: 0%, PR: 20.7%	DFS: 33% (1-Y), 13.3% (2-Y)	0.009	1-Y: 75.2%, 2-Y: 27.4%	<0.001
				82	Surgery alone	PVT				DFS: 14.9% (1-Y), 3.3% (2-Y)		1-Y: 43.1%, 2-Y: 9.4%	

Abbreviations: *R* retrospective, *P* prospective, *PS* propensity score, *IPTW* inverse probability of treatment weighting, *Tx* treatment, *RT* radiotherapy, *TACE* transarterial chemo-embolization, *CCRT* concurrent chemoradiotherapy, *HAIC* hepatic arterial infusion chemotherapy, *MVI* macroscopic vascular invasion, *PVT* portal vein thrombus, *IVCT* inferior vena cava thrombus, *3D-CRT* 3-dimensional conformal radiotherapy, *Gy* gray; *fx* fraction, *CR* complete response, *PR* partial response, *DFS* disease-free survival, *PFS* progression-free survival, *TTP* time-to-progression, *mo* months, *Y* year, *wk*, weeks.

14.4.4.2 TACE and Radiotherapy Combination Versus TACE

Koo et al. evaluated the efficacy of radiotherapy in combination with TACE compared with that of TACE alone in HCC patients with IVCTT [9]. The response rate in the TACE plus radiotherapy group was 42.9%, which is significantly better than 13.8% in the TACE group ($p < 0.01$). According to the responses of IVCTT to treatment, the overall survival rates of the responders were significantly higher than non-responders ($p = 0.02$), and the patients who were free of IVCTT progression had a significantly higher survival rate than those with IVCTT progression ($p < 0.01$). The median survival duration was significantly longer in the TACE plus radiotherapy group than in the TACE group (11.7 vs. 4.7 months; $p < 0.01$), and therefore they concluded that the combination of TACE and radiotherapy was more effective in control of IVCTT associated with HCC and improved survival outcomes compared with TACE alone [9]. Lu et al. also performed a similar retrospective study for 63 patients with PVTT and reported a significantly higher response and longer overall survival rates in the TACE plus radiotherapy group compared with in the TACE-only group [48].

Although the study design was a bit different, there was a recent retrospective study to compare the effectiveness of TACE plus radiotherapy ($n = 203$) with TACE plus sorafenib ($n = 104$) as a first-line treatment for HCC with PVTT [49]. The progression-free survival and overall survival rates were significantly longer in the TACE plus radiotherapy group than in the TACE plus sorafenib group in the entire study population; however, these oncologic outcomes were not significantly different between the two groups after propensity score matching [49].

14.4.4.3 Concurrent Radiotherapy with HAIC Versus HAIC Alone

Two retrospective studies evaluated the efficacy of concurrent HAIC plus radiotherapy in comparison with the results of HAIC alone for HCC with PVTT from Japan [50, 51]. The first study revealed that the objective response rate of PVTT was significantly higher in the combined treatment group than in the HAIC-alone group (45 vs. 18%; $p = 0.01$); the median survival time of the combined treatment group tended to be longer, but not significant, than in the HAIC group (12.4 vs. 5.7 months; $p = 0.14$) [50]. The other study found that the maximum treatment response of PVTT was also significantly higher in the combined treatment group than in the HAIC-alone group (56 vs. 33%; $p = 0.013$); the median survival time was not significantly different between the two groups (the combined treatment group: 12.1 months vs. the HAIC alone group: 7.2 months; $p = 0.308$) [51]. Although neither study showed the statistical differences on overall survival rate between the two groups, the combined HAIC and radiotherapy might be a promising treatment option for advanced stage HCC with PVTT, and needs to be clarified with a well-designed study in future.

14.4.4.4 Study Including Hepatic Resection as a Primary Treatment

Although most advanced HCC with MVI is unresectable disease as discussed above, hepatic resection can also be considered in very selected patients with resectable HCC having PVTT. Lee et al. compared retrospectively the treatment efficacy between resection and TACE plus radiotherapy in HCC patients with PVTT [52]. They included 43 patients who received hepatic resection as a primary treatment during the study period, then selected 43 patients who initially treated with TACE plus radiotherapy by matching the Child-Pugh class, tumor size, and the extent of PVTT. The demographic, clinical, and laboratory characteristics were similar between the two groups. The progression-free survival rates did not show significant differences between the two groups, but the overall survival was significantly longer in the resection group than in the TACE plus radiotherapy group (median survival: 26.9 vs. 14.2 months; $p = 0.04$) [52].

Recently, a randomized, multi-center, controlled study was done to evaluate the role of neoadjuvant radiotherapy in patients with resectable HCC and PVTT [47]. They prescribed a total dose of 18 Gy with a fraction size of 3 Gy and performed surgery in four weeks after completion of radiotherapy in the neoadjuvant radiotherapy arm ($n = 82$). For patients who were randomly assigned to the surgery-alone group ($n = 82$), surgery was carried out within five days after assignment. Both overall survival and disease-free survival rates were significantly better in the neoadjuvant radiotherapy arm compared with the surgery-alone arm ($p < 0.001$, each). Therefore, the authors concluded that neoadjuvant radiotherapy provided significantly better postoperative survival outcomes than surgery alone for patients with resectable HCC and PVTT [47].

14.4.4.5 Combined TACE and Radiotherapy Versus Sorafenib

Systemic therapies are currently the standard of care treatment for advanced HCC with or without MVI according to the recent treatment guidelines for HCC [10, 11]. Except for recent years, sorafenib has been the only first-line systemic therapy with a high level of clinical evidence, and therefore there have been some efforts to compare the results of combined TACE plus radiotherapy to sorafenib in patients with HCC showing MVI.

Cho et al. reported a retrospective study to determine the efficacy of TACE plus radiotherapy compared to sorafenib in a cohort of newly diagnosed advanced HCC patients between January 2007 and December 2011 [53]. Forty-nine patients were treated with sorafenib while 67 patients underwent combined TACE and radiotherapy. Because there were significant differences in performance status, tumor size, presence of lymph node metastasis, and the extent of PVTT in main portal vein between the two groups, the propensity score matching analysis was performed. The overall survival of the TACE plus radiotherapy group was significantly longer compared to the sorafenib treatment group (median survival: 8.9 vs. 3.1 months; $p < 0.001$) and multivariate analysis revealed that treatment modality of TACE plus radiotherapy versus sorafenib was the only independent prognostic factor associated with overall survival (the hazard ratio of the TACE plus radiotherapy group: 0.18; 95% CI: 0.088–0.378; $p < 0.001$) [53]. Kim et al. also reported a similar retrospective comparison study of the different specific treatments for HCC with PVTT [54]. They enrolled 557 patients who were initially treated with TACE alone ($n = 295$), TACE plus radiotherapy ($n = 196$), or sorafenib ($n = 66$) between 1997 and 2012, and performed rigorous adjustment for significant differences in all relevant baseline characteristics using inverse probability of treatment weighted (IPTW) and propensity score-based matching analyses. In the propensity score-matched cohorts, median time-to-progression was significantly longer in the TACE plus radiotherapy group than sorafenib group (5.1 vs. 1.6 months; $p < 0.001$), and median overall survival was also significantly longer in the TACE plus radiotherapy group than sorafenib group (8.2 vs. 3.2 months; $p < 0.001$), consistent with the results of IPTW adjustment. In addition, overall survival was longer for TACE-based treatment than sorafenib across most subgroups, including the Child-Pugh score, viral etiology, tumor type, the extent of tumor, number of the tumor, the extent of PVTT, and baseline alpha-fetoprotein level in subgroup analysis [54].

Based on these encouraging results, a randomized clinical trial to assess the efficacy and safety of TACE plus radiotherapy compared with sorafenib for patients with HCC and MVI was performed in Korea [38]. Between July 2013 and October 2016, all eligible patients ($n = 90$) were randomly assigned to receive sorafenib or TACE plus radiotherapy. Treatment crossover was permitted after confirming disease progression during the initially assigned treatment. The combined TACE plus radiotherapy was associated with a significantly higher rate of progression-free survival (86.7 vs. 34.3% at 12 weeks), a significantly higher radiologic response rate (33.3 vs. 2.2% at 24 weeks), a markedly longer median time to progression (31.0 vs. 11.7 weeks), and a significantly longer overall survival (55.0 vs. 43.0 weeks) [38]. This was the first randomized study to show the improved oncologic outcomes after a combined locoregional treatment over the current standard treatment of sorafenib in patients with HCC having MVI.

14.5 Additional Considerations

14.5.1 Definition of the Target Volume During Radiotherapy Planning

There is still a debate about target volume delineation regarding whether to include the entire HCC in radiotherapy planning. According to the extent of the tumors or the discretion of physicians, there may be three different scenarios in treating MVI (Fig. 14.3). If the tumor is a single HCC and confined within a lobe, both MVI and the entire HCC can be treated with radiotherapy. However, it is difficult to treat the whole HCC and MVI, if the viable HCCs are multiple, infiltrative tumor, bilateral involvements of the liver, or the extensive involvement of MVI (e.g., bilateral portal vein, multiple vascular invasions). Other host factors, including baseline hepatic function or the limited liver volume due to the cirrhosis, are also influenced on determining target volume. In addition, the focal field radiotherapy targeting the MVI can be used if the combined locoregional therapy is intended to treat HCC

outside radiation field. Therefore, some researchers intended to treat the entire HCC and MVI with radiotherapy [19, 23, 34, 37, 48], while others defined the focal field radiotherapy solely to treat MVI [33, 43, 50, 51]; however, most other studies adopted the radiation field from including the whole HCC to the focal field irradiation considering various clinical situations [8, 17, 18, 20–22, 28, 32, 35, 38, 49, 52–54].

It is difficult to define which is better—to treat the whole HCC and MVI or to irradiate the focal field around the MVI—because the target volume delineation may be influenced by the extent of HCC and MVI. In a Korean nationwide retrospective cohort of HCC patients with PVTT who received radiotherapy, the PVTT and primary tumor were irradiated simultaneously in 413 (41.9%) patients, and focal field of PVTT was targeted in 572 (58.1%) patients [46]. After propensity score matching, the median overall survival of the PVTT plus primary tumor and focal field of PVTT groups were 11.8 months and 10.4 months, respectively, and this was not significantly different ($p = 0.713$) [46]. Therefore, the focal field radio-

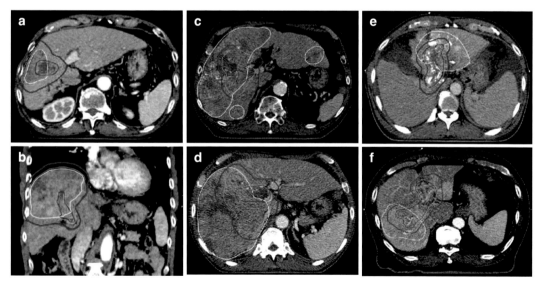

Fig. 14.3 Three different scenarios to define target volumes in treating macroscopic vascular invasion (MVI) with radiotherapy. Radiation field includes MVI and whole viable hepatocellular carcinoma (HCC) (**a**, **b**). Target volume covers MVI and a certain margin of adja-

cent viable HCC (**c**, **d**). Radiation field includes MVI-only without inclusion of adjacent viable HCC (**e**, **f**) (Red line: MVI, white line: viable HCC, orange line: gross tumor volume, magenta line: planning target volume) therapy targeting the MVI could be a suggested treatment strategy to reduce the risk of hepatic toxicity when performing the combined locoregional treatment for HCC.

14.5.2 Radiotherapy-Related Toxicities

Hepatic dysfunction is an important treatment-related toxicity and will be discussed in Chap. 21. Classic radiation-induced liver disease (RILD) represented as anicteric hepatomegaly, ascites, or elevated alkaline phosphatase between two weeks and three months after treatment was proposed in 1995 [55]. Non-classic RILD, however, involved elevated liver transaminases or a decline in liver function (measured by a worsening of Child-Pugh score by 2 or more), usually developed in HCC patients with hepatitis B virus infection between a week and three months after therapy [56]. Most previous studies reported an acceptable hepatic toxicity after radiotherapy for MVI; however, long-term liver damage has not been as well understood because of the poor prognosis of MVI. Moreover, subsequent repeated treatments (both locoregional and systemic therapies) are usually required in the management of advanced HCC with MVI; it is also difficult to discriminate the proportion of liver damage induced by radiotherapy. Therefore, it is necessary to interpret the results about hepatic toxicity in consideration of various clinical possibility.

Gastrointestinal structures such as the stomach or duodenum are radiosensitive organs in radiotherapy for HCC. According to the routine examination of esophagogastroduodenoscopy one to three months after radiotherapy, the overall incidence of gastrointestinal complications was as high as around 50% [57, 58]. Yu et al. reported that 25% of patients who experienced gastrointestinal bleeding were treated with endoscopic argon plasma coagulation therapy or blood transfusion, even though they modified the prescribed dose when the stomach or duodenum was irradiated during radiotherapy planning [57]. Because most patients have underlying liver cirrhosis, portal hypertension, and coagulopathy that can exacerbate the risk for gastrointestinal toxicities, it would be necessary to treat with more stringent constraints for gastrointestinal structures to minimize this toxicity.

14.5.3 Future Directions in Combination with New Immunotherapy and Systemic Therapies

In recent years, new results of both molecular targeted agents and immune checkpoint inhibitors (ICI) provided many new options for advanced HCC [59]. Moreover, combination of ICI with other systemic agents may be a new standard therapy in treatment of HCC with MVI [59, 60]. Radiotherapy has been used as a potent locoregional treatment option in this advanced HCC; it is also necessary to make efforts to establish the clinical evidence in combination with both ICIs and novel systemic agents for HCC with MVI. This subject will be discussed in more detail in Chap. 23.

14.6 Conclusions

Based on the results of previous studies, radiotherapy combined with or without locoregional treatments is tolerable and effective treatment modality for patients with advanced HCC having MVI. The reported response rates are promising for delaying intravascular tumor growth from MVI, the deterioration of liver function, and to facilitate the subsequent treatment of primary tumor. Therefore, the use of radiotherapy as an initial treatment can be a good treatment strategy to improve the oncologic outcomes in patients with advanced HCC having MVI. A more definite role of radiotherapy should be identified from future clinical trials.

References

1. Korean Liver Cancer Association, National Cancer Center. 2018 Korean Liver Cancer Association-National Cancer Center. Korea practice guidelines for the management of hepatocellular carcinoma. Gut Liver. 2019;13(3):227–99.
2. Forner A, Reig M, Bruix J. Hepatocellular carcinoma. Lancet. 2018;391(10127):1301–14.
3. Park HC, Seong J, Tanaka M, Zeng ZC, Lim HY, Guan S, et al. Multidisciplinary management of nonresectable hepatocellular carcinoma. Oncology. 2011;81(Suppl 1):134–40.
4. Bruix J, Cheng AL, Meinhardt G, Nakajima K, De Sanctis Y, Llovet J. Prognostic factors and predictors of sorafenib benefit in patients with hepatocellular carcinoma: analysis of two phase III studies. J Hepatol. 2017;67(5):999–1008.
5. Llovet JM, Bustamante J, Castells A, Vilana R, Ayuso Mdel C, Sala M, et al. Natural history of untreated nonsurgical hepatocellular carcinoma: rationale for the design and evaluation of therapeutic trials. Hepatology. 1999;29(1):62–7.
6. Katagiri S, Yamamoto M. Multidisciplinary treatments for hepatocellular carcinoma with major portal vein tumor thrombus. Surg Today. 2014;44(2):219–26.
7. Knox JJ, Cleary SP, Dawson LA. Localized and systemic approaches to treating hepatocellular carcinoma. J Clin Oncol. 2015;33(16):1835–44.
8. Yoon SM, Lim YS, Won HJ, Kim JH, Kim KM, Lee HC, et al. Radiotherapy plus transarterial chemoembolization for hepatocellular carcinoma invading the portal vein: long-term patient outcomes. Int J Radiat Oncol Biol Phys. 2012;82(5):2004–11.
9. Koo JE, Kim JH, Lim YS, Park SJ, Won HJ, Sung KB, et al. Combination of transarterial chemoembolization and three-dimensional conformal radiotherapy for hepatocellular carcinoma with inferior vena cava tumor thrombus. Int J Radiat Oncol Biol Phys. 2010;78(1):180–7.
10. European Association for the Study of the Liver. EASL Clinical Practice Guidelines: management of hepatocellular carcinoma. J Hepatol. 2018;69(1):182–236.
11. Marrero JA, Kulik LM, Sirlin CB, Zhu AX, Finn RS, Abecassis MM, et al. Diagnosis, staging, and management of hepatocellular carcinoma: 2018 practice guidance by the American Association for the Study of Liver Diseases. Hepatology. 2018;68(2):723–50.
12. Cheng AL, Kang YK, Chen Z, Tsao CJ, Qin S, Kim JS, et al. Efficacy and safety of sorafenib in patients in the Asia-Pacific region with advanced hepatocellular carcinoma: a phase III randomised, double-blind, placebo-controlled trial. Lancet Oncol. 2009;10(1):25–34.
13. Llovet JM, Ricci S, Mazzaferro V, Hilgard P, Gane E, Blanc JF, et al. Sorafenib in advanced hepatocellular carcinoma. N Engl J Med. 2008;359(4):378–90.
14. Kudo M, Finn RS, Qin S, Han KH, Ikeda K, Piscaglia F, et al. Lenvatinib versus sorafenib in first-line treatment of patients with unresectable hepatocellular carcinoma: a randomised phase 3 non-inferiority trial. Lancet. 2018;391(10126):1163–73.
15. Finn RS, Qin S, Ikeda M, Galle PR, Ducreux M, Kim TY, et al. Atezolizumab plus bevacizumab in unresectable hepatocellular carcinoma. N Engl J Med. 2020;382(20):1894–905.
16. Bang A, Dawson LA. Radiotherapy for HCC: ready for prime time? JHEP Rep. 2019;1(2):131–7.
17. Yu JI, Park HC, Lim DH, Park W, Yoo BC, Paik SW, et al. Prognostic index for portal vein tumor thrombosis in patients with hepatocellular carcinoma treated with radiation therapy. J Korean Med Sci. 2011;26(8):1014–22.
18. Zeng ZC, Fan J, Tang ZY, Zhou J, Wang JH, Wang BL, et al. Prognostic factors for patients with hepatocellular carcinoma with macroscopic portal vein or inferior vena cava tumor thrombi receiving external-beam radiation therapy. Cancer Sci. 2008;99(12):2510–7.
19. Han KH, Seong J, Kim JK, Ahn SH, Lee DY, Chon CY. Pilot clinical trial of localized concurrent chemoradiation therapy for locally advanced hepatocellular carcinoma with portal vein thrombosis. Cancer. 2008;113(5):995–1003.
20. Toya R, Murakami R, Baba Y, Nishimura R, Morishita S, Ikeda O, et al. Conformal radiation therapy for portal vein tumor thrombosis of hepatocellular carcinoma. Radiother Oncol. 2007;84(3):266–71.
21. Lin CS, Jen YM, Chiu SY, Hwang JM, Chao HL, Lin HY, et al. Treatment of portal vein tumor thrombosis of hepatoma patients with either stereotactic radiotherapy or three-dimensional conformal radiotherapy. Jpn J Clin Oncol. 2006;36(4):212–7.
22. Zeng ZC, Fan J, Tang ZY, Zhou J, Qin LX, Wang JH, et al. A comparison of treatment combinations with and without radiotherapy for hepatocellular carcinoma with portal vein and/or inferior vena cava tumor thrombus. Int J Radiat Oncol Biol Phys. 2005;61(2):432–43.
23. Kim DY, Park W, Lim DH, Lee JH, Yoo BC, Paik SW, et al. Three-dimensional conformal radiotherapy for portal vein thrombosis of hepatocellular carcinoma. Cancer. 2005;103(11):2419–26.
24. Yu JI, Park JW, Park HC, Yoon SM, Lim DH, Lee JH, et al. Clinical impact of combined transarterial chemoembolization and radiotherapy for advanced hepatocellular carcinoma with portal vein tumor thrombosis: An external validation study. Radiother Oncol. 2016;118(2):408–15.
25. Kim KM, Kim JH, Park IS, Ko GY, Yoon HK, Sung KB, et al. Reappraisal of repeated transarterial che-

moembolization in the treatment of hepatocellular carcinoma with portal vein invasion. J Gastroenterol Hepatol. 2009;24(5):806–14.

26. Sinn DH, Choi GS, Park HC, Kim JM, Kim H, Song KD, et al. Multidisciplinary approach is associated with improved survival of hepatocellular carcinoma patients. PLoS One. 2019;14(1):e0210730.

27. Lee DW, Yim HJ, Seo YS, Na SK, Kim SY, Suh SJ, et al. Prognostic assessment using a new substaging system for Barcelona clinic liver cancer stage C hepatocellular carcinoma: a nationwide study. Liver Int. 2019;39(6):1109–19.

28. Kim YJ, Jung J, Joo JH, Kim SY, Kim JH, Lim YS, et al. Combined transarterial chemoembolization and radiotherapy as a first-line treatment for hepatocellular carcinoma with macroscopic vascular invasion: necessity to subclassify Barcelona Clinic Liver Cancer stage C. Radiother Oncol. 2019;141:95–100.

29. Chen SC, Lian SL, Chang WY. The effect of external radiotherapy in treatment of portal vein invasion in hepatocellular carcinoma. Cancer Chemother Pharmacol. 1994;33(Suppl):S124–7.

30. Yamada K, Soejima T, Sugimoto K, Mayahara H, Izaki K, Sasaki R, et al. Pilot study of local radiotherapy for portal vein tumor thrombus in patients with unresectable hepatocellular carcinoma. Jpn J Clin Oncol. 2001;31(4):147–52.

31. Igaki H, Nakagawa K, Shiraishi K, Shiina S, Kokudo N, Terahara A, et al. Three-dimensional conformal radiotherapy for hepatocellular carcinoma with inferior vena cava invasion. Jpn J Clin Oncol. 2008;38(6):438–44.

32. Nakazawa T, Adachi S, Kitano M, Isobe Y, Kokubu S, Hidaka H, et al. Potential prognostic benefits of radiotherapy as an initial treatment for patients with unresectable advanced hepatocellular carcinoma with invasion to intrahepatic large vessels. Oncology. 2007;73(1–2):90–7.

33. Huang YJ, Hsu HC, Wang CY, Wang CJ, Chen HC, Huang EY, et al. The treatment responses in cases of radiation therapy to portal vein thrombosis in advanced hepatocellular carcinoma. Int J Radiat Oncol Biol Phys. 2009;73(4):1155–63.

34. Lee SU, Park JW, Kim TH, Kim YJ, Woo SM, Koh YH, et al. Effectiveness and safety of proton beam therapy for advanced hepatocellular carcinoma with portal vein tumor thrombosis. Strahlenther Onkol. 2014;190(9):806–14.

35. Xi M, Zhang L, Zhao L, Li QQ, Guo SP, Feng ZZ, et al. Effectiveness of stereotactic body radiotherapy for hepatocellular carcinoma with portal vein and/or inferior vena cava tumor thrombosis. PLoS One. 2013;8(5):e63864.

36. Sugahara S, Nakayama H, Fukuda K, Mizumoto M, Tokita M, Abei M, et al. Proton-beam therapy for hepatocellular carcinoma associated with portal vein tumor thrombosis. Strahlenther Onkol. 2009;185(12):782–8.

37. Hata M, Tokuuye K, Sugahara S, Kagei K, Igaki H, Hashimoto T, et al. Proton beam therapy for hepato-

cellular carcinoma with portal vein tumor thrombus. Cancer. 2005;104(4):794–801.

38. Yoon SM, Ryoo BY, Lee SJ, Kim JH, Shin JH, An JH, et al. Efficacy and safety of transarterial chemoembolization plus external beam radiotherapy vs sorafenib in hepatocellular carcinoma with macroscopic vascular invasion: a randomized clinical trial. JAMA Oncol. 2018;4(5):661–9.

39. Han K, Kim JH, Yoon HM, Kim EJ, Gwon DI, Ko GY, et al. Transcatheter arterial chemoembolization for infiltrative hepatocellular carcinoma: clinical safety and efficacy and factors influencing patient survival. Korean J Radiol. 2014;15(4):464–71.

40. Reynolds AR, Furlan A, Fetzer DT, Sasatomi E, Borhani AA, Heller MT, et al. Infiltrative hepatocellular carcinoma: what radiologists need to know. Radiographics. 2015;35(2):371–86.

41. Ishikura S, Ogino T, Furuse J, Satake M, Baba S, Kawashima M, et al. Radiotherapy after transcatheter arterial chemoembolization for patients with hepatocellular carcinoma and portal vein tumor thrombus. Am J Clin Oncol. 2002;25(2):189–93.

42. Tazawa J, Maeda M, Sakai Y, Yamane M, Ohbayashi H, Kakinuma S, et al. Radiation therapy in combination with transcatheter arterial chemoembolization for hepatocellular carcinoma with extensive portal vein involvement. J Gastroenterol Hepatol. 2001;16(6):660–5.

43. Yamada K, Izaki K, Sugimoto K, Mayahara H, Morita Y, Yoden E, et al. Prospective trial of combined transcatheter arterial chemoembolization and three-dimensional conformal radiotherapy for portal vein tumor thrombus in patients with unresectable hepatocellular carcinoma. Int J Radiat Oncol Biol Phys. 2003;57(1):113–9.

44. Yu JI, Park HC, Lim DH, Kim CJ, Oh D, Yoo BC, et al. Scheduled interval trans-catheter arterial chemoembolization followed by radiation therapy in patients with unresectable hepatocellular carcinoma. J Korean Med Sci. 2012;27(7):736–43.

45. Kim BK, Kim DY, Byun HK, Choi HJ, Beom SH, Lee HW, et al. Efficacy and safety of liver-directed concurrent chemoradiotherapy and sequential sorafenib for advanced hepatocellular carcinoma: a prospective phase 2 trial. Int J Radiat Oncol Biol Phys. 2020;107(1):106–15.

46. Im JH, Yoon SM, Park HC, Kim JH, Yu JI, Kim TH, et al. Radiotherapeutic strategies for hepatocellular carcinoma with portal vein tumour thrombosis in a hepatitis B endemic area. Liver Int. 2017;37(1):90–100.

47. Wei X, Jiang Y, Zhang X, Feng S, Zhou B, Ye X, et al. Neoadjuvant three-dimensional conformal radiotherapy for resectable hepatocellular carcinoma with portal vein tumor thrombus: a randomized, open-label, multicenter controlled study. J Clin Oncol. 2019;37(24):2141–51.

48. Lu DH, Fei ZL, Zhou JP, Hu ZT, Hao WS. A comparison between three-dimensional conformal radiotherapy combined with interventional treatment and

interventional treatment alone for hepatocellular carcinoma with portal vein tumour thrombosis. J Med Imaging Radiat Oncol. 2015;59(1):109–14.

49. Chu HH, Kim JH, Shim JH, Yoon SM, Kim PH, Alrashidi I. Chemoembolization plus radiotherapy versus chemoembolization plus sorafenib for the treatment of hepatocellular carcinoma invading the portal vein: a propensity score matching analysis. Cancers (Basel). 2020;12(5):1116.

50. Onishi H, Nouso K, Nakamura S, Katsui K, Wada N, Morimoto Y, et al. Efficacy of hepatic arterial infusion chemotherapy in combination with irradiation for advanced hepatocellular carcinoma with portal vein invasion. Hepatol Int. 2015;9(1):105–12.

51. Fujino H, Kimura T, Aikata H, Miyaki D, Kawaoka T, Kan H, et al. Role of 3-D conformal radiotherapy for major portal vein tumor thrombosis combined with hepatic arterial infusion chemotherapy for advanced hepatocellular carcinoma. Hepatol Res. 2015;45(6):607–17.

52. Lee D, Lee HC, An J, Shim JH, Kim KM, Lim YS, et al. Comparison of surgical resection versus transarterial chemoembolization with additional radiation therapy in patients with hepatocellular carcinoma with portal vein invasion. Clin Mol Hepatol. 2018;24(2):144–50.

53. Cho JY, Paik YH, Park HC, Yu JI, Sohn W, Gwak GY, et al. The feasibility of combined transcatheter arterial chemoembolization and radiotherapy for advanced hepatocellular carcinoma. Liver Int. 2014;34(5):795–801.

54. Kim GA, Shim JH, Yoon SM, Jung J, Kim JH, Ryu MH, et al. Comparison of chemoembolization with and without radiation therapy and sorafenib for advanced hepatocellular carcinoma with portal vein tumor thrombosis: a propensity score analysis. J Vasc Interv Radiol. 2015;26(3):320–9.e6.

55. Lawrence TS, Robertson JM, Anscher MS, Jirtle RL, Ensminger WD, Fajardo LF. Hepatic toxicity resulting from cancer treatment. Int J Radiat Oncol Biol Phys. 1995;31(5):1237–48.

56. Pan CC, Kavanagh BD, Dawson LA, Li XA, Das SK, Miften M, et al. Radiation-associated liver injury. Int J Radiat Oncol Biol Phys. 2010;76(3 Suppl):S94–100.

57. Yu JI, Cho JY, Park HC, Lim DH, Gwak GY, Paik SW. Child-Pugh score maintenance in cirrhotic hepatocellular carcinoma patients after radiotherapy: aspects of gastroduodenal complications. Tumori. 2014;100(6):645–51.

58. Chon YE, Seong J, Kim BK, Cha J, Kim SU, Park JY, et al. Gastroduodenal complications after concurrent chemoradiation therapy in patients with hepatocellular carcinoma: endoscopic findings and risk factors. Int J Radiat Oncol Biol Phys. 2011;81(5):1343–51.

59. Dong Y, Liu TH, Yau T, Hsu C. Novel systemic therapy for hepatocellular carcinoma. Hepatol Int. 2020;14(5):638–51.

60. Cheng AL, Hsu C, Chan SL, Choo SP, Kudo M. Challenges of combination therapy with immune checkpoint inhibitors for hepatocellular carcinoma. J Hepatol. 2020;72(2):307–19.

Neoadjuvant Radiotherapy Converting to Curative Resection

15

Gi Hong Choi

Abstract

With technical improvements, radiotherapy (RT) has been adopted as an initial treatment modality for locally advanced hepatocellular carcinoma (HCC). Even though assessment of the resectability of HCC is still a controversial issue, neoadjuvant RT should be differentiated from downstaging treatment with RT because the aim of RT and timing of liver resection differ between the two approaches. In this chapter, the roles of neoadjuvant and downstaging RT in treating locally advanced HCC are investigated through a review of the literature.

Keywords

Locally advanced hepatocellular carcinoma · Portal vein tumor thrombus · Neoadjuvant radiotherapy · Downstaging radiotherapy · Curative liver resection · Long-term outcomes

15.1 Introduction

Surgical resection is an important primary treatment option for hepatocellular carcinoma (HCC), and long-term surgical outcomes have been gradually improving [1]. However, a surgical approach is contraindicated in most patients due to either advanced stage HCC or poor liver function. Locally advanced HCC defined as BCLC stage C without extrahepatic spread can be treated by systemic therapy, including sorafenib and regorafenib [2]. Recently, multimodal treatments for locally advanced HCC based on three-dimensional conformal radiotherapy (RT) have been introduced. In this chapter, the roles of neoadjuvant and downstaging RT are investigated by a review of the relevant literature.

15.2 How to Assess Resectability in HCC

To deal with the role of preoperative RT, the process used to assess resectability should first be addressed. Like other solid cancers, the general condition of the patient, presence of comorbidities, and tumor stage are the main determinants of resectability. Eastern Cooperative Oncology Group performance status ≥ 2, chronic renal failure, and congestive heart failure are relative contraindications for surgery [3]. Another factor determining resectability is remnant liver volume after planned resection. According to the baseline

G. H. Choi (✉)
Division of Hepatobiliary and Pancreatic Surgery, Department of Surgery, Yonsei University College of Medicine, Seoul, South Korea
e-mail: CHOIGH@yuhs.ac

© Springer Nature Singapore Pte Ltd. 2021
J. Seong (ed.), *Radiotherapy of Liver Cancer*, https://doi.org/10.1007/978-981-16-1815-4_15

condition of the liver, at least 30–40% of the total liver volume should be preserved after resection in patients with normal liver and chronic liver disease, respectively [4].

Tumor stage, which is determined by the number of tumors, vascular invasion, and extrahepatic spread, has been used to assess the resectability of HCC, but remains controversial. Most guidelines consider a single HCC with well-preserved liver function optimal indications for surgical resection [2, 3]; a few guidelines have extended this to three or fewer HCC lesions [5, 6]. HCC with tumor thrombus in the major vessels is usually regarded as a contraindication for surgical resection due to low curability, despite the apparent resectability of the tumor. However, some centers still recommended surgical resection in locally advanced HCC without extrahepatic spread because it may provide better survival outcomes than other non-surgical treatments [7]. In addition, HCC with Cheng's III portal vein tumor thrombus (PVTT), which involves the main trunk of the portal vein, was considered resectable in a recent randomized multicenter study for neoadjuvant three-dimensional conformal RT [8]. Assessment of the initial resectability of locally advanced HCC remains controversial, but is critical for investigation of the preoperative role of RT as the planned RT dose and the timing and indications for surgical resection differ between neoadjuvant and downstaging RT.

15.3   Neoadjuvant RT in Locally Advanced HCC

Neoadjuvant therapy for solid cancers is usually attempted to reduce tumor mass, which can make curative surgery more feasible and reduce postoperative recurrence. The role of neoadjuvant therapy in HCC is still controversial, and there is no clear evidence supporting its routine use.

Recently, the results of a randomized multicenter study in China of neoadjuvant three-dimensional conformal RT for resectable HCC with PVTT were reported [8]. In this study, 166 patients who had a HCC with PVTT were ran-

domly assigned to receive neoadjuvant RT followed by hepatectomy ($n = 82$) or hepatectomy alone ($n = 82$). Patients with either Cheng's type IV PVTT (defined as extension of thrombosis to the superior mesenteric vein) or inferior vena cava tumor thrombus were not considered for surgery alone in addition to the conventional criteria for liver resection such as performance status greater than 2, Child-Pugh class B or C, and more than three nodules on an imaging study. In the neoadjuvant RT group, the planned total dose for the planning target volume was 18 Gy at five fractions per week to minimize radiation injury to the non-tumorous liver and to shorten the time interval between neoadjuvant treatment and surgery. After completion of RT, patients were reevaluated within four weeks. Among 82 initial neoadjuvant patients, nine patients (11%) developed contraindications to surgery: disease progression ($n = 7$), HBV reactivation ($n = 1$), and deteriorated liver function ($n = 1$). According to the modified Response Evaluation Criteria in Solid Tumors guidelines®, 17 (20.7%) had a partial response, 58 (70.7%) had stable disease, and seven (8.5%) had progressive disease. After intention-to-treat analysis at a median follow-up of 15.2 months, the one- and two-year overall survival rates were 75.2% and 27.4% for the neoadjuvant RT group, respectively, versus 43.1% and 9.4% for the surgery-alone group, respectively ($p < 0.001$). The one-year and two-year disease-free survival rates were 33% and 13.3% in the neoadjuvant RT group, respectively, and 14.9% and 3.3% in the surgery-alone group, respectively ($p < 0.001$). Multivariable Cox proportional hazards regression analysis indicated that neoadjuvant RT significantly decreased both HCC-related mortality and HCC recurrence compared with surgery alone (hazard ratio (HR) 0.35; $p < 0.001$ and HR 0.45; $p < 0.001$, respectively). The authors of this study suggested that RT-related improvement in survival outcomes was mainly due to the decrease in tumor volume and PVTT, which facilitated *en block* resection of the tumor, downsized the tumor thrombus, and reduced the possibility of residual tumor or spread in the portal vein during surgery. Even though this study demonstrated that adjuvant RT improved surgical outcomes in patients with HCC with PVTT, this result requires further validation at other centers. In addition, the low radiation dose of 18 Gy was used to avoid adverse effects in this study. However, the optimal neoadjuvant RT dose requires further evaluation because total irradiation dose is significantly correlated with local control of HCC [9, 10]. Finally, preoperative RT induces hypertrophy of the non-radiated liver parenchyma, which can improve indications for resectability in patients who have a small future liver remnant, as well as decrease the possibility of postoperative liver dysfunction [11, 12]. The optimal timing of surgery after neoadjuvant RT should be further investigated to determine both the maximal tumor response and hypertrophy of the future liver remnant.

15.4 Curative Resection After Downstaging RT

Downstaging treatment is usually applied in patients with unresectable HCC based on the decision of a multidisciplinary team. Generally accepted criteria for unresectability of HCC include huge HCCs with an insufficient remnant liver volume, extrahepatic spread, extensive and multifocal bilobar tumors, and a tumor thrombus in either the main portal vein or the inferior vena cava [13]. Prognoses of these patients is very poor. With improvement in local and systemic treatments, some patients who initially were considered to have unresectable HCC experienced a downstaging response through palliative treatment because of shrinkage of huge tumors, regression and disappearance of major vessel tumor thrombi, and compensatory hypertrophy of the future remnant liver. In these patients, liver resection with curative aim was attempted. The first series of curative resections following tumor downstaging was introduced in 1993 by Sitzmann and colleagues [14]. The combination of radiotherapy and chemotherapy downstaged tumors from initially unresectable to resectable in 13 patients. The five-year survival rate after curative

resection in these patients was 48%. This concept of tumor downstaging followed by curative liver resection was matured by Lau and colleagues [13]. They also reported a good long-term survival of 57% at five years after curative resection following down-staging in 49 patients with unresectable HCC who initially received systemic chemotherapy, intra-arterial yttrium-90 microspheres, or sequential treatment [15]. Various treatment modalities have been introduced for HCC downstaging, including transarterial chemoemobolization (TACE), hepatic artery infusion chemotherapy (HAIC), systematic chemotherapy, and intra-arterial or external beam irradiation therapy [13, 16].

Recent advances in RT technology have facilitated an increase in the three-dimensional conformal RT irradiation dosage without an increase in toxicity to the surrounding liver parenchyma, resulting in a higher response rate [9]. Using this approach, our institute introduced localized concurrent chemoradiotherapy (CCRT) followed by HAIC for locally advanced HCC [17]. Curative resection was attempted in patients with tumor downstaging, and initial results were reported in 2014 by Lee et al. [11]. In this study, 41 (16.9%) among 243 patients who received CCRT followed by HAIC underwent curative resection. Tumor downstaging and pathologically complete necrosis was noted in 32 (78%) and nine (22.0%) resected patients, respectively. RT induced compensatory hypertrophy of the future remnant liver from 47.5 to 69.9% before surgery in patients who underwent major liver resection. The five-year overall survival rate of patients with curative resection was 49.6%; this is significantly higher than the five-year survival rate of 9.8% reported for patients without curative resection ($p < 0.001$). The authors of that study concluded that CCRT followed by HAIC increased resectability by downstaging tumors and increasing the volume of the future remnant liver, providing better long-term survival outcomes in patients who underwent curative resection.

The most common presentation of locally advanced HCC is a tumor thrombus in the portal vein. A case of HCC with PVTT is illustrated in Fig. 15.1. A 37-year-old woman was diagnosed

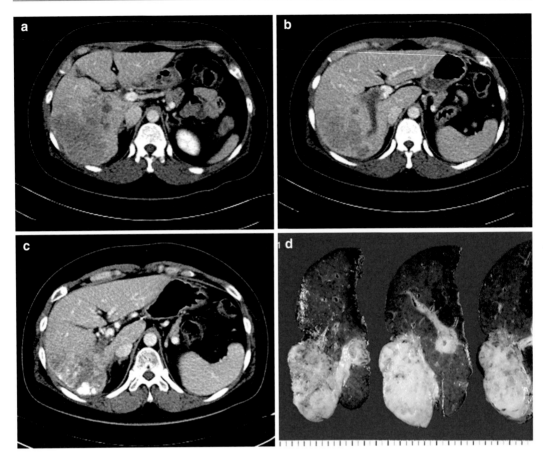

Fig. 15.1 Illustration of a patient with hepatocellular carcinoma with a portal vein tumor thrombus who underwent curative resection after tumor downstaging by concurrent chemoradiation (CCRT). Initial dynamic computed tomography showed a 12-cm infiltrative hepatocellular carcinoma with tumor thrombi in the right portal vein and the main portal vein (**a, b**). Initial left liver volume was 29% of the total liver volume. After CCRT followed by a second hepatic artery infusion chemotherapy and one-time transarterial chemoemobolization, the HCC and tumor thrombi showed a partial response (**c**). The portal vein tumor thrombus shrank, but did not disappear. The future remnant liver volume increased to 40% of the total liver volume. The patient underwent right hepatectomy and the tumor showed pathologically complete necrosis (**d**). The patient is still alive without recurrence seven years after surgery

with a 12-cm infiltrative HCC with tumor thrombus in the right portal vein and the main portal vein. The patient received CCRT as an initial treatment modality to downstage the tumor. After that, two HAIC regimens and one TACE regimen were initiated to treat the remaining tumor. Through these treatments, levels of tumor markers (α-fetoprotein [AFP] = 92,233.99 ng/mL and Protein Induced by Vitamin K absence or antagonist-II [PIVKA II] = 11,260 mAU/mL) normalized (AFP = 1.09 ng/mL and PIVKA II = 14 mAU/mL). The volume of the left liver increased

from 29 to 40%. The patient underwent right hepatectomy. The patient's postoperative course was uneventful and the tumor showed pathologically complete necrosis. The patient has been followed without recurrence for seven years since her surgery. As illustrated by this case, HCC with PVTT usually presents as a larger tumor with high levels of tumor markers. Curative resection is the only hope for cure; however, the selection of optimal surgical candidates is crucial to ensure curability. In addition, tumor biology is difficult to predict using clinical characteristics. In our institute, 98 patients who had HCC with PVTT and relatively well-preserved liver function received CCRT followed by HAIC as the initial treatment from 2005 to 2014 [18]. Among them, 26 patients (26.5%) underwent curative resection after downstaging. Their long-term outcomes were compared with 18 patients who underwent resection as the first treatment for HCC with PVTT during the same period. Based on intention-to-treat analysis, disease-specific survival for the CCRT group ($n = 98$) was comparable to that of the resection-first group ($n = 18$) (median 13 vs. 15 months, respectively; $p = 0.323$). However, disease-specific survival for the resection-after-CCRT group ($n = 26$) was significantly better than that of the resection-first group (median 62 vs. 15 months, respectively; $p = 0.006$). Therefore, CCRT followed by HAIC could be an effective tool to select optimal surgical candidates with a less aggressive tumor biology. Recently, Lee et al. analyzed factors predictive of conversion to curative surgery among 1078 patients who received liver-directed combined RT for locally advanced HCC [19]. In this study, 12.8% of all patients were converted to curative surgery. Based on multivariate logistic regression, age < 60 years, a single tumor, no treatment history, pre-treatment Child-Pugh class A, and lower treatment AFP and PIVKA II levels and radiologic response were associated with a higher probability of conversion to curative surgery.

After downstaging treatment, pathologically complete tumor necrosis occurs in 22–50% of patients [11, 13, 15]. One issue is whether liver resection is required in these patients. Pathologically complete necrosis after tumor downstaging may be associated with a complete radiologic response and normalization of initial tumor markers. However, there are no factors that can reliably predict pathologically complete necrosis. In addition, tumor recurrence rates and patterns in patients expected to have complete tumor necrosis without surgery remain to be elucidated. Therefore, liver resection is required in the majority of patients to induce complete remission and provide pathological information about the tumor.

15.5   Conclusions

Even though different institutes use different criteria to determine the resectability of locally advanced HCC, neoadjuvant RT and downstaging treatment with RT should be differentiated. A recent randomized controlled study demonstrated that neoadjuvant RT for HCC with PVTT improved long-term surgical outcomes compared with resection alone. However, this result should be validated in other centers. Downstaging treatment with RT can identify optimal surgical candidates with good tumor biology, and improve indications for resectability through tumor downstaging and hypertrophy of the future liver remnant. In patients with downstaging tumors expected to have pathologically complete necrosis, liver resection is still required until the prognoses of these patients without surgery has been determined.

References

1. Lim KC, Chow PK, Allen JC, Siddiqui FJ, Chan ES, Tan SB. Systematic review of outcomes of liver resection for early hepatocellular carcinoma within the Milan criteria. Br J Surg. 2012;99(12):1622–9.
2. European Association for the Study of the Liver. EASL clinical practice guidelines: management of hepatocellular carcinoma. J Hepatol. 2018;69(1):182–236.
3. Korean Liver Cancer Association, National Cancer Center. 2018 Korean Liver Cancer Association-National Cancer Center. Korea practice guidelines for the management of hepatocellular carcinoma. Gut Liver. 2019;13(3):227–99.
4. Guglielmi A, Ruzzenente A, Conci S, Valdegamberi A, Iacono C. How much remnant is enough in liver resection? Dig Surg. 2012;29(1):6–17.
5. Poon RT, Cheung TT, Kwok PC, Lee AS, Li TW, Loke KL, et al. Hong Kong consensus recommendations on the management of hepatocellular carcinoma. Liver Cancer. 2015;4(1):51–69.
6. Nakayama H, Takayama T. Role of surgical resection for hepatocellular carcinoma based on Japanese clinical guidelines for hepatocellular carcinoma. World J Hepatol. 2015;7(2):261–9.
7. Kokudo T, Hasegawa K, Matsuyama Y, Takayama T, Izumi N, Kadoya M, et al. Survival benefit of liver resection for hepatocellular carcinoma associated with portal vein invasion. J Hepatol. 2016;65(5):938–43.
8. Wei X, Jiang Y, Zhang X, Feng S, Zhou B, Ye X, et al. Neoadjuvant three-dimensional conformal radio-

therapy for resectable hepatocellular carcinoma with portal vein tumor thrombus: a randomized, open-label, multicenter controlled study. J Clin Oncol. 2019;37(24):2141–51.

9. Yu JI, Park HC, Lim DH, Kim CJ, Oh D, Yoo BC, et al. Scheduled interval trans-catheter arterial chemoembolization followed by radiation therapy in patients with unresectable hepatocellular carcinoma. J Korean Med Sci. 2012;27(7):736–43.

10. Kang JK, Kim MS, Cho CK, Yang KM, Yoo HJ, Kim JH, et al. Stereotactic body radiation therapy for inoperable hepatocellular carcinoma as a local salvage treatment after incomplete transarterial chemoembolization. Cancer. 2012;118(21):5424–31.

11. Lee HS, Choi GH, Choi JS, Kim KS, Han KH, Seong J, et al. Surgical resection after down-staging of locally advanced hepatocellular carcinoma by localized concurrent chemoradiotherapy. Ann Surg Oncol. 2014;21(11):3646–53.

12. Rim CH, Park S, Woo JY, Seong J. Compensatory hypertrophy of the liver after external beam radiotherapy for primary liver cancer. Strahlenther Onkol. 2018;194(11):1017–29.

13. Lau WY, Lai EC. Salvage surgery following downstaging of unresectable hepatocellular carcinoma--a strategy to increase resectability. Ann Surg Oncol. 2007;14(12):3301–9.

14. Sitzmann JV, Abrams R. Improved survival for hepatocellular cancer with combination surgery and multimodality treatment. Ann Surg. 1993;217(2):149–54.

15. Lau WY, Ho SK, Yu SC, Lai EC, Liew CT, Leung TW. Salvage surgery following downstaging of unresectable hepatocellular carcinoma. Ann Surg. 2004;240(2):299–305.

16. Akateh C, Black SM, Conteh L, Miller ED, Noonan A, Elliott E, et al. Neoadjuvant and adjuvant treatment strategies for hepatocellular carcinoma. World J Gastroenterol. 2019;25(28):3704–21.

17. Han KH, Seong J, Kim JK, Ahn SH, Lee DY, Chon CY. Pilot clinical trial of localized concurrent chemoradiation therapy for locally advanced hepatocellular carcinoma with portal vein thrombosis. Cancer. 2008;113(5):995–1003.

18. Chong JU, Choi GH, Han DH, Kim KS, Seong J, Han KH, et al. Downstaging with localized concurrent chemoradiotherapy can identify optimal surgical candidates in hepatocellular carcinoma with portal vein tumor thrombus. Ann Surg Oncol. 2018;25(11):3308–15.

19. Lee WH, Byun HK, Choi JS, Choi GH, Han DH, Joo DJ, et al. Liver-directed combined radiotherapy as a bridge to curative surgery in locally advanced hepatocellular carcinoma beyond the milan criteria. Radiother Oncol. 2020;152:1–7.

Bridging Therapy for Liver Transplantation

16

Pablo Munoz-Schuffenegger, Tommy Ivanics,
Marco P.A.W. Claasen, Laura A. Dawson,
and Gonzalo Sapisochin

Abstract

Liver transplantation represents the best treatment option for patients with early-stage hepatocellular carcinoma, but due to organ shortage, most regions place limits on the size and number of lesions that qualify for this treatment. Locoregional treatment is often used with the objective of controlling tumor growth and preventing waitlist dropout.

Historically, transarterial chemoembolization (TACE) and ablation techniques (radio-frequency ablation (RFA), among others) have been the most commonly used bridging techniques. Stereotactic body radiation therapy (SBRT), by delivering highly conformal radiation therapy, generally in 1–5 fractions, has emerged as a treatment modality with excellent local control and acceptable side effects, with similar outcomes following TACE or RFA, in similarly selected patients. The implementation of SBRT requires a multidisciplinary team that can address challenges in radiation treatment including liver motion, obtaining optimal imaging for planning, and image guidance.

Compared to other local-regional therapies, SBRT has generally been reserved for patients with a deeper impairment in liver function. Moreover, when compared with other forms of bridge to transplant therapies, such as RFA or TACE, there is no significant difference in the dropout rates, postoperative complications, disease-free, and overall survival after liver transplantation.

There are challenges regarding the use of SBRT as a bridge to transplant therapy. In addition to the need for advanced radiation therapy technologies, conventional imaging response assessment criteria such as RECIST and mRECIST have poor correlation with pathologic findings after SBRT in many reported series, and there is a need to develop more reliable radiologic response criteria in

P. Munoz-Schuffenegger
Radiation Oncology Unit, Department of Hematology – Oncology, Pontificia Universidad Catolica de Chile, Santiago, Chile

T. Ivanics · M. P.A.W. Claasen
Abdominal Transplant Surgery and HPB Surgical Oncology, University Health Network, Toronto, ON, Canada

L. A. Dawson
Radiation Medicine Program, Princess Margaret Cancer Centre, Toronto, ON, Canada

Department of Radiation Oncology, University of Toronto, Toronto, ON, Canada

G. Sapisochin (✉)
Abdominal Transplant Surgery and HPB Surgical Oncology, University Health Network, Toronto, ON, Canada

Department of Surgery, Faculty of Medicine, University of Toronto, Toronto, ON, Canada
e-mail: Gonzalo.sapisochin@uhn.ca

© Springer Nature Singapore Pte Ltd. 2021
J. Seong (ed.), *Radiotherapy of Liver Cancer*, https://doi.org/10.1007/978-981-16-1815-4_16

this setting. Promising technical advances such as adaptive radiotherapy, MRI image guidance, and proton beam therapy are being investigated in HCC patients with the goal of increasing the therapeutic ratio by reducing toxicity and improving tumor control.

Keywords

Hepatocellular carcinoma · Radiation therapy · Stereotactic body radiation therapy · Liver transplantation · Bridge to transplant

16.1   Introduction

Liver transplantation (LT) is the best treatment option for patients with early-stage hepatocellular carcinoma (HCC), as it treats both the tumor and the underlying liver disease. Given that the underlying liver disease is the leading risk factor for developing new tumors, patients receiving LT have the highest chance of cure and long-term overall survival compared to other HCC treatments [1].

Despite the effectiveness of LT as a treatment for HCC, due to organ shortage, most regions place limits on the size and numbers of lesions that qualify for this treatment. While waiting for LT, patients are at risk of disease progression and eventual dropout from the LT waiting list; also, after LT, patients remain at risk of tumor recurrence due to the presence of an active malignancy before LT. The best method to prevent dropout from the LT waiting list due to HCC progression and to reduce posttransplant HCC recurrence remains unknown. Locoregional treatment is frequently used with the objective of controlling tumor growth and reducing the risk of waitlist dropout. While evidence supporting "bridging" treatments in reducing waitlist dropout is limited [2], this approach is recommended by guidelines when the waiting time for LT is expected to be 6 months or more [3].

Radiation therapy (RT), either as external beam radiation therapy or Yttrium-90 radioembolization (Y90), has been slower to be investigated and adopted in HCC patients versus other solid malignancies, in part due to concerns about radiation-induced liver disease (RILD) [4]. Guidelines regarding how to avoid classic RILD and how to reduce the risk of non-classic RILD are now available, and RT is now a recognized treatment option in patients with HCC who are not well suited for or who progress following standard local therapies. Moreover, technological advances in imaging, treatment planning, and image guidance have allowed the implementation of stereotactic body radiation therapy (SBRT) to be used to deliver highly conformal RT in fewer fractions, with high geometric precision and accuracy. Several prospective and retrospective studies have been published showing that SBRT is associated with high rates of local control in early and advanced stage HCC [5–7]. On the other hand, Y90 has emerged over the past decade as a locoregional treatment with favorable efficacy, safety profile, and quality of life [8], and recently a phase II randomized controlled trial demonstrated significantly improved time to progression with Y90 over conventional TACE, leading to the adoption of Y90 as standard arterial therapy for HCC [9].

The purpose of this chapter is to review the current status of radiation therapy, particularly in the form of SBRT, as a bridging therapy for liver transplantation, highlighting the planning and treatment challenges specific to its use in this clinical scenario.

16.2   Bridge to Transplant Therapies for Hepatocellular Carcinoma

Local HCC treatment as a bridge to LT has been used by many institutions to decrease disease progression while patients await an available graft [3, 10]. In this regard, response to bridging and downstaging treatments significantly decreases dropout rates, and some studies have suggested a decrease in posttransplantation tumor recurrences [11, 12]; however, controversy still exists. Historically, transarterial chemoembolization (TACE) and ablation techniques (radiofrequency ablation, microwave ablation, or percutaneous ethanol injection) have been the most common techniques used as bridging therapies.

TACE is considered the standard treatment for patients with intermediate-stage HCC according to the Barcelona-Clinic Liver Cancer classification. It achieves a partial response in 15–55% of patients, and an improvement in overall survival (OS) over best supportive care [13, 14]. TACE has been extensively used as a bridging treatment to LT, with many retrospective and prospective studies reporting complete tumor necrosis ranging from 27 to 57% in patients within Milan Criteria [15, 16]; a good response to TACE (necrosis >60%) correlates with a low HCC recurrence rate and improved long-term survival after LT [17]. Recent series show dropout rates due to tumor progression ranging between 3.0 and 9.3%, with a mean waiting time on the LT list exceeding 6 months in the largest available studies.

Ablation techniques (radiofrequency ablation (RFA), microwave ablation, or percutaneous ethanol injection) have gained use as an effective treatment bridging treatment for small HCCs. Studies have reported complete tumor necrosis at pathological evaluation of the explanted liver in 47–75% of cases [18, 19], with a difference in effectiveness observed when separating according to size [20]. RFA has some complications and limitations. It should be avoided in subcapsular HCC and in nodules located near bowel loops or gallbladder. Also, due to the "heat sink" effect, its efficacy may be reduced for tumors near major vessels.

As many patients listed for LT would not be suitable candidates for these previously mentioned bridging therapies due to tumor location, size, progression after previous bridging therapy, or due to poor liver function, SBRT can provide an opportunity for bridging in a treatment population who may have been delisted in the past.

16.3 Clinical Evidence of Radiotherapy as a Bridge to Transplant Therapy

Several studies on the use of SBRT as a bridge to LT therapy have been published to this date and are summarized in Table 16.1. O'Connor et al. [21] published the first experience on the use of SBRT as a bridge to transplant therapy for HCC. In their study, 10 patients with 11 lesions were treated with Cyberknife-based SBRT to a median dose of 51 Gy in 3 fractions. Six patients had previous treatment with TACE. The median tumor size was 3.4 cm. No patients who were treated with SBRT with the intent of undergoing transplantation dropped off the waitlist because of progression.

Mannina et al. [22] reported a retrospective study of a subset of 38 patients from a phase 1–2 study that received SBRT and orthotopic LT. Sixteen percent of patients had radiographic evidence of segmental portal vein thrombus at the time of treatment. In this study, the most commonly used SBRT fractionation was 48 Gy in 3 fractions. The mean time from completion of SBRT until LT was 8.8 months. Pathologic response criterion (complete plus partial response) was 68%; furthermore, radiographic scoring criteria performed poorly, with modified RECIST having the highest concordance with complete pathologic response. Overall survival at 5 years after LT was 77%; no peritransplant death was attributed to SBRT. Disease-free survival (DFS) was 74% at 5 years; univariate analysis revealed an association between DFS and sum longest diameter of HCC.

Guarneri et al. [23] treated 8 patients with 13 lesions who were not suitable for other local therapies or had previously failed other local therapies as a bridge to LT. Viral hepatitis (either B or C) was the most common cause of liver cirrhosis. The median tumor size was 2.0 cm. One patient was previously treated with RFA prior to SBRT; all others had SBRT as their first local treatment. The mean interval between liver SBRT and LT was 3.2 months (range 0.4–6.9 months). Of the 13 lesions evaluated in the liver explant, 8 had a complete response, and none progressed. After liver SBRT, one patient developed an increase of 8 points in the MELD score. Intraoperative surgical complications were observed in 3 out of 8 patients; two patients experienced a sclerotic retraction within the retrohepatic region that involved the inferior vena cava, and one patient had a sclero-fibrotic fusion of the vena cava with the hepatic parenchyma at the level of the retrohepatic region.

Table 16.1 Selected studies of SBRT as a bridge to LT for HCC

Study, type of data	No. of patients	No. of lesions	Median follow-up (months)	CP class B or C (%)	Previous LDT (%)	Median GTV diameter (cm., range)	Median RT dose (Gy, range)	Median time from SBRT to LT (days, range)	Dropped off wait list for LT (%)	5-year DFS (%)	5-year OS (%)	Grade 2+ toxicity
O'Connor et al. [21], retrospective	10	11	62 (from the time of SBRT)	20%	40%	3.4 (2.5–5.5)	51 Gy (33–54) in 3 fractions	113 (8–794)	0%	Not reported	100% from the time of SBRT	Not reported
Sapisochin et al. [24], retrospective	36	Not reported	28.1	38%	11.1%	4.5 (2.9–5.8)	36 Gy (30–40) in 6 fractions	158 (88–274)	10.7% (due to tumor progression)	74%	75% (from the time of LT)	38.9% had an increase in CP score or was admitted due to deterioration of liver function[a]
Mannina et al. [22], subset of phase I/II	38	51	57.6 (from the time of LT)	55%	0%	3.1 (1.0–6.1)	40 Gy (36–45) in 5 fractions	263 (13–1220)	Not reported	74%	73% (3-year OS; from the time of LT)	Not reported
Guarneri et al. [23], retrospective	8	13	9.6	37%	10%	2.0 (0.9–4.3)	48 Gy (36–48) in 3 fractions	96 (12–207)	0%	Not reported	Not reported	One patient developed non-classic RILD

CP Child–Pugh score, *DFS* disease-free survival, *GTV* gross tumor volume, *Gy* Gray, *HCC* hepatocellular carcinoma, *LDT* liver-directed therapies, *LT* liver transplantation, *NCDB* National Cancer Database, *OS* overall survival, *RILD* radiation-induced liver disease, *SBRT* stereotactic body radiation therapy

[a]In the first 3 months post treatment

Sapisochin et al., at the University of Toronto, published a large cohort comparing SBRT with other forms of bridge to LT therapies [24]. In this study, from a total of 406 patients who received any form of bridging therapy, 36 (8.9%) were treated with SBRT. The most common reason for receiving SBRT as a bridge therapy was liver function impairment that precluded TACE (66.7%); 36% of patients in the SBRT cohort were beyond Milan criteria at the time of treatment. The median prescribed dose was 36 Gy in 6 fractions. Out of the 30 patients treated with SBRT who were finally transplanted, 26 (87%) had some degree of tumor necrosis and 4 (13%) had complete tumor necrosis. During the follow-up period after LT, the 3- and 5-year cumulative risk of recurrence was 26% and 26%; and the 3- and 5-year overall survival from the time of LT was 75% and 75%.

16.4 Radiotherapy Compared to Other Bridge to Transplant Therapies

In the study by Sapisochin et al., HCC patients treated with SBRT, RFA, or TACE as a bridge to transplant therapy were compared. In this cohort, patients treated with SBRT had worsening of liver function after SBRT more frequently than in patients treated with TACE or RFA groups in the first 3 months after treatment. The baseline calculated MELD score was higher in the SBRT group. No patients had to be urgently transplanted for further liver decompensation after treatment. No patients were delisted due to treatment-related toxicity, and there were no differences between patients treated with SBRT, RFA, and TACE in the need for transfusions or major postoperative complications. During follow-up post LT, tumor recurrence occurred in 23.3% of patients in the SBRT group vs. 30.4% in the TACE group vs. 13.3% in the RFA group. The 3- and 5-year survival from the time of transplant was 75% and 75% in the SBRT group vs. 75% and 69% in the TACE group vs. 81% and 73% in the RFA group.

Bush et al. reported the interim results of a randomized, clinical trial comparing proton beam therapy (PBT) and TACE in HCC. Eligible patients had either clinical or pathological diagnosis of HCC and met either Milan or San Francisco transplant criteria. This study evaluated 69 patients; 36 were randomized to TACE, and 33 to PBT to a dose of 70.2 GyE in 15 daily fractions. Ten TACE and twelve PBT patients underwent LT after treatment, and the pathologic complete response was 10% after TACE, and 25% after PBT. The median overall survival was 30 months. There was a trend toward improved 2-year local tumor control (88 vs. 45%) and progression-free survival (48 vs. 31%) favoring the PBT group [25].

Mohamed et al. reported on 60 patients who received a total of 79 treatments of either SBRT, Y-90, TACE, or RFA as a bridge to transplant treatment for HCC [26]. The median SBRT dose was 50Gy in 5 fractions, and the average dose of Y90 was 109Gy. In this cohort, 6 episodes of major toxicities which required in-house management were reported only after TACE and RFA, with none reported in patients who received SBRT or Y90. The number of patients who achieved a radiological response (complete or partial response) was 61% for TACE, 65% for SBRT, and 67% for Y90. Five-year OS for SBRT and TACE was 73% and 72%, respectively.

Currently, there is no standard of care treatment for bridging patients with HCC as they await LT. A randomized controlled clinical trial is being conducted at the Lahey Clinic (NCT03960008), comparing SBRT to TACE as a bridging therapy for patients with HCC undergoing LT. The primary objective of this study is to compare the duration of disease control in treated lesions when utilizing these treatment modalities at 1 year post treatment.

16.5 Toxicity

A decline in Child-Pugh (CP) score has been seen following SBRT in 10–30% of early and locally advanced HCC patients, respectively, within 3 months following SBRT [5]. In a prospective study analyzing clinical and dosimetric variables on 101 patients treated on a sequential phase I/II trial of SBRT for advanced HCC, worse baseline CP score, lower platelet count, and an increased liver dose were found to be the strongest variables associated with a worsening of CP score 3 months after SBRT. In patients with CP B7 or higher score, 54% experienced an increase in their CP score, emphasizing the role of baseline liver function in predicting its deterioration after SBRT [27]. Recently, Pursley et al. showed a stronger influence of low-dose bath on hepatic toxicity than those found in previous studies, further emphasizing that RT techniques which minimize the low-dose bath may be beneficial [28].

Treating centrally located HCC poses particular challenges regarding the tolerance of the main bile duct and other areas to SBRT and potential surgical complications at the time of LT. In the Guarneri et al. study, two patients developed a sclerotic retraction within the retrohepatic region which involved the inferior vena cava, leading to technical difficulties during its surgical isolation at the time of LT [23]. In the Sapisochin et al. study, 25% of the treated lesions were central, and there was no difference in the surgical complication rate at the time of LT [24]. However, numbers were small to draw strong conclusions. Surgical challenges at the time of LT can be encountered when treating central lesions close to the porta, and need of jump grafts can be required.

Recently, Hasan et al. investigated post-LT mortality and acute readmissions in HCC with and without preoperative RT using the National Cancer Database (NCDB) [29]; in this study, 11,091 LT patients were analyzed, 165 of whom received RT prior to transplant. The median RT dose was 40 Gy in 5 fractions. Although RT was more often delivered to larger tumors and advanced stages, it resulted in a 59% downstaging rate, 39% pathologic complete response rate. The time from diagnosis to LT was nearly 6 months longer on average with preoperative RT. In this study, the 30- and 90-day mortality rates for patients having undergone preoperative RT were both 1.2%, as compared to 2.7% and 4.4%, respectively, without preoperative RT. Following propensity matching, there were no differences in 30- or 90-day mortality rates with preoperative RT, compared with other therapies.

16.6 Radiology - Pathology Correlation After Stereotactic Body Radiation Therapy for Hepatocellular Carcinoma

The usual criteria for measuring residual disease after ablation or TACE, which immediately induces tumor necrosis and devascularization, does not apply well to HCC treated with SBRT. The variable post-SBRT imaging features of HCC and the adjacent liver parenchyma, along with potential pitfalls of imaging evaluation after SBRT for HCC have been reviewed elsewhere [30].

In the O'Connor et al. study, from 11 lesions that were treated with SBRT, the radiographic tumor response assessed with CT or MRI at 3 months revealed stable disease in 5 patients and a partial response in 3 patients; however, explant pathology revealed that in 3 of the 11 lesions there was no evidence of viable tumor. Residual tumor was seen in the other 8 tumors, and in 3 of these patients, only small foci of viable HCC were present after SBRT [21]. Also, in the Mannina et al. study there was a poor correlation between CT agreement (22–39%) and MRI agreement (31–39%) with pathologic findings, irrespective of radiographic criteria used; sensitivity ranged from 54% (RECIST) to 90% (mRECIST), whereas specificity ranged from 18% (EASL, mRECIST) to 50% (WHO, RECIST) [22].

Mendiratta-Lala et al. correlated imaging findings of HCC within the first 12 months after SBRT with explant pathology and alpha-fetoprotein response. In this study, 10 patients with successfully treated HCC (>90% necrosis and/or AFP normalization) were analyzed. In four out of ten patients, there was persistent central arterial enhancement 3–12 months after SBRT, and in 9 of 10 lesions, there was persistent washout up to 12 months. These findings suggest the enhancement pattern observed after SBRT is different from that expected after successful thermal ablation or TACE, and that freedom from local progression seems to be a better measure of HCC control after SBRT [31].

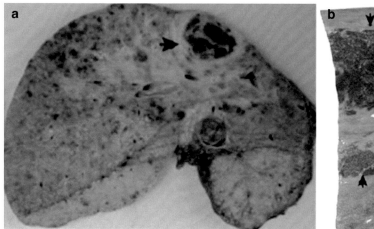
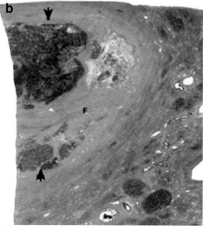

Fig. 16.1 Liver explant of a patient treated with SBRT. (**a**) Liver explant — subcapsular nodule corresponds to the SBRT site (arrow) surrounded by rim fibrous tissue with dark necrotic areas in the center. (**b**) Light-microscopic image from SBRT site containing necrotic areas (thin arrow), a small focus of residual HCC (thick arrow), and dense fibrous tissue between (F). Masson trichrome stain (Reprinted from Sapisochin et al. [24])

With the growing use of SBRT in HCC, response assessment after treatment represents a challenge in the bridge to transplant and downstaging populations. As diameter does not correlate with necrosis, particularly in the initial stages of follow-up post SBRT, the lack of reduction in diameter could prevent patients from being downstaged, reaching the diameter target required in order to be listed for LT, despite necrosis within the HCC (Fig. 16.1). This emphasizes the need for more reliable imaging biomarkers for post-SBRT response assessment.

16.7 Special Considerations for Stereotactic Body Radiation Therapy Planning

When planning SBRT for HCC as a bridge to transplant therapy, as the primary objective is stabilizing the treated lesion while minimizing the risk of serious toxicity (i.e., not complete ablation), doses no higher than 45 Gy in 5 fractions are recommended, and consideration should be given to lower doses in higher-risk patients (impaired liver function, central lesions where fibrosis may lead to a potential increased operative toxicity) (Fig. 16.2) [24]. Sometimes only

the largest highest-risk HCC is targeted, given the inherent poor liver function and the goal of bridging.

Contouring for liver lesions should be performed on a multi-phasic contrast-enhanced treatment-planning CT scan with the aid of diagnostic imaging, such as MRI, to identify the gross tumor volume (GTV). Ideally, both a planning multi-phasic CT and MRI should be used for contouring [32].

Dose prescription is based on the volume of normal tissues irradiated (correlated with the mean liver dose), as well as proximity to gastrointestinal luminal organs such as the stomach, duodenum, small and large bowel, to the target volumes. In CP B7 or higher patients, strong efforts should be made to keep the mean liver dose (MLD) as low as possible; an MLD < 6 Gy has been previously recommended [33]. Treatment every other day should also be considered.

Liver motion is complex owing to organ deformation and rotation with breathing motion. Craniocaudal liver motion, which may be as high as 2 cm, has adverse effects on RT planning and treatment including the introduction of artifacts on planning CT scans, altered dosimetry based on a static plan, increased volume of normal tissue radiation, with a potential to increase toxicity, which is critical in this setting. Different strate-

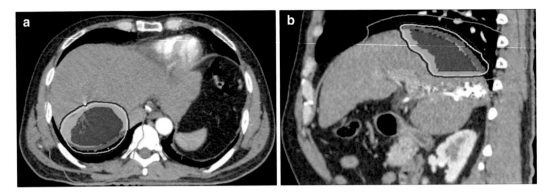

Fig. 16.2 Axial and sagittal images of a 45 Gy in six fraction SBRT plan of a bridge to transplant patient who had a significant pathological response (85%) of a segment VII/VIII HCC lesion (Reprinted from Sapisochin et al. [24])

gies have been used to address liver motion during RT and include controlling motion through abdominal compression, breath-hold techniques, respiratory gating, and real-time tumor tracking [34].

Daily image guidance is necessary for the treatment of liver cancer, as intra- and inter-fractional motion can be considerable. Image guidance using a soft tissue surrogate such as lipiodol following TACE, calcifications, surgical clips, the liver itself or portion of the liver adjacent to the tumor is needed. Cone-beam computed tomography (CBCT) liver matching has been suggested to be superior to orthogonal X-rays [35].

16.8   Future Directions

MRI-guided radiotherapy is a rapidly evolving technology that might enhance the benefits of HCC SBRT. MRI-based treatment and tracking confer advantages such as improved soft tissue target and organs at risk (OAR) delineation, real-time tumor tracking, requiring smaller volumes of normal tissues to be irradiated. In the setting of liver SBRT as a bridging therapy, with patients commonly having a poor baseline function and ascites, MRI-guided radiotherapy provides an ideal platform for decreasing toxicity and potential dose escalation by allowing for real-time MRI imaging and online treatment adaptation [36].

Strategies focusing on the adaptation of liver SBRT delivery based on the liver tolerance to

SBRT have been developed. Feng et al. published a phase II clinical trial of an adaptive liver SBRT approach where 90 patients with intrahepatic malignancies and prior liver-directed therapies (77% HCC), using indocyanine green retention at 15 minutes as a direct biomarker of liver function, underwent liver SBRT adaptation midway through the course of treatment with the objective of maintaining liver function. In this study, there was a lower than expected complication rate without adaptation; 7% of patients experienced a 2-point decline in the CP score 6 months post SBRT, with a 1-year local control rate of 100% [37]. Such an individualized adaptive RT strategy may be particularly well suited in patients with a high risk of decline in liver function.

Proton beam therapy (PBT), using charged particles that come to rest within the patient, have no exit dose because of the characteristic proton Bragg peak, allowing a potential decrease of unwanted dose to the non-target liver and other organs at risk. Small, single-arm studies have suggested that proton therapy may improve OS compared to photon therapy; however, patient selection is a potentially strong confounding factor. A single-institution retrospective study by Sanford et al. compared photon- with proton-based treatment in 133 patients with HCC; in this study, 59% of proton patients had Child–Pugh A5 liver function versus 36% of photon patients. After accounting for baseline imbalances, differences in non-classic RILD and OS persisted in favor of protons, which may be driven by the decreased incidence of posttreatment liver decompensation; however, there was no statistically significant difference in tumor local control, which was high for both treatment modalities [38]. Worldwide, the main barrier to use proton therapy remains that of access, so the generation of high-quality evidence supporting protons is essential to understand the patient populations most likely to benefit from PBT and to improve its global availability.

16.9 Summary

Locoregional treatment is often used to control tumor growth and to prevent LT waitlist dropout. SBRT has emerged as a treatment modality with excellent local control and acceptable side effects, with similar outcomes following TACE or RFA, in similarly selected patients. Compared to other local-regional therapies, SBRT has been reserved for patients with a more profound liver function impairment. Still, compared with other forms of bridge to transplant therapies, there is no significant difference in the dropout rates, postoperative complications, disease-free, and overall survival after LT.

There are challenges regarding the use of SBRT as a bridge to transplant therapy. Conventional imaging response assessment criteria have a poor correlation with pathologic findings after SBRT, and there is a need to develop more reliable radiologic response criteria in this setting. Promising technical advances such as adaptive radiotherapy, MRI image guidance, and proton beam therapy are being investigated to increase the therapeutic ratio by reducing toxicity and improving tumor control.

References

1. European Association for the Study of the Liver. EASL Clinical Practice Guidelines: management of hepatocellular carcinoma. J Hepatol. 2018;69(1):182–236.
2. Majno P, Lencioni R, Mornex F, Girard N, Poon RT, Cherqui D. Is the treatment of hepatocellular carcinoma on the waiting list necessary? Liver Transpl. 2011;17(Suppl 2):S98–108.
3. Clavien PA, Lesurtel M, Bossuyt PM, Gores GJ, Langer B, Perrier A, et al. Recommendations for liver transplantation for hepatocellular carcinoma: an international consensus conference report. Lancet Oncol. 2012;13(1):e11–22.
4. Munoz-Schuffenegger P, Ng S, Dawson LA. Radiation-induced liver toxicity. Semin Radiat Oncol. 2017;27(4):350–7.
5. Bujold A, Massey CA, Kim JJ, Brierley J, Cho C, Wong RK, et al. Sequential phase I and II trials of stereotactic body radiotherapy for locally advanced hepatocellular carcinoma. J Clin Oncol. 2013;31(13):1631–9.
6. Kang JK, Kim MS, Cho CK, Yang KM, Yoo HJ, Kim JH, et al. Stereotactic body radiation therapy for inoperable hepatocellular carcinoma as a local salvage treatment after incomplete transarterial chemoembolization. Cancer. 2012;118(21):5424–31.
7. Ohri N, Tome WA, Mendez Romero A, Miften M, Ten Haken RK, Dawson LA, et al. Local control after stereotactic body radiation therapy for liver tumors. Int J Radiat Oncol Biol Phys. 2018; https://doi.org/10.1016/j.ijrobp.2017.12.288.
8. Salem R, Lewandowski RJ, Mulcahy MF, Riaz A, Ryu RK, Ibrahim S, et al. Radioembolization for hepatocellular carcinoma using Yttrium-90 microspheres: a comprehensive report of long-term outcomes. Gastroenterology. 2010;138(1):52–64.
9. Salem R, Gordon AC, Mouli S, Hickey R, Kallini J, Gabr A, et al. Y90 radioembolization significantly prolongs time to progression compared with chemoembolization in patients with hepatocellular carcinoma. Gastroenterology. 2016;151(6):1155–63.e2.
10. Cescon M, Cucchetti A, Ravaioli M, Pinna AD. Hepatocellular carcinoma locoregional therapies for patients in the waiting list. Impact on transplantability and recurrence rate. J Hepatol. 2013;58(3):609–18.
11. Yao FY, Mehta N, Flemming J, Dodge J, Hameed B, Fix O, et al. Downstaging of hepatocellular cancer before liver transplant: long-term outcome compared to tumors within Milan criteria. Hepatology. 2015;61(6):1968–77.
12. Andreou A, Bahra M, Schmelzle M, Ollinger R, Sucher R, Sauer IM, et al. Predictive factors for extrahepatic recurrence of hepatocellular carcinoma following liver transplantation. Clin Transpl. 2016;30(7):819–27.
13. Llovet JM, Real MI, Montana X, Planas R, Coll S, Aponte J, et al. Arterial embolisation or chemoembolisation versus symptomatic treatment in patients with unresectable hepatocellular carcinoma: a randomised controlled trial. Lancet. 2002;359(9319):1734–9.
14. Lo CM, Ngan H, Tso WK, Liu CL, Lam CM, Poon RT, et al. Randomized controlled trial of transarterial lipiodol chemoembolization for unresectable hepatocellular carcinoma. Hepatology. 2002;35(5):1164–71.
15. Majno PE, Adam R, Bismuth H, Castaing D, Ariche A, Krissat J, et al. Influence of preoperative transarterial lipiodol chemoembolization on resection and transplantation

for hepatocellular carcinoma in patients with cirrhosis. Ann Surg. 1997;226(6):688–701. discussion 701-3

16. Nicolini A, Martinetti L, Crespi S, Maggioni M, Sangiovanni A. Transarterial chemoembolization with epirubicin-eluting beads versus transarterial embolization before liver transplantation for hepatocellular carcinoma. J Vasc Interv Radiol. 2010;21(3):327–32.

17. Allard MA, Sebagh M, Ruiz A, Guettier C, Paule B, Vibert E, et al. Does pathological response after transarterial chemoembolization for hepatocellular carcinoma in cirrhotic patients with cirrhosis predict outcome after liver resection or transplantation? J Hepatol. 2015;63(1):83–92.

18. Mazzaferro V, Battiston C, Perrone S, Pulvirenti A, Regalia E, Romito R, et al. Radiofrequency ablation of small hepatocellular carcinoma in cirrhotic patients awaiting liver transplantation: a prospective study. Ann Surg. 2004;240(5):900–9.

19. Rodriguez-Sanjuan JC, Gonzalez F, Juanco C, Herrera LA, Lopez-Bautista M, Gonzalez-Noriega M, et al. Radiological and pathological assessment of hepatocellular carcinoma response to radiofrequency. A study on removed liver after transplantation. World J Surg. 2008;32(7):1489–94.

20. DuBay DA, Sandroussi C, Kachura JR, Ho CS, Beecroft JR, Vollmer CM, et al. Radiofrequency ablation of hepatocellular carcinoma as a bridge to liver transplantation. HPB (Oxford). 2011;13(1):24–32.

21. O'Connor JK, Trotter J, Davis GL, Dempster J, Klintmalm GB, Goldstein RM. Long-term outcomes of stereotactic body radiation therapy in the treatment of hepatocellular cancer as a bridge to transplantation. Liver Transpl. 2012;18(8):949–54.

22. Mannina EM, Cardenes HR, Lasley FD, Goodman B, Zook J, Althouse S, et al. Role of stereotactic body radiation therapy before orthotopic liver transplantation: retrospective evaluation of pathologic response and outcomes. Int J Radiat Oncol Biol Phys. 2017;97(5):931–8.

23. Guarneri A, Franco P, Romagnoli R, Trino E, Mirabella S, Molinaro L, et al. Stereotactic ablative radiation therapy prior to liver transplantation in hepatocellular carcinoma. Radiol Med. 2016;121(11):873–81.

24. Sapisochin G, Barry A, Doherty M, Fischer S, Goldaracena N, Rosales R, et al. Stereotactic body radiotherapy vs. TACE or RFA as a bridge to transplant in patients with hepatocellular carcinoma. An intention-to-treat analysis. J Hepatol. 2017;67(1):92–9.

25. Bush DA, Smith JC, Slater JD, Volk ML, Reeves ME, Cheng J, et al. Randomized clinical trial comparing proton beam radiation therapy with transarterial chemoembolization for hepatocellular carcinoma: results of an interim analysis. Int J Radiat Oncol Biol Phys. 2016;95(1):477–82.

26. Mohamed M, Katz AW, Tejani MA, Sharma AK, Kashyap R, Noel MS, et al. Comparison of outcomes between SBRT, yttrium-90 radioembolization, tran-

sarterial chemoembolization, and radiofrequency ablation as bridge to transplant for hepatocellular carcinoma. Adv Radiat Oncol. 2016;1(1):35–42.

27. Velec M, Haddad CR, Craig T, Wang L, Lindsay P, Brierley J, et al. Predictors of liver toxicity following stereotactic body radiation therapy for hepatocellular carcinoma. Int J Radiat Oncol Biol Phys. 2017;97(5):939–46.

28. Pursley J, El Naqa I, Sanford NN, Noe B, Wo JY, Eyler CE, et al. Dosimetric analysis and normal tissue complication probability modeling of Child-Pugh score and Albumin-Bilirubin grade increase after hepatic irradiation. Int J Radiat Oncol Biol Phys. 2020;107(5):986–95.

29. Hasan S, Abel S, Uemura T, Verma V, Koay EJ, Herman J, et al. Liver transplant mortality and morbidity following preoperative radiotherapy for hepatocellular carcinoma. HPB (Oxford). 2019;22(5):770–8.

30. Mastrocostas K, Jang HJ, Fischer S, Dawson LA, Munoz-Schuffenegger P, Sapisochin G, et al. Imaging post-stereotactic body radiation therapy responses for hepatocellular carcinoma: typical imaging patterns and pitfalls. Abdom Radiol (NY). 2019;44(5):1795–807.

31. Mendiratta-Lala M, Gu E, Owen D, Cuneo KC, Bazzi L, Lawrence TS, et al. Imaging findings within the first 12 months of hepatocellular carcinoma treated with stereotactic body radiation therapy. Int J Radiat Oncol Biol Phys. 2018;102(4):1063–9.

32. Voroney JP, Brock KK, Eccles C, Haider M, Dawson LA. Prospective comparison of computed tomography and magnetic resonance imaging for liver cancer delineation using deformable image registration. Int J Radiat Oncol Biol Phys. 2006;66(3):780–91.

33. Pan CC, Kavanagh BD, Dawson LA, Li XA, Das SK, Miften M, et al. Radiation-associated liver injury. Int J Radiat Oncol Biol Phys. 2010;76(3 Suppl):S94–100.

34. Brandner ED, Chetty IJ, Giaddui TG, Xiao Y, Huq MS. Motion management strategies and technical issues associated with stereotactic body radiotherapy of thoracic and upper abdominal tumors: a review from NRG oncology. Med Phys. 2017;44(6):2595–612.

35. Hawkins MA, Brock KK, Eccles C, Moseley D, Jaffray D, Dawson LA. Assessment of residual error in liver position using kV cone-beam computed tomography for liver cancer high-precision radiation therapy. Int J Radiat Oncol Biol Phys. 2006;66(2):610–9.

36. Witt JS, Rosenberg SA, Bassetti MF. MRI-guided adaptive radiotherapy for liver tumours: visualising the future. Lancet Oncol. 2020;21(2):e74–82.

37. Feng M, Suresh K, Schipper MJ, Bazzi L, Ben-Josef E, Matuszak MM, et al. Individualized adaptive stereotactic body radiotherapy for liver tumors in patients at high risk for liver damage: a phase 2 clinical trial. JAMA Oncol. 2018;4(1):40–7.

38. Sanford NN, Pursley J, Noe B, Yeap BY, Goyal L, Clark JW, et al. Protons versus photons for unresectable hepatocellular carcinoma: liver decompensation and overall survival. Int J Radiat Oncol Biol Phys. 2019;105(1):64–72.

Palliative Radiotherapy

17

Zhao-Chong Zeng and Qian-Qian Zhao

Abstract

Palliative radiotherapy (RT) is a relative term, which refers to the use of RT in situations when it is impossible to completely eliminate all visible lesions. It contrasts with radical RT, in which the goal is complete elimination of visible tumors. One or both of the following conditions are regarded as palliative RT: (1) the radiation dose fails to achieve radical goals unless combined with other radical treatments, such as surgical resection; and (2) visible lesions exist beyond the radiation fields. Since radical goals cannot be achieved, palliative RT aims to relieve cancer symptoms and slightly prolong survival.

A considerable proportion of patients with hepatocellular carcinoma (HCC) have intrahepatic lesions that may be converted to sequential surgical resection after the combination of RT and transarterial chemoembolization (TACE). We classify this type of RT as consolidation RT, not palliative RT. This chapter discusses the use of RT for portal vein (PV)/ inferior vena cava (IVC) tumor thrombi, as well as extrahepatic metastatic lesions, including lymph node (LN), bone, pulmonary, and adrenal metastases.

Keywords

Liver Cancer · Palliative therapy · External beam radiotherapy · Tumor thrombi · Lymph node metastases

17.1 Radiotherapy for Treating HCC with Venous Tumor Thrombi

The incidence of PV or IVC tumor thrombi is high in patients with HCC: up to 44–84% according to autopsy data [1] and 31.4–50% based on clinical data [2, 3]. Most patients with these thrombi have a poor prognosis, with a median survival of only 2.4–2.7 months without treatment [4–6]. The therapeutic effectiveness of various treatment strategies for PV tumor thrombi (PVTT) in patients with HCC is summarized in Table 17.1. When patients with PV or IVC tumor thrombi received systemic chemotherapy, the median survival time ranged from 3.9 to 9.2 months [20]. TACE can be administered via a catheter placed in hepatic arteries, but it has relatively poor efficacy for tumor thrombi. Investigators have reported median survival times of only 10–13.4 months for patients with tumor thrombosis in the first branch or trunk of the PV [21, 22]. Patients with early (type I or II) resectable tumor thrombi may have a longer survival time [23]. However, both TACE and surgical

Z.-C. Zeng (✉) · Q.-Q. Zhao
Department of Radiation Oncology, Zhongshan Hospital, Fudan University, Shanghai, China
e-mail: zeng.zhaochong@zs-hospital.sh.cn

© Springer Nature Singapore Pte Ltd. 2021
J. Seong (ed.), *Radiotherapy of Liver Cancer*, https://doi.org/10.1007/978-981-16-1815-4_17

Table 17.1 Overall survival of HCC patients with PVTT treated with different modalities

First author	Year	Type of PVTT	Resection		TACE or TAC*		TACE + RT		TACE, HAIC* or CT + Sorafenib#	Sorafenib#	Sorafenib alone		HAIC + RT		RT alone		P value
			N	OS (months)	N	OS (months)	N	OS (months)	N	OS (months)	N	OS (months)	N	OS (months)	N	OS (months)	
Wei [7]	2019	II–III	82 / 82 (adjuvant RT)	11 / 17	–	–	–	–	–	–	–	–	–	–	–	–	<0.01
Abou-Alfa [8]	2019	All	–	–	–	–	–	–	180#	9.3	176	9.4	–	–	–	–	n.s.
He [9]	2019	All	–	–	–	–	–	–	124*	13.4	123	7.1	–	–	–	–	<0.001
Yoon [10]	2018	I–II	–	–	–	–	45	**12.8**	–	–	44	10.0	–	–	–	–	0.04
Kodama [11]	2018	III	–	–	–	–	–	–	–	–	36	5.3	36	9.9	–	–	0.002
Hou [12]	2016	I–III	–	–	–	–	54 / 64	**15.5** / **10.5**	–	–	–	–	–	–	–	–	0.005
Wang [13]	2016	I	236	15.9	47	9.3	8	**12.2**	31	12	–	–	–	–	–	–	<0.001
		II	315	12.5	288	4.9	54	**10.6**	45	8.9	–	–	–	–	–	–	<0.001
		III	194	6.0	269	4.0	56	**8.9**	37	7.0	–	–	–	–	–	–	0.001
Kim [14]	2016	II	–	–	102	7.4	102	**11.4**	–	–	–	–	–	–	–	–	<0.001
		III	–	–	–	–	30	**8.2**	–	–	30	3.2	–	–	–	–	<0.001
Onishi [15]	2015	II–III	–	–	–	–	34	**12.4**	–	–	33	5.7	–	–	–	–	0.14
Lu [16]	2015	No state	–	–	33	9	30	**13**	–	–	–	–	–	–	–	–	0.047
Nakazawa [17]	2014	II–III	–	–	–	–	–	–	–	–	28	4.8	–	–	28	10.9	0.025
Tang [18]	2013	I–III	186	10.0	–	–	185	**12.3**	–	–	–	–	–	–	–	–	0.029
Chuma [19]	2011	No state	–	–	20*	9.1*	–	–	–	–	–	–	20	12	–	–	0.041

CT chemotherapy, *HAIC* hepatic artery infusion chemotherapy, *N* number of patients, *n.s.* not stated, *OS* overall survival, *PVTT* portal vein tumor thrombi, *RT* radiotherapy, *TAC* transarterial chemotherapy, *TACE* transarterial chemoembolization resection are not indicated when the PV trunk is occluded by tumor thrombus because if the hepatic artery is embolized for therapeutic purposes when the PV is completely blocked by tumor and portal-systemic collaterals have not developed, then the entire hepatic blood supply will be interrupted, producing widespread liver necrosis and liver failure. Some studies conducted approximately 20 years ago reported survival benefit after external-beam RT (EBRT) in patients with PV thrombi [24, 25]. This section discusses more recent evidence regarding the efficacy of EBRT for patients with HCC who have PV and/or IVC tumor thrombi.

17.1.1 Survival of HCC Patients with PV and/or IVC Tumor Thrombi Treated with 2- or 3-Dimensional Conformal RT Versus no RT

Table 17.2 shows data from four studies performed approximately 12 years ago, which retrospectively compared the efficacy of EBRT versus no RT in HCC patients with PV/IVC tumor thrombi. Univariate and multivariate analysis of all studies indicated that RT prolonged survival. In a retrospective review conducted at Zhongshan Hospital, Fudan University, involving 44 patients with HCC and tumor thrombosis in the PV and/or IVC, median survival was much longer in the EBRT

group than in the no RT group [26]. In a review of data from 32 patients with HCC and PVTT, Japanese researchers reported that median survival of patients treated with EBRT was 7 months longer than in those who did not receive RT [27]. This result was consistent with the results of a Korean study based on data from 71 HCC patients with PVTT, 42 of whom received TACE and RT and 29 of whom who received TACE alone [28]. Similarly, Chen et al. reported that RT significantly improved median survival time of patients with HCC and PVTT ($n = 34$), compared with patients who did not receive RT ($n = 29$) [29].

17.1.2 Combined TACE and 3-Dimensional Conformal RT

17.1.2.1 Retrospective Studies

In general, both intrahepatic lesions and tumor thrombi should be considered when determining treatment for patients with PV and/or IVC tumor thrombi. If all intrahepatic tumors and tumor thrombi are included in the same target volume, radiation fields will often be so large that the radiation dose will be inadequate and treatment outcomes will be poor. It is often advised that intrahepatic lesions be treated mainly with TACE, while tumor thrombi be treated with RT. If treatment efficacy of intrahepatic lesions is unsatisfactory with TACE, these lesions may then be included in radiation fields, depending on the

Table 17.2 Retrospective comparisons of efficacy of EBRT versus no EBRT in patients with HCC and PV or IVC tumor thrombi[a]

First author	Location	Year	Treatment	No. of patients	Efficacy (%)	Survival Median (months)	1 year (%)	2 years (%)	P value
Zeng [26]	PV or IVC	2005	EBRT	44	45.5	8	34.8	–	<0.001
			No EBRT	114	–	4	11.4	–	
Nakazawa [27]	PV	2007	EBRT	32	48.0	10	38.0	20.7	<0.001
			No EBRT	36	–	3.6	8.3	2.7	
Koo [28]	IVC	2010	EBRT	42	42.9	11.7	47.7	–	<0.01
			No EBRT	29	13.8	4.7	17.2	–	
Chen [29]	PV	2010	EBRT	34	–	7.0	–	–	<0.01
			No EBRT	29	–	3.9	–	–	

EBRT external-beam radiotherapy, *IVC* inferior vena cava, *No.* number, *PV* portal vein
[a]In all studies, patients in the EBRT and no EBRT groups were treated at the same institution and over the same time period

Table 17.3 Outcomes of various therapies combined with EBRT for patients with HCC and PVTT

First author	Year	No. of patients	Radiation dose (Gy), median (range)	Treatment for intrahepatic tumor before RT	Efficacy (%)	Survival Median (months)	1 year (%)	2 years (%)
Kim [30]	2005	59	39–70	TACE: 59%; untreated: 39%	45.8	10.7	40.7	20.7
Nakagawa [31]	2005	52	57 (39–60)	TACE: 77%; sonographically-guided alcohol injection or microwave ablation: 60%; both: 42%	50.0	1031	45.1	25.3
Lin [32]	2006	43	45 (37–51)	Surgical resection: 16.3%; TACE: 41.9%; untreated: 41.8%	83	6.7	–	–
Toya [33]	2007	38	50.7 (23–59)	TACE or surgical resection: 79%; untreated: 21%	44.7	9.6	39.6	–
Yoon [34]	2012	412	40 (21–60)	Surgical resection: 3.4%; TACE after RT: 69.9%	39.6	10.6	42.5	22.8
Hou [35]	2012	144	50 (30–60)	TACE: 85%	54.1	9.7	41.7	17.4
Rim [36]	2012	45	61.2 (38–65)	TACE: 93.3%; untreated: 6.7%	62.3	13.9	51.5	–

No. number, *TACE* transarterial chemoembolization

individual patient's situation. TACE for intrahepatic primary tumors should be performed before EBRT for PV and/or IVC tumor thrombi if the PV trunk is incompletely occluded by tumor thrombi; otherwise, EBRT should be administered before TACE. At present, the combination of EBRT and TACE is widely available internationally. Table 17.3 lists treatment outcomes of EBRT plus TACE for patients with HCC and PV or IVC tumor thrombi from studies reported more than eight years ago. TACE was usually performed for intrahepatic lesions before and after RT. In Lin et al.'s study, only 41% of all patients underwent TACE [32]. The survival of this patient population was much shorter than in study populations in which more than 70% of patients underwent TACE [31, 34–36].

17.1.2.2 Prospective Randomized Studies

In a prospective randomized study conducted by Yoon and colleagues at the Asan Medical Center of Korea and published in 2018, 90 treatment-naive patients with liver-confined HCC and macroscopic vascular invasion were randomly assigned to receive sorafenib (400 mg twice daily; $n = 45$) or TACE (every 6 weeks) plus RT

(within 3 weeks after the first TACE, maximum 45 Gy with the fraction size of 2.5 to 3 Gy; $n = 45$). Overall survival (OS) was significantly longer in the TACE-RT group than in the sorafenib group (55.0 vs 43.0 weeks; $P = 0.04$) [10].

One must be wary of using TACE in patients with HCC who have complete main PV obstruction: if the PV is completely blocked and portal collateral vessels have not developed, when the arterial supply to the liver is embolized, liver failure can result. In approximately 50% of patients, the embolus does not shrink after EBRT because of concomitant thrombosis of the PV [26]. There are no treatment options for intrahepatic lesions in these cases because of the unshrinkable embolus, and these patients will die of uncontrolled intrahepatic lesions. At our hospital, 45 patients with HCC complicated by main PVTT were treated first with percutaneous transhepatic PV stenting to maintain blood flow, followed by TACE for intrahepatic lesions and then EBRT for PVTT. Follow-up data showed a median survival of 16.5 months for patients who received EBRT versus 4.8 months for those who did not undergo EBRT ($P < 0.01$) [37]. Thus, EBRT of PVTT is of particular importance in the treatment of HCC.

Liver failure caused by intrahepatic tumor extension is the main cause of death of patients with HCC. Clinical manifestations of patients with liver failure include abdominal fullness, jaundice, ascites, and gastrointestinal bleeding. It is extremely difficult to distinguish liver failure caused by intrahepatic tumor from that caused by PV thrombosis progression. In our retrospective study of 158 patients with PV or IVC thrombi, the incidence of liver failure was lower in patients who received EBRT (71.4%) than in those who did not receive RT (93.4%) [26]. The EBRT group had a higher incidence of death from extrahepatic disease because of their prolonged survival. Patients with PVTT almost always had larger tumors than those without thrombi. The main cause of death in the EBRT group was liver failure secondary to uncontrolled growth of intrahepatic tumors (71.4%). TACE is the best way to control intrahepatic tumors among current nonsurgical treatments, unless patients have a completely obstructed PV without collateral vessels.

In our study, we also observed a strong relationship between survival and tumor type (unifocal or multifocal/diffuse) in patients with HCC who did not have PV or IVC tumor thrombi. This is because patients with multifocal/diffuse tumors were less likely to undergo surgery; intrahepatic dissemination developed rapidly and they ultimately died from liver failure. Of note, survival was not related to tumor type in patients with PV or IVC tumor thrombosis when patients were not treated with EBRT, which was because most of these patients died from thrombosis and not because of their intrahepatic tumors. After EBRT, patients experienced prolonged survival, and the failure pattern returned to that of intrahepatic tumors rather than tumor thrombosis. If tumor thrombosis is relieved after EBRT, it is recommended that treatment with TACE be provided as soon as possible. In our institution, many patients with tumor thrombi in both PV branches and trunk first receive EBRT, which is then followed by TACE when the occlusion has resolved. Iodized oil is deposited in "satellite" lesions outside the EBRT fields. Therefore, TACE is not performed prior to EBRT in all cases.

HCC has a natural history that results in multiple satellite lesions in both lobes of the liver. If these lesions are <1 cm, they are usually difficult to detect by regular computed tomography (CT). Therefore, TACE also plays an important role in treating small lesions beyond the radiation fields, allowing EBRT to be focused on the PVTT and larger intrahepatic lesions. Therefore, combinations of EBRT and TACE are important for treating multiple intrahepatic lesions. EBRT is usually administered before TACE if the PV trunk is completely obstructed by tumor thrombi; otherwise, TACE is generally performed before EBRT.

17.1.3 Combined EBRT and Chemotherapy

Han et al. reported a median OS time of 13.1 months and actuarial three-year OS rate of 24.1% for patients with locally advanced HCC and PVTT treated with hepatic arterial infusion chemotherapy combined with RT [38], although chemotherapy alone does not prolong survival. This result is the best outcome among all reports of RT efficacy for tumor thrombi at that time, but the study contained no control group. Another study reported that concomitant chemoradiation therapy (CCRT) did not prolong survival, but it did relieve complications of PVTT, such as esophageal variceal bleeding and ascites [39]. Recently, phase 2 clinical trial has been issued [40]. Forty-seven patients with portal vein tumor thrombi were recruited, including portal vein main trunk in 10 patients, the first branch in 13 patients, the second branch or less in 24 patients. All of them received liver-directed concurrent chemoradiotherapy (LD-CCRT). Four weeks after completing LD-CCRT, 34 patients received sequential sorafenib. The median overall survival was 24.6 months. Phase 3 clinical integration and research is required to determine the efficacy of CCRT for HCC with PVTT.

17.1.4 Neoadjuvant RT

Only a small minority of patients with PVTT who undergo hepatic resection have prolonged survival; most patients die of intrahepatic recurrence or metastasis in a short period of time. In patients with HCC, RT alone for PVTT is just palliative care. Japanese researchers [41] reported that outcomes were better with preoperative RT of PVTT combined with surgical resection, compared with surgical resection alone. In their study, RT for PVTT was administered as 30–36 Gy in 10–12 fractions, which was then followed within two weeks by hepatectomy. TACE, percutaneous ethanol injection (PEI), or radiofrequency ablation (RFA) was performed postoperatively, according to specific criteria. Median survival time was 19.6 months in the hepatectomy plus preoperative RT group, in contrast to 9.1 months in the hepatectomy without preoperative RT group ($P = 0.036$). Pathological examination revealed complete necrosis of the PVTT in 83% (5/6) of patients who underwent hepatectomy with preoperative RT. These results indicate that the main purpose of surgery is to improve the control rate of primary lesions rather than PVTT. Preoperative RT combined with surgical resection is a new and effective combined mode of therapy for PVTT.

Kim et al. [42] from Yonsei University College of Medicine analyzed outcomes after concurrent CCRT for locally advanced HCC. A total of 264 patients with HCC were treated with CCRT when surgery was not feasible because of PVTT or inadequate non-tumor liver volume. Most patients received 45 Gy with a fractional dose of 1.8 Gy. Intra-arterial 5-fluorouracil was administered during the first and fifth weeks of RT. One month after CCRT, intra-arterial 5-fluorouracil and cisplatin were administered every four weeks for 3–12 cycles. Hepatic resection was performed in 18 patients. On pathologic review of resection specimens, four patients (22.2%) exhibited total necrosis and seven patients (38.9%) had 70–99% necrosis of the tumor. Median OS was 40 months and median disease-free survival (DFS) was 24 months in patients who underwent surgery. Four patients (22.2%) were free of disease for a median of 54.6 months postoperatively. The authors concluded that, in selected patients, originally unresectable HCC may become resectable after CCRT.

In a randomized, open-label, multicenter controlled study published in 2019 [7], patients with resectable HCC and PVTT were randomly assigned to receive neoadjuvant RT followed by hepatectomy ($n = 82$) or hepatectomy alone ($n = 82$). The planned total dose to the intrahepatic tumor and PVTT was 18 Gy, with a fraction size of 3.0 Gy. For patients randomly assigned to the surgery-alone group, surgery was performed within five days after assignment. Patients randomized to the neoadjuvant RT group were re-evaluated four weeks after completing RT, after which surgery was performed within five days if they had no new contraindication to surgery. OS rates for the neoadjuvant RT group were 75.2% and 27.4% at one and two years, respectively, compared with 43.1% and 9.4% in the surgery-alone group ($P < 0.001$).

The goals of adjuvant RT following hepatectomy are to destroy remaining tumor cells and at least part of any remaining organized thrombi. However, outcomes of patients who received preoperative RT were not as satisfactory, when compared with palliative RT. The median survival was only 17 months, which is similar to the results of patients receiving palliative RT. Studies comparing TACE combined with RT versus neoadjuvant preoperative RT are required in the future. Chapter 15, "Neoadjuvant RT Converting to Curative Resection," discusses this concept in further detail.

17.1.5 EBRT for IVC Tumor Thrombosis

HCC often invades or metastases to the IVC through the hepatic vein, producing IVC tumor thrombosis. If the tumor thrombus dislodges, severe and lethal complications, such as pulmonary embolus and infarction, can occur. IVC tumor thrombosis progresses rapidly and is associated with a very poor prognosis if left untreated. IVC tumor thrombi have been successfully removed in a few patients with cardiopulmonary bypass and hypothermic circulatory arrest [43–45]. However, treatment strategies depend on the patient's general condition and whether the intrahepatic lesions are controlled. Our retrospective clinical data showed that survival in patients with

IVC tumor thrombi was significantly worse in patients who did not undergo EBRT, with a median survival of only two months versus 17.4 months in those who received EBRT [26]. Data from a multicenter trial in Korea (KROG 17–10) revealed that the median survivals were 12.1 months for IVC tumor thrombi alone, and 9.3 months for IVC combination with PV tumor thrombi [46]. Researchers from Japan reported that the combination of EBRT and chemotherapy was more effective for treating advanced HCC with venous tumor thrombosis in the PV or IVC, when compared with chemotherapy alone [47]. Combination therapy significantly improved OS according to multivariate analysis.

EBRT appears to produce better outcomes for IVC tumor thrombosis than for PVTT. Based on our clinical data, EBRT was associated with a median survival of 9.7 months for patients with PVTT and 17.4 months for those with IVC tumor thrombi alone [35]. There are at least two possible explanations for this difference. One explanation is that compared to patients with PVTT, patients with IVC thrombi had a higher rate of solitary intrahepatic lesions and well-controlled intrahepatic tumors, as well as a better response to EBRT. The other explanation relates to PV characteristics. Not only does this vessel have a narrower lumen than the IVC, but the PV also carries nutritional substances (e.g., including fat, amylum) from the gastrointestinal tract, which could slow blood flow to the liver and thereby lead to platelet accumulation because of eddy currents. Therefore, PV tumor thrombi are more often mixed with hemostatic thrombi, and EBRT does not affect hemostatic thrombi. Patients with IVC thrombi would have a greater chance to receive further treatment (TACE) for intrahepatic tumors than those with PV thrombi. Thus, local control of intrahepatic tumors was better for patients with IVC than for those with PVTT [35].

17.1.6 Image-Guided Intensity Modulated RT

In general, both intrahepatic lesions and tumor thrombi should be considered concurrently when developing treatment plans for patients with HCC and PV and/or IVC tumor thrombi. These patients often have multiple intrahepatic lesions. Dose distribution of 3-dimensional conformal RT (3D-CRT) for irregular multiple lesions is generally unsatisfactory. Image-guided intensity modulated radiotherapy (IGRT) can deliver a higher radiation dose than 3D-CRT, with more accuracy and better dose distribution in the tumor and remaining liver tissue. In our retrospective study of 118 patients with HCC and PV and/or IVC tumor thrombi referred for EBRT at Zhongshan Hospital, Fudan University, 64 received 3D-CRT and 54 received IGRT. Baseline demographic, clinical, and laboratory characteristics were similar between groups. Overall average radiation fractions were 19.44 ± 4.09 (IGRT) with a biologically effective dose $(BED)_{10}$ of 72.3 Gy versus 25.48 ± 3.80 (3D-CRT) with BED_{10} of 61.5 Gy ($P < 0.001$). IGRT provided a significantly higher dose of radiation to the tumor, with no increase in mean dose to the whole liver. Median survival was 15.5 months in patients treated with IGRT versus 10.5 months in those treated with 3D-CRT ($P = 0.005$) [12]. Chapter 8, "Image Guided Radiotherapy," discusses this concept in further detail.

17.1.7 Prognostic Factors

In a cohort of 136 patients with a median OS of 9.7 months, we identified several prognostic factors for patients with HCC and tumor thrombi treated with EBRT [48]. Based on the results of multivariate analysis, we categorized unfavorable predictors into three groups: (1) tumor-related factors (γ-glutamyltransferase [γ-GT], alphafetoprotein [AFP], tumor size, intrahepatic tumor number, tumor thrombi status, LN involvement, and distant metastases); (2) liver function-related factors (total bilirubin, albumin, hepatic enzymes, and Child–Pugh classification); and (3) treatment-related factors (response to EBRT). As for RT technique, 2D-RT was not as effective as 3D-CRT, and 3D-CRT was not as effective as IGRT.

Interestingly, platelet count was a simple and important prognostic factor on univariate analysis, which was difficult to classify into the above three groups [48]. Higher platelet counts were significantly associated with a higher cumulative incidence of hemostatic thrombosis and poorer survival, which contrasts with observations in the setting of HCC without PVTT, in which patients with normal platelet counts had a better prognosis than those with reduced platelet counts ($<100 \times 10^9$/L). However, platelet counts were not associated with survival on multivariate analysis, possibly because both higher and lower counts may be associated with reduced survival. Poorer survival in patients with higher platelet counts may be attributed to their increased risk of hemostatic thrombus. Although tumor cells in a tumor thrombus would be destroyed by radiation, a hemostatic thrombus would not be dissipated as easily. Occluded venous channels are difficult to recanalize and make further treatment difficult. Poorer outcomes in people with lower platelet counts may be attributed to concomitant hypersplenism and poor liver function, which were negative prognostic factors in our study.

Case 1 (described in the Sect. 17.4) was a patient with HCC who had a PVTT that resolved completely after IGRT. RT, as a component of the comprehensive treatment of PVTT, is usually performed in combination with other treatment approaches, including TACE, surgery, and/or RFA, before or after RT.

17.1.8 RT Techniques

Before initiating EBRT, patients receive breathing training to reduce the amplitude and increase the frequency of breaths with the goal of minimizing tumor movement. Liver movement is estimated during simulation, and if it is >0.4 cm, pressure is applied to the patient's abdomen to minimize tumor movement. Parallel-opposed portals are frequently used, and combinations of three or more ports are applied, depending on the tumor's location. Wedges or compensation devices are used if necessary.

Whether the tumor thrombus is located in the main PV, PV branches, or IVC, EBRT is used as palliative treatment or neoadjuvant therapy, despite recent advanced RT techniques. When used for tumor thrombus alone, the median total dose is 50 Gy, which is administered in daily doses of 2 Gy per fraction, five times per week. If IGRT is used, dose uniformity of the tumor and liver can be improved with a relatively small planning tumor volume (PTV), and a higher radiation dose and hypofractionation can also be achieved. Depending on the field size and anatomic location, all or part of the right kidney may be within the radiation field. In these situations, intravenous pyelography should be performed before RT to ensure adequate left kidney function. When the duodenum is within the radiation field, the full radiation dosage should be limited to ≤ 54 Gy. Other factors that suggest the need for a reduced dose include severe side effects during EBRT (e.g., nausea, vomiting, lack of appetite), exacerbation of tumor thrombus symptoms (e.g., ascites), and distant metastasis during EBRT. Conversely, if EBRT is tolerated without undue side effects, increasing the radiation dosage should be considered to improve tumor local control.

The design of radiation fields is of great importance. Making full use of the regenerative ability of normal liver is the basic principle. When designing radiation fields, a portion of normal liver tissue must be preserved from radiation to ensure that it is able to regenerate when most of the liver is damaged by radiation. Since helical tomotherapy (HT) can be applied to multiple targets at the same time, this technique allows concurrent RT of both primary tumor sites and tumor thrombi with higher radiation doses to improve survival. The results of our study and a South Korean study showed that median survival was 15 months in HCC patients with PVTT treated with HT [12, 49].

17.2 Lymph Node Metastases

17.2.1 Introduction

HCCs are primarily confined to the liver. Hematogenous spread (to lungs, bones, and adrenal glands) is the main mode of distant metastases, and regional LN metastasis (LNM) is uncommon. The incidence of LN involvement in patients with HCC ranges between 0.8 and 7.4% in series of patients with resectable tumors [50, 51], but the incidence is as high as 25.5 and 32.9% in autopsy series [52, 53]. In series of unresectable cases, determination of LN status is generally neglected. Furthermore, death from LN involvement is usually caused by local mechanical obstruction, which is difficult to distinguish from liver failure caused by intrahepatic tumors.

Although LNM is clinically uncommon, it may become more frequent in the future with further development of diagnostic imaging techniques, advances in treatment, prolonged survival of patients, and improved understanding of LNM.

Figure 17.1 depicts four common lethal patterns of metastatic LNs from HCC observed at our institution: (1) biliary obstruction, which produces jaundice; (2) pyloric (or duodenal) obstruction, which results in abdominal pain; (3) IVC obstruction, which is usually followed by

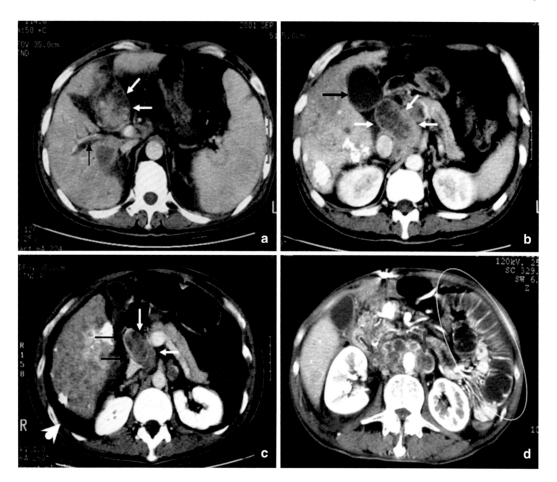

Fig. 17.1 Four lethal patterns of metastatic lymph nodes (LNs) from hepatocellular carcinoma. (**a–d**) Axial abdominal computed tomography scans obtained during (**a–c**) portal venous phase and (**d**) hepatic arterial phase. (**a**) Enlarged portal LNs (white arrows) causing jaundice and dilation of the intrahepatic bile duct (black arrow). (**b**) Peripancreatic LN metastasis resulting in pyloric obstruction and jaundice. Gallbladder (black arrow) dilation is caused by obstruction of common bile duct. (**c**) Enlarged peripancreatic LNs (white arrows) compressing the infe-

rior vena cava (black arrows), which is distorted to appear linear. The patient presented with ascites (white arrowhead) and edema of the lower extremities secondary to inferior vena cava compression. (**d**) Compression of the celiac nerve plexus by paraaortic LN metastasis (red arrows), which produced abdominal fullness and severe pain. Intestinal distention from nerve paralysis is shown within the white oval (Obtained from Zeng et al. Int J Radiation Oncology Boil Phys, 2005:63:1067–1076)

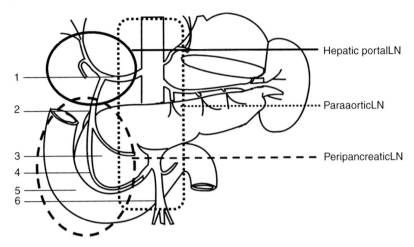

Fig. 17.2 Abdominal lymph node (LN) metastases from hepatocellular carcinoma grossly classified as hepatic portal, peripancreatic, and paraaortic nodes, reflecting increasing distance from the liver following the natural flow of lymph. Numbers identify the following structures: 1, Common hepatic artery; 2, Gastroduodenal artery; 3, Pancreas; 4, Superior pancreaticoduodenal artery; 5, Duodenum; 6, Superior mesenteric artery (Obtained from Zeng et al. Int J Radiation Oncology Boil Phys, 2005:63:1067–1076)

ascites and lower extremity edema; and (4) motility (paralytic) intestinal obstruction, which occurs occasionally and is likely due to compression of the celiac plexus. As jaundice, abdominal pain, lower extremity edema, and abdominal distension are all symptoms of intrahepatic tumor or thrombus progression in patients with HCC, without imaging studies, it is difficult to differentiate these signs and symptoms from those resulting from LNM.

Patterns of abdominal LNM from HCC can be grossly classified as hepatic portal, peripancreatic, and paraaortic LNs, which reflect increasing distance from the liver, following the natural flow of lymph (Fig. 17.2). Portal LNs include hepatoduodenal ligament and common hepatic artery nodes. Right gastric LNs are classified as portal nodes if HCC involves the left lobe. Peripancreatic LNs consist of posterior pancreaticoduodenal and anterior pancreaticoduodenal nodes. Paraaortic LNs are composed of the celiac trunk, superior mesenteric artery, and middle colic artery nodes. If positive nodes are located in more than one area, the pattern of LN spread is classified according to the higher station following the natural lymph flow.

The most common sites of LNM from HCC are the three aforementioned intra-abdominal areas. Metastasis may also involve LNs in the left supraclavicular, mediastinal (e.g., paratracheal, inferior tracheal protuberance), cardiophrenic angle, internal mammary, or retrosternal areas. From the abdominal LNs, tumor cells may travel retrogradely, spreading caudally to the lumbar or sacral vertebrae LNs. They may then flow into the cisterna chyli through the lymphatic vessels and finally into the central thoracic veins through the thoracic duct.

We analyzed 125 HCC patients with abdominal LNM [54] in our institution more than 10 years ago. Metastases followed the natural flow of lymph in 120 patients, whereas in the remaining five patients, they skipped to a remote LN station (i.e., metastases occurred in the aortic or peripancreatic LNs with no portal node metastasis). Of these five patients, two underwent surgical resection with portal lymphadenectomy, and three had large (>12-cm) tumors at the hepatic hilum, which were unresectable or involved the hepatic capsule.

There are not only few patients with LNM from HCC, but there are also few effective treatments for these patients. Prognosis is poor, even after radical resection by experienced surgeons [55]. Sun et al. from Zhongshan Hospital, Fudan University, reported outcomes of 49 patients with

HCC and LNM. They found that one-, three-, and five-year OS rates in patients who underwent complete lymphadenectomy ($n = 26$) were similar to those of patients who received RT ($n = 23$) (68.0%, 31.0%, and 31.0% vs. 57.0%, 33.0%, and 26.0%, respectively; $P = 0.944$) [50]. This lack of difference reflects observations that LN involvement is generally not the only or main factor determining symptoms or survival in patients with HCC. Hepatic parenchymal involvement and distant metastases are more important factors affecting survival. TACE and PEI are not suitable treatments for patients with HCC and LNM. Some patients undergo palliative therapy, such as biliary decompression using self-expanding metal stents, to relieve obstructive jaundice, but obstruction commonly recurs in ≤6 months because of tumor ingrowth and biliary sludge [56]. Sorafenib, as a form of molecular targeted therapy, was delivered to 46 HCC patients with LNM. Median OS was only 5.6 months in these patients, although it was slightly longer than the OS of patients who received placebo (3.2 months) [57]. Use of EBRT for LNM in patients with HCC has been reported in several articles, from case reports [58, 59] to prognostic analyses of large patient samples. This section discusses the role of EBRT for LNM from HCC.

17.2.2 Efficacy of EBRT

Researchers from Zhongshan Hospital, Fudan University, identified 125 patients with HCC metastasis to regional LNs treated with or without EBRT and evaluated the role of EBRT in these patients [54]. Of these, 62 patients received locoregional EBRT focused on the metastatic LNs (with intrahepatic lesions included in six patients), and 63 (who were hospitalized at the same time as the EBRT group) did not receive EBRT. Of the patients who received EBRT, 23 (37.1%) achieved a complete response (CR) and 37 (59.7%) had a partial response (PR), resulting in an objective regression rate of 96.8%. Symptoms caused by enlarged LNs were completely relieved after EBRT. Median survival and

OS rates at one and two years for patients treated with EBRT versus no EBRT were 9.4 versus 3.3 months, 42.1% versus 3.4%, and 19.9% versus 0%, respectively. These survival times and rates were significantly different between groups ($P < 0.001$). LNM location and primary intrahepatic tumor size had virtually no effect on survival in the non-EBRT group, but they significantly affected survival in the EBRT group. Median survival times in patients with hepatic portal, peripancreatic, and para-aortic LNM were 24.1, 9.4, and 6.0 months, respectively, in the EBRT group and 3.6, 3.8, and 3.2 months, respectively, in the non-EBRT group. EBRT was noted to be a protective factor in both univariate and multivariate Cox survival analyses (relative risk, 0.15; $P < 0.001$).

Table 17.4 summarizes the survival of patients with HCC and LNM treated with EBRT in studies conducted by researchers in China, Japan, and Korea. The median survival in most studies was approximately 10 months [60–64]. These patients survived longer (and with significant pain relief) than individuals in the Asia-Pacific Trial, who had a median survival of 3.2 months if they received no treatment or 5.6 months if they were treated with sorafenib [65].

In the study from Zhongshan Hospital, Fudan University, described above [54], 43.5% (27/62) of patients in the non-EBRT group died of LN-related complications, whereas only 8.0% (4/50) of patients in the EBRT group died of these complications. Thus, EBRT can reduce mortality resulting from nodal involvement. However, the incidence of gastrointestinal bleeding was greater in the EBRT group. The main side effects of EBRT were moderate-to-acute gastrointestinal and hepatic toxicity, frequently presenting as loss of appetite and nausea. Thirteen patients (21%) had mild heartburn relieved by histamine-2 blockers or omeprazole. Heartburn usually resolved within three months after completing EBRT. These side effects did not affect the timing or delivery of EBRT. All patients who had fatal gastrointestinal bleeding received EBRT with a dose >56 Gy, and no fatal gastrointestinal bleeding occurred in patients receiving <56 Gy. Eight patients (12.9%) devel-

Table 17.4 Treatment outcomes of EBRT for HCC with LNM

Author	Year	No. of patients	Radiation dose (Gy), median (range)	Response to EBRT		Survival		
				Complete response (%)	Partial response (%)	Median (months)	1 year (%)	2 years (%)
Park [60]	2006	45	50 (39–58.5)	25.6	53.8	10	35.2	21.7
Yamashita [61]	2007	28	50 (46–60)	17.9	64.3	13	53	33
Toya [62]	2009	23	58.5 (36–67.2)	21.7	60.9	19	–	–
Kim [63]	2010	38	59 (43.7–67.2)	24.1	41.4	10	–	–
Chen [64]	2013	191	50 (40–60)	31.4	47.6	8.0	39.3	18.9

EBRT external-beam radiotherapy

oped elevated liver enzymes, but they generally remained less than twofold higher than the upper limit of normal. Park et al. also reported that approximately 20% of patients (9/45) developed RT-induced gastric or duodenal ulcers when receiving >50 Gy in conventional fractions [60]. Kim et al. described four patients with Grade 2 gastrointestinal bleeding among 38 patients with HCC and LNM who received EBRT. Three of the four patients received >64.8 Gy in conventional fractions [63].

Although EBRT induced LNM shrinkage, 76% of patients died of uncontrolled intrahepatic tumors or extrahepatic relapse in our study [54]. Few patients died as a direct result of LN involvement. Similar results were reported by researchers from South Korea. Among 45 patients with LNM from HCC, 35 patients died during follow-up, 23 of whom died of liver failure caused by intrahepatic relapse [60].

Abdominal metastatic LNs are usually surrounded by gastrointestinal tract organs, which limits dose escalation to radical doses and the dose administered per fraction. Image-guided radiotherapy (IGRT) can achieve a higher conformal dose distribution, allowing higher radiation doses in some situations and thereby improving treatment outcomes. Researchers from Zhongshan Hospital, Fudan University, evaluated responses and toxicities in 85 patients with HCC and abdominal LNM treated with either IGRT ($n = 43$) or non-IGRT ($n = 42$) [65]. Mean doses were 56 Gy/21 fractions with a BED_{10} of 67.2 Gy for the IGRT group and 52 Gy/26 fractions with a BED_{10} of 63.4 Gy for the non-IGRT group. Median OS time was 15.3 months for the IGRT

group and 9.7 months for the non-IGRT group ($P = 0.098$). One-year OS was 69.1% versus 38.1% ($P = 0.006$) and two-year OS was 19.3% versus 14.5% ($P = 0.066$) for the IGRT group versus non-IGRT groups, respectively. These results, therefore, indicate that IGRT improves short-term survival but not longer-term outcomes. The rate of hepatic toxicity was lower in the IGRT group, but there were no differences in cause of death from intrahepatic tumor or extrahepatic metastasis between groups. Even with IGRT, a radical dose is not achieved and only short-term, local control of LNM or intrahepatic tumor occurs [65].

Case 1 (see the Sect. 17.4) illustrates a typical example of LN involvement in the peripancreatic nodes, as well as cardiophrenic angle LNs. Metastatic LNs showed a good response to EBRT; however, gastrointestinal toxicity from EBRT was the main factor limiting the delivered radiation dose.

17.2.3 Prognostic Factors

The few studies that have analyzed prognostic factors of HCC patients with LNM treated with EBRT have reported similar findings. Prognostic factors can be categorized into three groups: patient factors, tumor factors, and treatment factors. Liver function is considered the main index of liver-related patient factors. Patients with Child-Pugh class B liver function have a poorer prognosis than those with class A function.

Data from our institution [64] and South Korea [60] suggested that LNM response to

EBRT was significantly related to survival. The prognosis of patients with reduced size of LNs was better than that of patients with no reduction. Radiation dose was not a prognostic factor of survival because the dosage administered to metastatic LNs was a palliative dose. Good intrahepatic tumor control and LNM restricted to the abdomen were associated with a better prognosis. Neither the number of involved LNs nor intrahepatic tumor size was associated with survival. Authors of the study from Korea identified LN-related symptoms as a poor prognostic factor. Our results showed that the abdominal location of LNM (classified grossly as hepatic portal, peripancreatic, or paraaortic) had virtually no effect on survival of patients who did not receive EBRT but significantly affected survival in those who underwent EBRT. These observations suggest a change in the natural course of LN involvement when EBRT is used. After EBRT for LNM, intrahepatic tumors have a much more important effect on prognosis than LNM. EBRT also reduced mortality attributed to nodal involvement from 43 to 8%. Most deaths were due to liver failure or systemic metastases in patients receiving EBRT, whereas LN-related complications were the cause of death in approximately one-half of patients who did not undergo EBRT.

The TNM classification system is an important reference index for predicting prognosis, determining treatment strategies, and evaluating outcomes. There are several staging systems for HCC, such as the International Union Against Cancer, American Joint Committee on Cancer, Marsh [66], China, and Asia-Pacific systems. However, all these staging systems simply categorize LNs as positive or negative. LNs have not been distinguished by site, such as hepatic portal, peripancreatic, or paraaortic, or by number. The reasons for this simple categorization may be the lack of clinical data (including treatment) for patients with HCC and LNM and the poor prognosis (only three months) of patients with LNM in the absence of RT. Recent advances in imaging techniques have enabled more accurate nonsurgical diagnosis of locoregional LNM. In our study, CT was used to evaluate abdominal LN involve-

ment, which was classified into three anatomic groups [54]. Median survival time after EBRT consistently decreased as the distance of LN involvement from the liver increased, following the natural flow of lymph. Thus, it is important to recognize the role of the anatomic site of metastatic LNs in patients with HCC. This contrasts with the number and size of metastatic LNs, which were not associated with survival in our study.

17.2.4 RT Techniques

If Lipiodol uptake is defective in the intrahepatic primary tumor, both the primary tumor and metastatic LNs should be included in the radiation field as much as possible. Otherwise, EBRT should focus on only the metastatic LNs. It is recommended that patients receive gastrointestinal contrast agents before CT simulation. LNs are contoured as GTV during the venous phase, which clearly distinguishes arteriovenous blood flow in the gastrointestinal tract. CTV includes the involved LNs, as well as electively irradiated LNs. For example, when the portal LNs are involved, we enlarge the irradiated volume to include the peripancreatic area, and when the peripancreatic LNs are involved, we cover the paraaortic area (to the level of the renal hilum) as well. Anterior (AP) and posterior (PA) fields are frequently used, and combinations of lateral fields are applied when using 3D-CRT. With the popularity of intensity-modulated RT (IMRT) and IGRT, it is recommended that these techniques be used as much as possible. We try to avoid including the gastrointestinal tract, especially the descending duodenum, in the radiation fields. Radiation dosage depends on intrahepatic tumor control, whether TACE is used, the field size, and the dose to organs at risk. For patients estimated to have a longer survival with good and stable intrahepatic tumor control, radiation dosage to GTV can be increased to 60 Gy, in conventional fractions, dosage to CTV can be increased to 45 Gy, and gastroduodenal dosage maintained at $\leq$54 Gy. Radiation dosage should be reduced considerably if the field size exceeds 150 cm^2 or if patients have severe nausea, vomiting, or poor liver function. Silver clips placed around metastatic LNs during previous resection can provide a reference for delineating GTV and act as markers during IGRT. Molecular targeted agents should be used with caution, as they can aggravate radiation damage of gastrointestinal and liver.

Patients with obstructive jaundice are first referred to radiologists for decompression with percutaneous transhepatic catheters or self-expanding metal stents to relieve jaundice, after which they begin EBRT. We do not consider here the patients who develop obstructive jaundice as the terminal stage of their malignancy, because these patients could be treated solely with stents for decompression and then following EBRT. Overall, obstructive jaundice is completely relieved, and the biliary tract is reopened in most patients following EBRT for LNM.

17.3 EBRT for Non-lymphatic Extrahepatic Metastasis

17.3.1 Bone and Soft Tissue Metastasis

A clinical retrospective analysis of 342 patients with HCC and extrahepatic metastasis found that bone (25.4%) was the third most common site of extrahepatic tumor metastases following the lungs (39.5%) and lymph nodes (34.2%) [67]. Bone metastases (BM) have been detected much more frequently in recent years because of improved imaging. Previously, BM were detected only when they produced symptoms, but whole-body positron emission tomography (PET) or emission computed tomography (ECT) scans are now able to detect BM in asymptomatic individuals. The frequency of BM from HCC was noted to be 19% (49 of 257 patients) using dual-tracer (carbon 11 acetate and fluorine 18 fluorodeoxyglucose) PET/CT [68]. With ongoing improvements in HCC treatment, patient survival rates and the incidence of BM from HCC are expected to continue to rise.

17.3.1.1 Diagnosis of Bone Metastases from HCC

Diagnosing BM from many malignancies often does not require biopsy. BM usually produce osteolytic and osteoblastic lesions, and it is often difficult to detect tumor cells under a microscope. Furthermore, some BM, such as vertebral metastasis, occur in areas where biopsy material is difficult to obtain. Therefore, clinical diagnostic criteria are often used. With HCC, the usual diagnostic criteria for bone metastasis are as follows: (1) history of HCC; (2) accompanying clinical manifestations, such as pain or numbness, the location of which are consistent with the site of the BM; (3) imaging evidence, including bone scans, PET-CT, MRI, CT, or x-ray plain films (with the axial skeleton being the most common site of BM); and (4) relief of symptoms after EBRT, as any clinical diagnosis of BM must be confirmed by treatment efficacy.

With increasing use of PET-CT or ECT for bone scanning as routine examinations for cancer staging, some BM from HCC are detected by their typical abnormal appearance but are not accompanied by symptoms. Because of this, the clinical diagnostic criteria may not be met. However, these criteria apply only to patients receiving RT. Indications of EBRT for BM include pain, risk of pathologic fracture, neurologic complications arising from spinal cord compression, and nerve root pain. EBRT is used only as palliative treatment to relieve BM symptoms; there is no evidence that RT prolongs survival in these patients.

17.3.1.2 Clinical Features of BM from HCC

BM from different malignancies have general characteristics, as well as specific characteristics. There are three specific characteristics of BM from HCC, which have relevance for the diagnosis and treatment of BM from HCC.

One characteristic is that the BM from HCC are predominantly osteolytic. Osteolytic destruction is detected by imaging at the BM site and by the presence of uneven or no increased isotope uptake at the corresponding area on a bone scan. These findings are due to active osteoclasts and inactive osteoblasts in the metastasis area. In our retrospective analysis of 205 patients with BM from HCC, 200 (97.6%) had a combination of both osteolytic and osteoblastic components, with predominantly osteolysis, and five patients (2.4%) had purely osteolytic lesions [69].

Another specific characteristic of BM from HCC is that these lesions are usually accompanied by a soft tissue mass. Almost half of HCC patients have a large or small soft tissue mass around their BM, especially around flat BM. These masses also consist of metastatic tumor cells. In our retrospective analysis of 205 patients, BM with expansile soft-tissue masses were detected in 80 patients (39.0%) [69].

Decreased leucocyte count, hemoglobin, and platelet count are a third characteristic of BM from HCC. Liver cirrhosis exists in the majority of patients with BM from HCC. Cirrhosis is further aggravated during treatment for HCC, which can lead to hypersplenism and reductions in leukocytes, platelets, and hemoglobin. Of note, hypersplenism can also occur in patients with HCC who have metastases in other (non-bone) sites. Radionuclide brachytherapy should not be offered to patients with HCC and BM, as it will exacerbate bone marrow depression and further aggravate decreases in leukocytes, platelets, and hemoglobin.

17.3.1.3 Treatment of BM from HCC

Surgery

Surgery is a form of local therapy for BM from malignancies, which should be performed as early as possible for patients with pathological fractures or spinal cord compression (present or impending). In addition, surgery may also be used for patients with a well-controlled primary tumor and a single bone metastasis. Cho et al. [70] conducted a retrospective study of 42 patients with HCC and vertebral metastases who underwent surgery (including internal fixation): 30 had a pathological fracture and 12 had a high-risk fracture. Median survival time was 10 months after surgery. Using Cox regression analysis, the number of BM and the Child-Pugh class were identified as independent prognostic factors for survival.

RFA

BM can be controlled by heating malignant cells. Kashima et al. [71] reported the outcomes of 40 consecutive HCC patients with 54 BM treated with RFA. The average maximum diameter of the BM was 4.8 cm (range, 1.0–12.0 cm). Technical success was 100% and pain relief rate was 96.6%; one patient had a transient nerve injury. Median survival time was 7.1 months. A single bone lesion, normal AFP level, and absence of viable intrahepatic lesions were identified as factors significantly associated with a better prognosis.

TACE

In theory, TACE should be effective for BM from HCC because HCC is a generally hypervascular tumor. However, clinical reports regarding the use of TACE for BM from HCC are rare and primarily consist of case reports. Japanese researchers [72] reported the efficacy of TACE for BM from malignancies in 24 patients, 12 of whom had HCC. The patients obtained satisfactory pain relief the day after TACE, but more than half (66.7%; 4/6) of the patients with complete pain relief had also received EBRT. The clinical efficacy of TACE for BM remains a question. Uemura et al. [73] compared the efficacy of TACE, a combination of TACE and EBRT, or EBRT alone for BM from HCC. Thirty-nine BM from HCC in 33 patients were retrospectively reviewed in their study. TACE alone was effective, with 90% of patients achieving pain relief. However, the combination of TACE and EBRT provided the best effects and was recommended for permanent pain relief. Nevertheless, TACE does not provide ideal pain relief for BM from HCC in our clinical experience.

Internal RT

Radioisotopes currently used for internal radiation of BM are chemical elements located in the second major group of the periodic table of elements. This is because active osteoblasts in bone lesions will take up substances containing these elements. While internal RT is effective for BM from prostate and breast cancers, which contain mainly osteoblasts, they have poor therapeutic efficacy for BM consisting of primarily osteoclasts. Therefore, before considering internal RT, bone scan results should be reviewed to select patients for whom the treatment may be effective. As metastases to bone from HCC are primarily osteolytic and present with an accompanying soft-tissue mass, they generally respond poorly to internal RT. Clinical reports of BM from HCC treated with internal RT are rare and primarily consist of case reports. Relative contraindications to internal RT for BM include the following: solitary bone metastasis, pathologic fracture, vertebral metastases (risk of spinal cord paralysis), false negative on bone scan, accompanying soft-tissue mass, hypersplenism (as systemic myelosuppression will dramatically reduce blood cell production), and estimated patient survival time < 3 months.

Bisphosphonates

As bisphosphonates inhibit osteoclast-mediated bone destruction, they are suitable for BM from HCC because active osteoclasts are present in these lesions. Bisphosphonates do not, however, destroy tumor cells. Treatment outcomes are better when bisphosphonates are combined with EBRT, compared with EBRT alone, but these drugs cannot be combined with internal RT. Katamura et al. [74] conducted a retrospective cohort study to investigate the efficacy of combined EBRT and zoledronic acid for BM from HCC. In this study, all 31 patients received RT for BM: 12 also received zoledronic acid, whereas 19 were treated with RT alone. The patients receiving zoledronic acid plus EBRT had 23 BM sites: 14 received RT and nine sites did not. Cumulative pain progression rate at six months was 0% at irradiated sites and 20% at non-irradiated sites ($P = 0.005$). There were 38 BM sites in the patients who were not treated with zoledronic acid: 22 sites received RT and 16 sites did not. In these patients, cumulative pain progression rate at six months was 34% at irradiated sites and 66% at non-irradiated sites ($P = 0.045$). The authors concluded that zoledronic acid delayed pain progression in both irradiated and non-irradiated BM.

Analgesic Medications

There are many mechanisms of BM-related pain, including mechanical damage, pain receptor activation induced by endosteum or periosteum injury caused by inflammatory cytokines released by the interaction between normal bone tissue and tumor cells, and tumor extension to adjacent soft tissue or peripheral nerves. Analgesic drugs will inhibit inflammatory cytokines or increase the pain threshold, but they do not destroy tumor cells. Use of analgesics can reduce pain and help patients maintain an appropriate body position during EBRT.

EBRT

EBRT can be used as local therapy for BM. Radiation damage is limited to only the tissue immediately surrounding the BM sites, and the degree and effects of injury depend on the radiosensitivity and importance of the surrounding tissues. Patients may develop radiation myelitis if metastases are located in the spine and radiation-induced gastrointestinal injury if metastases are located between the T10 vertebra and sacrum. RT relieves pain because the cytotoxic effects of irradiation on bone tissue affect neural depolarization, interfere with signaling processes, and further inhibit the secretion of pain mediators, such as bradykinin and prostaglandin. Pain is usually relieved within 48 hours after EBRT, but it is delayed in patients with osteolytic destruction and soft-tissue extension because pain is reduced only after tumor lesions have decreased in size and pressure on the periosteum and bone marrow cavity has been reduced. The goals of EBRT are to relieve pain, control growth of BM, and maintain bone structure and function.

Table 17.5 summarizes the outcomes of various treatment strategies for BM from HCC. EBRT is generally accepted as a palliative form of pain relief for these metastases.

17.3.1.4 Efficacy of EBRT

Effectiveness of EBRT for BM from HCC

In our review of data from 205 patients with BM from HCC who received EBRT, CR for pain pal-

Table 17.5 Effects of different treatment strategies for BM from HCC

Treatments	First author	Year	No. of patients	Symptom relief	Survival Median (months)	1 year (%)	2 years (%)
Surgical resection	Cho [70]	2009	42	Functional evaluation in 36 patients who survived >2 months postoperatively: Mean score = 23.4; 30-day postoperative mortality: 11.9% (5/42)	10	42.2	25.8
Radiofrequency ablation	Kashima [71]	2010	40	96.6% (28/29)	7.1	34.2	19.9
Bisphosphonates	Montella [75]	2010	17	Mean VAS pain score of patients receiving ≥3 doses (15/17 patients) of zoledronic acid: 7.1 before treatment and 5.3 after 3 months	10.2	30.7	–
TACE	Koike[72]	2011	12	Complete pain relief: 6 patients (4 also received EBRT); partial pain relief: 4 patients; no relief: 2 patients	Not reported because of few patients		
Radionuclide internal radiotherapy	Suzawa [76]	2010	1	Complete regression	Patient lived for 1 year without bone metastasis recurrence		
EBRT	He [69]	2009	205	Complete pain relief: 29.8%; partial pain relief: 69.7%	7.4	32.4	13.2

EBRT external-beam radiotherapy, *No.* number, *TACE* transarterial chemoembolization, *VAS* visual analogue scale

liation (i.e., complete pain relief) was observed in 61 patients (29.8%), PR for pain palliation (i.e., partial pain relief) occurred in 143 patients (69.7%), and pain remained stable in one patient (0.5%). Overall, pain improved in 99.5% of patients. The radiation dose was not significantly different between patients with CR and those with PR ($P = 0.068$). There was also no consistent dose-response relationship for pain palliation (Table 17.6). The results, however, did show that higher radiation doses could achieve higher CR rates for pain. Thus, there are two possible mechanisms for the pain-relieving effects of EBRT in BM: 1) initial pain relief by inhibiting pain mediators, which is independent of dosage; and 2) reduction in tumor burden, which depends on the dosage [69].

Radiation toxicity was mild or absent in all study participants. If the radiation field involved the gastrointestinal area (e.g., when BM were between T10 and the sacrum), some patients had mild loss of appetite and nausea. Local hair loss occurred in patients who received RT for skull

Table 17.6 Radiation dose-response relationship for pain palliation of BM from HCC in 204 patients with pain relief from EBRT

Total dose (Gy)	No. of patients	Response, % (number) CR	PR	P value
≤38	29	20.7 (6/29)	79.3 (23/29)	0.068
38–50	145	28.3 (41/145)	71.7 (104/145)	
≥50	30	46.7 (14/30)	53.3 (16/30)	
Total	204	61	143	

CR complete response for pain, *No.* number, *PR* partial response for pain

metastasis. Local pigmentation changes occurred in all radiation fields. No adverse effects influenced the timing or delivery of EBRT, and no medical management was required for any radiation-associated toxicity.

By the end of the study, 31 (15.6%) patients were alive and 174 (84.4%) patients had died. The one-year, two-year, and median survival for

Table 17.7 Pain improvement and survival in patients with BM from HCC

First author	Year	No. of patients	Radiation dosage (Gy), median (range)	Symptom relief	Survival Median (months)	1 year (%)
Kaizu [77]	1998	57	43 (20–65)	CR: 43%; PR: 42%	6	20.7
Seong [78]	2005	51	30 (12.5–50)	Pain relief rate: 73%	5.0	15
Nakamura [79]	2007	24	44.8 (39–50.7)	Symptom relief: 87.5%; spinal cord compression relief: 80% of patients (without decompressive surgery)	5.1	18
He [69]	2009	205	50 (32–66)	CR: 29.8%; PR: 69.7%	7.4	32.4
He [80]	2011	30[a]	40 (8–60)	CR: 30%; PR: 66.7%	8.6	39.7

CR complete response for pain; *No.* number, *PR* partial response for pain
[a]Bone metastases after liver transplantation

all 205 study participants were 32.4%, 13.2%, and 7.4 months, respectively. The causes of death were liver failure in 154 (88.5%) patients, secondary to hepatic decompensation, tumor progression, or both; brain metastases in nine (5.2%) patients; lung metastases in six (3.4%) patients; BM-related complications in two (1.1%) patients, both of whom had pulmonary failure induced by high-level paraplegia; heart failure in one patient (0.6%); myocardial infarction in one patient; and stroke in one patient.

Outcomes reported by other authors for patients with BM from HCC treated with EBRT are summarized in Table 17.7. Common findings are the relatively high rate of pain relief and short patient survival time.

Efficacy of EBRT for BM Following Liver Transplantation for HCC

Approximately 70% of liver transplantation recipients with HCC will develop extrahepatic tumor metastases, primarily in the lungs and bones [81]. We analyzed outcomes in 30 patients with HCC who underwent EBRT for BM after liver transplantation. The total radiation dose ranged from 8 to 60 Gy, with a median of 40.0 Gy. Median survival time and one-year and two-year OS rates after BM diagnosis were 8.6 months, 39.7%, and 24.4%, respectively. Overall pain relief from EBRT occurred in 96.7% of patients (29/30). No consistent dose-response relationship was found for palliation of pain with doses between 30 and 56 Gy ($P = 0.670$). The clinical features and efficacy of RT for BM in these patients were similar to those of our previously reported patients who did not undergo liver transplantation [80].

Differentiating Between Needle Tract Seeding and BM in Patients with Soft-Tissue Masses

Expansile soft-tissue masses are a typical clinical feature of BM from HCC. Needle tract seeding after percutaneous invasive procedures, such as PEI or RFA therapy, usually spread to the ribs and must be distinguished from BM accompanying soft-tissue masses. The overall incidence of HCC needle tract seeding secondary to invasive procedures has been estimated as 0.13% (17/11350) [82] to 0.14% (6/441) [83]. There is no doubt that BM from HCC represent an advanced tumor stage, classified as M1 according to the TNM system. By contrast, needle tract seeding is not a type of distant metastasis. There is currently no clear classification for needle tract seeding, but it may be reasonable to classify it as T4. A clinical study showed that one-year, two-year, and three-year OS rates were 76.5%, 47.1%, and 29.4%, respectively, for patients with needle tract seeding, in contrast to 31.8%, 13.6%, and 13.6% for patients with bone and soft-tissue metastases ($P = 0.049$) [82]. Thus, the prognosis appears to be much better for patients with needle tract seeding than for individuals with distant metastasis. Figure 17.3 provides information to help differentiate between needle tract seeding and BM. Needle tract seeding is always located around the intrahepatic lesion or along RFA pathways. BM usually present as multiple lesions in the axial skeleton.

Comparison Between Conventional Fractionation and Hypofractionated RT for BM from HCC

A single-center randomized controlled trial conducted at Zhongshan Hospital, Fudan University, between January 2009 and December 2014 compared the efficacy of conventional fractionation versus hypofractionation schedules for BM from HCC. The conventional fractionation group (*n* = 92) received either 40 Gy in 20 fractions or 60 Gy in 30 fractions, for patients without or with soft tissue involvement, respectively. The hypofractionation group (*n* = 91) received either 28 Gy in 7 fractions or 40 Gy in 10 fractions, for patients without or with soft tissue involvement, respectively. Pain relief rate was 96.7% in the conventional fractionation group and 91.2% in the hypofractionation group (*P* = 0.116). Response times were 6.7 ± 3.3 fractions in the conventional group and 4.1 ± 1.2 fractions in the hypofractionation group (*P* < 0.001). Time to treatment failure was significantly longer in the conventional group than in the hypofractionation group (*P* = 0.025). Median OS time of both groups was eight months. Thus, for patients with a shorter predicted survival time, hypofractionated RT is a safe and effective therapeutic option [84].

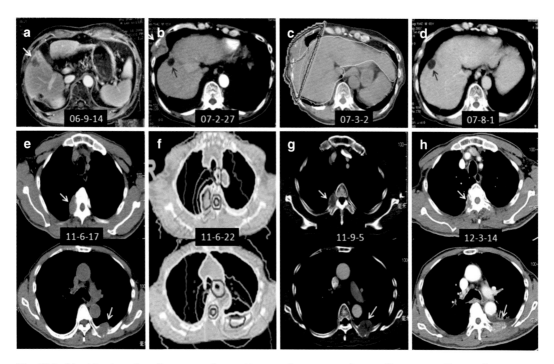

Fig. 17.3 Identification of needle tract seeding and bone metastases. (**a–d**) Series of images from a patient with hepatocellular carcinoma who developed needle tract seeding after radiofrequency ablation (RFA). (**a**) A subcapsular intrahepatic tumor (white arrow) in the right lobe located close to the gallbladder. (**b**) Computed tomography (CT) scan five months after RFA completion showing needle tract seeding in the right rib (consistent with the patient's symptom of right chest pain) and a residual intrahepatic cavity (violet arrow). (**c**) The radiation treatment plan was 3-dimensional conformal radiotherapy (RT), with 60 Gy/30 fractions. (**d**) Complete response of the needle tract seeding lesion four months after completing RT, which eliminated the patient's pain. The residual cavity (violet arrow) is unchanged. The patient survived three years after needle tract seeding (**e–f**). Series of images from a patient with multiple bone metastases from hepatocellular carcinoma. (**e**) Bone metastases accompanied by a soft tissue mass in the right paravertebral body (top) and left posterior rib (bottom), as indicated by white and yellow arrow, respectively. The patient had chest and back pain. (**f**) Treatment involved helical tomotherapy-based image-guided radiotherapy, with 40 Gy/10 fractions. (**g**) The bone lesions (arrows) remained stable two months after completing RT, but the patient had complete pain relief. (**h**) Follow-up CT scan eight months after completing RT showing complete response of the bone masses. This patient survived 1.5 years after the bone metastases were diagnosed. (Numbers on the images represent dates in year-month-day format.)

17.3.1.5 Prognostic Factors

We performed a retrospective analysis of 205 patients to identify independent predictors of survival in patients with BM from HCC. On univariate analysis, better survival was significantly associated with a better Karnofsky Performance Status (KPS); higher serum albumin; lower alkaline phosphatase (ALP), γ-GT, and AFP levels; intrahepatic tumor dimension ≤ 5 cm; well-controlled intrahepatic tumor; solitary bone metastasis beyond the spine; BM only; and longer interval from time of HCC diagnosis to BM diagnosis. On multivariate analysis, pre-treatment predictors of an unfavorable prognosis were lower KPS, higher AFP and γ-GT levels, and uncontrolled intrahepatic tumor [69].

Another study [85] also showed that patients with well-controlled intrahepatic tumors survived longer. A total of 37 patients with HCC and BM were stratified into two groups: untreated intrahepatic tumors as control group ($n = 16$) and treated group who underwent TACE for their intrahepatic tumor ($n = 21$). Baseline characteristics, including intrahepatic tumor stage, liver function, and metastases features, were similar between groups. Median survival was longer in the treated group (9.7 months) than in the untreated group (2.9 months), although the difference did not reach statistical significance ($P = 0.081$). These results are consistent with our previous data showing that approximately 84% of patients with BM from HCC died from liver failure because of intrahepatic tumor progression. To date, there is no evidence that EBRT for BM prolongs life span.

Estimating the prognosis of BM from HCC may aid selection of appropriate therapeutic strategies, especially palliative RT, for individual patients. At present, the optimal fractionated dose scheme for patients with BM from HCC remains unclear. In general, short-term hypofractionation should be considered for patients with a shorter predicted survival time to quickly relieve pain, whereas longer-term palliative RT is more appropriate for patients with a longer life expectancy to reduce radiation effects on adjacent normal tissues.

17.3.1.6 RT Techniques

A whole-body PET/CT or bone scan or an MRI/CT scan of metastasis sites must be performed before EBRT to estimate the extent of bone destruction and whether soft-tissue extension is present. RT should focus mainly on painful area(s), as the primary goal is to relieve pain. Radiation fields involve the macroscopic tumor volume plus 3-cm margins if non-IGRT is used. For vertebral BM, radiation fields usually encompass one normal vertebra above and below the metastatic lesion. Radiation fields involve only the macroscopic tumor volume when IGRT is used, especially for vertebral BM. The majority of therapy is provided with 6-megavolt (MV) to 15-MV photons. Conventional fractionation or hypofractionated RT with a total dose of 28–60 Gy is used, based on the adjacent organs at risk and the predicted survival time of the patient. Radiation dosage depends on the prognosis of patients with BM and whether soft-tissue extension exists. Tumor doses as high as possible are used for patients with a good prognosis, and moderately reduced doses are used for patients with a poor prognosis. Radiation dosage should also be increased for lesions accompanied by soft-tissue extension, as this represents a heavy tumor burden. Irradiation with a dosage within 50 Gy in conventional fractions is delivered through parallel opposed fields (AP and PA) for vertebral lesions, depending on the depth of the lesion between the surface of the back and the anterior edge of the vertebra. Hypofractionated RT should be considered in patients with shallow lesions, such as BM in the skull, ribs, or extremities. Precise RT is recommended for patients with spinal metastases.

17.3.2 Adrenal Gland Metastases

17.3.2.1 Introduction

The adrenal gland is a site of extrahepatic metastases from HCC, with an incidence of 8% according to autopsy data [86, 87]. Similarly, adrenal gland metastases accounted for 8.8% of all extrahepatic metastasis according to clinical follow-up data. However, limited clinical data are available regarding treatment strategies for adrenal gland metastases, and optimal treatment remains unclear. Case reports have described the use of various methods, including surgical resection [88, 89], TACE [90], PEI, RFA [91, 92], and EBRT [93]. It has also been reported that patients with adrenal gland metastases may survive long-term after surgical resection of metastases. However, HCC is classified as advanced stage when adrenal gland metastases are present. In a considerable proportion of these patients, surgical resection is not considered because they also have unresectable intrahepatic tumors, tumor thrombi, LN involvement, and/or synchronous distant metastases to bones or lungs. Theoretically, TACE should be beneficial because adrenal metastases, like primary HCC, are hypervascular. However, it is often anatomically difficult to perform TACE for adrenal gland metastases through the adrenal or renal arteries. PEI may be useful for small lesions, but it is not sufficiently effective for larger tumors, and the location of the adrenal gland produces technical challenges. There have been some published reports describing EBRT for adrenal gland metastases from HCC.

17.3.2.2   RT Effects

We retrospectively investigated 55 patients with adrenal metastases from HCC, which were treated with EBRT [94]. The patients' characteristics are summarized in Table 17.8. Radiation doses to the adrenal lesions ranged from 26 to 60 Gy. Before EBRT, 42 patients had a chief complaint of pain in the back or flank, secondary to the adrenal metastasis, and one patient had lower extremity edema, secondary to IVC compression. After completing EBRT, all patients experienced at least some symptom relief; visual analogue scale (VAS) pain scores were reduced >3 points (out of 10); and the lower extremity edema (in the one patient) was completely resolved.

In total, 63 lesions in 55 patients received EBRT [94]. PR was achieved in 68.4%. In four patients, the adrenal lesions (total of four lesions) relapsed after RT, with the time of relapse ranging from 6 to 14 months. Because their intrahe-patic primary tumors were well controlled, all four patients received a second course of RT, using the same radiation fields as before and a prescribed dose of 40 Gy. PR was again achieved in these patients. Serum AFP levels were above normal before EBRT in 40 patients and decreased by >50% in 19 (47.5%) patients after treatment.

By the time of the retrospective analysis, 42 (76.4%) of the 55 patients had died, and the median survival time was 13.6 months. Liver failure secondary to primary tumor progression was the cause of 35 deaths. Other causes of death were lung metastasis (four patients; 9.5%), abdominal LN metastasis and related complications (two patients; 4.8%), and brain metastasis (one patient). No deaths were attributed to adrenal metastasis-related complications. Adverse effects included grade I or II gastrointestinal side effects and grade III thrombocytopenia, which occurred in 12.5% patients. No renal toxicity was observed.

Table 17.9 lists the survival outcomes of various therapies for metastatic adrenal tumors from HCC. Most of these outcomes are based on reports involving a small number of patients. It is difficult to directly compare outcomes of different strategies because of differences in patient characteristics; in particular, patients who underwent surgery had more features associated with a good prognosis. However, these data show that survival was longer in patients who underwent some treatment than in patients at a similar stage who did not receive any treatment. As good palliative therapy for adrenal metastases from HCC, EBRT is relatively safe and easy to perform and has obvious beneficial effects on relieving compression symptoms caused by adrenal metastasis.

17.3.2.3   Prognostic Factors

In our study of 55 patients with adrenal metastasis from HCC treated with EBRT, univariate analysis revealed several variables that were associated with shorter OS: uncontrolled or multiple intrahepatic tumors, higher serum AFP and γ-GT levels, Child-Pugh class B or higher, metastasis to additional organ(s), and poor response to EBRT (Table 17.8). On multivariate analysis, the

Table 17.8 Univariate and multivariate associations between characteristics and survival in patients with adrenal gland metastases from HCC treated with EBRT

Clinical variables	No. of patients	Median survival (months)	P value Univariate analysis	Multivariate analysis
Age (years)			0.114	n.s.
≤50	23	12.63		
>50	32	13.63		
Sex			0.411	n.s.
Male	52	13.63 ± 1.48		
Female	3	7.27 ± 1.63		
γ-GT (U/L)[a]			0.008	0.326
≥150	16	17.80 ± 6.51		
<150	33	5.57 ± 3.53		
AFP level (μg/mL)			0.027	0.719
<400	33	15.90 ± 2.62		
≥400	22	5.57 ± 2.01		
Child-Pugh classification			0.043	0.420
A	45	15.27 ± 1.63		
B	10	5.53 ± 2.43		
Maximal diameter of intrahepatic tumors (mm)			0.074	0.180
≤80	33	15.13 ± 3.32		
>80	22	8.87 ± 1.46		
No. of intrahepatic tumors			<0.001	0.012
Solitary	45	15.90 ± 2.61		
Multiple (≥2)	10	5.57 ± 3.30		
Interval			0.422	n.s.
Synchronous	8	8.87 ± 1.22		
Metachronous	47	13.63 ± 1.52		
Resection, including liver transplantation, for intrahepatic tumors			0.483	n.s.
Yes	35	15.90 ± 2.38		
No	20	10.53 ± 3.17		
Additional organ metastasis			0.001	0.013
Yes	9	15.27 ± 1.63		
No	46	4.47 ± 0.45		
Metastatic adrenal tumor size (mm)			0.476	n.s.
<50	21	15.13 ± 4.40		
≥50	34	13.20 ± 2.02		
Location of adrenal lesions			0.614	n.s.
Unilateral	47	13.63 ± 1.42		
Bilateral	8	9.27 ± 5.33		
Radiation dose (Gy)			0.102	0.073
≥54	18	21.27 ± 8.46		
<54	37	12.93 ± 2.15		
Primary HCC			<0.001	0.003
Controlled	38	17.80 ± 4.77		
Uncontrolled	17	9.77 ± 2.94		
Response to radiotherapy[b]			0.017	0.478
Partial response	32	17.80 ± 8.28		
Stable disease	18	12.63 ± 2.79		

[a]Data missing for 6 patients
[b]Data missing for 5 patients
HCC hepatocellular carcinoma, *n.s.* not significant, *No.* number

Table 17.9 Effects of various therapies for metastatic adrenal tumors from HCC

Treatment	First author	Year	No. of patients	Tumor	Survival time (from treatment of adrenal metastases)		
					Median or individual (months)	1 year (%)	2 years (%)
Surgery	Momoi	2002	13	8/13 had additional organ metastases	–	51.3	42
	Park	2007	5	Well-controlled intrahepatic foci; no additional organ metastases; single adrenal metastasis	21.4	100	50
TACE	Momoi	2002	4	Tumor thrombus or additional organ metastases	5.9, 6.5, 16.1, and 21.3	–	–
	Taniai	1999	2	Single adrenal metastases; well-controlled intrahepatic foci	At least 3 and 8 (still alive)	–	–
PEI	Momoi	2002	4	Additional organ metastases: 1 patient; intrahepatic tumor: 3 patients	7.6, 8.5, 21.4, and 32	–	
PEI + TACE	Park	2007	19	Well-controlled intrahepatic foci; no additional organ metastases	10.5	43	0
RFA + TACE	Yamakado	2009	6	Intrahepatic tumor: 3 patents; additional organs metastases: 3 patients; size of metastatic adrenal tumor: 3–8 cm	24.9	–	–
No treatment	Park	2007	6	Well-controlled intrahepatic foci; no additional organ metastases	5.6	0	–
EBRT	Jung	2016	134	No evidence of disease 22%, stable disease 46%, uncontrol 32%	12.8	53.1	23.9
	Yuan	2017	81	Intrahepatic tumor controlled in 59%, uncontrolled in 41%	13.5	59.9	35.0

EBRT external-beam radiotherapy, *PEI* percutaneous ethanol injection, *RFA* radiofrequency ablation, *TACE* transarterial chemoembolization

presence of uncontrolled or multiple intrahepatic tumors and metastasis to additional organ(s) remained as pretreatment predictors of poor OS. Of note, radiation dosage is an important factor affecting survival, although statistical significance was not achieved when considering the whole study population. However, in subgroup analysis of patients with well-controlled primary tumors, high-dose RT ($\geq$54 Gy) was associated with a significantly longer OS time. If the dose is reduced because of a patient's poor general condition, the effectiveness of EBRT may be decreased, leaving survival to be influenced by other factors.

17.3.2.4 RT Techniques

In our basic EBRT technique for adrenal metastases from HCC, we use 6- to 15-MV photon beams, the selection of which is based on tumor location and depth. Each patient is immobilized in the supine position with arms folded overhead using a custom-made cradle mold. A CT simulation scan without contrast can be performed because adrenal gland metastases are clearly visible on plain CT images. However, if intrahepatic lesions are simultaneously treated with RT, the CT simulation should be contrast-enhanced. GTV is defined as the volume of radiographically visible adrenal lesion(s). CTV construction is generally unnecessary because the vast majority of adrenal gland metastases are isolated lesions, but if adhesions are present around the kidney, CTV is created by adding 0.4-cm margins around the visible tumor. Although the adrenal gland is a retroperitoneal organ, intra-adrenal tumors are affected by respiratory motion [95]. PTV is determined as GTV plus 1 cm in the craniocaudal direction and 0.4 cm in other directions, without 4D-CT. Two posterior oblique fields are often used for isocentric irradiation. This combination of fields helps protect the liver, spinal cord, intestines, and contralateral kidney from radiation. The radiation dosage can be increased because the intestines usually do not appear in two radiation fields at the same time during EBRT; however, the right adrenal gland is located near the lower pole of the liver. We generally schedule a full dosage of up to 50–60 Gy in conventional fractions, but some factors indicate the need for a reduced dose. These factors include the occurrence of adverse effects and the status of intrahepatic tumors and distant metastases.

Image-guided hypofractionated RT or stereotactic body RT (SBRT) could be used for metastases when the gastrointestinal tract is not included in the radiation field. All or part of the ipsilateral kidney is included in the radiation field, depending on the field size and anatomic location of the adrenal tumor. Intravenous pyelography should be performed prior to RT to ensure that the contralateral kidney has adequate function. In rare patients with bilateral adrenal metastases, it is generally better to choose IGRT. HT is the best option for patients with synchronous extrahepatic or intrahepatic lesions [96].

Residual cancer cells may lead to recurrent tumors after palliative RT because of the relatively long survival time of patients with adrenal gland metastases from HCC. Repeat irradiation of adrenal gland metastases is common, and the surrounding organs, such as the intestines, are easy to protect from radiation. Even if one kidney is damaged by radiation, serious consequences will not occur because of compensatory increased function of the contralateral kidney.

Case 1 (see the Sect. 17.4) illustrates a typical patient with an adrenal gland metastasis from HCC, which was treated with IGRT using HT. The patient lived for 42 months after this.

17.3.3 Pulmonary Metastases from HCC

17.3.3.1 Introduction

With recent developments in diagnostic and therapeutic modalities for HCC, well-controlled intrahepatic tumors have become more common, and patient survival times have increased. Hence, the incidence of distant metastases is increasing. Lungs are the most common site of extrahepatic metastases. The incidence of pulmonary metastases from HCC is as high as 46.3% in autopsy cases [97–99] and 13.8% (12/87) in PET/CT examinations of patients with newly diagnosed HCC [100]. Pulmonary metastases account for 39.5–53.8% of extrahepatic metastases [101]. Once extrahepatic metastasis develops, the survival time of patients is much lower than that of patients without extrahepatic metastasis [102]. Pulmonary metastases from HCC usually occur in patients with tumor thrombi. Based on data from our institution, lung metastases were observed during the entire treatment period in 53% of patients with IVC tumor thrombi but only 18.1% of patients with PVTT [48]. These results suggest that tumor cells from IVC tumor thrombi travel directly through the heart to the pulmonary circulation.

Up to 77.6% of patients with advanced HCC present with multiple (≥2) metastatic lung nodules, and 46.1% present with bilateral metastatic lung nodules [103]. Local treatment for multiple pulmonary metastases is difficult, and pulmonary metastases easily travel to other areas, such as the brain. Approximately 60–70% of patients with HCC and brain metastases have been previously diagnosed with pulmonary metastases. As 20% of patients with pulmonary metastases from HCC die from respiratory failure [104], pulmonary lesions require aggressive treatment.

The probability of metastasis or recurrence of HCC after liver transplantation depends on the HCC stage before transplantation. Pulmonary metastases are the most common extrahepatic metastases after liver transplantation. In our study of 95 patients with HCC who underwent liver transplantation, 42 developed recurrence or metastasis, with pulmonary metastasis accounting for 50% of these outcomes [105]. The risk of metastases may be at least partly attributed to post-transplantation immunosuppressive therapy. Cyclosporin A can increase the activity of matrix metalloproteinases, potentially enhancing metastasis of HCC cells [106].

17.3.3.2 Treatment

Although many therapeutic options exist for pulmonary metastases from HCC, the most appropriate standard treatment remains unclear. Surgery appears to be the best strategy for patients with a single metastatic lesion or oligometastasis, but it is probably not the best option for multiple pulmonary metastases from HCC. Chemotherapy and molecular targeted treatments have not been shown to be effective. At present, EBRT is recognized as an important local treatment for pulmonary metastases from HCC. HT has distinct advantages over conventional linear accelerator therapy for treating multiple pulmonary metastases.

Surgical Resection

At present, reports of surgical resection of pulmonary metastases from HCC have only involved patients with well-controlled intrahepatic tumors, no metastatic area except the lungs, a small number of pulmonary lesions (usually <2 and not >5), metastases located in the same lung, and a pulmonary mass that can be completely resected during one operation. Table 17.10 summarizes the available literature reporting survival after surgical resection of patients with pulmonary metastases. The prognosis is better for these patients than for those with distant metastasis of other sites, with three-year OS rates of approximately 50% and five-year OS rates of approximately 40%.

Interventional Therapy

Interventional therapy for pulmonary metastases from HCC mainly involves the delivery of che-motherapy drugs through pulmonary artery infusion or bronchial artery embolization. Data from our institution showed that survival of patients with pulmonary metastases was significantly longer in patients who received interventional therapy than in patients who received no treatment [104]. The combination of systemic therapy using sorafenib, local treatment with TACE for intrahepatic lesions, and bronchial transarterial chemoinfusion for pulmonary lesions has also been reported to be effective. Among 52 treated patients, pulmonary lesions completely resolved in one patient and partially resolved in eight cases after treatment. Median OS time was 12 months [107]. Unfortunately, there was no control group in this study.

Molecular Targeted Therapy

Molecular targeted therapy for pulmonary metastases from HCC has been associated with different survival rates, compared with other types of extrahepatic metastases. The phase III Asia-Pacific trial provided good evidence that sorafenib improves OS and is safe for patients with advanced HCC. Sorafenib consistently improved median OS compared with placebo (5.6 vs. 4.2 months) for patients with pulmonary metastases [57]. These data are very similar to our reported median survival time of untreated patients with pulmonary metastases (5.4 months), suggesting that while molecular targeted therapy may improve survival, the effects are small [104].

Chemotherapy

When extrahepatic metastasis is present, HCC is classified as stage IV according to the TNM classification, which necessitates the use of systemic therapy. Nevertheless, the effectiveness of chemotherapy for extrahepatic metastasis is currently disputed. A recent report described the use of an intravenous infusion of arsenic trioxide combined with TACE for the treatment of HCC with pulmonary metastasis [108]. Most other publications regarding the use of chemotherapy for lung metastasis from HCC have been case reports (usually involving just a single patient). Systemic 5-fluorouracil plus interferon-alpha

Table 17.10 Survival of HCC patients with pulmonary metastases treated with surgical resection

First author	Year	No. of patients	Tumor	Survival Median (months)	1 year (%)	2 years (%)	3 years (%)	5 years (%)
Hwang	2012	23	LT for primary liver cancer; pulmonary metastatic foci ≤4: 56.5% of patients; single metastasis: 13 patients	24	77.4%	43.5%	30.6%	–
Ohba	2012	20	Intrahepatic lesions well controlled after surgical resection ($n = 15$) or microwave ablation ($n = 5$); number of pulmonary metastases: 1 ($n = 11$), 2 ($n = 4$), or ≥ 3 ($n = 5$)	60	–	–	–	46.9
Kitano	2012	45	Intrahepatic lesions treated with surgical resection ($n = 39$) or RFA or PEI ($n = 6$); no additional organ metastases	26.5	–	53.9	–	40.9
Yoon	2010	45	Well-controlled intrahepatic foci; no additional organs metastases; total of 52 pulmonary lesions	40.7	86.0	–	56.3	37.0
Han	2010	41	Intrahepatic foci treated with surgical resection ($n = 28$), LT ($n = 12$), or interventional therapy ($n = 1$); pulmonary masses completely resected during 1 operation	–	92.4	–	74.3	56.9
Lee	2010	32	Intrahepatic foci well controlled after surgical resection ($n = 21$), LT ($n = 1$), or interventional or alcohol injection ($n = 10$); ≤2 pulmonary metastases: 26 (81%) patients	10.7	–	–	–	–
Kawamura	2008	61	All intrahepatic lesions well controlled after surgical resection; pulmonary metastases identified at time of HCC diagnosis ($n = 6$), <1 year after surgery ($n = 15$ patients), or >1 year after surgery ($n = 40$); ≤2 pulmonary metastases: 47 (77%) patients	30.0	69.8	–	46.9	32.2

HCC hepatocellular carcinoma, *LT* liver transplantation, *PEI* percutaneous ethanol injection, *RFA* radiofrequency ablation

[109], oral S-1[110], and transcatheter arterial infusion chemotherapy with zinostatin [111] have been described, but the overall efficacy of chemotherapy in this setting requires further investigation.

Microwave Ablation or RFA

As minimally invasive techniques, the use of microwave ablation or RFA for pulmonary metastases has been reported extensively for a variety of tumors. However, these techniques can only be used when there are at most a few pulmonary metastases and the maximal axial diameter is 5 cm (and preferably <3 cm). Accordingly, thoracic surgeons usually choose surgical resection for patients who meet these criteria, so ablation therapies have seldom been reported for the treatment of pulmonary metastases from HCC. Reports of successful use of microwave ablation therapy and RFA for unresectable pulmonary metastases have been published in small case series of 10 cases [112] and two cases [113], respectively. While these reports suggest that ablation techniques are safe, they involve too few patients to confirm the efficacy of these treatments for pulmonary metastases from HCC.

EBRT

Most pulmonary metastases from HCC present as multiple lesions. Coupled with respiratory motion, it is difficult to treat multiple lesions using linear accelerator radiation. In addition, pulmonary metastases from HCC are not usually fatal. Previously, palliative RT was offered only to patients with pulmonary symptoms or complications such as hemoptysis, pain, or atelectasis. With the development of RT facilities and further understanding of the radiosensitivity of pulmonary metastases from HCC, RT for multiple pulmonary lesions is now receiving increasing attention not only for palliation but also as potentially curative therapy, as described in Case 2 in the Sect. 17.4. This case illustrates that not all patients with distant metastases should be treated with purely palliative goals. Radical RT may be possible for patients with oligometastases involving the lungs.

17.3.3.3 RT Effects

We retrospectively analyzed data from 13 patients with symptomatic pulmonary metastases from HCC who were treated with EBRT at our institution [114]. Their intrahepatic lesions were well controlled with surgery ($n = 9$) or TACE ($n = 4$). These patients had a total of 31 pulmonary metastatic nodules, 23 of which received EBRT using a linear accelerator with 6-MV photons focused on the pulmonary nodules. Significant symptoms were completely or partially relieved in 12 patients (92.3%), and an objective response was observed on CT imaging in 10 patients (76.9%). Median progression-free survival for all patients was 13.4 months. Patient one-year, two-year, and three-year survival rates from pulmonary metastasis were 82.0%, 70.7%, and 70.7%, respectively. Pulmonary lesions that did not receive RT remained stable for a long time or disappeared spontaneously. Although the patients in this study were a select group, these preliminary results showed that pulmonary metastases from HCC are sensitive to RT. The survival of these patients was similar to the survival reported in other studies of individuals who underwent surgical resection for HCC pulmonary metastases.

Because of limitations of lung tolerance to radiation dosage, RT was only administered to some of the pulmonary metastases in the aforementioned study. With the development of advanced RT facilities, HT could simultaneously technically treat multiple tumors, as described for Case 2 (see the Sect. 17.4). In a recent study, we reviewed data from a cohort of 45 patients at our institution who received HT alone or in combination with sorafenib for pulmonary metastases from HCC [115]. CR was achieved in one patient (2.2%), PR in 29 patients (64.4%), and stable disease in 14 patients (31.1%). A total of 195 pulmonary metastatic lesions were detected in these 45 patients, all of which were treated with HT. CR was achieved in 13 lesions (6.7%), and PR was achieved in 137 lesions (70.3%). Median OS after diagnosis of pulmonary metastases was 26.40 months, and the two-year survival rate was 46.7%. Patients treated with the combination of HT and sorafenib ($n = 23$) had a median OS of 29.6 months. This was longer than the median

OS of patients who received only HT ($n = 22$; 23.0 months; $P = 0.031$) or of patients who received only sorafenib ($n = 18$; 25.0 months; $P = 0.018$). Thus, these results showed that HT was useful for treating pulmonary metastases, and treatment outcomes were improved when combined with sorafenib. Efficacy of HT for pulmonary metastases from HCC was also reported by South Korea researchers, who noted a median survival time > 12 months [116, 117]. HT therefore appears to be safe and effective for treating pulmonary metastases from HCC.

After large pulmonary metastases are treated with radiation, some small, distant lesions outside the local RT field disappear. This clinical observation is known as the abscopal effect, in which radiation reduces tumor growth outside the radiation field [118]. An increasing body of evidence suggests that this is an immune-mediated phenomenon. Tumor cell death resulting from local high-dose RT enhances antigen-presenting capacities. In cooperation with other immunotherapies, this produces strong anti-tumor immunity, which leads to effects similar to those seen with systemic therapy. As more research has been conducted, the exact mechanism of the abscopal effect is gradually being clarified [119]. Furthermore, along with recent advances in immunotherapy, the combination of RT and immunotherapy may become a new treatment strategy, altering traditional therapeutic patterns.

17.3.3.4 RT Techniques

Unlike with primary lung cancer, it is unnecessary to consider preventive RT for lymphatic drainage when treating pulmonary metastases from HCC. RT with 50–60 Gy in conventional fractions can achieve reasonable local control and palliative effects.

It is preferable to perform pulmonary function tests before RT, and if possible, PET/CT should be obtained to exclude distant metastasis beyond the lung. Before RT, each patient undergoes basic respiratory training regarding how to take shallow breaths to reduce the effects of respiratory motion on the target tumor. Patients are immobilized using a vacuum bag. Abdominal compression is used for all patients to reduce uncertainty

bias caused by respiratory movements. Heavy compression, however, is avoided because it would reduce abdominal breathing and thereby increase chest breathing movements. We suggest that 4D-CT simulation be acquired during the four phases of each respiratory cycle to generate the internal target volume (ITV). Digital CT images with ≥3-mm thick slices are more appropriate if multiple small lesions are present. GTV is defined as the volume of macroscopic tumor delineated on pulmonary windows of the chest CT. CTV is created by adding a 0.4-cm margin around the metastatic tumor. PTV is determined by the RT equipment and quality control of each hospital. If 4D-CT is not available, the range of ITV depends on the degree of respiratory movement under the simulator. When determining the dosage limit, one must consider whether the esophagus, liver, spinal cord, and/or heart are in the radiation field. The incidence and degree of radiation esophagitis should be estimated. Hypofractionated RT should not be used if the esophagus is included in the radiation field. The mean lung dose should be limited to <25 Gy and the V25 to <35% for patients with good pulmonary function. Dose limits should be reduced for patients with poor pulmonary function, as exemplified by a forced expiratory volume in one second and diffusion capacity of carbon monoxide ≤50–60% of predicted. We recommend a mean lung dose <15 Gy and V25 < 25% when using conventional RT.

SBRT with a radical dosage may be considered for patients with ≤5 pulmonary metastases, no distant metastasis beyond the lung, and well-controlled intrahepatic tumors. Case 2 (described in the Sect. 17.4) is an example of a patient with three pulmonary metastases treated with SBRT. Multiple pulmonary metastases accompanied by uncontrolled intrahepatic tumors or extrapulmonary metastases should be followed conservatively, then treated with palliative RT when patients develop symptoms. However, RT can be considered for multiple pulmonary metastases in the setting of well-controlled intrahepatic tumors and no extrapulmonary metastases, with HT being especially advantageous for multiple metastases.

Lung metastases from HCC differ from primary lung cancers in several ways: (1) pulmonary function of patients with pulmonary metastases is often better than in patients with primary lung cancer; (2) patients with pulmonary metastases from HCC often receive chest RT alone, while patients with primary lung cancer often receive concurrent chemoradiotherapy; and (3) preventive RT for lymphatic drainage is not necessary for pulmonary metastases from HCC. Because of these differences, dosage limits to organs at risk when treating primary lung cancer are not applicable when treating pulmonary metastases from HCC. Researchers from Zhongshan Hospital, Fudan University, analyzed clinical data of 62 patients with 407 pulmonary metastases from HCC who were treated with HT. The median radiation dose was 50 Gy, administered as 4.0 Gy/fraction. Multivariate analysis showed that the percentage of non-target normal lung volume receiving a BED > 20 Gy (V_{BED20}) and the number of pulmonary metastatic lesions were the two significant predictors of radiation pneumonitis ($P < 0.001$) [120].

17.3.4 Brain metastasis

17.3.4.1 Characteristics of Brain Metastasis from HCC

The overall incidence of brain metastasis from HCC is very low, especially when compared with primary lung and breast cancer, which have brain metastasis rates of 20–40%. However, the incidence of brain metastasis from HCC appears to be rising. Originally, the incidence was only 0.3–0.6%, but it increased to 0.9% with more widespread use of brain CT or magnetic resonance imaging (MRI) and with increased resolution and improved diagnostic accuracy of these scanning techniques. The incidence further increased to approximately 7% with improvements in clinical treatment, prolongation of survival, and extended intervals from diagnosis of HCC to brain metastasis (as illustrated in Table 17.11).

When brain metastasis from HCC occurs, the prognosis is very poor. Most reports suggest that median OS is only one to two months after diagnosis, as shown in Table 17.12. Our data [127] showed a median survival time of 4.5 months for patients treated with EBRT, in contrast to only 20 days for patients whose poor condition prevented them from undergoing EBRT. Brain metastasis is associated with such a poor prognosis because most of these patients have advanced HCC and often die from uncontrolled intrahepatic lesions. As they are often in the terminal stage of HCC, hepatic function of patients with brain metastasis is typically very poor, with a prolonged prothrombin time and thrombocytopenia induced by hypersplenism. The incidence of stroke from intracranial tumors is very high. Strokes are associated with rapid progression of HCC and deterioration of coagulation function, which prevent many patients from receiving RT.

Table 17.11 Emerging time and incidence of brain metastasis from HCC

First author	Time period	Median interval from diagnosis of HCC to brain metastasis (months)	Incidence of brain metastasis, % (number)
Kim [121]	1987–1991	13	0.6 (19/3100)
Chang [122]	1986–2002	10.5	–
Chen [123]	1993–2003	–	0.28 (42/15088)
Choi [124]	1995–2006	18.2	0.9 (62/6919)
Shao [125]	2005–2009	9.6	7.0 (11/158)
Jiang [126]	1994–2009	15.0	0.47 (41/8676)
Qiu [127]	2004–2011	14.5	–
Han [128]	2001–2012	18.3	0.65 (33/5015)
Nam [129]	1995–2017	–	0.6 (86/13581)
Mean	–	–	0.56 (294/52537)

HCC hepatocellular carcinoma

Table 17.12 Survival of patients with brain metastasis from HCC

First author (year)	No. of Patients	Median survival time (months)
Chang (2004) [122]	45	1.0
Choi (2009) [124]	62	1.6
Shao (2011) [125]	11	4.6
Jiang (2012) [126]	41	3.0
Qiu (2013) [127]	32	4.5
Hsieh (2009) [130]	42	1.2
Hsiao (2011) [131]	46	2.0
Han (2013) [128]	33	2.4
Nam (2019) [129]	86	1.7

No. number

Table 17.13 Incidence of stroke-like presentation in patients with brain metastasis from HCC

First author (year)	Incidence of stroke-like presentation, % (number)
Choi (2009) [124]	54.8 (34/62)
Kim (1998) [121]	36.8 (7/19)
Hsieh (2009) [130]	42.9 (18/42)
Chang (2004) [122]	40.0 (18/45)
Han (2013) [128]	51.5 (17/33)
Nam (2019) [129]	39.5 (34/86)
Total	44.6 (128/287)

Table 17.14 Incidence of lung metastasis at the time of brain metastasis diagnosis in patients with HCC

First author (year)	Incidence of brain metastasis accompanied by lung metastasis, % (number)
Kim (1998) [121]	75.0 (6/8)
Chen (2007) [123]	61.9 (26/42)
Choi (2009) [124]	69.4 (43/62)
Shao (2011) [125]	91.0 (10/11)
Jiang (2012) [126]	75.6 (31/41)
Qiu (2013) [127]	62.5 (20/32)
Han (2013) [128]	72.7 (24/33)
Nam (2019) [129]	87.2 (75/86)
Total	74.6 (235/315)

Another key issue regarding brain metastases is that they are often neglected in patients with HCC. Brain imaging (especially MRI) is generally not included in routine or follow-up examinations because brain metastasis is uncommon. In addition, symptom onset is often sudden and clinical deterioration is usually rapid, with a very short survival time. Patients are often unconscious or dead before further medical tests can be obtained. Furthermore, symptoms of brain metastasis are difficult to differentiate from those of hepatic encephalopathy.

When brain metastases from HCC become apparent clinically, they usually present like a stroke, with motor weakness, mental change, and headache (Table 17.13). Intracranial hemorrhage can be seen on imaging tests, especially MRI scans. Hemorrhage occurs because intracranial metastatic tumors from HCC, like the primary tumors, are generally hypervascular, and these patients usually have severe hepatic dysfunction, with coagulopathy and thrombocytopenia.

Most patients have already developed extracranial (especially lung) metastasis at the time of brain metastasis diagnosis. According to most published data, 61.9–91% of patients have lung metastases when brain metastases are diagnosed (Table 17.14). We found a relative lower rate in our study of 32 patients with brain metastasis from HCC, in whom 20 patients had lung metastasis [127]. The frequent presence of lung metastasis in people with brain metastases from HCC can be attributed to the widely anastomosing blood supply between intracerebral vessels and the vertebral artery and venous plexus of the brain. Intrapulmonary tumor cells directly enter the brain by traveling through the heart, carotid artery, and intracranial circulation without pulmonary capillary filtering. Therefore, patients with extrahepatic metastasis, especially in the lungs, require imaging examinations for early detection of brain metastasis. In the abovementioned study of 32 patients with brain metastasis from HCC, the lesions were detected by follow-up brain MRI in only five asymptomatic patients, and survival time was clearly longer in these patients than in individuals with symptoms. Thus, early detection of brain metastasis is important in patients with HCC.

17.3.4.2 Management of Brain Metastasis from HCC

Management of brain metastasis from HCC is similar to that of brain metastasis from other tumors. Surgery and/or RT is the mainstay of therapy for intracranial lesions. However, unlike with brain metastasis from other tumors, emergency RT should be performed upon diagnosis of HCC brain metastasis because life-threatening intratumoral hemorrhage may occur at any time. HCC is not sensitive to chemotherapy, and there are no reports describing the use of molecular targeted agents for intracranial lesions from HCC. We can only follow current recommended treatment options for brain metastasis, as there are no persuasive clinical trials with high-level evidence comparing the efficacy of surgical resection versus RT for intracranial metastasis from HCC because of the low number of patients with these lesions.

Single Intracranial Metastasis

When a single brain metastasis from HCC is detected, surgical resection or SBRT (both with or without whole brain RT) is appropriate for patients with an estimated survival time ≥ 3 months and a completely resectable metastasis with a maximum axial diameter ≤ 3–4 cm. Postoperative RT is required when the maximum diameter is >3–4 cm. SBRT combined with whole brain RT or IMRT is administered to patients with unresectable metastases with a maximal axial diameter > 3–4 cm. In this way, metastatic nodules receive a high dose of radiation, while normal brain tissue concurrently receives a prophylactic dosage. Palliative RT is administered to patients with a poor prognosis (estimated survival <3 months).

Multiple Intracranial Metastases

When multiple intracranial metastases from HCC are present, SBRT with or without whole brain RT or whole brain RT alone is used for patients with an estimated survival time ≥3 months and tumors confined to one location and with a maximal axial

diameter ≤3–4 cm. Whole brain RT is used for patients with diffuse brain metastases. Surgery combined with postoperative RT are used for patients with tumor-related symptoms (e.g., tumor-induced apoplexy). Whole brain RT or supportive therapy should be offered to patients with a poor prognosis (estimated survival <3 months).

If treatment strategies for intracranial metastases are initiated promptly, death rates from intracranial metastases will decrease. Tables 17.15 and 17.16 show the results of two studies examining the causes of death among patients with HCC and brain metastasis treated by different methods. These results show that treatment of intracranial metastases can control the lesions and prolong survival [124].

There are various regimens for radiation dosage to brain metastasis, including 40 Gy in 20 fractions over four weeks, 37.5 Gy in 15 fractions over three weeks, 30 Gy in 10 fractions over

Table 17.15 Deaths due to brain metastases in patients with HCC treated with steroids alone or various other treatments [124]

Cause of death	Treatment		
	Steroids alone (n = 25)	Resection, Whole brain RT, or γ-knife[a] (n = 32)	Resection + Whole brain RT (n = 5)
Nervous system	21 (84.0%)	10 (33.3%)	0 (0%)
Extracranial lesion progression	4 (16.0%)	17 (56.7%)	2 (100%)
Unknown	0	3 (10.0%)	0 (0%)
Patients alive at follow-up	0	2	3

[a]Patients were treated with resection alone (6), Whole brain RT alone (16), or γ-knife radiosurgery alone (10)

Table 17.16 Deaths due to brain metastases in patients with HCC treated with conservative therapy, whole brain radiotherapy, or surgery and/or γ-knife radiosurgery [129]

Cause of death	Treatment		
	Conservative therapy (n = 24)	Whole brain RT (n = 30)	Surgery and/or radiosurgery (n = 32)
Nervous system	24 (44.4%)		5 (15.6%)
Extracranial lesion progression	27 (50.0%)		20 (62.5%)
Survivors or patients lost to follow-up	3 (5.6%)		7 (21.9%)
Median survival (weeks)	3.9	6.9	16

two weeks, and 20 Gy in five fractions over five days. The literature contains no evidence of differences in efficacy between different fractionated dose schemes. Fractionation and dosing schemes are determined by individual RT facility protocols, preferences of the treating physician, and convenience to the patient. There is also no clinical evidence indicating that RT should be combined with chemotherapy or targeted drug treatment.

17.3.4.3 Prognostic Factors

Recursive partitioning analysis (RPA) is a statistical methodology that has been used to identify prognostic factors of brain metastasis from any type of primary tumor. Brain metastases have been categorized into three classes based on RPA: Class 1, which includes patients with a KPS score > 70, age < 65 years, controlled primary disease, and no evidence of extracranial metastasis; Class 3, which includes patients with a KPS score < 70; and Class 2, which includes all patients who do not fit into Class 1 or 3. Prognosis is best for patients with Class 1 metastases and worst for those with Class 3 lesions.

Because of the rarity of brain metastasis from HCC, data regarding its prognostic factors are limited. In a retrospective review of 62 patients, researchers from South Korea [124] reported that Eastern Cooperative Oncology Group performance score, number of brain lesions, serum AFP, RPA class, Child-Pugh class, and treatment modality had a statistically significant impact on survival, based on univariate analysis. In our study [127] of the clinical characteristics and prognosis of 31 HCC patients with brain metastasis, univariate analysis revealed that RPA class (which includes KPS), Child-Pugh class, and central nervous system symptoms were significantly associated with survival. Multivariate analysis showed that, in addition to central nervous system symptoms, the number of intracranial metastases and whether patients received focal RT also affected prognosis. The differences between univariate and multivariate analysis results may reflect the small sample size. In contrast to the Korean study, we did not detect an association between survival and AFP level, but we did note an association between survival and

well-controlled intrahepatic lesions. Uncontrolled intrahepatic lesions are the leading cause of death in patients with brain metastasis from HCC. As HCC cells are quite sensitive to irradiation, whole brain RT combined with a boost dose to local lesions will generally control intracranial lesions. As long as patients receive RT with > 50 Gy in conventional fractions, intracranial lesions should be effectively controlled.

17.3.5 Peritoneal Implantation of HCC

Rupture of hepatic tumors and needle tract seeding after percutaneous procedures are the most common risk factors for peritoneal implantation (PI) in patients with HCC. Among 68 HCC patients with PI, 34 (50%) had a documented history of intrahepatic tumor rupture, puncture, or both [132]. The incidence of PI in patients with HCC has been reported to range from 3 to 15% based on clinical data, with rates as high as 52.9% obtained from autopsy data [132]. However, few reports have been published regarding PI, and this phenomenon is often ignored clinically. It is often difficult to differentiate hepatic tumor rupture from needle tract seeding, although doing so is important because of the large difference in prognosis between the two conditions. Hepatic tumor rupture is usually indicative of a large tumor and widespread metastases, whereas needle tract seeding is often the result of RFA, PEI, or biopsy for small focal liver lesions. However, no clinical data comparing these two PI causes have been published.

PI may lead to various complications, including bowel obstruction, hemorrhage from implanted lesions, and hydronephrosis from ureteral obstruction. These complications are not fatal, but they seriously affect quality of life. Recent reports suggested that survival of patients with PI controlled with treatment was not better than survival of patients in whom PI was not controlled. In 2012, Kwak et al. reported the results of a study examining prognosis of patients with PI from HCC [132]. Median survival of patients with PI was only three months, but propensity score matching analysis showed no significant difference in median OS from the time of HCC diagnosis between patients with or without PI. This result indicates that PI is not an independent risk factor of death in HCC patients; it is simply an indicator of advanced HCC. Multivariable analysis did identify elevated AFP, advanced Child-Pugh class, and progressive intrahepatic tumors as independent predictors for early death after PI diagnosis in patients with HCC. These findings reflect the lethality of hepatic dysfunction secondary to progression of intrahepatic tumors [132].

Current treatment for PI primarily focuses on surgical resection of implanted metastatic lesions, based on the literature. Researchers from Taiwan reported that OS of 16 HCC patients with PI after selective resection for peritoneal implant masses was similar to OS of patients without PI. Patients with PI from HCC have a much better prognosis than individuals with extrahepatic metastases at other sites because PI does not represent distant blood metastasis [133]. In another group of 16 patients who underwent resection for PI from HCC, median DFS was 7.9 months and median OS was 16.0 months [134].

Intrahepatic tumor rupture can spread to the entire abdominal cavity, and the median duration from HCC diagnosis to PI has been reported as 11 months (0–64 months) [132]. After rupture, the time for HCC tumor cells to grow into a mass is relatively long. Many case reports have described the presence of multiple implanted intraperitoneal metastases detected after resection of a ruptured large HCC. A case reported by South Korea researchers [135] is typical. This patient presented with intrahepatic tumor rupture and underwent emergency hepatic angiography and TACE. Ten days after TACE, a tumor located in the right lobe of the liver was resected successfully. Four months later, follow-up CT showed a 2-cm, irregularly-shaped mass at the right greater omentum. During a second surgery, omentectomy with mass excision was performed. Three months later, the patient underwent splenectomy and segmental resection of the colon for additional PI sites. Five months later, a metastatic LN was detected around the head of the pancreas, which was excised surgically. All resected tumors were histologically confirmed to represent metastatic HCC. After three operations to resect multiple intraperitoneal metastases within one year after initial resection of ruptured HCC, the patient was disease free at 15-month follow-up.

PI occurs successively, with or without multiple lesions. Like surgery, precise RT is a form of local therapy, which is technically difficult when multiple implantation sites or metastases are present. RT with a linear accelerator is more difficult for multiple lesions than for a single lesion. Furthermore, radiation dosage is difficult to increase because of the various organs at risk, including intestines, kidneys, and liver, around the intra-abdominal implantation sites. Thus, RT has been rarely reported for PI from HCC. In the past 10 years, we have used RT for 11 patients with HCC rupture and PI. The longest-surviving patient has lived for 15 years, after undergoing multiple operations and RT (Fig. 17.4). With the emergence of HT, RT for multiple implanted intraperitoneal metastases is no longer difficult. HT allows the delivery of radiation to multiple lesions simultaneously, while avoiding damage to the intestines.

17.3.6 Rare Types of Metastases

Bile duct tumor thrombi (BDTT) from HCC are unique in that the primary tumor usually has no capsule and the surrounding tissue often shows direct invasion from the primary tumor. BDTT may occur when the primary tumor is still very small. The development of BDTT does not depend on tumor size but rather on the pathologic behavior of HCC and the physical relationship between the tumor and bile duct.

Based on the combined results of several studies, 127 of 6287 patients with HCC developed BDTT after surgical resection of their intrahepatic primary lesion, representing an incidence of 2% [136–139]. Authors of these studies indicated that after surgical resection (especially R0 resection), patients with BDTT have a relatively long survival time, which is similar to the survival time of patients without BDTT. As study of 69 HCC patients with BDTT from South Korea reported survival rates of 76.5%, 41.4%, 32.0%, and 17.0% at one, three, five, and ten years after surgery, respectively [136]. In a study from Henan

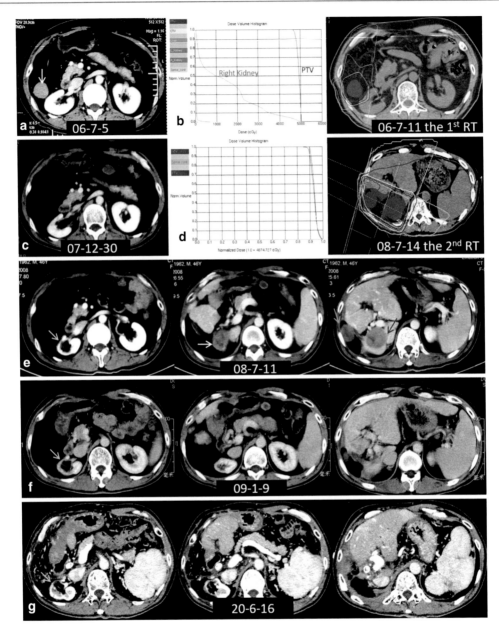

Fig. 17.4 A 43-year-old male with abdominal pain, who was diagnosed with hepatocellular carcinoma and hepatic tumor rupture in August 2005. He underwent transarterial chemoembolization for the intrahepatic tumor in September 2005 and hepatectomy in March 2006. Peritoneal implantation was found on follow-up. (**a**) Computed tomography (CT) image in July 2006 showing peritoneal implantation at the anterior right kidney (white arrow). (**b**) First course of 3-dimensional conformal radiotherapy (3D-CRT) for peritoneal implantation tumor with 50 Gy/25 fractions, which began in July 2006. *PTV* planning target volume. (**c**) CT showing complete response of the peritoneal implant 1.5 years after completing radiotherapy (RT). (**d**) A second course of 3D-CRT was delivered for successive peritoneal implantation, using 46 Gy/23 fractions. (**e**) CT images of successive peritoneal implantation sites treated as in D, with the three masses indicated by green, red, and white arrows. Atrophy of the right kidney is seen, two years after the first course of 3D-CRT (yellow arrow). (**f–g**) Complete response of peritoneal implantation lesions to the second course of RT during follow-up at (**f**) six months and (**g**) 12 years. The patient remains alive and well 15 years after the original tumor rupture. (Numbers on the images represent dates in year-month-day format.)

Provincial People's Hospital in China, one-, three- and five-year survival rates were 89.3%, 46.4%, and 21.4%, respectively, in 28 patients with BDTT who underwent radical hepatectomy [138].

Along with improvements in RT technology, images can accurately guide radiation to the tumor thrombus. We analyzed the efficacy of RT for treating BDTT in five patients with HCC at our institution. Of these, three patients with well-controlled intrahepatic tumors had long-term survival, whereas two individuals with intrahepatic tumor progression died in the short term. BDTT is sensitive to radiation, but obstructive jaundice secondary to thrombus requires drainage before RT. Figure 17.5 shows a patient who developed BDTT after interventional therapy for HCC. Complete remission of BDTT was achieved after RT, and the patient survived >10 years.

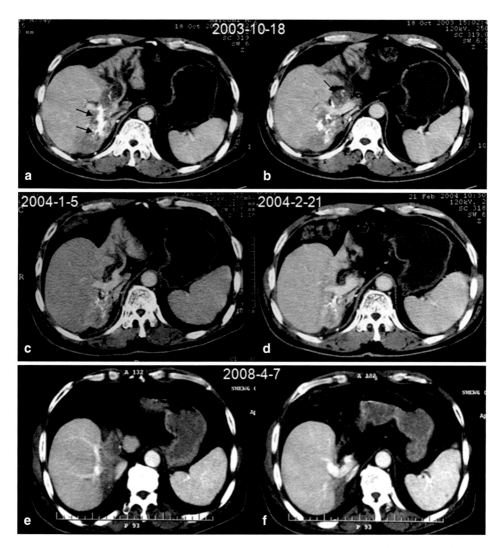

Fig. 17.5 A patient with hepatocellular carcinoma who developed obstructive jaundice after transarterial chemo-embolization. Series of follow-up computed tomography (CT) venous phase images. (**a**) Partial Lipiodol (black arrows) deposition in a right lobe tumor. Bile duct dilation is present in the left lobe. (**b**) Intrabiliary tumor thrombus (black arrow). (**c**) CT image 1.5 months after completing external-beam radiotherapy (EBRT). The intrahepatic lesion shows partial regression, but bile duct dilatation remains obvious. (**d**) Partial regression of the intrahepatic lesion and partial atrophy of left liver three months after completing EBRT. (**e–f**) Completion regression of both the intrahepatic lesion and intrabiliary tumor thrombus 4.5 years after completing EBRT. (Numbers on the images represent dates in year-month-day format.)

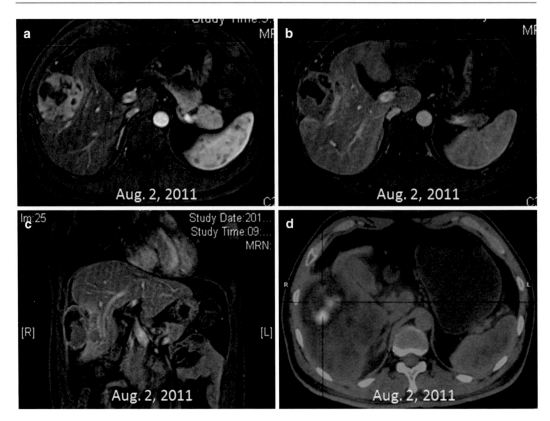

Fig. 17.6 A 49-year-old male (Case 1) with an approximately 7.0 × 6.5 cm mass with intratumoral hemorrhage located in the right lobe of the liver. (**a**) Axial arterial phase magnetic resonance (MR) image showing hyperenhancement of a mass in the right hepatic lobe. (**b**) Image showing washout in the portal venous phase. (**c**) Sagittal MR images showing the tumor invading the diaphragm and peritoneum. (**d**) Positron emission tomography/computed tomography image demonstrating hypermetabolic activity in the region, consistent with viable tumor

A limited number of clinical reports have been published regarding the use of RT for HCC metastases to the pancreas, spleen, ovary, diaphragm, or subcutaneous tissue. Indeed, RT can be considered for any unresectable metastatic lesion to alleviate symptoms. However, whether RT improves survival in these situations is unclear because of the small number of reported cases.

17.4   Typical Cases: Description and Discussion

17.4.1 Case 1

17.4.1.1   Description

A 49-year-old male was diagnosed with HCC (7.0 × 6.5 × 6.5 cm), as shown in Fig. 17.6, and underwent extensive local excision of the tumor in August 2011. His serum AFP level was negative after surgery. In February 2012, multiple recurrent intrahepatic nodules were detected on MRI (Fig. 17.7a–d), and the patient underwent TACE in March and May 2012. Follow-up CT in August 2012 revealed an enlarged cardiophrenic angle LN (Fig. 17.7e); intrahepatic lesions, which had responded to TACE with Lipiodol deposition (Fig. 17.7f); recurrent HCC at the resection margin in the right abdominal wall (Fig. 17.7g); and costophrenic angle and peripancreatic LNM (Fig. 17.7h). The LNs were subsequently confirmed to be metastatic by PET/CT (Fig. 17.7i–l). Routine blood test results were normal. The patient was treated with IGRT, with treatment fields covering all extrahepatic lesions, including the LNs and abdominal wall lesion, as shown in Fig. 17.8.

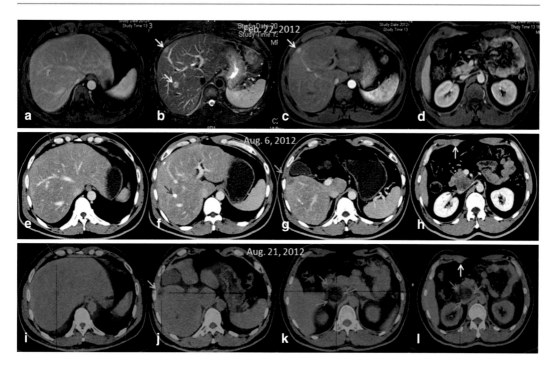

Fig. 17.7 Follow-up imaging of Case 1 after hepatectomy. (**a–d**) Magnetic resonance imaging six months after hepatectomy. (**a**) Enlargement of a right cardiophrenic angle lymph node, shown with a pink arrow. (**b**) Two lesions located in the right lobe in T2-weighted imaging, as indicated by white arrows. (**c**) Only one lesion is seen in the arterial phase. (**d**) No tumor is seen in this image. (**e–h**) Computed tomography (CT) scans one year after hepatectomy and transarterial chemoembolization. (**e**) The enlarged right cardiophrenic angle lymph node is again visualized (pink arrow). (**f**) Deposition of Lipiodol is present in both right lobe lesions (red arrows). (**g**) Low-density lesion between the resection margin and diaphragm, as indicated by the green arrow. (**h**) Compared with D, new lesions are seen in the right lower abdominal wall (belongs to cardiophrenic angle lymph node; white arrow) and inferior pancreatic lymph nodes (between the portal vein and inferior vena cava; orange arrows). (**i–l**) Positron emission tomography/CT images. (**i**) Right cardiophrenic angle lymph node without radioactivity uptake (pink arrow). (**j**) This image corresponds to G and shows slightly increased radioactivity uptake in the intrahepatic lesion (green arrow). (**k**) Radioactivity uptake is increased in an inferior pancreatic lymph node (orange arrows), indicative of lymph node metastasis. (**l**) This image corresponds to H and shows increased radioactivity uptake in the right lower abdominal wall lesion (white arrow) and peripancreatic lymph node (orange arrows)

After IGRT, the patient was followed as an outpatient from November 2012 to April 2014 (Fig. 17.9). The LNs and abdominal wall lesion both exhibited a partial response to RT; however, a de novo right lobe intrahepatic lesion was detected in April 2014 (Fig. 17.9j, k). The patient underwent TACE in April 2014, June 2014, and January 2015 for this hepatic lesion. Unfortunately, the lesion progressed and invaded the umbilical portion of the PV (Fig. 17.10a, b) and metastasized to right adrenal gland in September 2015 (Fig. 17.10c). The patient then received a second course of IGRT, in which the radiation fields included the right lobe intrahepatic lesion, PVTT, right adrenal metastasis, and peripancreatic LNs, as shown in Fig. 17.11. The PTV received 55 Gy in 25 fractions. The only adverse effect was mild nausea. The right lobe lesion, PVTT, right adrenal metastasis, and LNM responded partially to IGRT, according to follow-up MR images in March and December 2016. However, these images showed de novo nodules in the left lobe of the liver (Fig. 17.10e–l). The patient underwent TACE for these nodules, but the intrahepatic tumor gradually progressed, and the patient died of liver failure in March 2019.

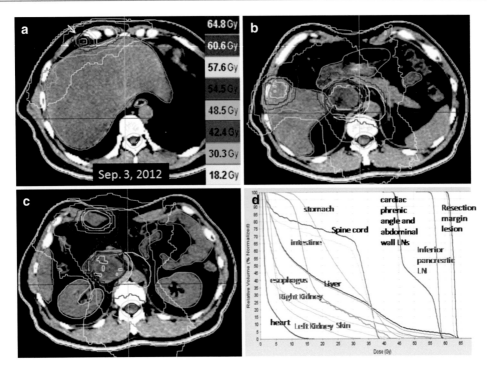

Fig. 17.8 Dose distribution of image-guided radiotherapy for Case 1. (**a**) Planning target volume (PTV) with 44 Gy/20 fractions for the right cardiophrenic angle lymph node (LN). (**b**) PTV with 60 Gy/20 fractions for the resection margin lesion and 56 Gy/20 fractions for the inferior pancreatic LN. (**c**) PTV with 44 Gy/20 fractions for the right lower abdominal wall lesion and 56 Gy/20 fractions for the inferior pancreatic LN. (**d**) Dose–volume histogram

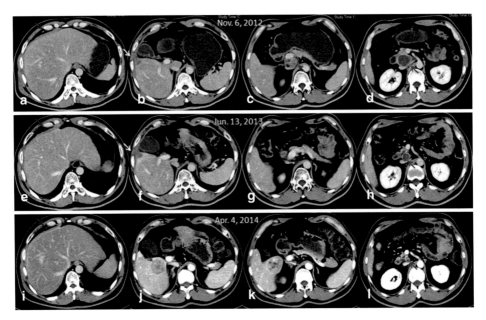

Fig. 17.9 Follow-up computed tomography (CT) scans after the first course of radiotherapy (RT) of Case 1. (**a–d**) Images 40 days after completing RT. (**e–h**) Images eight months after completing RT. (**i–l**) Images 18 months after completing RT. The right cardiophrenic angle metastatic lymph node (pink arrows), resection margin lesion (white arrows), and inferior pancreatic lymph node metastasis (blue arrows) became gradually smaller over time, and the right lower abdominal wall lesion exhibited a complete response to RT. A de novo nodule (red arrows) is seen in the right lobe of the liver on follow-up CT images (**j** and **k**) in April 2014

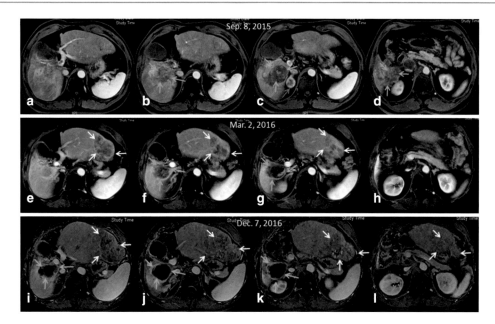

Fig. 17.10 Later follow-up imaging results of Case 1. (**a–d**) Three years after the first course of radiotherapy (RT), the intrahepatic tumor (green arrows) is shown invading the portal vein (pink arrows), and adrenal metastasis (orange arrow) is seen in magnetic resonance images. The inferior pancreatic lymph node (LN) (blue arrow) is larger than in April 2014. (**e–h**) Images four months and (**i–l**) 13 months after completing a second course of RT. As shown, the portal vein tumor thrombus had a complete response to RT, and the right lobe intrahepatic nodule (green arrows), adrenal metastasis (orange arrows), and inferior pancreatic LN became smaller (green arrows). However, a new mass is visualized in the left lobe of the liver (white arrows)

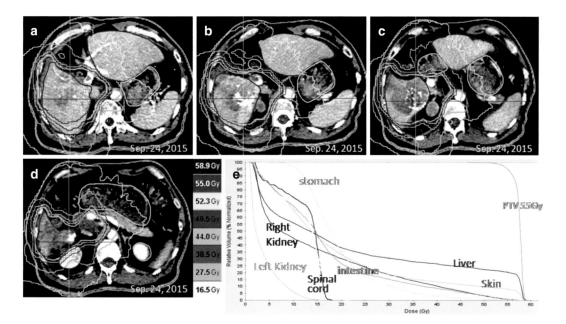

Fig. 17.11 Dose distribution of the second course of image-guided radiotherapy for Case 1. (**a–d**) The right lobe intrahepatic tumor, portal vein tumor thrombi, right adrenal metastasis, and inferior pancreatic lymph node metastasis are all covered in the radiation fields, with the planning target volume (PTV) receiving 55 Gy in 25 fractions. (**e**) Dose–volume histogram showing doses to the tumors (PTV) and organs at risk

17.4.1.2 Discussion

Does RT Decrease Mortality of Patients with HCC Who Have Abdominal LNM?

Most patients with LNM from HCC are no longer eligible for surgical resection, TACE, PEI, or RFA. We analyzed patients with HCC and abdominal LNM who either were or were not treated with EBRT over the same time period at our institution. The effect on survival was significant, with EBRT reducing mortality secondary to nodal involvement [52]. Our latest data from 191 patients with LNM treated with EBRT revealed a median OS of 8.0 months [64]. A similar result was obtained by researchers from Korea [60].

What Dosage Can Be Delivered to Abdominal LNM?

Radiation complications consistently increase as radiation dose increases, and gastrointestinal bleeding is a major potential complication of abdominal RT. With EBRT doses of 55 Gy to the duodenum or stomach, the risk of severe gastrointestinal complications varies from 5 to 10%, depending on the parameter evaluated. At doses > 55 Gy, approximately one-third of patients have been reported to develop severe gastrointestinal adverse effects [140]. These findings regarding gastric and duodenal tolerance to EBRT are consistent with our results. In our study, we divided patients receiving EBRT for abdominal LNM into two groups, based on the radiation dose: one group received ≥5 6 Gy, and the other group received <56 Gy. The incidence of gastrointestinal bleeding was greater in the higher dose group (44.4%; 4/9), and this complication was clearly related to radiation dose [54]. A total dose between 50 and 56 Gy is possibly effective as palliative treatment. We recommend <56 Gy as the most appropriate radiation dose based on our experience.

Can RT Improve Survival in Patients with HCC Who Have PV or IVC Tumor Thrombi?

HCC patients with PVTT have a poor prognosis, with a median survival time of only 2.4–2.7 months without treatment. Our retrospective data showed that the median survival of 181 patients with PV and/or IVC tumor thrombi referred for EBRT was 10.7 months [48]. A comparative study of patients treated at our institution over the same period showed that median and one-year survival were 8.9 months and 34.4% in the EBRT group, in contrast to 4 months and 11.4% in the non-EBRT group [26]. As shown in Table 17.2, which summarizes a series of published reports comparing outcomes with or without EBRT, RT improves survival of HCC patients with PV/IVC tumor thrombi.

What Dosage Can Be Delivered to PV and/or IVC Tumor Thrombi?

Local control rates consistently increase as the radiation dose increases. However, radiation doses to PV and/or IVC tumor thrombi are limited by organs at risk, such as the gastrointestinal tract and liver, which typically dictate the need for a reduced dose. We usually schedule a full radiation dosage of up to 50 Gy, but reduced doses are considered based on tolerance of the gastrointestinal tract and liver to EBRT.

Does RT Shrink Adrenal Metastatic HCC Lesions?

The most effective treatment modality for adrenal metastases from HCC remains unclear. Based on case reports, various treatment approaches have included surgical resection, TACE, and PEI. Surgical resection is usually not considered because unresectable intrahepatic tumors, tumor thrombi, LN involvement, and/or synchronous distant metastases to bone or lungs are often present upon diagnosis of adrenal metastasis. Theoretically, TACE should be effective for treating adrenal metastases because metastatic lesions (like primary HCC) are hypervascular. However, TACE is usually not performed because catheterization of the adrenal arteries and complete embolization of the adrenal gland is anatomically and technically challenging. In two studies of 134 and 81 patients with adrenal gland metastases from HCC who were treated with RT, median

Table 17.17 Comparison of survival after IGRT versus non-IGRT

BCLC stage	First author and year	Median overall survival (months) Non-IGRT[a]	IGRT	P value
B (confined to liver)	Jiang T, 2017 [141]	24.0	44.7	0.009
C (portal vein tumor thrombi)	Hou JZ, 2016 [12]	10.5	15.5	0.05
C (lymph node metastases)	Zhang HG, 2019 [142]	9.7	15.3	0.098
C (lung metastases)	Jiang W, 2012 [114] Sun TW, 2016 [115]	16.7	29.6	<0.001

BCLC Barcelona-Clinic Liver Cancer, *IGRT* image-guided radiotherapy
[a]Treated with 3-dimensional conformal radiotherapy

survival times were 12.8 and 13.5 months, respectively (Table 17.9).

Is IGRT Superior to Non-IGRT for Overall Survival and Local Control?

Yes, IGRT is superior to non-IGRT for treatment outcomes. Table 17.17 shows the results of studies comparing survival after IGRT versus non-IGRT (i.e., treatment with 3D-CRT). We treated Case 1 with two courses of HT-based IGRT because this allowed the delivery of a higher radiation dose than 3D-CRT, with more accuracy and superior dose distribution around the tumor and liver. This patient survived 79 months after LNM, and 42 months after both PVTT and adrenal metastasis, which was likely attributable to the IGRT.

Why Was the Tumor in the Left Hepatic Lobe Not Treated with a Third Course of RT?

The patient underwent local hepatectomy and two courses of RT to the right liver. Right liver atrophy was revealed on CT scans from March and December 2016. As the normal liver volume was estimated to be <600 mL, the risk of radiation-induced liver disease was too high to consider another course of RT.

17.4.2 Case 2

17.4.2.1 Case Description

A 57-year-old female was diagnosed in February 2018 with HCC based on MRI results and an elevated AFP and abnormal prothrombin. The mass was approximately 12.3 × 7.5 cm and located in the right lobe of the liver, as shown in Fig. 17.12a. The patient was diagnosed with HCC, Barcelona-Clinic Liver Cancer stage B. She received TACE in March and April 2018, and follow-up MRI in May 2018 showed that most of the tumor was necrotic except for a small lesion at the edge of capsule (Fig. 17.12b). The patient was referred to our department for consolidation RT in May 2018 and received 55 Gy in 22 fractions, as shown in Fig. 17.12c, f. She had mild anorexia during RT, which resolved within one month after completing treatment. A CR to RT was achieved for the intrahepatic tumor, based on European Association for the Study of the Liver (EASL) criteria (Fig. 17.12d, e).

The patient was followed as an outpatient and, after transiently decreasing, her AFP and abnormal prothrombin levels both rose again in August 2018, as shown in Fig. 17.12g. Chest CT in August 2018 revealed a total of four lesions distributed between her lungs (Fig. 17.13A1–A4), which were suggestive of lung metastases. Upon repeat chest CT three months later, all lung nodules were larger (Fig. 17.13B) except for one nodule in the right upper lung (Fig. 17.13B1). At that time, both the AFP and abnormal prothrombin were further increased. Thus, we assumed that the nodules increasing its size were metastases from HCC, but the stable lesions were calcification foci. We delivered SBRT (60 Gy in 10 fractions) to three metastatic lesions, as shown in Fig. 17.13C1–C4. Follow-up CT revealed CR of the lung metastatic lesions (Fig. 17.13D2–D4, E2–E4) and continued stability of the calcification foci (Fig. 17.13D1, E1). Increases in AFP and abnormal prothrombin mirrored the imaging findings (Fig. 17.12g) and returned to normal level after SBRT. CR to SBRT was achieved for the lung metastases, according to the modified Response Evaluation Criteria in Solid Tumors. The patient experienced no symptoms during

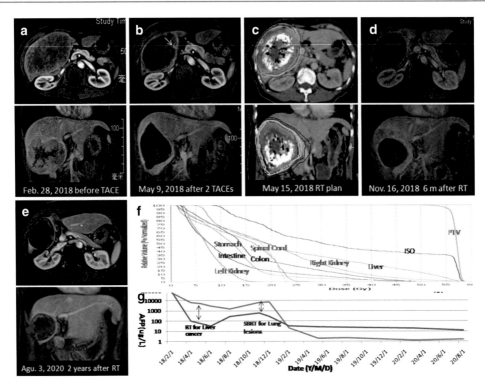

Fig. 17.12 Changes in intrahepatic tumor before and after conventional external-beam radiotherapy

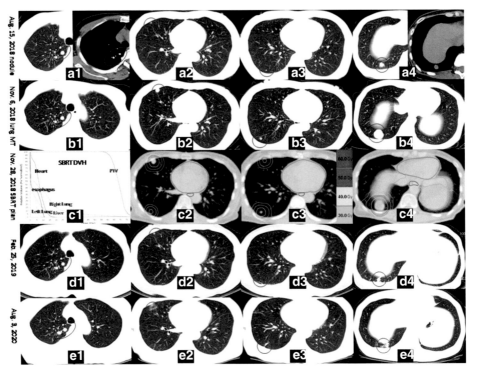

Fig. 17.13 Changes in lung nodules (including calcification foci) before and after stereotactic body radiotherapy

SBRT except mild weakness. After SBRT, she began treatment with sorafenib 400 mg, twice daily, but discontinued it after one month because of intolerable toxicity.

17.4.2.2 Discussion

Diagnosis
This patient was diagnosed clinically with HCC based on her MR images and tumor markers (elevated AFP and abnormal prothrombin). Use of clinical examinations to diagnose HCC is common practice in Asian countries. With respect to the pulmonary masses, no criteria are available to clearly differentiate benign pulmonary nodules from metastatic lesions from HCC. Thus, we followed this patient with chest CT and found that the nodules enlarged in parallel with an increase in tumor markers. Thus, they were presumed to represent metastases. These nodules responded completely to SBRT, confirming the diagnosis of pulmonary metastasis from HCC.

Treatments
When a physician considers RT, six fundamental questions must be answered:

What Is the Indication for RT?
TACE is unable to induce complete necrosis of HCC tumors > 5 cm in diameter. Because larger tumors have both arterial and portal blood supply allowing tumor cells to remain viable, even following complete arterial embolization by TACE, these cells become the source of recurrence and metastasis after treatment. However, combining TACE with EBRT is a promising strategy to overcome this problem. Our retrospective study suggested that median OS of patients treated with TACE plus RT was 23.1 months, which was significantly better than that observed in patients who received TACE alone [143]. Similar findings have been reported by other investigators, with TACE plus RT providing more therapeutic benefit than TACE alone when treating HCC. Thus, the combination is recommended for suitable patients with unresectable HCC [144]. Chapter 13 "Adjuvant RT for incomplete TACE" discusses this concept in further detail. In Case 2, a residual nodule was present on follow-up MR images (Fig. 17.12b) after initial treatment with TACE, and subsequent addition of EBRT resulted in a CR, based on EASL evaluation criteria.

The lung is the organ most affected by extrahepatic metastases from HCC. Pulmonary metastases tend to be multiple, but they progress more slowly than primary intrahepatic lesions. Thus, death from lung metastases occurs in no more than 20% of patients with HCC [145]. In our review of data from 45 patients who received HT combined with sorafenib for the treatment of pulmonary metastases from HCC [115], median OS after diagnosis of pulmonary metastases was 26.4 months and two-year survival was 46.7%. Thus, RT may be beneficial for pulmonary metastases from HCC. As demonstrated in Case 2, RT can improve local tumor control and increase DFS.

What Is the Goal of RT?
In Case 2, RT was regarded as adjuvant or consolidation treatment after an incomplete response was achieved with TACE. RT is not simply a form of palliative treatment, as use of RT may completely eliminate visible intrahepatic lesion. Similarly, the goal of RT for pulmonary metastases may also be curative. Because pulmonary oligometastases were observed in this case, we performed RT with curative intent, administering 60 Gy in 10 fractions (which is an absolutely radical dose).

What Is the Treatment Volume?
In Case 2, we treated the gross tumor visualized on MRI or CT images. There was no need to prevent potential LN metastases in either the liver or lungs.

What Is the Planned Treatment Technique?
In patients with HCC, outcomes are much better with IGRT than without IGRT (see Table 17.17). Therefore, we selected IGRT for intrahepatic tumors and SBRT for pulmonary oligometastases in Case 2.

What Is the Planned Treatment Dose?
As the goal of RT for intrahepatic HCC was adjuvant or consolidation treatment, the higher the

radiation dose, the better would be the local control rate. Although the whole liver mean dose was only 13 Gy in Case 2, the colon was close to the tumor (Fig. 17.12f). Thus, we limited the dose to the colon to <45 Gy. Similarly, the goal of RT for pulmonary metastases was curative treatment, so we used radical doses for the metastatic lesions. SBRT with 60 Gy in 10 fractions completely controls small pulmonary metastases from HCC.

What Types of Treatment Could Be Combined with RT to Improve Patient Outcomes?

TACE can decrease tumor burden by inducing ischemic necrosis. Use of TACE permits the radiation dose to be reduced to a safe level, while achieving a higher response rate. Thus, combining TACE with RT is recommended to improve outcomes related to intrahepatic HCC.

When considering pulmonary metastases, the combination of helical tomotherapy (HT) and sorafenib ($n = 23$) has been shown to increase median OS to 29.6 months, which is longer than OS with HT alone ($n = 22$; 23.0 months; $P = 0.031$) or sorafenib alone ($n = 18$; 25.0 months; $P = 0.018$). These results indicate that HT is beneficial for treating pulmonary metastases, especially when combined with sorafenib [115]. Thus, we recommend combining sorafenib with HT, although the drug was not tolerated by Case 2.

References

1. Pirisi M, Avellini C, Fabris C, et al. Portal vein thrombosis in hepatocellular carcinoma: age and sex distribution in an autopsy study. J Cancer Res Clin Oncol. 1998;124:397–400.
2. Stuart KE, Anand AJ, Jenkins RL. Hepatocellular carcinoma in the United States. Prognostic feature, treatment outcome, and survival. Cancer. 1996;77:2217–22.
3. Fong Y, Sun RL, Jarnagin W, Blumgart LH. An analysis of 412 cases of hepatocellular carcinoma at a Western Center. Ann Surg. 1999;229:790–800.
4. Rabe C, Pilz T, Klostermann C, et al. Clinical characteristics and outcome of a cohort of 101 patients with hepatocellular carcinoma. World J Gastroenterol. 2001;7:208–15.
5. Ando E, Yamashita F, Tanaka M, Tanikawa K. A novel chemotherapy for advanced hepatocellular carcinoma with tumor thrombosis of the main trunk of the portal vein. Cancer. 1997;79:1890–6.
6. The Cancer of the Liver Italian Program Investigators. A new prognostic system for hepatocellualr carcinoma: a retrospective study of 435 patients. Hepatology. 1998;28:751–5.
7. Wei X, Jiang Y, Zhang X, et al. Neoadjuvant three-dimensional conformal radiotherapy for resectable hepatocellular carcinoma with portal vein tumor thrombus: a randomized, open-label, multicenter controlled study. J Clin Oncol. 2019;37(24):2141–51.
8. Abou-Alfa GK, Shi Q, Knox JJ, et al. Assessment of treatment with sorafenib plus doxorubicin vs sorafenib alone in patients with advanced hepatocellular carcinoma: phase 3 CALGB 80802 randomized clinical trial. JAMA Oncol. 2019;5(11):1582–8.
9. He M, Li Q, Zou R, et al. Sorafenib plus hepatic arterial infusion of oxaliplatin, fluorouracil, and leucovorin vs sorafenib alone for hepatocellular carcinoma with portal vein invasion: a randomized clinical trial. JAMA Oncol. 2019;5(7):953–60.
10. Yoon SM, Ryoo BY, Lee SJ, Kim JH, Shin JH, An JH, Lee HC, Lim YS. Efficacy and safety of transarterial chemoembolization plus external beam radiotherapy vs sorafenib in hepatocellular carcinoma with macroscopic vascular invasion: a randomized clinical trial. JAMA Oncol. 2018;4(5):661–9.
11. Kodama K, Kawaoka T, Aikata H, et al. Comparison of outcome of hepatic arterial infusion chemotherapy combined with radiotherapy and sorafenib for advanced hepatocellular carcinoma patients with major portal vein tumor thrombosis. Oncology. 2018;94(4):215–22.
12. Hou JZ, Zeng ZC, Wang BL, Yang P, Zhang JY, Mo HF. High dose radiotherapy with image-guided hypo-IMRT for hepatocellular carcinoma with portal vein and/or inferior vena cava tumor thrombi is more feasible and efficacious than conventional 3D-CRT. Jpn J Clin Oncol. 2016;46(4):357–62.
13. Wang K, Guo WX, Chen MS, et al. Multimodality treatment for hepatocellular carcinoma with portal vein tumor thrombus: a large-scale, multicenter, propensity matthcing score analysis. Medicine (Baltimore). 2016;95(11):e3015.
14. Kim GA, Shim JH, Yoon SM, et al. Comparison of chemoembolization with and without radiation therapy and sorafenib for advanced hepatocellular carcinoma with portal vein tumor thrombosis: a propensity score analysis. J Vasc Interv Radiol. 2015;26(3):320–9.e6.
15. Onishi H, Nouso K, Nakamura S, et al. Efficacy of hepatic arterial infusion chemotherapy in combination with irradiation for advanced hepatocellular carcinoma with portal vein invasion. Hepatol Int. 2015;9(1):105–12.
16. Lu DH, Fei ZL, Zhou JP, et al. A comparison between three-dimensional conformal radiotherapy combined with interventional treatment and interventional treatment alone for hepatocellular carcinoma with portal vein tumour thrombosis. J Med Imaging Radiat Oncol. 2015;59(1):109–14.

17. Nakazawa T, Hidaka H, Shibuya A, et al. Overall survival in response to sorafenib versus radiotherapy in unresectable hepatocellular carcinoma with major portal vein tumor thrombosis: propensity score analysis. BMC Gastroenterol. 2014;14:84.

18. Tang QH, Li AJ, Yang GM, et al. Surgical resection versus conformal radiotherapy combined with TACE for resectable hepatocellular carcinoma with portal vein tumor thrombus: a comparative study. World J Surg. 2013;37(6):1362–70.

19. Chuma M, Taguchi H, Yamamoto Y, et al. Efficacy of therapy for advanced hepatocellular carcinoma: intra-arterial 5-fluorouracil and subcutaneous interferon with image-guided radiation. J Gastroenterol Hepatol. 2011;26(7):1123–32.

20. Chung YH, Song IIH, Song BC, et al. Combined therapy consisting of intraarterial cisplatin infusion and systemic interferon-α for hepatocellular carcinoma patients with major portal vein thrombosis or distant metastasis. Cancer. 2000;88:1986–91.

21. Ando E, Tanaka M, Yamashita F, et al. Hepatic arterial infusion chemotherapy for advanced hepatocellular carcinoma with portal vein tumor thrombosis: analysis of 48 cases. Cancer. 2002;95:588–95.

22. Yen FS, Wu JC, Kuo BI, et al. Transcatheter arterial embolization for hepatocellular carcinoma with portal vein thrombosis. J Gastroenterol Hepatol. 1995;10:237–40.

23. Minagawa M, Makuuchi M, Takayama TK, et al. Selection criteria for hepatectomy in patients with hepatocellular carcinoma and portal vein tumor thrombus. Ann Surg. 2001;233:379–84.

24. Cheng SH, Lin YM, Chuang VP, et al. A pilot study of three dimensional conformal radiotherapy in unresectable hepatocellular carcinoma. J Gastroenterol Hepatol. 1999;14:1025–33.

25. Ishikura S, Ogino T, Furuse J, et al. Radiotherapy after transcatheter arterial chemoembolization for patients with hepatocellular carcinoma and portal vein tumor thrombus. Am J Clin Oncol. 2002;25:189–93.

26. Zeng ZC, Fan J, Zhou J, et al. A comparison of treatment combinations with and without radiotherapy for hepatocellular carcinoma with portal vein and/or inferior vena cava tumor thrombus. Int J Radiation Oncology Boil Phys. 2005;61:432–43.

27. Nakazawa T, Adachi S, Kitano M, et al. Potential prognostic benefits of radiotherapy as an initial treatment for patients with unresectable advanced hepatocellular carcinoma with invasion to intrahepatic large vessels. Oncology. 2007;73:90–7.

28. Koo JE, Kim JH, Lim YS, et al. Combination of transarterial chemoembolization and three-dimensional conformal radiotherapy for hepatocellular carcinoma with inferior vena cava tumor thrombus. Int J Radiat Oncol Biol Phys. 2010;78:180–7.

29. Chen LW, Chien RN, Fang KM, et al. Elucidating therapeutic effects on patients with hepatocellular carcinoma and main portal vein thrombosis. Hepato-Gastroenterology. 2010;57(98):228–31.

30. Kim DY, Park W, Lim DH, et al. Three-dimensional conformal radiotherapy for portal vein thrombosis of hepatocellular carcinoma. Cancer. 2005;103:2419–26.

31. Nakagawa K, Yamashita H, Shiraishi K, et al. Radiation therapy for portal venous invasion by hepatocellular carcinoma. World J Gastroenterol. 2005;11:7237–41.

32. Lin CS, Jen YM, Chiu SY, et al. Treatment of portal vein tumor thrombosis of hepatoma patients with either stereotactic radiotherapy or three-dimensional conformal radiotherapy. Jpn J Clin Oncol. 2006;36:212–7.

33. Toya R, Murakami R, Baba Y, et al. Conformal radiation therapy for portal vein tumor thrombosis of hepatocellular carcinoma. Radiother Oncol. 2007;84:266–71.

34. Yoon SM, Lim YS, Won HJ, et al. Radiotherapy plus transarterial chemoembolization for hepatocellular carcinoma invading the portal vein: long-term patient outcomes. Int J Radiat Oncol Biol Phys. 2012;82:2004–11.

35. Hou JZ, Zeng ZC, Zhang JY, et al. Influence of tumor thrombus location on the outcome of external-beam radiation therapy in advanced hepatocellular carcinoma with macrovascular invasion. Int J Radiat Oncol Biol Phys. 2012;84:362–8.

36. Rim CH, Yang DS, Park YJ, et al. Effectiveness of high-dose three-dimensional conformal radiotherapy in hepatocellular carcinoma with portal vein thrombosis. Jpn J Clin Oncol. 2012;42:721–9.

37. Zhang XB, Wang JH, Yan ZP, et al. Hepatocellular carcinoma with main portal vein tumor thrombus. Treatment with 3-D conformal radiotherapy after portal vein stenting and transarterial chemoembolization. Cancer. 2009;115:1245–52.

38. Han KH, Seong J, Kim JK, et al. Pilot clinical trial of localized concurrent chemoradiation therapy for locally advanced hepatocellular carcinoma with portal vein thrombosis. Cancer. 2008;113:995–1003.

39. Katamura Y, Aikata H, Takaki S, et al. Intra-arterial 5-Fu/interferon combination therapy for advanced hepatocellular carcinoma with or without 3-dimensional conformal radiotherapy for portal vein tumor thrombosis. J Gastroenterol. 2009;44:492–502.

40. Kim BK, Kim DY, Byun HK, et al. Efficacy and safety of liver-directed concurrent chemoradiotherapy and sequential sorafenib for advanced hepatocellular carcinoma: a prospective phase 2 trial. Int J Radiat Oncol Biol Phys. 2020;107(1):106–15.

41. Kamiyama T, Nakanishi K, Yokoo H, et al. Efficacy of preoperative radiotherapy to portal vein tumor thrombus in the main trunk or first branch in patients with hepatocellular carcinoma. Int J Clin Oncol. 2007;12:363–8.

42. Kim J, Lee I, Kim J, et al. Clinical features of hepatocellular carcinoma patients undergoing resection after concurrent chemoradiation therapy. Int J Radiat Oncol Biol Phys. 2012;84:S336–7.

43. Shirabe K, Shimada M, Tsujita E, et al. Thrombectomy before hepatic resection for hepatocellular carcinoma with a tumor thrombus extending to the inferior vena cava. Int Surg. 2001;86:141–3.

44. Yogita S, Tashiro S, Harada M, et al. Hepatocellular carcinoma with extension into the right atrium: report of a successful liver resection by hepatic vascular exclusion using cardiopulmonary bypass. J Med Investig. 2000;47:155–60.

45. Wu CC, Hseih S, Ho WM, et al. Surgical treatment for recurrent hepatocellular carcinoma with tumor thrombi in right atrium: using cardiopulmonary bypass and deep hypothermic circulatory arrest. J Surg Oncol. 2000;74:227–31.

46. Rim CH, Jeong BK, Kim TH, Hee Kim J, Kang HC, Seong J. Effectiveness and feasibility of external beam radiotherapy for hepatocellular carcinoma with inferior vena cava and/or right atrium involvement: a multicenter trial in Korea (KROG 17-10). Int J Radiat Biol. 2020;96(6):759–66.

47. Murakami E, Aikata H, Miyaki D, et al. Hepatic arterial infusion chemotherapy using 5-fluorouracil and systemic interferon-α for advanced hepatocellular carcinoma in combination with or without three-dimensional conformal radiotherapy to venous tumor thrombosis in hepatic vein or inferior vena cava. Hepatol Res. 2012;42:442–53.

48. Zeng ZC, Fan J, Tang ZY, et al. Prognostic factors for hepatocellular carcinoma with macroscopic portal vein or inferior vena cava tumor thrombi receiving radiotherapy. Cancer Sci. 2008;99:2510–7.

49. Kim JY, Yoo EJ, Jang JW, Kwon JH, Kim KJ, Kay CS. Hypofractionated radiotherapy using helical tomotherapy for advanced hepatocellular carcinoma with portal vein tumor thrombosis. Radiat Oncol. 2013;8:15.

50. Sun HC, Zhuang PY, Qin LX, et al. Incidence and prognostic values of lymph node metastasis in operable hepatocellular carcinoma and evaluation of routine complete lymphadenectomy. J Surg Oncol. 2007;96:37–45.

51. Kobayashi S, Takahashi S, Kato Y, et al. Surgical treatment of lymph node metastases from hepatocellular carcinoma. J Hepatobiliary Pancreat Sci. 2011;18:559–66.

52. Watanabe J, Nakashima O, Kojiro M. Clinicopathologic study on lymph node metastasis of hepatocellular carcinoma: a retrospective study of 660 consecutive autopsy cases. Jpn J Clin Oncol. 1994;24:37–41.

53. Yuki K, Hirohashi S, Sakamoto M, et al. Growth and spread of hepatocellular carcinoma: a review of 240 consecutive autopsy cases. Cancer. 1990;66:2174–9.

54. Zeng ZC, Tang ZY, et al. Consideration of the role of radiotherapy for lymph node metastases in patients with HCC-A retrospective analysis for prognostic factors from 125 patients. Int J Radiation Oncology Boil Phys. 2005;63:1067–76.

55. Uenishi T, Hirohashi K, Shuto T, et al. The clinical significance of lymph node metastases in patients undergoing surgery for hepatocellular carcinoma. Surg Today. 2000;30:892–5.

56. Prat F, Chapat O, Ducot B, et al. A randomized trial of endoscopic drainage methods for inoperable malignant strictures of the common bile duct. Gastrointest Endosc. 1998;47:1–7.

57. Cheng AL, Guan Z, Chen Z, et al. Efficacy and safety of sorafenib in patients with advanced hepatocellular carcinoma according to baseline status: subset analyses of the phase III Sorafenib Asia-Pacific trial. Eur J Cancer. 2012;48(10):1452–65.

58. Chen SC, Lian SL, Chuang WL, et al. Radiotherapy in the treatment of hepatocellular carcinoma and its metastases. Cancer Chemother Pharmacol. 1992;31(suppl):103–5.

59. Omuraya M, Beppu T, Ishiko T, et al. Lymph node excision with laparotomy and chemo-radiation therapy for a hepatocellular carcinoma patient with multiple lymph node metastases. Gan To Kagaku Tyoho. 2001;28:1699–703.

60. Park YJ, Lim DH, Paik SW, et al. Radiation therapy for abdominal lymph node metastasis from hepatocellular carcinoma. J Gastroenterol. 2006;41:1099–106.

61. Yamashita H, Nakagawa K, Shiraishi K, et al. Radiotherapy for lymph node metastases in patients with hepatocellular carcinoma: retrospective study. J Gastroenterol Hepatol. 2007;22:523–7.

62. Toya R, Murakami R, Yasunaga T, et al. Radiation therapy for lymph node metastases from hepatocellular carcinoma. Hepato-Gastroenterology. 2009;56:476–80.

63. Kim K, Chie EK, Kim W, et al. Absence of symptom and intact liver function are positive prognosticators for patients undergoing radiotherapy for lymph node metastasis from hepatocellular carcinoma. Int J Radiat Oncol Biol Phys. 2010;78:729–34.

64. Chen YX, Zeng ZC, Fan J, et al. Defining prognostic factors of survival after external beam radiotherapy treatment of hepatocellular carcinoma with lymph node metastases. Clin Transl Oncol. 2013;15(9):732–40.

65. Zhang HG, Chen YX, Hu Y, et al. Image-guided intensity-modulated radiotherapy improves short-term survival for abdominal lymph node metastases from hepatocellular carcinoma. Ann Palliat Med. 2019;8(5):717–27.

66. Marsh JW, Dvorchik I, Bonham CA, et al. Is the pathologic TNM staging system for patients with hepatoma predictive of outcome? Cancer. 2000;88:538–43.

67. Uchino K, Tateishi R, Shiina S, et al. Hepatocellular carcinoma with extrahepatic metastasis: clinical features and prognostic factors. Cancer. 2011;117:4475–83.

68. Ho CL, Chen S, Cheng TK, Leung YL. PET/CT characteristics of isolated bone metastases in hepatocellular carcinoma. Radiology. 2011;258:515–23.

69. He J, Zeng ZC, Tang ZY, et al. Clinical features and prognostic factors in patients with bone metastases

from hepatocellular carcinoma receiving external-beam radiotherapy. Cancer. 2009;115:2710–20.

70. Cho HS, Oh JH, Han I, Kim HS. Survival of patients with skeletal metastases from hepatocellular carcinoma after surgical management. J Bone Joint Surg Br. 2009;91:1505–12.

71. Kashima M, Yamakado K, Takaki H, et al. Radiofrequency ablation for the treatment of bone metastases from hepatocellular carcinoma. AJR Am J Roentgenol. 2010;194:536–41.

72. Koike Y, Takizawa K, Ogawa Y, et al. Transcatheter arterial chemoembolization (TACE) or embolization (TAE) for symptomatic bone metastases as a palliative treatment. Cardiovasc Intervent Radiol. 2011;34(4):793–801.

73. Uemura A, Fujimoto H, Yasuda S, et al. Transcatheter arterial embolization for bone metastases from hepatocellular carcinoma. Eur Radiol. 2001;11:1457–62.

74. Katamura Y, Aikata H, Hashimoto Y, et al. Zoledronic acid delays disease progression of bone metastases from hepatocellular carcinoma. Hepatol Res. 2010;40:1195–203.

75. Montella L, Addeo R, Palmieri G, et al. Zoledronic acid in the treatment of bone metastases by hepatocellular carcinoma: a case series. Cancer Chemother Pharmacol. 2010;65:1137–43.

76. Suzawa N, Yamakado K, Takaki H, et al. Complete regression of multiple painful bone metastases from hepatocellular carcinoma after administration of strontium-89 chloride. Ann Nucl Med. 2010;24:617–20.

77. Kaizu T, Karasawa K, Tanaka Y, et al. Radiotherapy for osseous metastases from hepatocellular carcinoma: a retrospective study of 57 patients. Am J Gastroenterol. 1998;93:2167–71.

78. Seong J, Koom WS, Park HC. Radiotherapy for painful bone metastases from hepatocellular carcinoma. Liver Int. 2005;25:261–5.

79. Nakamura N, Igaki H, Yamashita H, et al. A retrospective study of radiotherapy for spinal bone metastases from hepatocellular carcinoma (HCC). Jpn J Clin Oncol. 2007;37:38–43.

80. He J, Zeng ZC, Fan J, et al. Clinical features and prognostic factors in patients with bone metastases from hepatocellular carcinoma after liver transplantation. BMC Cancer. 2011;11:492.

81. Kneuertz PJ, Cosgrove DP, Cameron AM, et al. Multidisciplinary management of recurrent hepatocellular carcinoma following liver transplantation. J Gastrointest Surg. 2012;16:874–81.

82. Tung WC, Huang YJ, Leung SW, et al. Incidence of needle tract seeding and responses of soft tissue metastasis by hepatocellular carcinoma postradiotherapy. Liver Int. 2007;27:192–200.

83. Szpakowski JL, Drasin TE, Lyon LL. Rate of seeding with biopsies and ablations of hepatocellular carcinoma: a retrospective cohort study. Hepatol Commun. 2017;1(9):841–51.

84. He J, Shi S, Ye L, Ma G, Pan X, Huang Y, Zeng Z. A randomized trial of conventional fraction versus hypofraction radiotherapy for bone metastases from hepatocellular carcinoma. J Cancer. 2019;10(17):4031–7.

85. Kim SU, Kim DY, Park JY, et al. Hepatocellular carcinoma presenting with bone metastasis: clinical characteristics and prognostic factors. J Cancer Res Clin Oncol. 2008;134:1377–84.

86. Katyal S, Oliver JH III, Peterson MS, Ferris JV, Carr BS, Baron RL. Extrahepatic metastases of hepatocellular carcinoma. Radiology. 2000;216:698–703.

87. Nakashima T, Okuda K, Kojiro M, Jimi A, Yamaguchi R, Sakamoto K, et al. Pathology of hepatocellular carcinoma in Japan. 232 consecutive cases autopsied in ten years. Cancer. 1983;51:863–77.

88. Momoi H, Shimahara Y, Terajima H, et al. Management of adrenal metastasis from hepatocellular carcinoma. Surg Today. 2002;32:1035–41.

89. Park JS, Yoon DS, Kim KS, et al. What is the best treatment modality for adrenal metastasis from hepatocellular carcinoma? J Surg Oncol. 2007;96:32–6.

90. Taniai N, Egami K, Wada M, Tajiri T, Onda M. Adrenal metastasis from hepatocellular carcinoma: report of 3 cases. Hepato-Gastroenterology. 1999;46:2523–8.

91. Shibata T, Maetani Y, Ametani F, et al. Percutaneous ethanol injection for treatment of adrenal metastasis from hepatocellular carcinoma. Am J Roentgenol. 2000;174:333–5.

92. Yamakado K, Anai H, Takaki H, et al. Adrenal metastasis from hepatocellular carcinoma: radiofrequency ablation combined with adrenal arterial chemoembolization in six patients. Am J Roentgenol. 2009;192:300–5.

93. Zeng ZC, Tang ZY, Fan J, et al. Radiation therapy for adrenal gland metastases from hepatocellular carcinoma. Jpn J Clin Oncol. 2005;35:61–7.

94. Zhou LY, Zeng ZC, Fan J, et al. Radiotherapy treatment of adrenal gland metastases from hepatocellular carcinoma: clinical features and prognostic factors. BMC Cancer. 2014;14:878.

95. Chen B, Hu Y, Liu J, Cao AN, Ye LX, Zeng ZC. Respiratory motion of adrenal gland metastases: analyses using four-dimensional computed tomography images. Phys Med. 2017;38:54–8.

96. Yuan BY, Hu Y, Zhang L, Chen YH, Dong YY, Zeng ZC. Radiotherapy for adrenal gland metastases from hepatocellular carcinoma. Clin Transl Oncol. 2017;19(9):1154–60.

97. Liver Cancer Study Group of Japan. Primary liver cancer in Japan. Clinicopathologic features and results of surgical treatment. Ann Surg. 1990;211:277–87.

98. Kakumu S. Trends in liver cancer researched by the Liver Cancer Study Group of Japan. Hepatol Res. 2002;24:S21–7.

99. Ikai I, Itai Y, Okita K, et al. Report of the 15th follow-up survey of primary liver cancer. Hepatol Res. 2004;28:21–9.

100. Yoon KT, Kim JK, Kim DY, et al. Role of 18F-fluorodeoxyglucose positron emission tomogra-

phy in detecting extrahepatic metastasis in pretreatment staging of hepatocellular carcinoma. Oncology. 2007;72:104–10.

101. Natsuizaka M, Omura T, Akaike T, et al. Clinical features of hepatocellular carcinoma with extrahepatic metastases. J Gastroenterol Hepatol. 2005;20:1781–7.

102. Taketomi A, Toshima T, Kitagawa D, et al. Predictors of extrahepatic recurrence after curative hepatectomy for hepatocellular carcinoma. Ann Surg Oncol. 2010;17:2740–6.

103. Yang T, Lu JH, Lin C, et al. Concomitant lung metastasis in patients with advanced hepatocellular carcinoma. World J Gastroenterol. 2012;18:2533–9.

104. Zhang SM, Zeng ZC, Tang ZY, et al. Prognostic analysis of pulmonary metastases from hepatocellular carcinoma. Hepatol Int. 2008;2:237–43.

105. Zheng SS, Chen J, Wang WL, et al. Recurrence and metastasis of hepatocellular carcinoma after liver transplantation: single center experiences. Zhonghua Wai Ke Za Zhi. 2008;46:1609–13.

106. Zhang M, Dai C, Zhu H, et al. Cyclophilin A promotes human hepatocellular carcinoma cell metastasis via regulation of MMP3 and MMP9. Mol Cell Biochem. 2011;357:387–95.

107. Duan F, Wang MQ, Liu FY, et al. Sorafenib in combination with transarterial chemoembolization and bronchial arterial chemoinfusion in the treatment of hepatocellular carcinoma with pulmonary metastasis. Asia Pac J Clin Oncol. 2012;8:156–63.

108. Hu HT, Yao QJ, Meng YL, Li HL, Zhang H, Luo JP, Guo CY, Geng X. Arsenic trioxide intravenous infusion combined with transcatheter arterial chemoembolization for the treatment of hepatocellular carcinoma with pulmonary metastasis: long-term outcome analysis. J Gastroenterol Hepatol. 2017;32(2):295–300.

109. Katamura Y, Aikata H, Kimura Y, et al. Successful treatment of pulmonary metastases associated with advanced hepatocellular carcinoma by systemic 5-fluorouracil combined with interferon-alpha in a hemodialysis patient. Hepatol Res. 2009;39:415–20.

110. Tomokuni A, Marubashi S, Nagano H, et al. A case of complete response to S-1 therapy for multiple pulmonary recurrences of hepatocellular carcinoma after hepatic resection. Gan To Kagaku Ryoho. 2009;36:2383–5.

111. Koyama J, Honjo S, Morizono R, et al. Hepatocellular carcinoma with multiple lung metastasis resulting in long-term disease-free survival by transcatheter arterial infusion chemotherapy of SMANCS. Gan To Kagaku Ryoho. 2011;38:461–4.

112. Vogl TJ, Naguib NN, Gruber-Rouh T, et al. Microwave ablation therapy: clinical utility in treatment of pulmonary metastases. Radiology. 2011;261:643–51.

113. Hiraki T, Gobara H, Mimura H, et al. Long-term survival after radiofrequency ablation for pulmonary metastasis from hepatocellular carcinoma: report of two cases. J Vasc Interv Radiol. 2009;20:1106–7.

114. Jiang W, Zeng ZC, Zhang JY, et al. Palliative radiation therapy for pulmonary metastases from hepatocellular carcinoma. Clin Exp Metastasis. 2012;29:197–205.

115. Sun TW, He J, Zhang SM, Sun J, Zeng MS, Zeng ZC. Simultaneous multitarget radiotherapy using helical tomotherapy and its combination with sorafenib for pulmonary metastases from hepatocellular carcinoma. Oncotarget. 2016;7(30):48586–99.

116. Jang JW, Kay CS, You CR, et al. Simultaneous multitarget irradiation using helical tomotherapy for advanced hepatocellular carcinoma with multiple extrahepatic metastases. Int J Radiat Oncol Biol Phys. 2009;74:412–8.

117. Kim JY, Kay CS, Kim YS, et al. Helical tomotherapy for simultaneous multitarget radiotherapy for pulmonary metastasis. Int J Radiat Oncol Biol Phys. 2009;75:703–10.

118. Okuma K, Yamashita H, Niibe Y, et al. Abscopal effect of radiation on lung metastases of hepatocellular carcinoma: a case report. J Med Case Rep. 2011;5:111.

119. Hodge JW, Sharp HJ, Gameiro SR. Cancer Abscopal regression of antigen disparate tumors by antigen cascade after systemic tumor vaccination in combination with local tumor radiation. Biother Radiopharm. 2012;27:12–22.

120. Lin G, Xiao H, Zeng Z, Xu Z, He J, Sun T, Liu J, Guo G, Ji W, Hu Y. Constraints for symptomatic radiation pneumonitis of helical tomotherapy hypofractionated simultaneous multitarget radiotherapy for pulmonary metastasis from hepatocellular carcinoma. Radiother Oncol. 2017;123(2):246–50.

121. Kim M, Na DL, Park SH, et al. Nervous system involvement by metastatic hepatocellular carcinoma. J Neuro-Oncol. 1998;36:85–90.

122. Chang L, Chen YL, Kao MC. Intracranial metastasis of hepatocellular carcinoma: review of 45 cases. Surg Neurol. 2004;62:172–7.

123. Chen SF, Tsai NW, Lui CC, et al. Hepatocellular carcinoma presenting as nervous system involvement. Eur J Neurol. 2007;14:408–12.

124. Choi HJ, Cho BC, Sohn JH, et al. Brain metastases from hepatocellular carcinoma: prognostic factors and outcome: brain metastasis from HCC. J Neuro-Oncol. 2009;91:307–13.

125. Shao YY, Lu LC, Cheng AL, Hsu CH. Increasing incidence of brain metastasis in patients with advanced hepatocellular carcinoma in the era of antiangiogenic targeted therapy. Oncologist. 2011;16:82–6.

126. Jiang XB, Ke C, Zhang GH, et al. Brain metastases from hepatocellular carcinoma:clinical features and prognostic factors. BMC Cancer. 2012;12:49.

127. Qiu SJ, Zeng ZC, Chen J, et al. Clinical features and prognosis of patients with brain metastasis from hepatocellular carcinoma. Chin J Cancer Prev Treat. 2013;20:1924–7.

128. Han MS, Moon KS, Lee KH, et al. Brain metastasis from hepatocellular carcinoma: the role of surgery as a prognostic factor. BMC Cancer. 2013;13:567.

129. Nam HC, Sung PS, Song DS, et al. Control of intracranial disease is associated with improved survival in patients with brain metastasis from hepatocellular carcinoma. Int J Clin Oncol. 2019;24:666–76.

130. Hsieh MJ, Lu CH, Tsai NW, et al. Prediction, clinical characteristics and prognosis of intracerebral hemorrhage in hepatocellular carcinoma patients with intracerebral metastasis. J Clin Neurosci. 2009;16:394–8.

131. Hsiao SY, Chen SF, Chang CC, et al. Central nervous system involvement in hepatocellular carcinoma: clinical characteristics and comparison of intracranial and spinal metastatic groups. J Clin Neurosci. 2011;18:364–8.

132. Kwak MS, Lee JH, Yoon JH, et al. Risk factors, clinical features, and prognosis of the hepatocellular carcinoma with peritoneal metastasis. Dig Dis Sci. 2012;57:813–9.

133. Yeh CN, Chen MF. Resection of peritoneal implantation of hepatocellular carcinoma after hepatic resection: risk factors and prognostic analysis. World J Surg. 2004;28:382–6.

134. Yeh CN, Chen MF, Jeng LB. Resection of peritoneal implantation from hepatocellular carcinoma. Ann Surg Oncol. 2002;9:863–8.

135. Ryu JK, Lee SB, Kim KH, Yoh KT. Surgical treatment in a patient with multiple implanted intraperitoneal metastases after resection of ruptured large hepatocellular carcinoma. Hepato-Gastroenterology. 2004;51:239–42.

136. Moon DB, Hwang S, Wang HJ, et al. Surgical outcomes of hepatocellular carcinoma with bile duct tumor thrombus: a korean multicenter study. World J Surg. 2013;37:443–51.

137. Liu QY, Lai DM, Liu C, et al. A special recurrent pattern in small hepatocellular carcinoma after treatment: bile duct tumor thrombus formation. World J Gastroenterol. 2011;17:4817–24.

138. Wang YD, Xue HZ, Jiang QF, et al. Surgical operation and re-operation for hepatocellular carcinoma with bile duct thrombosis. Chin Med J. 2010;123:2163–70.

139. Yu XH, Xu LB, Liu C. Clinicopathological characteristics of 20 cases of hepatocellular carcinoma with bile duct tumor thrombi. Dig Dis Sci. 2011;56:252–9.

140. Buskirk SJ, Gunderson LL, Schild SF. Analysis of patterns of failure following curative irradiation of extrahepatic bile duct carcinoma. Ann Surg. 1992;215:125–31.

141. Jiang T, Zeng ZC, Yang P, Hu Y. Exploration of superior modality: safety and efficacy of hypofractioned image-guided intensity modulated radiation therapy in patients with unresectable but confined intrahepatic hepatocellular carcinoma. Can J Gastroenterol Hepatol. 2017;2017:6267981.

142. Zhang HG, Yang P, Jiang T, Zhang JY, Jin XJ, Hu Y, Sun J, Du SS, Zeng ZC. Lymphopenia is associated with gross target volumes and fractions in hepatocellular carcinoma patients treated with external beam radiation therapy and also indicates worse overall survival. Can J Gastroenterol Hepatol. 2019;2019:9691067.

143. Zeng ZC, Tang ZY, et al. A comparison of chemoembolization combination with and without radiotherapy for unresectable hepatocellular carcinoma. Cancer J. 2004;10:307–16.

144. Huo YR, Eslick GD. Transcatheter arterial chemoembolization plus radiotherapy compared with chemoembolization alone for hepatocellular carcinoma: a systematic review and meta-analysis. JAMA Oncol. 2015;1(6):756–65.

145. Kitano K, Murayama T, Sakamoto M, et al. Outcome and survival analysis of pulmonary metastasectomy for hepatocellular carcinoma. Eur J Cardiothorac Surg. 2012;41:376–82.

Part IV

Specific Issues

Multidisciplinary Team Approaches for the Management of Hepatocellular Carcinoma

18

Kwang-Hyub Han

Abstract

Hepatocellular carcinoma (HCC) is one of the most common malignancies worldwide. With the advancement of diagnostic tools and therapeutic options, the management of HCC has improved remarkably. However, the majority of patients with HCC are diagnosed at an advanced stage and overall prognosis is still grave. Major milestones have occurred in the management of advanced HCC after the introduction of the molecular targeted therapy (MTX). Owing to emerging new targeted therapeutic agents in first-line and second-line settings, HCC seemed to be manageable. In addition, immune checkpoint inhibitors (ICI) are also an attractive choice for the treatment of HCC. Although emerging systemic therapeutic agents may have shifted the treatment paradigm for HCC, there is still an unmet need for effective systemic therapy as monotherapy. Recently, ICI-based combination therapy is expected to improve therapeutic efficacy for HCC. Given the complex nature of the treatment strategy of advanced HCC, optimal treatment of HCC remains complex despite the treatment guidelines for HCCs. Although there are guidelines for the management of HCC, optimal care of HCC remains complex because of the complexity of managing HCC. Multidisciplinary team approaches using multimodality treatment are therefore used in the management of HCC.

Keywords

Hepatocellular carcinoma · Molecular target therapy · Immunotherapy · Multidisciplinary team approach · Multimodal treatment

18.1 Introduction

Hepatocellular carcinoma (HCC) is one of the most common malignancies worldwide and there has been a marked increase in HCC-related annual death rates over the past two decades. With the advancement of diagnostic tools and therapeutic options such as surgical or locoregional therapy (LRT), the management of HCC has improved remarkably [1, 2]. However, the majority of patients with HCC are still diagnosed at advanced stage and overall prognosis is grave despite recent advances in therapy.

Major milestones in the treatment of HCC have been reached after the development of molecular targeted therapy (MTX). HCC seemed to be treatable with the emergence of novel tar-

K.-H. Han (✉)
Department of Internal Medicine, Yonsei University College of Medicine, Seoul, Republic of Korea
e-mail: gihankhys@yuhs.ac

geted therapeutic agents such as sorafenib and lenvatinib in the first-line setting, and regorafenib, cabozantinib, and ramucirumab in the second-line setting [3–7]. In addition, immunotherapy using immune checkpoint inhibitors (ICI) such as anti-PD-1/PD-L1 or CTLA-4 antibodies is also an attractive and alternative treatment option for HCC with promising outcomes [8, 9]. However, the therapeutic effect of immunotherapy on overall survival (OS) of patients in advanced stage was not confirmed in the large-scale controlled trials [10, 11]. Although emerging systemic therapeutic agents may have shifted the treatment paradigm for HCC, there is still an unmet need for effective systemic therapy as monotherapy. Recently, ICI-based combination therapy improved therapeutic efficacy in HCC, but not ICI monotherapy [12].

In real clinical practice, the loco-regional therapy (LRT) could be an alternative option for locally advanced HCC. Given the complex nature of the treatment of advanced HCC, it is crucial to adopt multidisciplinary team (MDT) approach, which consist of hepatologists, medical oncologists, surgeons, interventional radiologists, radiation oncologists, and pathologists.

18.2   What Is the Hurdle of Current Systemic Therapy?

Despite recent advances in the treatment for advanced HCC, there are still hurdles to overcome. After sorafenib was approved as the first systemic MTX for patients with inoperable HCC [3], there have been many clinical trials using new molecular target agents. However, most clinical trials using new target agents were not successful for the past 10 years. After struggling with negative clinical trials for HCC, there are approved MTX for HCC, including sorafenib and lenvatinib for the first-line therapy, and regorafenib, cabozantinib, and ramucirumab for the second-line therapy [3–7]. In spite of recent achievements of new emerging approved targeted agents, there are still unsolved hurdles of current MTX. Median OS of patients with advanced HCC using systemic MTX remains unsatisfactory due to not durable, low objective response rate (ORR) and frequent toxicity [11, 13].

Immunotherapy in the management of HCC is likely to have a large impact on HCC management. With the success of anti-PD therapy, immunotherapy has already shown promising results. However, a large portion of patients do not benefit from the immunotherapy, and a fraction of responders relapsed. Although ICI therapy could be an attractive approach for new drug development in HCC, randomized trials of anti-PD-1 monotherapy in both first-line and second-line settings did not have statistically significant improvement in OS [10, 11]. In order to improve treatment efficacy for HCC, development of combination strategies has become an alternative option. Preliminary results from early-phase clinical trials indicated better response rates and duration of response when ICI was combined with other agents. Recently, a combination of atezolizumab (anti-PD-L1 antibody) plus bevacizumab (antiangiogenic agent) has a superior OS and PFS compared to sorafenib in the first-line treatment of advanced HCC [12].

18.3   Can Combination Therapy Overcome the Hurdle of Current Systemic Therapy?

In the era of immuno-oncology-based combination therapies, there are promises and challenges of immuno-oncology-based combination therapy for HCC. Treatment with atezolizumab plus bevacizumab is associated with significantly better OS and PFS outcomes than sorafenib in patients with unresectable HCC patients who have not been treated with systemic therapy previously [12]. After them, combinations of ICI and anti-angiogenic therapy have become the mainstream of combination therapy trials for HCC. Combinations of ICI with other MTX, immune modulators, or cytotoxic agents are promising, but require further study. Combination therapies have led to specific challenges in study design and management of adverse events, which need to be overcome in order to optimize treatment for HCC [11].

LRT, including ablation therapy, transarterial chemoembolisation (TACE), internal or external radiation therapy, and hepatic arterial infusion chemotherapy, has been widely used for HCC management [14]. LRT has been shown to induce immune responses in patients with HCC. With the advent of immunotherapy in HCC, there is increasing interest in determining the best way to combine immunotherapy with LRT. Based on positive results from previous studies evaluating ICI in HCC, a number of studies have been initiated to test the combination of ICI plus LR [15, 16]. However, many questions, such as the precise immunologic effects of LRT, remain unanswered [15]. Most of the previous randomized trials that tested the combination of systemic therapy and LRT for HCC failed to demonstrate a survival benefit of combination therapy. However, a recent phase 2 trial of concurrent LRT and sequential sorafenib demonstrated a survival benefit of combination therapy for advanced HCC [17].

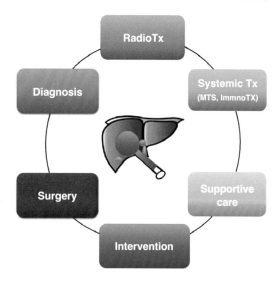

Fig. 18.1 Multidisciplinary team approach for the management of HCC using multimodality

18.4 Multidisciplinary Team Approach to Patients with HCC

Cancer treatment requires the cooperation of a multidisciplinary team (MDT) approach to coordinate the delivery of the appropriate treatment such as surgery, chemotherapy, radiotherapy, and other supportive or symptomatic care, including psychological support. Multidisciplinary teams coordinate and work together to offer a comprehensive approach for providing the best care, tailored to the specific needs of each patient. This collaborative approach to patients with cancer offers the most balanced and objective understanding of available options, provides best chance for cure, catalyzes patient engagement, and improves quality of care.

Why Is MDA Needed in the Management of HCC? Although there are guidelines for the management of HCC, optimal care of HCC is not simple owing to the complexity of managing HCC [18–20]. The management of HCC may have many challenges such as multifocal occurrence, high recurrence rate, frequent vascular invasion and intra and extra-hepatic metastasis, rapid growth, and frequent metastasis after incomplete treatment and underlying cirrhosis (80%) with/without active hepatitis. Therefore, many specialists are required to manage patients with HCC according to the disease status. Multidisciplinary collaboration and multimodal treatment approaches are important in the management of HCC and improve survival [21–28]. In addition, a multidisciplinary team (MDT) composed of specialists may offer more options and better outcomes for HCC patients (Fig. 18.1).

Moreover, a focused MDT approach using multimodality may offer curative surgery followed by downstaging in patients with inoperable stage [29–32]. LRTs (Fig. 18.2) or systemic therapies can induce tumor downstaging by achieving tumor size reduction to meet current selection criteria for liver transplantation or resection.

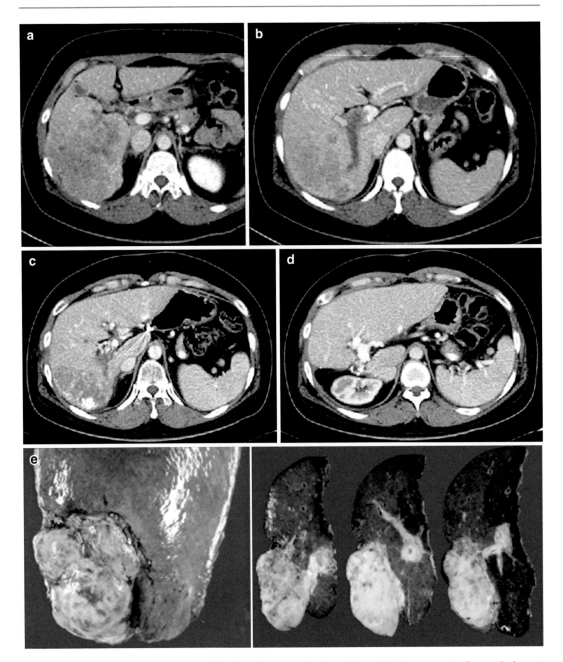

Fig. 18.2 Illustration showing 34-year-old female patient with hepatocellular carcinoma with portal vein tumor thrombosis (PVTT) who underwent liver resection after successful conversion to resectable status by concurrent chemoradiation (CCRT). Computed tomography images recorded (**a**, **b**) before CCRT and (**c**) at six months after CCRT before surgical resection and (**d**) at one month after surgical resection. PVTT before CCRT is indicated by the yellow arrow. (**e**) Surgical specimen showing complete tumor necrosis. The patient was disease-free for five years. Tumor marker became WNL at six months after CCRT (AFP 92233 ng/ml to 1.15 ng/ml, PIVKA II 11260 mAU/ml to 15 mAU/ml)

18.5 Localized Concurrent Chemoradiation Therapy for Locally Advanced HCC

Macrovascular invasion (MVI) is a quite common finding in advanced HCC. HCC with portal vein tumor thrombus (PVTT) is usually inoperable and is associated with poor prognosis in spite of standard targeted treatment according to international guidelines. The recently updated AASLD guidelines point out that the selection of treatment may vary depending on the extent of MVI, but there was still no recommendation [18]. Many studies suggest alternative or more aggressive LRT approaches could benefit selected patients with MVI [26–30]. There are many alternative trial reports for HCC with MVI using hepatic arterial infusion chemotherapy, external radiation therapy or selective internal radiation therapy. However, the level of evidence is not strong enough to adopt any alternative strategy as international guidelines yet. The ideal strategy can be multimodal treatment using a combination of LRT and personalized systemic therapy. Therefore, a focused MDT approach using multimodality is needed in those.

External beam radiotherapy (EBRT) has become a feasible and safe technique against HCC, delivering high tumoricidal radiation doses with minimal risk of damage to non-tumorous liver and adjacent organs [33]. So, recently, it has been listed in the National Comprehensive Cancer Network guidelines as one of feasible LRT for inoperable HCC [27, 29]. In order to make up for the issue of local or systemic failure outside the radiation field, a combination of other LRT or systemic treatments with EBRT has been widely evaluated with some promising results. By MDT approach, **localized concurrent chemoradiotherapy (CCRT)** demonstrated favorable survival outcomes with acceptable tolerability in patients with locally advanced stage HCC [26–29, 34]. Furthermore, remarkable tumor reduction by initial localized CCRT enabled downstaging and subsequent curative treatment in 16.9% with initially inoperable HCC and overall survival of the subsequent curative resection group was remarkably longer than in the without-resection group after CCRT [32].

Based on a recent report, liver-directed combined radiotherapy (LDCRT) can provide substantial tumor control and convert locally advanced tumor larger than 5 cm or macrovascular invasion to within the Milan criteria by successful down-staging, and could perform liver transplantation or curative surgery in selected patients. Clinicians should consider LDCRT followed by curative surgery for younger patients who are treatment-naïve and have good liver reserve function with favorable tumor characteristics showing radiologic response to LDCRT. This study indicated that LDCRT not only provides favorable survival outcomes in locally advanced HCC, but it also could be a bridge to curative surgery by converting the unresectable tumors to within the Milan criteria [29].

18.6 Summary and Conclusion

Significant advances have been made in the development of surgical, LRT, and systemic treatment modalities for HCC. Nevertheless, in the face of the global disease burden and the limited survival in advanced stages, further research is fundamental to improve the prognosis of patients with HCC. Emerging molecular targeted drugs approved not only first-line but second-line may bring significant changes in the treatment paradigm for the management of HCC. With the success of anti-PD therapy, cancer immunotherapy has already shown great promise. In spite of recent achievements of systemic treatment for HCC, there are still hurdles to overcome. To optimize management of HCC, the MDT approach can help to select the best options for each patient by tailoring approach according to tumor status and characteristics beyond guidelines.

References

1. Nault JC, Cheng AL, Sangro B, Llovet JM. Milestones in the pathogenesis and management of primary liver cancer. J Hepatol. 2020;72(2):209–14.

2. Kudo M, Han KH, Ye SL, Zhou J, Huang YH, et al. A changing paradigm for the treatment of intermediate-stage hepatocellular carcinoma: Asia-Pacific primary liver cancer expert consensus statements. Liver Cancer. 2020;9(3):245–60.

3. Llovet JM, Ricci S, Mazzaferro V, Hilgard P, Gane E, et al. Sorafenib in advanced hepatocellular carcinoma. N Engl J Med. 2008;359:378–90.

4. Kudo M, Finn RS, Qin S, Ikeda M, Han KH, Ikeda K, Piscaglia F, et al. Lenvatinib versus sorafenib in first-line treatment of patients with unresectable hepatocellular carcinoma: a randomised phase 3 non-inferiority trial. Lancet. 2018;391:1163–73.

5. Bruix J, Qin S, Merle P, Granito A, Huang YH, Bodoky G, et al. Regorafenib for patients with hepatocellular carcinoma who progressed on sorafenib treatment (RESORCE): a randomised, double-blind, placebo-controlled, phase 3 trial. Lancet. 2017;389:56–66.

6. Zhu AX, Kang YK, Yen CJ, Finn RS, et al. Ramucirumab after sorafenib in patients with advanced hepatocellular carcinoma and increased α-fetoprotein concentrations (REACH-2): a randomised, double-blind, placebo-controlled, phase 3 trial. Lancet Oncol. 2019;20:282–96.

7. Abou-Alfa GK, Meyer T, Cheng AL, El-Khoueiry AB, Rimassa L, Ryoo BY, et al. Cabozantinib in patients with advanced and progressing hepatocellular carcinoma. N Engl J Med. 2018;379:54–63.

8. El-Khoueiry AB, Sangro B, Yau T, Crocenzi TS, Kudo M, Hsu C, et al. Nivolumab in patients with advanced hepatocellular carcinoma (CheckMate 040): an open-label, non-comparative, phase 1/2 dose escalation and expansion trial. Lancet. 2017;389:2492–502.

9. Zhu AX, Finn RS, Edeline J, Cattan S, Ogasawara S, et al. Pembrolizumab in patients with advanced hepatocellular carcinoma previously treated with sorafenib (KEYNOTE-224): a non-randomised, open-label phase 2 trial. Lancet Oncol. 2018;19:940–52.

10. Finn RS, Ryoo BY, Merle P, Kudo M, Bouattour M, Lim HY, et al. Pembrolizumab as second-line therapy in patients with advanced hepatocellular carcinoma in KEYNOTE-240: a randomized, double-blind, phase III trial. J Clin Oncol. 2020;38(3):193–202.

11. Cheng A-L, Hsu C, Chan SL, Choo S-P, Kudo M. Challenges of combination therapy with immune checkpoint inhibitors for hepatocellular carcinoma. J Hepatol. 2020;72:307–19.

12. Finn RS, Qin S, Ikeda M, Galle PR, Ducreux M, Kim TY, Kudo M, Breder V, Merle P, Kaseb AO, Li D, Verret W, Xu DZ, Hernandez S, Liu J, Huang C, Mulla S, Wang Y, Lim HY, Zhu AX, Cheng AL. IMbrave150 investigators. Atezolizumab plus Bevacizumab in unresectable hepatocellular carcinoma. N Engl J Med. 2020;382(20):1894–905.

13. Kim DY, Kim HJ, Han KH, Han SY, Heo J, Woo HY, Um SH, Kim YH, Kweon YO, Lim HY, Yoon JH, Lee WS, Lee BS, Lee HC, Ryoo BY, Yoon SK. Real-life experience of sorafenib treatment for hepatocellular carcinoma in Korea: from GIDEON data. Cancer Res Treat. 2016;48(4):1243–52.

14. Bruix J, Han KH, Gores G, Llovet JM, Mazzaferro VJ. Liver cancer: approaching a personalized care. J Hepatol. 2015;62(1 Suppl):S144–56.

15. Greten TF, Mauda-Havakuk M, Heinrich B, Korangy F, Wood BJ. Combined locoregional-immunotherapy for liver cancer. J Hepatol. 2019;70(5):999–1007.

16. Greten TF, Lai CW, Li G, Staveley-O'Carroll KF. Targeted and immune-based therapies for hepatocellular carcinoma. Gastroenterology. 2019;156:510–24.

17. Kim BK, Kim DY, Byun HK, Choi HJ, Beom SH, Lee HW, Kim SU, Park JY, Ahn SH, Seong J, Han KH. Efficacy and safety of liver-directed concurrent chemoradiotherapy and sequential sorafenib for advanced hepatocellular carcinoma: a prospective phase 2 trial. Int J Radiat Oncol Biol Phys. 2020;107(1):106–15.

18. Heimbach JK, Kulik LM, Finn RS, Sirlin CB, Abecassis MM, et al. AASLD guidelines for the treatment of hepatocellular carcinoma. Hepatology. 2018;67:358–80.

19. Omata M, Cheng AL, Kokudo N, Kudo M, Lee JM, Jia J, et al. Asia-Pacific clinical practice guidelines on the management of hepatocellular carcinoma: a 2017 update. Hepatol Int. 2017;11:317–70.

20. Kim BK, Kim DY, Han KH, Seong JS. Changes in real-life practice for hepatocellular carcinoma patients in the Republic of Korea over a 12-year period: a nationwide random sample study. PLoS One 2019;17;14(10).

21. Agarwal PD, Phillips P, Hillman L, et al. Multidisciplinary management of hepatocellular carcinoma improves access to therapy and patient survival. J Clin Gastroenterol. 2017;51(9):845–9.

22. Serper M, Taddei TH, Mehta R, et al. Association of provider specialty and multi-disciplinary care with hepatocellular carcinoma treatment and mortality. Gastroenterology. 2017;152:1954–64.

23. Yopp AC, Mansour JC, Beg MS, et al. Establishment of a multidisciplinary hepatocellular carcinoma clinic is associated with improved clinical outcome. Ann Surg Oncol. 2014;21:1287–95.

24. Guy J, Kelley RK, Roberts J, et al. Multidisciplinary management of hepatocellular carcinoma. Clin Gastroenterol Hepatol. 2012;10(4):354–62.

25. Chang TT, Sawhney R, Monto A, et al. Implementation of a multidisciplinary treatment team for hepatocellular cancer at a Veterans Affairs Medical Center improves survival. HPB (Oxford). 2008;10(6):405–11.

26. Han HJ, Kim MS, Cha J, Choi JS, Han KH, Seong J. Multimodality treatment with radiotherapy for huge hepatocellular carcinoma. Oncology. 2014;87(Suppl 1):82–9.

27. Byun HK, Kim HJ, Im YR, Kim DY, Han KH, Seong J. Dose escalation by intensity modulated radiotherapy in liver-directed concurrent chemoradiotherapy for locally advanced BCLC stage C hepatocellular carcinoma. Radiother Oncol. 2019;133:1–8.

28. Yoon HI, Song KJ, Lee IJ, Kim DY, Han KH, Seong J. Clinical benefit of hepatic arterial infusion concur-

rent chemoradiotherapy in locally advanced hepatocellular carcinoma: a propensity score matching analysis. Cancer Res Treat. 2016;48(1):190–7.

29. Lee WH, Byun HK, Choi JS, Choi GH, Han DH, Joo DJ, Kim DY, Han KH, Seong J. Liver-directed combined radiotherapy as a bridge to curative surgery in locally advanced hepatocellular carcinoma beyond the Milan criteria. Radiother Oncol. 2020;152:1–7.

30. Chong JU, Choi GH, Han DH, Kim KS, Seong J, Han KH, Choi JS. Downstaging with localized concurrent chemoradiotherapy can identify optimal surgical candidates in hepatocellular carcinoma with portal vein tumor thrombus. Ann Surg Oncol. 2018;25(11):3308–15.

31. Han DH, Joo DJ, Kim MS, Choi GH, Choi JS, Park YN, Seong J, Han KH, Kim SI. Living donor liver transplantation for advanced hepatocellular carcinoma with portal vein tumor thrombosis after

concurrent chemoradiation therapy. Yonsei Med J. 2016;57(5):1276–81.

32. Lee HS, Choi GH, Choi JS, Kim KS, Han KH, Seong J, Ahn SH, Kim DY, Park JY, Kim SU, Kim BK. Surgical resection after down-staging of locally advanced hepatocellular carcinoma by localized concurrent chemoradiotherapy. Ann Surg Oncol. 2014;21(11):3646–53.

33. Choi Y, Kim JW, Cha H, Han KH, Seong J. Overall response of both intrahepatic tumor and portal vein tumor thrombosis is a good prognostic factor for hepatocellular carcinoma patients receiving concurrent chemoradiotherapy. J Radiat Res. 2014;55(1):113–20.

34. Han KH, Seong J, Kim JK, Ahn SH, Lee DY, Chon CY. Pilot clinical trial of localized concurrent chemoradiation therapy for locally advanced hepatocellular carcinoma with portal vein thrombosis. Cancer. 2008;113(5):995–1003.

Response Evaluation After Radiotherapy

19

Cheng-Hsiang Lo, Jen-Fu Yang, Po-Chien Shen, and Wen-Yen Huang

Abstract

Accurate assessment of the response to radiotherapy is essential to avoid missing the opportunity for early salvage treatment for residual tumors as well as overtreatment in complete responders. The evaluation of radiotherapy response in liver tumors mainly involves the interpretation of imaging studies. Dynamic contrast-enhanced computed tomography (CT) or magnetic resonance imaging (MRI) are the most widely used image evaluation tools. Enhancement-based imaging response evaluation criteria, such as the European Association for Study of the Liver (EASL) and the modified Response Evaluation Criteria in Solid Tumors (mRECIST), are more sensitive than the size change-based RECIST and World Health Organization (WHO) criteria. However, early assessment of the tumor response is challenging. Understanding the time frame of imaging changes of the tumor and surrounding irradiated liver parenchyma is essential for accurate assessment. The typical imaging changes of the tumor are gradual reduction in size of the enhancing part and increase of necrosis over time. The focal liver reaction of the irradiated peritumoral liver tissue also changes

over time from hyperemia in acute phase to gradual returning to normal enhancement pattern in chronic phase. Thus, accurate response interpretation requires a series of follow-up contrast-enhanced images with careful assessment of consecutive changes. In this chapter, we describe the imaging assessment of radiotherapy response in liver tumors, focusing on hepatocellular carcinoma (HCC).

Keywords

Liver cancer · Hepatocellular carcinoma · Radiotherapy · Stereotactic body radiotherapy · Response evaluation · Computed tomography · Magnetic resonance imaging

19.1 Histopathological Changes After Liver Radiotherapy

19.1.1 Changes in the Liver Parenchyma

The hepatic lobules are the anatomical and functional units of the liver, composed of the central vein, portal vein triad, and the hepatocytes arranged linearly between the capillary network (Fig. 19.1). The classical lobule is hexagonal and can be divided into periportal, midzonal, and cen-

C.-H. Lo · J.-F. Yang · P.-C. Shen · W.-Y. Huang (✉)
Department of Radiation Oncology, Tri-Service
General Hospital, National Defense Medical Center,
Taipei, Taiwan

© Springer Nature Singapore Pte Ltd. 2021
J. Seong (ed.), *Radiotherapy of Liver Cancer*, https://doi.org/10.1007/978-981-16-1815-4_19

Fig. 19.1 Schematic presentation of the anatomical and functional units of the liver. Zone I, II, and III refer to the periportal, transition, and pericentral areas, respectively. *CV* central vein, *PT* portal tract

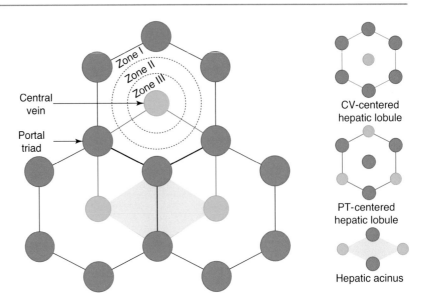

trilobular areas, referred to as zones I, II, and III, respectively [1, 2].

There are limited studies of the histopathological change after liver radiotherapy, because most patients who receive radiotherapy are inoperable. Post-radiotherapy histopathological changes are mainly present in the liver parenchyma surrounding the irradiated tumor. In the past, the surrounding reaction was called radiation hepatitis. However, little or no inflammatory response was observed. The peritumoral liver parenchyma was more hyperemic and swollen compared to the nonirradiated liver tissue [1]. These changes are mainly due to endothelial cell damage, which leads to the formation of thin fibrin deposits trapping red blood cells, resulting in obstruction of the outer cavity of hepatic veins. Therefore, central vascular damage with central congestion, venous fibrosis, terminal hepatic venule stenosis, sinusoidal artery congestion, regional parenchymal atrophy, and collagen deposition in the subendothelial space may be observed [1, 3].

Typically, these events mainly occur around zone III, and their histopathological features are similar to those of veno-occlusive disease caused by high-dose chemotherapy or viral infections [1, 3]. These features include congestion with extravasation of red blood cells, intrahepatic vein occlusive fibrosis, and alternating areas of hepatocyte atrophy and regeneration. The sub-lobular veins

may still be patent in the early period after radiotherapy, but become thrombosed later [3]. Yellow necrosis may appear at the center of the irradiation lesion [4]. The above pathological changes can appear in a part of the liver, a lobe, or rarely the whole liver. If the lesion involves most areas of the liver, such as an entire liver lobe, it may lead to a significant reduction in volume, accompanied by a wrinkled or granular capsule [4].

19.1.2 Changes in the Tumor Tissue

After radiotherapy, the tumor cells gradually die, and the tumor may undergo a partial or complete fibrotic change. The effect of radiotherapy on liver tumors is somewhat similar to that of radiofrequency ablation (RFA), which induces liquefaction or coagulation necrosis at the target [1, 5]. There would be a paucicellular collagenized zone with focal collections of lipid-laden macrophages at the target center that receives the highest dose [6].

19.2 Image Response Evaluation Criteria

In 1979, the WHO published the first tumor response criteria, which used bidimensional measurements to evaluate the tumor response. The

RECIST based on unidimensional measurements were published in 2000 [7] and later revised to RECIST version 1.1 in 2009 [8]. These criteria were initially created for systemic treatment response assessment. They might not apply well to HCC due to the lack of consideration of necrosis caused by targeted agents or loco-regional treatment.

In 2001, the EASL criteria introduced a concept of bidimensional response evaluation that takes into account the tumor enhancement as an indicator of a viable tumor tissue, not just the overall tumor size reduction [9]. In 2010, in order to adapt the concept proposed by the EASL criteria, specific modified RECIST (mRECIST) for HCC were developed [10], which became more commonly used over time. Table 19.1 summarizes the differences between the respective criteria.

19.3 Image Evaluation Tools

As with other locoregional therapies, the response to radiotherapy for HCC is predominantly assessed by dynamic contrast-enhanced CT or MRI. Specific for hypervascular tumors, the imaging response is based on diminishment of arterial enhancement as a marker of tumor necrosis. In tumors that lack arterial enhancement at baseline, the size change would indicate response as determined by the RECIST or the WHO criteria.

While no consensus guidelines exist on the ideal imaging modality for evaluating radiotherapy response in HCC, MRI may provide additional advantages in some scenarios. Given the beam-hardening artifact from the radiodense Lipiodol, it is challenging on CT to distinguish viable tumor enhancement from retained Lipiodol in tumors previously treated with transarterial chemoembolization (TACE). Similarly, metal artifacts from fiducial markers used for image-guided radiotherapy may preclude CT evaluation. In this respect, contrast-enhanced MRI is useful given that the signal intensity is less affected by Lipiodol and fiducial markers compared with CT [11].

Diffusion-weighted imaging (DWI) with apparent diffusion coefficient (ADC) map is an MRI technique that measures the water mobility within tissues, which could function as a biomarker of cellularity and aid in the discrimination of viable tumors (lower ADC level) from necrosis (higher ADC level). Decreased signal on DWI with corresponding increase in the ADC

Table 19.1 Comparison of imaging response evaluation criteria

Response	WHO	RECIST 1.0 and 1.1	EASL	mRECIST
Complete response	Disappearance of all target lesions	Disappearance of all target lesions	Disappearance of intratumoral arterial enhancement in all target lesions	Disappearance of intratumoral arterial enhancement in all target lesions
Partial response	≥50% decrease in the sum of the products of bidimensional diameters of the target lesions	≥30% decrease in the sum of the greatest unidimensional diameters of the target lesions	≥50% decrease in the sum of the product of bidimensional diameters of the target enhancing area	≥30% decrease in the sum of the greatest unidimensional diameters of the target enhancing area
Stable disease	Neither PR nor PD	Neither PR nor PD	Neither PR nor PD	Neither PR nor PD
Progressive disease	≥25% increase in the sum of the products of bidimensional diameters of the target lesions or development of new lesions	≥20% increase in the sum of the greatest unidimensional diameters of the target lesions or development of new lesions	≥25% increase in the sum of the product of bidimensional diameters of the target enhancing area or development of new lesions	≥20% increase in the sum of the greatest unidimensional diameters of the target enhancing area or development of new lesions

CR complete response, *PR* partial response, *SD* stable disease, *PD* progressive disease value in the locoregionally treated lesions reflects hypocellularity change, predictive of a favorable response that occurs earlier than the usual assessments of tumor response [12, 13]. In addition, DWI with an ADC map could improve the detection of viable tumors in patients with HCC postradiotherapy [14, 15], and the increment in the tumor ADC value was correlated with the radiation response and local progression-free survival [15–17]. Considering the ADC increment within the irradiated tumor, the diagnostic performance of the RECIST is comparable to that of the mRECIST [14]. These features make DWI an attractive and useful modality for evaluation of the response to radiotherapy, as well as other liver-directed therapy in HCC, particularly in patients with renal dysfunction or other contraindications to contrast agents. However, the absence of standardization of DWI acquisition and interpretation limits its use as a standard measure of response evaluation at present.

MRI with hepatobiliary contrast agents, such as gadoxetate disodium (Gd-EOB-DTPA; Primovist/Eovist, Bayer), is an emerging imaging modality for liver tumor diagnosis, particularly for the detection of small HCCs [18]. Because of the feature of internalization by functional hepatocytes, these contrast agents are used as surrogate markers of hepatocellular function. The focal liver reaction to SBRT presents as a well-demarcated hypointense area around the irradiated tumor in the hepatobiliary phase of Gd-EOB-DTPA-enhanced MRI, reflecting the extent of damaged liver volume [19]. Thus, this technique can potentially provide quantitative information about radiation-induced liver disease.

Positron emission tomography (PET) using ^{18}F-fluorodeoxyglucose (^{18}F-FDG-PET) has been applied widely for tumor detection, staging, and early treatment response evaluation in various malignancies [20]. Given its poor sensitivity of approximately 50–55% in the detection of HCC, particularly for small and/or well-differentiated tumors, ^{18}F-FDG-PET is not considered mandatory in the management of HCC [21, 22]. Complementary to CT or MRI, ^{18}F-FDG-PET may be helpful in assessing non-shrinking

tumors after radiotherapy with a response being evident by the metabolic activity of the tumor (maximum standardized uptake value [SUV$_{max}$]), which declines and reaches values similar to those of the background normal liver [1]. In an orthotopic HCC model, irradiation resulted in a rapid increase in ^{18}F-FDG uptake on day one and sustained until day six, which differed from the pattern of gradual increase in ^{18}F-FDG levels in accordance with the tumor development in non-irradiated tumors. This spatiotemporal information regarding the tumor metabolism may help to illustrate the early tumor microenvironment change and immune response in relation to radiation [23]. However, no clinical study has investigated the application of ^{18}F-FDG-PET for radiotherapy response assessment in primary HCC.

PET with ^{18}F-fluorocholine (^{18}F-FCH-PET) is an emerging functional imaging modality for HCC detection, with a high sensitivity approaching 90% [24]. A decrease of > 45% in the ^{18}F-FCH SUV$_{max}$ obtained at 6–12 weeks post-locoregional therapies, including SBRT, was identified as a predictor of a longer progression-free survival and a favorable response by the mRECIST in early-stage HCCs [25].

19.4 Imaging Changes

19.4.1 Tumor Imaging Changes

Following locoregional therapies, treated HCC tumors would present with one of the three imaging changes: response, progression, or stable disease. For responding tumors, reduced postcontrast enhancement is usually the first feature with subsequent reduction in size and replacement by fibrotic tissue or regenerative hepatic parenchyma. In contrast to RFA or TACE, the immediate loss of tumor enhancement is not seen after radiotherapy, which precludes an effective early evaluation and warrants a long-term imaging follow-up. In fact, Price et al. demonstrated little change in the tumor size of HCC during the first three months after SBRT and concluded that decreased tumor enhancement on CT or MRI was

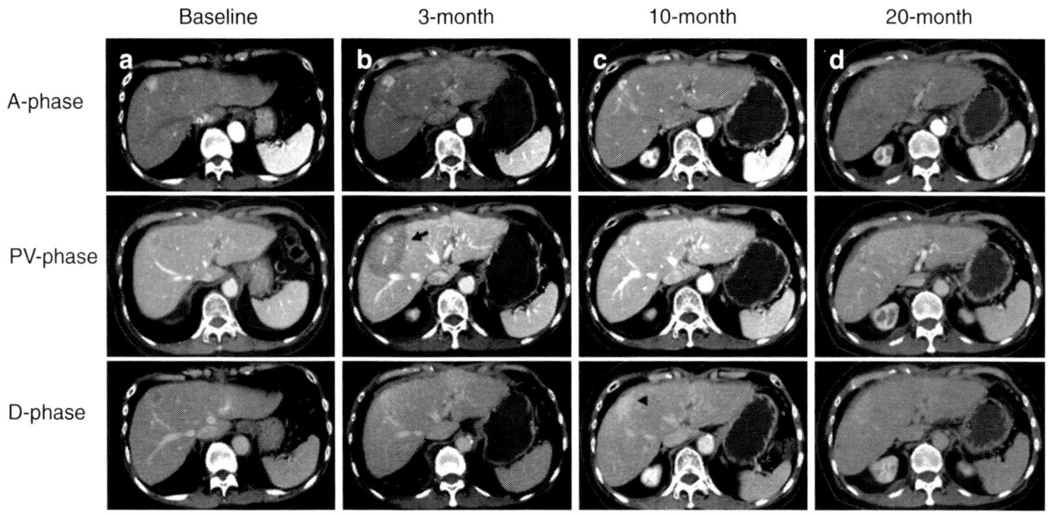

	Baseline	3-month	10-month	20-month
A-phase				
PV-phase				
D-phase				

Fig. 19.2 Multiphase contrast-enhanced CT of a 71-year-old man with HCC. (**a**) Pretreatment arterial phase (A-phase) shows a 1.8 cm hypervascular HCC at segment 8 with wash-out at portal venous and delayed phases (PV- and D-phase). The patient received 55 Gy delivered in 5 fractions. (**b**) Imaging three months post SBRT shows stable size of the enhancing tumor by mRECIST. Note the surrounding wedge-shaped hypoenhancement (arrow) of liver parenchyma in PV-phase (focal liver reaction), which does not persist into D-phase. (**c**) Imaging at 10 months shows decreased enhancement size of the tumor (1.2 cm), considered as partial response. The hypoenhancement at PV-phase resolves but hyperenhancement develops at D-phase (arrowhead). (**d**) Imaging at 20 months shows no enhancement of the tumor, indicating complete response. Continuous volume loss of the overlying liver parenchyma was observed at 10 and 20 months

a better indicator of SBRT response within the first 6–12 months [26]. Of note, the percentage of necrosis (nonenhancement) within the tumor increased with time, from 59% at 3 months to 92% at 12 months. Similar observations were obtained by Sanuki et al. in a series of 277 HCC hypervascular tumors after SBRT. On contrast-enhanced CT, the complete response as evaluated by the mRECIST increased gradually from 24% to 67% to 71% at 3, 6, and 12 months after SBRT, respectively, and the median time to complete response was 5.9 months with a wide range of 1.2 to 34.2 months. Another study from the University of Michigan focused on MRI changes in HCC following SBRT. Of the 67 HCC lesions, 58% had persistent arterial hyperenhancement and 54% had a washout appearance at 3–6 months [27]. These features of viable tumors disappeared over time without disease progression, resulting in a continuous response from 25% at 3–6 months to 70% at 12 months. These data suggest that persistent arterial enhancement is common and does not necessarily indicate viable lesions, particularly in the early phase after radiotherapy. Radiation response may take many months to manifest as decreased enhancement or size on images (Fig. 19.2). This partly accounts for the poor concordance between the pathological response and the available radiological criteria in HCC following SBRT [28].

On MRI, signal intensity changes within the treated tumor may be seen after SBRT, including decreased signal intensity on T1-weighted images, less hyperintensity on T2-weighted images, and reduced signal intensity on DWI with corresponding increased ADC values on ADC maps. As mentioned in Sect. 19.3, DWI and ADC changes at the microscopic level usually appear earlier than decreased enhancement or size in responding tumors (Fig. 19.3). An increment in ADC values of 20–25% was found to be an early indicator of response to hypofractionated radiotherapy or SBRT [14, 16].

In summary, a series of follow-up contrast-enhanced images (> 6–12 months) is essential to define the response of HCC to radiotherapy.

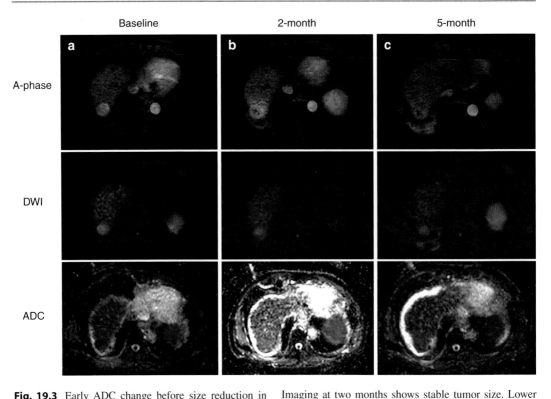

| Baseline | 2-month | 5-month |

Fig. 19.3 Early ADC change before size reduction in HCC on diffusion-weighted MRI. A 71-year-old man with a 2.8 cm HCC in segment 7. He received 45 Gy in 5 fractions. At baseline (**a**), the tumor shows strong enhancement in the arterial phase (A-phase) with moderate hyperintensity on DWI (b = 500) and a corresponding ADC value of 1.37×10^{-3} mm^2/s. (**b**) Imaging at two months shows stable tumor size. Lower hyperintensity at DWI with an ADC of 2.00×10^{-3} mm^2/s (a 46% increased ADC level) were noted. (**c**) Partial response (tumor 1.9 cm) was observed on the imaging five months after SBRT. Reactive hyperemia was noted in A-phase at two months, and resolved at five months after SBRT

Even the mRECIST or the EASL criteria might be insufficient to define the radiotherapy effect, particularly during the early period (< 3 months). Salvage treatment should be considered cautiously, only in case of definite evidence of disease progression as increased tumor size/enhancement.

19.4.2 Liver Parenchyma Imaging Changes

In contrast to the nonirradiated normal liver parenchyma, the irradiated peritumoral liver tissue shows unique and distinctive imaging features. This phenomenon is referred to as focal liver reaction (FLR). After radiotherapy, the imaging appearance of the FLR changes over time. Based on the corresponding pathophysi-ological findings, the FLR timeframe can generally be divided into acute, subacute, and chronic stages [29].

The acute stage is defined as 1–3 months after radiotherapy. Pathologically, the dominant features are severe sinusoidal congestion with perisinusoidal hyperemia and hemorrhage. Before contrast administration, the irradiated liver shows hypoattenuation relative to the background liver on CT [29]. On MRI, there may be low signal intensity on T1-weighted images, high signal intensity on T2-weighted images, and mildly restricted diffusion on DWI with an ADC increase. Arterial phase hyperenhancement caused by compensatory inflow increase from the hepatic artery is commonly seen on post-contrast images. The irradiated liver in the portal venous phase can show hyper- or hypoenhancement, which depends on whether sinusoid congestion in

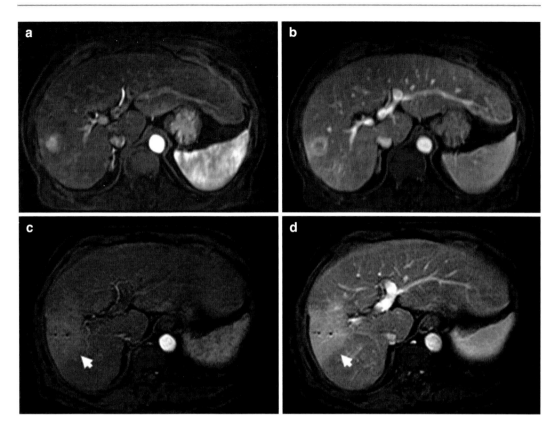

Fig. 19.4 Contrast-enhanced MR imaging of tumor response and focal liver reaction in a 77-year-old woman with HCC treated by stereotactic body radiotherapy (SBRT). The patient received 50 Gy in 5 fractions. Axial arterial phase at baseline (**a**) demonstrates an enhancing mass arising from segment 6 with subsequent wash-out at portal venous phase (**b**). (**c** and **d**) Imaging three months post SBRT shows reduction of enhancement of the mass without subsequent wash-out. Note the wedge-shaped enhancement at the irradiated non-tumorous liver parenchyma adjacent to HCC, indicative of reactive hyperemia (arrow)

the irradiated liver leads to slower contrast inflow than that in the nonirradiated liver (Fig. 19.4). In the delayed phase, the irradiated liver has similar attenuation to that of the non-irradiated liver due to unimpaired contrast-clearing ability after irradiation [1].

The subacute stage is defined as 3–6 months after radiotherapy. The pathological features are similar to those seen in the acute stage, except for progressive obstruction of the sublobular veins, which reduces their ability to clear the contrast. On CT and MRI, it is manifested as hypoenhancement during the arterial and portal venous phases, while the stasis of contrast leads to hyperenhancement in the delayed phases [29].

The chronic stage, defined as more than 6 months after radiotherapy, is characterized by central vein occlusion, loss of hepatocytes with irreversible fibrosis replacement, or collapse of the lobules with architecture distortion. The liver parenchyma may progress to atrophy and volume reduction, resulting in capsular contraction depending on the liver regeneration capacity [29]. MRI is better for detecting fibrosis, which displays low signal intensity on T1- and T2-weighted images. Generally, the presentation is the same as that in the subacute stage with a possible gradual transition to a normal enhancement pattern. Diffuse hypoenhancement may be seen during the hepatobiliary phase of MRI since permanently non-functioning hepatocytes exist [27]. One uncommon finding is low signal intensity on in-phase MRI, probably due to accumulation of Kupffer cells loaded with hemosiderin [1].

Table 19.2 Characteristics of the focal liver reaction

Time from radiotherapy	Pathological findings	Imaging appearance
Acute (1–3 months)	– Sinusoidal congestion and fibrin thrombi within sinusoids – Perisinusoidal hemorrhages and reactive hyperemia – Atrophy and degeneration of hepatocytes in zone 3	*Precontrast*: – CT: hypoattenuation relative to the background liver – MRI: T1: low signal intensity; T2: high signal intensity; DWI: mildly restricted; ADC: increased *Postcontrast*: – Arterial phase: band-like or wedge-shaped enhancement – Portal venous phase: reduced or persistent enhancement – Delayed phase: isoenhancement relative to the background liver
Subacute (3–6 months)	– Further obstruction or occlusion of sublobular veins compared with the acute stage findings – Obstructed small portal veins in the triad due to dense proliferation of collagen	*Precontrast*: – the same findings as in the acute stage *Postcontrast*: – Arterial and portal venous phase: hypoenhancement – Delayed phase: hyperenhancement
Chronic (≥ 6 months)	– Fibrosis and/or occlusion of central veins – Collapse of lobules and architecture distortion – Little congestion and rebuilt hepatocyte plate – Accumulation of Kupffer cells with/without hemosiderin	*Precontrast*: – MRI: T1: low signal intensity; T2: low signal intensity *Postcontrast*: – Generally, the same findings as in the subacute stage with gradual returning to normal enhancement pattern – Volume loss

CT computed tomography, *MRI* magnetic resonance imaging, *DWI* diffusion-weighted imaging, *ADC* apparent diffusion coefficient

The characteristics of pathological findings and imaging appearance of the FLR are summarized in Table 19.2.

The dynamic changes of the FLR should be differentiated from residual or recurrent tumors. For example, the rim-like enhancement seen on the arterial and portal venous phases typically occurs in the early stage and resolves beyond 6 months following radiotherapy [30–32]. The presence of contrast washout and vessel displacement may indicate suspicious tumors.

19.5   Potential Pitfalls in Tumor Response Evaluation

With the concept of considering enhancement as an indicator of viable tumors, the EASL and mRECIST correlate better with survival than do the RECIST v1.1 and WHO guidelines [33, 34]. However, concerns remain regarding inaccurate interpretation by the current imaging response criteria. Since radiotherapy inevitably delivers a radiation dose to the normal hepatic parenchyma adjacent to the treated tumor, an FLR with a post-radiotherapy enhancement pattern that mimics the presence of a tumor can be observed in the irradiated non-tumorous area [32, 35]. In addition, persistent arterial enhancement of the irradiated tumor can be observed within the first 12 months after radiotherapy in patients with HCC who remain disease-free. All these phenomena could easily be misinterpreted as disease persistence or local recurrence. Given that post-radiotherapy changes with much slower tumor shrinkage and necrosis formation differ from the immediate coagulative and devascularization changes resulting from RFA or TACE, many studies have found poor concordance between the post-radiotherapy imaging response and the pathological response evaluated by examining explant specimens [28, 36]. This indicates that refinement of the response evaluation criteria for HCC is required in the near future.

19.6   Conclusion

Assessing tumor response is challenging and requires evaluating image changes of both tumor and surrounding liver parenchyma over time. In early follow-up (3–6 months) after radiotherapy, the irradiated area can show hyperemia change. This does not necessarily indicate viable tumor or tumor progression. The typical follow-up images of the responders can show decreased size of the enhancing tumor over time for one year or longer. Thus, accurate response interpretation requires a series of follow-up contrast-enhanced images with careful assessment of consecutive changes.

References

1. Haddad MM, Merrell KW, Hallemeier CL, Johnson GB, Mounajjed T, Olivier KR, et al. Stereotactic body radiation therapy of liver tumors: post-treatment appearances and evaluation of treatment response: a pictorial review. Abdom Radiol (NY). 2016;41(10):2061–77.
2. Fu X, Sluka JP, Clendenon SG, Dunn KW, Wang Z, Klaunig JE, et al. Modeling of xenobiotic transport and metabolism in virtual hepatic lobule models. PLoS One. 2018;13(9):e0198060.
3. Takamatsu S, Kozaka K, Kobayashi S, Yoneda N, Yoshida K, Inoue D, et al. Pathology and images of radiation-induced hepatitis: a review article. Jpn J Radiol. 2018;36(4):241–56.
4. Lawrence TS, Robertson JM, Anscher MS, Jirtle RL, Ensminger WD, Fajardo LF. Hepatic toxicity resulting from cancer treatment. Int J Radiat Oncol Biol Phys. 1995;31(5):1237–48.
5. Maturen KE, Feng MU, Wasnik AP, Azar SF, Appelman HD, Francis IR, et al. Imaging effects of radiation therapy in the abdomen and pelvis: evaluating "innocent bystander" tissues. Radiographics. 2013;33(2):599–619.
6. Olsen CC, Welsh J, Kavanagh BD, Franklin W, McCarter M, Cardenes HR, et al. Microscopic and macroscopic tumor and parenchymal effects of liver stereotactic body radiotherapy. Int J Radiat Oncol Biol Phys. 2009;73(5):1414–24.
7. Therasse P, Arbuck SG, Eisenhauer EA, Wanders J, Kaplan RS, Rubinstein L, et al. New guidelines to evaluate the response to treatment in solid tumors. European Organization for Research and Treatment of Cancer, National Cancer Institute of the United States, National Cancer Institute of Canada. J Natl Cancer Inst. 2000;92(3):205–16.
8. Eisenhauer EA, Therasse P, Bogaerts J, Schwartz LH, Sargent D, Ford R, et al. New response evaluation criteria in solid tumours: revised RECIST guideline (version 1.1). Eur J Cancer. 2009;45(2):228–47.
9. Bruix J, Sherman M, Llovet JM, Beaugrand M, Lencioni R, Burroughs AK, et al. Clinical management of hepatocellular carcinoma. Conclusions of the Barcelona-2000 EASL conference. European Association for the Study of the Liver. J Hepatol. 2001;35(3):421–30.
10. Lencioni R, Llovet JM. Modified RECIST (mRECIST) assessment for hepatocellular carcinoma. Semin Liver Dis. 2010;30(1):52–60.
11. De Santis M, Alborino S, Tartoni PL, Torricelli P, Casolo A, Romagnoli R. Effects of lipiodol retention on MRI signal intensity from hepatocellular carcinoma and surrounding liver treated by chemoembolization. Eur Radiol. 1997;7(1):10–6.
12. Tsien C, Cao Y, Chenevert T. Clinical applications for diffusion magnetic resonance imaging in radiotherapy. Semin Radiat Oncol. 2014;24(3):218–26.
13. Hamstra DA, Rehemtulla A, Ross BD. Diffusion magnetic resonance imaging: a biomarker for treatment response in oncology. J Clin Oncol. 2007;25(26):4104–9.
14. Yu JI, Park HC, Lim DH, Choi Y, Jung SH, Paik SW, et al. The role of diffusion-weighted magnetic resonance imaging in the treatment response evaluation of hepatocellular carcinoma patients treated with radiation therapy. Int J Radiat Oncol Biol Phys. 2014;89(4):814–21.
15. Park HJ, Kim SH, Jang KM, Lim S, Kang TW, Park HC, et al. Added value of diffusion-weighted MRI for evaluating viable tumor of hepatocellular carcinomas treated with radiotherapy in patients with chronic liver disease. AJR Am J Roentgenol. 2014;202(1):92–101.
16. Lo CH, Huang WY, Hsiang CW, Lee MS, Lin CS, Yang JF, et al. Prognostic significance of apparent diffusion coefficient in hepatocellular carcinoma patients treated with stereotactic ablative radiotherapy. Sci Rep. 2019;9(1):14157.
17. Eccles CL, Haider EA, Haider MA, Fung S, Lockwood G, Dawson LA. Change in diffusion weighted MRI during liver cancer radiotherapy: preliminary observations. Acta Oncol. 2009;48(7):1034–43.
18. Choi JY, Lee JM, Sirlin CB. CT and MR imaging diagnosis and staging of hepatocellular carcinoma: part II. Extracellular agents, hepatobiliary agents, and ancillary imaging features. Radiology. 2014;273(1):30–50.
19. Sanuki N, Takeda A, Oku Y, Eriguchi T, Nishimura S, Aoki Y, et al. Threshold doses for focal liver reaction after stereotactic ablative body radiation therapy for small hepatocellular carcinoma depend on liver function: evaluation on magnetic resonance imaging

with Gd-EOB-DTPA. Int J Radiat Oncol Biol Phys. 2014;88(2):306–11.

20. Juweid ME, Cheson BD. Positron-emission tomography and assessment of cancer therapy. N Engl J Med. 2006;354(5):496–507.

21. Trojan J, Schroeder O, Raedle J, Baum RP, Herrmann G, Jacobi V, et al. Fluorine-18 FDG positron emission tomography for imaging of hepatocellular carcinoma. Am J Gastroenterol. 1999;94(11):3314–9.

22. Khan MA, Combs CS, Brunt EM, Lowe VJ, Wolverson MK, Solomon H, et al. Positron emission tomography scanning in the evaluation of hepatocellular carcinoma. J Hepatol. 2000;32(5):792–7.

23. Chung YH, Yu CF, Chiu SC, Chiu H, Hsu ST, Wu CR, et al. Diffusion-weighted MRI and (18)F-FDG PET correlation with immunity in early radiotherapy response in BNL hepatocellular carcinoma mouse model: timeline validation. Eur J Nucl Med Mol Imaging. 2019;46(8):1733–44.

24. Talbot JN, Fartoux L, Balogova S, Nataf V, Kerrou K, Gutman F, et al. Detection of hepatocellular carcinoma with PET/CT: a prospective comparison of 18F-fluorocholine and 18F-FDG in patients with cirrhosis or chronic liver disease. J Nucl Med. 2010;51(11):1699–706.

25. Wallace MC, Sek K, Francis RJ, Samuelson S, Ferguson J, Tibballs J, et al. Baseline and post-treatment 18F-fluorocholine PET/CT predicts outcomes in hepatocellular carcinoma following locoregional therapy. Dig Dis Sci. 2020;65(2):647–57.

26. Price TR, Perkins SM, Sandrasegaran K, Henderson MA, Maluccio MA, Zook JE, et al. Evaluation of response after stereotactic body radiotherapy for hepatocellular carcinoma. Cancer. 2012;118(12):3191–8.

27. Mendiratta-Lala M, Masch W, Shankar PR, Hartman HE, Davenport MS, Schipper MJ, et al. Magnetic resonance imaging evaluation of hepatocellular carcinoma treated with stereotactic body radiation therapy: long term imaging follow-up. Int J Radiat Oncol Biol Phys. 2019;103(1):169–79.

28. Mannina EM, Cardenes HR, Lasley FD, Goodman B, Zook J, Althouse S, et al. Role of stereotactic body radiation therapy before orthotopic liver transplantation: retrospective evaluation of pathologic response and outcomes. Int J Radiat Oncol Biol Phys. 2017;97(5):931–8.

29. Mastrocostas K, Jang HJ, Fischer S, Dawson LA, Munoz-Schuffenegger P, Sapisochin G, et al. Imaging post-stereotactic body radiation therapy responses for hepatocellular carcinoma: typical imaging patterns and pitfalls. Abdom Radiol (NY). 2019;44(5):1795–807.

30. Fajardo LF. The pathology of ionizing radiation as defined by morphologic patterns. Acta Oncol. 2005;44(1):13–22.

31. Oldrini G, Huertas A, Renard-Oldrini S, Taste-George H, Vogin G, Laurent V, et al. Tumor response assessment by MRI following stereotactic body radiation therapy for hepatocellular carcinoma. PLoS One. 2017;12(4):e0176118.

32. Park MJ, Kim SY, Yoon SM, Kim JH, Park SH, Lee SS, et al. Stereotactic body radiotherapy-induced arterial hypervascularity of non-tumorous hepatic parenchyma in patients with hepatocellular carcinoma: potential pitfalls in tumor response evaluation on multiphase computed tomography. PLoS One. 2014;9(2):e90327.

33. Edeline J, Boucher E, Rolland Y, Vauleon E, Pracht M, Perrin C, et al. Comparison of tumor response by Response Evaluation Criteria in Solid Tumors (RECIST) and modified RECIST in patients treated with sorafenib for hepatocellular carcinoma. Cancer. 2012;118(1):147–56.

34. Gillmore R, Stuart S, Kirkwood A, Hameeduddin A, Woodward N, Burroughs AK, et al. EASL and mRECIST responses are independent prognostic factors for survival in hepatocellular cancer patients treated with transarterial embolization. J Hepatol. 2011;55(6):1309–16.

35. Sanuki-Fujimoto N, Takeda A, Ohashi T, Kunieda E, Iwabuchi S, Takatsuka K, et al. CT evaluations of focal liver reactions following stereotactic body radiotherapy for small hepatocellular carcinoma with cirrhosis: relationship between imaging appearance and baseline liver function. Br J Radiol. 2010;83(996):1063–71.

36. Mendiratta-Lala M, Gu E, Owen D, Cuneo KC, Bazzi L, Lawrence TS, et al. Imaging findings within the first 12 months of hepatocellular carcinoma treated with stereotactic body radiation therapy. Int J Radiat Oncol Biol Phys. 2018;102(4):1063–9.

Liver Hypertrophy Following Radiotherapy

20

Chai Hong Rim and Jinsil Seong

Abstract

Success of hepatic resection depends on procuring adequate volume of future liver remnant (FLR), which prevents postoperative hepatic failure and renders surgery feasible. Several methods have traditionally been utilized for FLR procurement: portal vein ligation/embolization. More recently, the effect of transarterial radioembolization using yttrium-90 on hypertrophy of non-involved liver has been reported. External beam radiotherapy can produce the same results. By achieving both tumor downstaging and compensatory liver hypertrophy, surgery might ultimately be possible for initially unresectable patients, which opens a chance for cure with long-term survival. In this chapter, EBRT-induced liver hypertrophy will be discussed while further active investigation is warranted.

Keywords

Liver hypertrophy · Radiotherapy · Radiation therapy · Portal vein ligation · Portal vein embolization

20.1 Portal Vein Ligation or Embolism to Achieve an Adequate Future Liver Remnant

Surgical liver resection is performed as a primary curative option for intrahepatic malignancies including hepatocellular carcinoma (HCC). To maintain adequate hepatic function and avoid postoperative hepatic failure, the future liver remnant (FLR) needs to be at least 25–30% of the original liver volume [1]. A more generous FLR of up to 40% is recommended for safe resection in patients who have impaired liver function owing to cirrhosis, steatosis, or other causes [2, 3].

Contralateral liver hypertrophy following liver atrophy by portal vein ligation was first reported in 1920 by Rous and Larimore using a rabbit model [4]. Honjo et al. [5] first reported the use of portal vein ligation (PVL) in humans as part of two-stage hepatectomy. Portal vein embolization (PVE) is a less invasive procedure that can similarly cause an atrophy-hypertrophy complex in the liver, and its application in humans was first reported by Kinoshita et al. in 1986 [6]. Given its

C. H. Rim
Korea University Medical College,
Seoul, South Korea

J. Seong (✉)
Department of Radiation Oncology, Yonsei Cancer Center, Yonsei University College of Medicine,
Seoul, South Korea
e-mail: jsseong@yuhs.ac

advantage of being less invasive, there have been numerous reports on the clinical efficacy of PVE in management of primary or metastatic liver neoplasms [7–9]. According to a recent meta-analysis that encompassed 21 studies involving up to 2000 patients, the rates of FLR hypertrophy following PVL (38.5%) and PVE (43.2%) were not significantly different ($p = 0.39$), with a similar level of serious morbidity rates, that ranged between 4% and 5% ($p = 0.397$). Although PVL has the disadvantage requiring surgery with general anesthesia, it can be a good alternative when radiological facilities for PVE are lacking, when staging laparotomy is required, or as a part of staged hepatectomy [10].

Either preoperative PVE or PVL causes the redistribution of portal blood flow which concentrates it in the non-embolized or ligated lobe [11]. Together with shear stress, it further triggers release of various factors involving hepatocyte growth factor, epidermal growth factor, transforming growth factor α, insulin, noradrenaline, as well as cytokines such as interleukin-6 and tumor necrosis factor-α. All these contribute to pro-proliferative signaling that leads to mitosis, increased transcription, and hepatocyte proliferation [12, 13]. The clinical factors associated with liver hypertrophy after PVE or PVL are still unclear; clinical studies on PVE have found that the disease status of the liver (including cirrhosis and steatosis) was not correlated with this phenomenon [14–17]. Lee et al. [18] induced cirrhosis in rats using carbon tetrachloride and found that both cirrhotic and noncirrhotic hepatocytes had comparable elevations in their mitotic indices after PVE. Similarly, Mizuno et al. [19] reported that the expression of DNA polymerase α, a marker of hepatocyte replication, was also induced in unoccluded lobes of the cholestatic livers of rats.

Rather, liver hypertrophy after PVE or PVL appears to be affected by anatomical consideration. It has been consistently reported that liver volume hypertrophy is more pronounced when the initial FLR is small [15, 17, 20]. This might be because the larger the liver volume affected by embolization, the greater the portal blood flow redistribution, which can affect release of growth factors and cytokines. Extended PVE, including in segment IV, might induce a higher level of contralateral volume hypertrophy, although this observation hasn't been reproduced in the studies [17, 21–23]. Collateral vascular formations were found to be negatively correlated with contralateral liver hypertrophy [24, 25]. In clinical practice, PVE or PVL is usually performed by embolizing or ligating, respectively, the blood flow of the right lobe, thereby inducing hypertrophy of the left lobe. These procedures are rarely applied to the left, because a relatively small volume of left lobe may result in a lesser degree of blood flow redistribution and release of the related factors, causing FLR increase that is less than satisfactory [13, 26, 27].

20.2 Liver Hypertrophy Following Internal Radiotherapy

Selective internal radiotherapy (SIRT), also known as radioembolization, is a transarterial intervention therapy delivering the radioisotope yttrium-90 through glass beads or resin microspheres to cancer-feeding arteries. It has been increasingly used for the treatment of unresectable HCC [28–30]. In a recent randomized study of patients with Barcelona Clinic of Liver Cancer stages A or B HCC, those treated with SIRT had longer times to progression than—and comparable survival rates to—those who underwent conventional transarterial chemoembolization [31]. The recent National Cancer Comprehensive Network guidelines also recommend SIRT as one of the primary locoregional modalities for unresectable HCC [29]. Along with favorable tumor responses ranging from 40–70% [28, 29, 32], certain degrees of contralateral hypertrophy were consistently reported after unilateral radio-embolization [33–36]. While PVE has long been utilized for liver hypertrophy prior to liver resection, a major drawback is that tumor growth can continue during the time waiting for contralateral hypertrophy. For tumors close to major biliary or vascular structures, such growth might preclude planned surgical resections [7, 37, 38]. In SIRT, however, these limitations can be overcome by eliciting contralateral liver hypertrophy while also controlling and possibly downstaging the tumor.

Most of the studies published to date are single-arm observational investigations of changes in the FLR after SIRT. A study by Vouche et al. [34], which was one of the largest series to date, found that contralateral hypertrophy increased steadily and that the median maximal %FLR hypertrophy (FLR post-treatment—FLR pre-treatment/FLR pre-treatment) was 26%. The tumor burden in the right lobe gradually decreased up to the last follow-up visit > 9 months later. Among the clinical features including cirrhosis, liver function, and radiation dose, the presence of right PVT was the only significant factor affecting contralateral hypertrophy. Fernandez-Ros et al. [35] also reported a temporal increase in the size of the spared hemiliver, with a mean absolute increase of 230 mL after 26 weeks. The degree of hypertrophy was negatively associated with cirrhosis and elevated bilirubin levels with borderline statistical significance.

Garlipp et al. [33] attempted a head-to-head comparison between preoperative PVE and SIRT. They found that PVE yielded a significantly higher FLR increase than SIRT (61.5% vs. 29%, $p < 0.001$) as well as a shorter median time interval for FLR increase (33 days vs. 46 days). Serious complications were rare in both arms. The authors concluded that PVE had a significantly higher potential inducing contralateral hypertrophy, whereas SIRT notably minimized the risk of tumor progression in certain patients. In a recent systematic review of seven observational clinical series, SIRT induced contralateral liver hypertrophy between 26% and 47% during a period ranging from 44 days to 9 months; the extent of hypertrophy was similar to that induced by PVE (10–46%), although PVE induced hypertrophy faster (2–8 weeks) [37].

SIRT is an attractive local treatment that can both control the tumor and induce FLR hypertrophy, thereby rendering surgery more feasible. Since the current literature is mostly limited to single-arm observational studies, future research should investigate its efficacy, including in comparison to PVE; moreover, clinical factors that can predict the degree of contralateral liver hypertrophy should be identified.

20.3 Liver Hypertrophy Following External Beam Radiotherapy (EBRT)

Compensatory liver hypertrophy after EBRT has been frequently observed in radiation oncology clinical practice. However, this issue hasn't been well reported when compared to that concerning PVE, PVL, and internal radiotherapy [39]. This lack of interest might come because most radiation oncologists focus more on the intended purpose of EBRT, while liver hypertrophy after EBRT is an unintended consequence. Another reason is that many patients with locally advanced HCC who are referred for EBRT have major vessel invasion, such as PVT, which is deemed a contraindication for consequent therapeutic surgery [30, 40, 41].

A recent study from our group appears to be the only investigation to date aiming to evaluate liver hypertrophy after EBRT using X-ray [39]. Eighty-two patients with primary hepatic neoplasms were included; 63 had disease in the right lobe and 19 had disease in the left lobe. Among patients with right lobe tumors, %FLR hypertrophy (FLR at follow-up–FLR at baseline/FLR at baseline) continued to increase until the last follow-up (median: 396 days); the median maximal %FLR hypertrophy was 49.6%. Tumor volume also continued to shrink until the third follow-up visit (median: 211 days). Clinical factors affecting liver hypertrophy were analyzed involving liver function in Child-Pugh score, PVT, and treatment modalities, showing that tumor extent as the only one; the %FLR for tumors extending to both the upper and lower lobes was 77.4% whereas that for tumors extending to only one of the lobes was 49.4% ($p = 0.022$). Liver volume receiving less than 30 Gy was inversely correlated with %FLR hypertrophy at the first (median: 50 days) and second follow-ups (median: 120 days). No significant compensatory hypertrophy was observed in patients with tumors in the left lobe.

Table 20.1 Summary of the studies on liver hypertrophy after external beam radiotherapy

Author Type of RT	Dose	BED_{10Gy}	Tumor size (ml)	Child-Pugh score (%)	%FLR[a] hypertrophy at 1 year	Factors related to hypertrophy	Hypertrophy and survival
Rim et al. [39] Conventional 72%; SBRT 28%	M50Gy/25F (conventional) M52 Gy/4F (SBRT)	M60; M119.6	GTV: M63.6 (0.9–1529.2)	5 (71%); ≥6 (29%)	M51.5% (−3–196.1)	Tumor extent (extending both upper and lower lobe) V30Gy (first and second f/u)	Not significant
Imada et al. [42] Carbon ion	48–79.5 GyE in 4–15F	65.8–122.5	GTV: M35.2 (4.6–861.9)	Class A (81.3%)	M35.9%	Platelet count (MVA) PTV volume (UVA)	Larger hypertrophy group showed higher OS and better liver function profiles (albumin, PT, bilirubin, platelet)
Kim et al. [44] SBRT	M50Gy/10F	M75	CTV: mean 14.7	5 (69%); 6 (31%)	Not significant		

Uppercase M prefixes denote median value

Abbreviations: *RT* radiotherapy, *BED* biologically equivalent dose, *FLR* future liver remnant ratio, *SBRT* stereotactic body radiotherapy, *GTV* gross tumor volume, *CTV* clinical target volume, *V30Gy* volume irradiated with <30Gy of irradiation, *PTV* planning target volume, *PT* prothrombin, *MVA* multivariate analysis, *UVA* univariate analysis, *OS* overall survival

%FLR hypertrophy: FLR at follow-up–FLR at baseline/FLR at baseline

aFLR was calculated as non-irradiated region (left lobe)/non-irradiated and irradiated regions in the study by Imada et al., and left lobe volume/whole normal liver volume in the study by Rim et al.

Imada et al. [42] investigated the hypertrophy of the unirradiated contralateral liver after carbon ion radiotherapy (CIRT); their study included 43 patients who underwent CIRT to the right lobe of the liver but not to the left lobe. On serial follow-up visits at three, six, and 12 months, hypertrophy of the unirradiated lobe showed the most significant increase three months post-CIRT. The patient subgroup with larger hypertrophy demonstrated better liver function profiles one year later, including higher serum albumin, lower total bilirubin, and higher platelet counts. Patient subgroups with greater hypertrophy also achieved better overall survival, which suggested a consequence of the relatively favorable liver function profile achieved after CIRT. The only clinical variable affecting hypertrophy on multivariate analysis was platelet count, which the authors suggested as a marker of chronic liver

disease [43]. The radiotherapy target volume was a factor that significantly affected hypertrophy on univariate analysis. In a small case series by Kim et al. [44], no significant change in liver volume was noted after 12 months of follow-up in patients who underwent stereotactic body radiation therapy with a mean target volume of 14.7 cm³, which seems to be caused by the small volume of treatment.

The results of the aforementioned studies are summarized in Table 20.1.

As summarized in Table 20.1, treatment volume was found to be the most significant factor for liver hypertrophy. Our group reported that tumors extending to both the upper and lower right lobes and those with larger V_{30Gy} volumes (volume of liver irradiated < 30 Gy) were positively correlated with compensatory hypertrophy [39]. Imada et al. [42] also reported that the

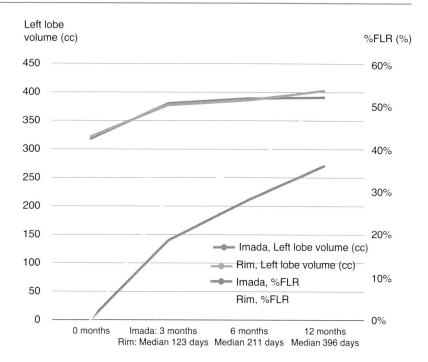

Fig. 20.1 Temporal change of non-irradiated volumes (left lobes) and %FLR increase in the study by Imada et al. [42] and Rim et al. [39]

planning target volume was a significant factor in hypertrophy ($p = 0.013$), although it was not found to be a significant factor in multivariate analysis ($p = 0.147$). Importance of irradiated volume is repeatedly proved as seen in the study of Kim et al. showing lack of hypertrophy in small target volume [44]. This finding was also observed in the PVE studies, which showed that a small initial FLR led to more liver hypertrophy after PVE [15, 17, 20], because of greater blood flow redistribution and correlating cytokines. Additionally, %FLR hypertrophy increased steadily till the one-year follow-up, and the non-irradiated left lobe volume increased maximally in the first 3–4 months (Fig. 20.1). The relationship between liver function profiles and compensatory hypertrophy should be further investigated, since platelet count was correlated with the degree of hypertrophy in the study by Imada et al. [42], whereas none of the liver function tests were correlated with hypertrophy in the study by Rim et al. [39].

In summary, to achieve a substantial level of compensatory hypertrophy in clinical practice, the key point is to irradiate a moderate-to to-large target volume in the right lobe while minimizing bystander irradiation to the normal liver (lowering V30Gy in planning). Substantial hypertrophy was found to occur in the first three to four months after EBRT, whereas %FLR hypertrophy steadily increased for up to one year with a mild increase in the volume of the non-irradiated left lobe and a decrease in the volume of the irradiated lobe.

It is also noteworthy that compensatory hypertrophy will play a significant role when curative resection can be performed following EBRT-induced downsizing and or downstaging (Fig. 20.2). Lee et al. [18] reported that 16.9% of initially inoperable patients underwent successful surgery after downstaging induced by EBRT and hepatic arterial infusion chemotherapy; moreover, half of these patients survived for more than five years. In his study, compensatory hypertrophy was one of the key factors in making surgery feasible.

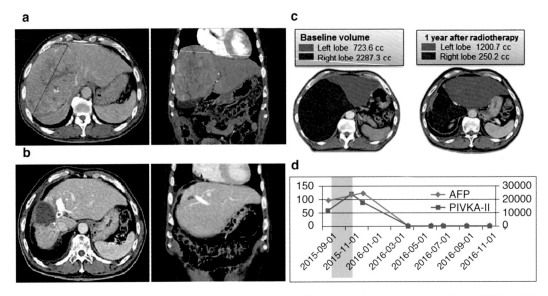

Fig. 20.2 Marked volumetric decrease with necrotic change (downstaging) as well as compensatory hypertrophy of the left liver one year after external beam radiotherapy (EBRT) (**a**, **b**). Volumetry of the atrophy-hypertrophy complex after EBRT (**c**). Normalization of tumor markers after EBRT (red shadow, **d**). AFP, alpha-fetoprotein; PIVKA-II, Protein Induced by Vitamin K Absence (Referenced from: Rim et al. [39])

20.4 Summary and Conclusions

Based on the accumulated evidence and clinical experience, PVE is currently accepted as a standard modality for producing hypertrophy of the FLR. More recently, SIRT has been increasingly investigated and applied given its merits; i.e., it can be used to achieve both contralateral hypertrophy and tumor control within the irradiated lobe. EBRT can also produce the same results. As discussed above, involving a moderate-to-large target volume for radiation in the right lobe while protecting the normal liver from bystander irradiation seems necessary to result in a significant level of compensatory hypertrophy. The greatest increase in the volume of the non-irradiated left lobe occurred in the first three to four months, whereas an increase in %FLR hypertrophy and a decrease in irradiated liver and tumor volume continued until the one-year follow-up. By achieving both tumor downstaging and compensatory liver hypertrophy, surgery might ultimately be possible for initially unresectable patients, which opens a chance for cure with long-term survival.

References

1. Goh BK. Measured versus estimated total liver volume to preoperatively assess the adequacy of future liver remnant: which method should we use? Ann Surg. 2015;262(2):e72.
2. Tanaka K, Shimada H, Matsuo K, Ueda M, Endo I, Togo S. Remnant liver regeneration after two-stage hepatectomy for multiple bilobar colorectal metastases. Eur J Surg Oncol (EJSO). 2007;33(3):329–35.
3. Hemming AW, Reed AI, Howard RJ, Fujita S, Hochwald SN, Caridi JG, et al. Preoperative portal vein embolization for extended hepatectomy. Ann Surg. 2003;237(5):686.
4. Rous P, Larimore LD. Relation of the portal blood to liver maintenance: a demonstration of liver atrophy conditional on compensation. J Exp Med. 1920;31(5):609–32.
5. Honjo I, Kozaka S. Extensive resection of the liver in two stages. Revue internationale d'hepatologie. 1965;15:309–19.
6. Kinoshita H, Sakai K, Hirohashi K, Igawa S, Yamasaki O, Kubo S. Preoperative portal vein embolization for hepatocellular carcinoma. World J Surg. 1986;10(5):803–8.
7. Azoulay D, Castaing D, Krissat J, Smail A, Hargreaves GM, Lemoine A, et al. Percutaneous portal vein embolization increases the feasibility and safety of major liver resection for hepatocellular carcinoma in injured liver. Ann Surg. 2000;232(5):665.

8. de Baere T, Roche A, Elias D, Lasser P, Lagrange C, Bousson V. Preoperative portal vein embolization for extension of hepatectomy indications. Hepatology. 1996;24(6):1386–91.

9. Kawasaki S, Makuuchi M, Kakazu T, Miyagawa S, Takayama T, Kosuge T, et al. Resection for multiple metastatic liver tumors after portal embolization. Surgery. 1994;115(6):674–7.

10. Schnitzbauer AA, Lang SA, Goessmann H, Nadalin S, Baumgart J, Farkas SA, et al. Right portal vein ligation combined with in situ splitting induces rapid left lateral liver lobe hypertrophy enabling 2-staged extended right hepatic resection in small-for-size settings. Ann Surg. 2012;255(3):405–14.

11. Goto Y, Nagino M, Nimura Y. Doppler estimation of portal blood flow after percutaneous transhepatic portal vein embolization. Ann Surg. 1998;228(2):209.

12. Yuceturk H, Yagmurdur M, Gur G, Demirbilek M, Bilezikci B, Turan M, et al. Role of heparin on TNF-α and IL-6 levels in liver regeneration after partial hepatic resection. Eur Surg Res. 2007;39(4):216–21.

13. Kim RD, Kim JS, Watanabe G, Mohuczy D, Behrns KE, editors. Liver regeneration and the atrophy-hypertrophy complex. Seminars in interventional radiology; 2008: © Thieme Medical Publishers.

14. Ribero D, Abdalla E, Madoff D, Donadon M, Loyer EM, Vauthey JN. Portal vein embolization before major hepatectomy and its effects on regeneration, resectability and outcome. Br J Surg Incorp Eur J Surg Swiss Surg. 2007;94(11):1386–94.

15. Cazejust J, Bessoud B, Le Bail M, Menu Y. Preoperative portal vein embolization with a combination of trisacryl microspheres, gelfoam and coils. Diagn Interv Imaging. 2015;96(1):57–64.

16. Giraudo G, Greget M, Oussoultzoglou E, Rosso E, Bachellier P, Jaeck D. Preoperative contralateral portal vein embolization before major hepatic resection is a safe and efficient procedure: a large single institution experience. Surgery. 2008;143(4):476–82.

17. de Baere T, Teriitehau C, Deschamps F, Catherine L, Rao P, Hakime A, et al. Predictive factors for hypertrophy of the future remnant liver after selective portal vein embolization. Ann Surg Oncol. 2010;17(8):2081–9.

18. Lee KC, Kinoshita H, Hirohashi K, Kubo S, Iwasa R. Extension of surgical indications for hepatocellular carcinoma by portal vein embolization. World J Surg. 1993;17(1):109–15.

19. Mizuno S-i, Nimura Y, Suzuki H, Yoshida S. Portal vein branch occlusion induces cell proliferation of cholestatic rat liver. J Surg Res. 1996;60(1):249–57.

20. Imamura H, Shimada R, Kubota M, Matsuyama Y, Nakayama A, Miyagawa S, et al. Preoperative portal vein embolization: an audit of 84 patients. Hepatology. 1999;29(4):1099–105.

21. Nagino M, Ando M, Kamiya J, Uesaka K, Sano T, Nimura Y. Liver regeneration after major hepatectomy for biliary cancer. Br J Surg. 2001;88(8):1084–91.

22. Kishi Y, Madoff DC, Abdalla EK, Palavecino M, Ribero D, Chun YS, et al. Is embolization of segment 4 portal veins before extended right hepatectomy justified? Surgery. 2008;144(5):744–51.

23. Massimino KP, Kolbeck KJ, Enestvedt CK, Orloff S, Billingsley KG. Safety and efficacy of preoperative right portal vein embolization in patients at risk for postoperative liver failure following major right hepatectomy. HPB. 2012;14(1):14–9.

24. Van Lienden K, Hoekstra L, Bennink R, van Gulik T. Intrahepatic left to right portoportal venous collateral vascular formation in patients undergoing right portal vein ligation. Cardiovasc Intervent Radiol. 2013;36(6):1572–9.

25. Zeile M, Bakal A, Volkmer JE, Stavrou GA, Dautel P, Hoeltje J, et al. Identification of cofactors influencing hypertrophy of the future liver remnant after portal vein embolization—the effect of collaterals on embolized liver volume. Br J Radiol. 2016;89(1068):20160306.

26. May BJ, Madoff DC, editors. Portal vein embolization: rationale, technique, and current application. Seminars in interventional radiology; 2012: Thieme Medical Publishers.

27. Abdalla EK, Denys A, Chevalier P, Nemr RA, Vauthey J-N. Total and segmental liver volume variations: implications for liver surgery. Surgery. 2004;135(4):404–10.

28. Salem R, Lewandowski RJ, Mulcahy MF, Riaz A, Ryu RK, Ibrahim S, et al. Radioembolization for hepatocellular carcinoma using Yttrium-90 microspheres: a comprehensive report of long-term outcomes. Gastroenterology. 2010;138(1):52–64.

29. Kulik LM, Carr BI, Mulcahy MF, Lewandowski RJ, Atassi B, Ryu RK, et al. Safety and efficacy of 90Y radiotherapy for hepatocellular carcinoma with and without portal vein thrombosis. Hepatology. 2008;47(1):71–81.

30. Rim CH, Kim CY, Yang DS, Yoon WS. Comparison of radiation therapy modalities for hepatocellular carcinoma with portal vein thrombosis: a meta-analysis and systematic review. Radiother Oncol. 2018;129(1):112–22.

31. Salem R, Gordon AC, Mouli S, Hickey R, Kallini J, Gabr A, et al. Y90 radioembolization significantly prolongs time to progression compared with chemoembolization in patients with hepatocellular carcinoma. Gastroenterology. 2016;151(6):1155–63.e2.

32. Khor AY-K, Toh Y, Allen JC, Ng DC-E, Kao Y-H, Zhu G, et al. Survival and pattern of tumor progression with yttrium-90 microsphere radioembolization in predominantly hepatitis B Asian patients with hepatocellular carcinoma. Hepatol Int. 2014;8(3):395–404.

33. Garlipp B, de Baere T, Damm R, Irmscher R, van Buskirk M, Stübs P, et al. Left-liver hypertrophy after therapeutic right-liver radioembolization is substantial but less than after portal vein embolization. Hepatology. 2014;59(5):1864–73.

34. Vouche M, Lewandowski RJ, Atassi R, Memon K, Gates VL, Ryu RK, et al. Radiation lobectomy: Time-dependent analysis of future liver remnant volume in unresectable liver cancer as a bridge to resection. J Hepatol. 2013;59(5):1029–36.

35. Fernandez-Ros N, Silva N, Bilbao JI, Inarrairaegui M, Benito A, D'Avola D, et al. Partial liver volume radioembolization induces hypertrophy in the spared hemiliver and no major signs of portal hypertension. HPB. 2014;16(3):243–9.

36. Theysohn J, Ertle J, Müller S, Schlaak J, Nensa F, Sipilae S, et al. Hepatic volume changes after lobar selective internal radiation therapy (SIRT) of hepatocellular carcinoma. Clin Radiol. 2014;69(2):172–8.

37. Teo JY, Allen JC Jr, Ng DC, Choo SP, Tai DW, Chang JP, et al. A systematic review of contralateral liver lobe hypertrophy after unilobar selective internal radiation therapy with Y90. HPB (Oxford). 2016;18(1):7–12.

38. Di Stefano DR, de Baere T, Denys A, Hakime A, Gorin G, Gillet M, et al. Preoperative percutaneous portal vein embolization: evaluation of adverse events in 188 patients. Radiology. 2005;234(2):625–30.

39. Rim CH, Park S, Woo JY, Seong J. Compensatory hypertrophy of the liver after external beam radiotherapy for primary liver cancer. Strahlenther Onkol. 2018;194(11):1017–29.

40. Galle PR, Forner A, Llovet JM, Mazzaferro V, Piscaglia F, Raoul J-L, et al. EASL clinical practice guidelines: management of hepatocellular carcinoma. J Hepatol. 2018;69(1):182–236.

41. Rim CH, Kim CY, Yang DS, Yoon WS. External beam radiation therapy to hepatocellular carcinoma involving inferior vena cava and/or right atrium: a meta-analysis and systemic review. Radiother Oncol. 2018;129(1):123–9.

42. Imada H, Kato H, Yasuda S, Yamada S, Yanagi T, Hara R, et al. Compensatory enlargement of the liver after treatment of hepatocellular carcinoma with carbon ion radiotherapy–relation to prognosis and liver function. Radiother Oncol. 2010;96(2):236–42.

43. Karasu Z, Tekin F, Ersoz G, Gunsar F, Batur Y, Ilter T, et al. Liver fibrosis is associated with decreased peripheral platelet count in patients with chronic hepatitis B and C. Dig Dis Sci. 2007;52(6):1535–9.

44. Kim YI, Park HC, Do Hoon Lim HJP, Kang SW, Park SY, Kim JS, et al. Changes of the liver volume and the Child-Pugh score after high dose hypofractionated radiotherapy in patients with small hepatocellular carcinoma. Radiat Oncol J. 2012;30(4):189.

Hepatic Dysfunction Following Radiotherapy and Management

21

Do Young Kim

Abstract

Although proper selection of patients with liver cancer minimizes the probability of occurrence of hepatic dysfunction, radiotherapy for patients with underlying liver diseases such as cirrhosis or chronic hepatitis B might lead to classic or non-classic radiation-induced liver disease. Clinically, hepatic dysfunction includes ascites, jaundice, variceal hemorrhage, hepatorenal syndrome and hepatic encephalopathy. Several factors such radiation dose, residual liver function, and treatment other than radiotherapy are involved in the development of hepatic dysfunction. Ascites is the most common manifestation of hepatic dysfunction after radiotherapy in patients with liver cancer. A strict adherence to a low-salt diet and medical therapies including diuretics and therapeutic paracentesis can control ascites. In patients with refractory ascites, liver transplantation should be considered if tumor extent after radiotherapy is decreased within usual criteria for transplantation. When patients develop jaundice during or after radiotherapy, radiation oncologists or hepatologists differentiate between obstructive jaundice and hepatocelluar jaundice, which often implies poor prognosis. Esophageal or gastric variceal bleeding is a medical emergency requiring intensive fluid resuscitation and endoscopic or interventional treatment. To prevent rebleeding from esophageal varices, endoscopic variceal ligation combined with pharmacologic therapy is necessary. Hepatic encephalopathy is a neurological or psychiatric manifestation of hepatic dysfunction resulting from inability to detoxify endogenous or exogenous compounds. Hepatic encephalopathy usually occurs late during hepatic dysfunction, requiring liver transplantation when tumor control is enough. It is essential for radiation oncologists and hepatologists to cooperate to properly manage liver cancer patients with radiation therapy.

Keywords

Radiation · Liver cancer · Hepatic dysfunction

D. Y. Kim (✉)
Department of Internal Medicine, Yonsei University College of Medicine, Seoul, South Korea
e-mail: DYK1025@yuhs.ac

21.1 Introduction

The survival of patients with liver cancer is substantially affected by not only tumor status but also liver function. Therefore, physicians and radiation oncologists should be alert to hepatic dysfunction that might occur during and after radiation treatment for liver cancer. This is because the liver is often not healthy, i.e., infected by hepatitis B virus (HBV) or hepatitis C virus (HCV) or cirrhotic, even though it is known to have a high regenerative potential. In spite of pretreatment selection of patients with liver cancer who are feasible for radiotherapy, a proportion of patients develop hepatic dysfunction including jaundice, ascites, variceal hemorrhage, and so on. In addition to appropriate selection of patients for radiotherapy, close monitoring during treatment and optimal management for patients with hepatic dysfunction are essential to improve patient survival. For successful radiation therapy for liver cancer patients, a multidisciplinary team approach and collaboration between radiation oncologists and hepatologists are crucial. Antiviral therapy for patients with HBV infection must be considered before radiation therapy since radiation might cause reactivation of HBV, resulting in liver injury and hepatic dysfunction [1].

21.1.1 Radiation-Induced Liver Disease

Traditionally, radiation therapy has not been frequently applied because of the relatively low tolerance of the whole liver to radiation [2]. However, technological advances including intensity-modulated radiotherapy (IMRT), image-guided radiotherapy (IGRT), and stereotactic body radiotherapy (SBRT) have made it possible for high doses of radiation to conform to the target volume safety [3]. Nevertheless, patients may experience liver damage such as transaminase elevation, jaundice, prolongation of prothrombin time, and aggravation of portal hypertension during or after radiation therapy. Radiation therapy causes these liver injuries for various reasons. The most important factors in avoiding radiation toxicity are the estimation of pretreatment residual liver function indicated by Child-Pugh score, accurate calculation of radiation dose, and precise targeting. Radiation-induced liver disease (RILD) is the terminology used to assess liver toxicity caused by radiation when there is an association between radiation therapy and liver disease, and it is diagnosed mainly based on clinical manifestations or laboratory findings.

21.1.1.1 Pathogenesis of RILD

The pathogenesis of RILD includes complex and multicellular responses related to vascular changes, increased collagen synthesis, and sequential activation of key growth factors and cytokines, such as tumor necrosis factor-alpha (TNF-α), transforming growth factor-beta (TGF-β), and hedgehog (Hh), which are important regulators in repair responses to liver damage [4]. Upon irradiation to the liver, subendothelial cells (SECs) are injured, undergo apoptosis and release TFN-α, which promotes hepatocyte apoptosis and Kupffer cell activation. Furthermore, injured SECs induce the penetration of red blood cells and activate fibrin deposition in central veins, resulting in sinusoidal obstruction. The ensuing hypoxic environment leads to the death of hepatocytes and the activation of Kupffer cells. Activated Kupffer cells release TGF-β, the major profibrogenic cytokine, which promotes the transdifferentiation of quiescent hepatic stellate cells (HSCs) into myofibroblast-like HSCs (MF-HSC). Apoptotic hepatocytes also produce Hh ligands, which trigger the proliferation of Hh-responsive cells, such as HSCs. MF-HSCs accumulate and promote the deposition of extracellular matrix proteins, leading to liver fibrosis [5].

21.1.1.2 Classification of RILD

RILD can be classified into two kinds of radiation toxicity. The first is classic RILD, which was historically the dose-limiting complication of liver radiation with onset two weeks to four months after whole hepatic radiation to 30–35 Gy using conventionally fractionated regimens. The underlying mechanism of liver damage is veno-occlusive disease secondary to fibrosis [6]. The clinical manifestations are comprised of anicteric hepatomegaly, ascites, and elevated liver enzymes, particularly alkaline phosphatase. Risk factors related with classic RILD are known to be high mean liver dose, primary liver cancer, male gender, and hepatic intra-arterial chemotherapy [6]. With technological advances, classic RILD is currently rare. Non-classical RILD is much more common, and the signs and symptoms are markedly elevated serum transaminases (>5× upper limit of normal) and jaundice. The most vulnerable populations affected by non-classic RILD are patients with underlying liver disease such as chronic hepatitis B or cirrhosis [7–9]. The mechanism of non-classic RILD is less well-understood but may involve the loss of regenerating hepatocytes and reactivation of hepatitis [8]. The most commonly used criteria for non-classic RILD are an increase in Child-Pugh score ≥2 in cirrhotic patients and a ≥5× increase in transaminases or change in albumin–bilirubin (ALBI) score in noncirrhotic patients. Table 21.1 shows the comparisons of several characteristics between classic and non-classic RILD.

Table 21.1 Characteristics of classic and non-classic RILD

Characteristics	Classic RILD	Nonclassic RILD
Onset	2 weeks to 4 months	
Underlying mechanism	Veno-occlusive disease	Loss of regenerating hepatocytes
Clinical manifestations	Anicteric hepatomegaly, liver enzyme elevation	Transaminase elevation, jaundice
Risk factors	High mean liver dose, male, primary liver cancer	Cirrhosis, Hepatitis B virus infection

21.1.2 Hepatic Dysfunction Following Radiation Therapy

21.1.2.1 Ascites

Ascites is the most common complication of cirrhosis, with 5–10% of patients with cirrhosis developing this complication. As a significant proportion of patients who receive radiation therapy for liver cancer have underlying cirrhosis, ascites manifests as the most frequent hepatic dysfunction following radiotherapy (Fig. 21.1). Development of ascites is due to portal hypertension according to progressive loss of functioning hepatocytes and aggravated liver fibrosis. Excessive accumulation of sodium, i.e., renal sodium retention, is explained by arterial splanchnic vasodilation. The resulting decrease in effective arterial volume activates vasoconstrictor and sodium-retaining systems such as sympathetic nervous system and renin-angiotensin-aldosterone system. Finally, renal sodium retention leads to expansion of extracellular fluid volume and formation of ascites [10]. When ascites develops, patients complain of abdominal discomfort, increase in abdominal girth, weight gain, and reduced food intake. With increasing amount of ascites, edema of the lower legs or scrotum in males might occur. The mainstays of first-line treatments for patients with ascites which occurs following radiotherapy include education regarding dietary sodium restriction (80–120 mmol/day) and oral diuretics

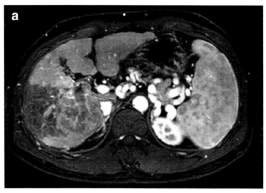
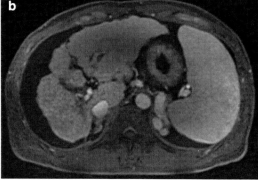

Fig. 21.1 Occurrence of ascites after radiotherapy for a 43-year-old patient with hepatocellular carcinoma. (**a**) Contrast-enhanced MRI showing advanced liver cancer with portal vein thrombosis. (**b**) Following concurrent chemoradiation therapy viable tumor substantially decreased with liver atrophy and ascites formation.

[11, 12]. More stringent dietary sodium restriction is not recommended to prevent a reduced caloric intake, which could aggravate malnutrition already present in patients with liver cancer. Fluid loss and weight change are directly related to sodium balance in patients with portal hypertension-associated ascites. It is sodium restriction, not fluid restriction, that results in weight loss, as fluid follows sodium passively [13]. It is not easy for patients with liver cancer and ascites to eat a low-salt diet because they have decreased appetite related with cancer and treatment.

21.1.2.2 Diuretics

The usual strategy of using diuretics consists in the simultaneous administration of spironolactone and furosemide starting with 100 mg/day 40 mg/day, respectively [11, 12]. Previously, single-agent spironolactone was advocated, but hypokalemia and the long half-life of this drug have resulted in its use as a single agent only in patients with minimal fluid overload [14]. Eventually most patients require combination treatment of spironolactone and furosemide. Starting both drugs appears to be the preferred approach in achieving rapid natriuresis and maintaining normokalemia. The doses of both oral diuretics can be increased simultaneously every three to five days (maintaining 100 mg:40 mg ratio) if weight loss and natriuresis are inadequate. Usual maximum doses are 400 mg/day of spironolactone and 160 mg/day of furosemide [11, 12]. Patients with parenchymal renal disease or post-liver transplantation may tolerate less spironolactone than usual because of hyperkalemia. Single morning dosing maximizes compliance. Dosing more than once daily reduces compliance and can cause nocturia. Amiloride (10–40 mg/day) can be substituted for spironolactone in patients with tender gynecomastia. Other diuretics such as torasemide must be proven to be superior to current drugs before the expense can be justified. The goal of diuretic treatment is to achieve a loss of body weight between 300 and 500 mg/day in patients without peripheral edema. Greater weight loss may be safe in patients with concomitant peripheral edema but may be asso-

ciated with complications in patients without edema [15].

21.1.2.3 Measures to Maintain Blood Pressure

Since blood pressure in patients with ascites is supported by elevated levels of vasoconstrictors such as vasopressin, angiotensin, and aldosterone, which compensate for the vasodilatory effect of nitric oxide (NO) [16], drugs that inhibit the effect of these vasoconstrictors would be expected to lower blood pressure, which might worsen survival. Angiotensin converting enzyme (ACE) inhibitors and angiotensin receptor blockers should be avoided or used with caution in patients with cirrhosis and ascites. In the unusual situations in which they are used, blood pressure and renal function must be monitored carefully to avoid rapid development of renal failure. Propranolol, which is used for reducing portal pressure, has been shown to shorten survival in patients with refractory ascites in a prospective study [17]. This could be due to its negative impact on blood pressure and the increase in the rate of paracentesis-induced circulatory dysfunction that is seen in patients who are taking propranolol in the setting of refractory ascites. Prostaglandin inhibitors such as nonsteroidal anti-inflammatory drugs (NSAIDs) can reduce urinary sodium excretion in patients with cirrhosis and can induce azotemia [18]. Thus, NSAIDS should be cautiously used in cirrhotic patients who are receiving various treatments including radiation for liver cancer.

21.1.2.4 Therapeutic Paracentesis

A prospective study has demonstrated that a single 5-liter paracentesis can be performed safely without post-paracentesis colloid infusion in patients with diuretic-resistant tense ascites [19]. Larger volumes (>5 L) of fluid have been safely removed with the administration of intravenous albumin (8 g/L of fluid removed) in patients with tense ascites whether it was diuretic-resistant or not [20]. A single large-volume paracentesis followed by diet and diuretic therapy is appropriate treatment for patients with tense ascites [19, 20]. In the outpatient clinic, body weight, blood pres-

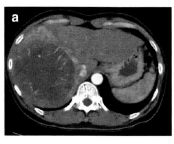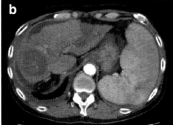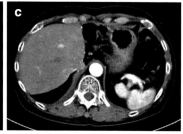

Fig. 21.2 A case of patient who underwent liver transplantation after radiotherapy for hepatocellular carcinoma. (**a**) contrast-enhanced CT scan showing a huge tumor with thrombus in inferior vena cava. (**b**) The tumor markedly decreased after concurrent chemoradiation therapy, but ascites and liver dysfunction developed. (**c**) Living donor liver transplantation was performed and there was no recurrence of tumor.

sure, orthostatic symptoms, serum electrolytes, urea, and creatinine are monitored. If weight loss is inadequate, a random spot urine sodium/potassium ratio or 24-h urine sodium can be measured. Patients who are excreting urine sodium/potassium greater than 1 or 24-h urine sodium greater than 78 mmol/day and not losing weight are consuming more sodium in their diet than 88 mmol/day (2000 g/day) and should be counseled further about dietary sodium restriction [21].

21.1.2.5 Management of Refractory Ascites

Refractory ascites is defined as fluid overload that is unresponsive to a sodium-restricted diet and high-dose diuretic treatment (400 mg/day of spironolactone and 160 mg/day of furosemide), or that recurs rapidly after therapeutic paracentesis [22]. Once ascites becomes refractory to medical treatment, the median survival of cirrhotic patients is approximately six months [23]. Therefore, the survival is expected to be much less than six months in patients with liver cancer and refractory ascites. There are several options in these patients. Serial therapeutic paracenteses are effective in controlling ascites. Even in patients with no urine excretion, paracentesis performed approximately every two weeks controls ascites [11, 12]. The treatment options for cirrhotic patients with refractory ascites are: large-volume paracentesis (LVP), defined by drainage of more than five liters of ascites, insertion of transjugular intrahepatic portosystemic shunt (TIPS), and liver transplantation (LT). In patients with liver cancer and ascites who received radiotherapy,

LT might be an effective and life-saving treatment if tumor burden does not exceed the usual criteria defined, for example, by the Milan criteria (Fig. 21.2). Frequently, TIPS is technically unavailable in these patients because of portal vein tumor thrombosis, which is contraindication of this procedure.

21.1.3 Spontaneous Bacterial Peritonitis

Spontaneous bacterial peritonitis (SBP) is an acute ascitic fluid infection, and clinically suspected when patients with cirrhosis and ascites have symptoms of fever and abdominal pain. SBP is the most frequent bacterial infection in cirrhotic patients. Diagnosis is based on paracentesis with a polymorphonuclear leukocyte count $\geq$250 cell/mm^3 in ascitic fluid, with or without positive ascitic culture, in the absence of other causes of peritonitis [24]. Patients diagnosed as SBP should receive empirical antibiotic therapy. Meanwhile, the ascitic fluid needs to be cultured in a blood culture bottle. Delaying treatment until the ascitic fluid culture grows bacteria may result in the death of the patient from overwhelming infection. Relatively broad-spectrum antibiotic therapy is warranted in patients with suspected ascitic fluid infection until the results of susceptibility testing are available. Cefotaxime or a similar third-generation cephalosporin appears to be the best choice for suspected SBP; it used to cover 95% of the flora, including the three most common isolates: *Escherichia coli*, *Klebsiella*

Pneumoniae, and *Streptococcal pneumoniae* [25]. After sensitivities are known, the spectrum of coverage can usually be narrowed. Oral oflox-acin (400 mg bid for an average of eight days) has been reported in a randomized controlled trial to be as effective as parenteral cefotaxime in the treatment of SBP in patients without vomit-ing, shock, grade II (or higher) hepatic encepha-lopathy, or serum creatinine greater than 3 mg/dl [26]. Norfloxacin 400 mg/day orally has been reported to successfully prevent SBP in patients with low-protein (<15 g/L) ascites and patients with prior SBP [27, 28].

21.1.4 Jaundice

Jaundice (from the French *jaune* meaning yel-low), refers to the yellowish discoloration of the skin, sclera, and mucous membranes that accompanies deposition of bilirubin in tissues [29]. It develops when serum bilirubin levels are elevated above 34 mmol/L (2 mg/dl), with yellow discoloration of the sclera being the site where jaundice is detected earliest due to high elastin content of sclera and its strong binding affinity for bilirubin [30]. Clinically and patho-physiologically, jaundice is classified as either hepatocellular jaundice or obstructive jaundice. Hepatocellular jaundice is due to hepatocyte dysfunction, resulting in failure of secretion of bilirubin into the bile duct. Obstructive jaun-dice, previously known as surgical jaundice, is a manifestation of cholestasis. Cholestasis is defined as impairment in the formation of bile or bile flow out of the porta hepatis through the biliary ducts into the duodenum. Cholestasis often results in conjugated hyperbilirubinemia and may or may not be accompanied by clini-cal jaundice. The main symptoms of cholestasis or jaundice are fatigue, pruritus, and indiges-tion. When physicians or radiation oncologists observe jaundice in patients who underwent radiotherapy, the first step is to differentiate hepatocellular jaundice (intrahepatic cholesta-sis) from obstructive jaundice (extrahepatic cho-lestasis). Cholestasis from bile duct obstruction is generally identified by abnormal findings on biochemical tests of the liver, such as elevated alkaline phosphatase (ALP) and γ-glutamyl transferase (γ-GT) levels and variable levels of bilirubin and prothrombin time. However, ele-vated ALP levels are not completely specific for cholestasis; the levels are often elevated even in patients with hepatocellular jaundice. The lev-els of enzyme can be elevated by less than three times the normal limit in virtually any type of liver disease. Once cholestasis is identified by the liver function tests, it should be determined whether the cholestasis is intrahepatic or extra-hepatic. Radiologic imaging plays an important role in evaluating the etiology of cholestasis and determining treatment strategies. In patients with liver cancer, extrahepatic cholestasis can be caused by extrinsic compression of bile ducts or invasion by tumors. Causes of intrahepatic cholestasis in patients with liver cancer who received radiotherapy include reactivation of hepatitis B or significant damage or lost of func-tioning hepatocytes.

21.1.4.1 Management of Jaundice

When patients with liver cancer develop intra or extrahepatic cholestasis due to compression of bile duct by mas, radiation therapy itself is sometimes useful for relieving obstructive jaun-dice. If other treatment modalities are not avail-able because of jaundice or poor liver function, radiation therapy might be optimal. In liver can-cer patients who underwent radiation therapy, the management of jaundice depends on the etiology of cholestasis. However, since patients usually have a significant tumor burden and underlying liver disease, manifestation of jaundice implies a dismal prognosis irrespective of the etiology of cholestasis. Supportive care with liver pills including ursodeoxycholic acid (UDCA) or sily-marin is recommended in patients with intrahe-patic cholestasis. Interventional or endoscopic palliation, such as percutaneous transhepatic bili-ary drainage (PTBD) or endoscopic retrograde cholangiopancreatography (ERCP) with stent-ing, might be provided to patients with obstruc-tive jaundice (Fig. 21.3).

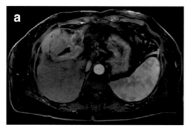 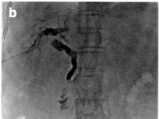 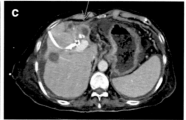

Fig. 21.3 Recurrent hepatocellular carcinoma after resection obstructing bile duct treated with radiotherapy. (**a**) A 2.7 cm recurrent tumor with bile duct dilatation at the margin of resection is observed. (**b**) Percutaneous transhepatic biliary drainage (PTBD) was performed to decompress biliary trees. (**c**) Post-radiation follow-up CT scan showing stable tumor and decompressed bile duct.

21.1.5 Portal Hypertension and Variceal Hemorrhage

Portal hypertension (PH) is defined as an increase of blood pressure in the portal venous system. Hepatic venous pressure gradient (HVPG) measurement is the gold-standard method to assess the presence of PH [31]. Based on portal pressure, patients with compensated cirrhosis can be divided into those with mild portal hypertension (HVPG >5 but <10 mmHg) and those with clinically significant PH (CSPH), defined by an HVPG ≥10 mmHg. CSPH is associated with an increased risk of developing varices and other cirrhotic complications [32–34]. As described above, radiation therapy may increase portal pressure by increasing deposition of extracellular matrix from hepatic stellate cells. Patients with gastroesophageal varices have, by definition, CSPH, because patients with GEV have an HVPG of at least 10 mmHg [35, 36]. Portal pressure increases initially as a consequence of increased intrahepatic resistance to portal flow attributed to structural mechanisms. This "structural" component, which explains around 70% of the increased intrahepatic resistance, could be targeted by treating the etiology of cirrhosis, the use of antifibrotic agents, and even anticoagulants [37]. However, at least one-third of the increased intrahepatic resistance is attributed to increased intrahepatic vascular tone, which, in turn, is attributed to endothelial dysfunction resulting mostly from reduced nitric oxide (NO) bioavailability [38]. Another factor that has been shown to contribute to the worsening of PH is the translocation of bacterial or bacterial products from the intestinal lumen into the systemic circulation [39].

21.1.5.1 Management of Acute Esophageal Variceal Bleeding

In patients with liver cancer who underwent radiation therapy, esophageal variceal hemorrhage (VH) implies poor prognosis because it is closely associated with HVPG ≥20 mmHg. Moreover, it is a life-threatening complication if hemostasis is not done urgently and completely. The precise prognosis of a patient with esophageal varices depends on whether the patient presents as an isolated decompensating event or whether the patient presents with other complications of cirrhosis such as ascites or encephalopathy [40]. New-onset or aggravation of portal vein thrombosis accompanied by hepatocellular carcinoma (HCC) could increase portal pressure and lead to VH. Therefore, imaging studies should be considered after emergent management for VH. The immediate goal of therapy in these patients is to control bleeding, to prevent early recurrence (within five days) and prevent six-week mortality, which is considered the main treatment outcome [41]. Acute VH is a medical emergency requiring intensive care. As in any patient with any hemorrhage, it is essential to first assess and protect the circulatory and respiratory status of the patient. Volume resuscitation should be initiated to restore and maintain hemodynamic stability. Packed red blood cell transfusion should be performed with a target hemoglobin level of between 7 and 8 g/dl [42]. Regarding correction of coagulopathy, correcting the international normalized ratio (INR) by the use of fresh frozen plasma or factor VIIa is not recommended. No recommendations can be given regarding platelet transfusion in patients with VH. Patients with cirrhosis presenting with GI hemorrhage are at a high risk of developing bacterial infections, and the use of antibiotic prophylaxis has been shown, in randomized controlled trials, to lead to a decrease in development of infections, recurrent hemorrhage, and death [43, 44]. Regarding the type of antibiotic, intravenous ceftriaxone has been shown to be more effective in preventing infection compared to oral norfloxacin [45]. Therefore, the antibiotic of choice is intravenous ceftriaxone at a dose of 1 g every 24 h. Duration of antibiotic prophylaxis is short term, for a maximum of seven days. Vasoactive drugs should be started as soon as variceal bleeding is suspected, ideally before endoscopy. Vasoactive drugs (terlipressin, somatostatin, octreotide) should be used in combination with endoscopic therapy and continued for up to five days [46]. Endoscopy is done as soon as possible and not more than 12 h after presentation. Endoscopic variceal ligation (EVL) is the recommended form of endoscopic therapy for acute esophageal variceal hemorrhage. Endoscopic therapy with a tissue adhesive (e.g., N-butylcyanoacrylate) is recommended for acute bleeding from gastric varices. The diagnosis VH is considered certain when active bleeding from a varix is observed or when a sign of recent bleeding, such as a "cherry red," is observed (Fig. 21.4). Early TIPS placement within 72 h improves survival in high-risk patients with acute variceal bleeding. However, in most patients with liver cancer who underwent radiotherapy, TIPS procedure is not technically available because of tumor or portal vein thrombosis. If rebleeding is modest, a second session of endoscopic therapy can be attempted. Up to 20% of VH episodes can be refractory to standard therapy and are associated with a high mortality. A "bridge" therapy may be necessary to acutely control hemorrhage until a more definitive therapy, such as TIPS, can be performed. Balloon tamponade is still used as bridge therapy and provides hemostasis in up to

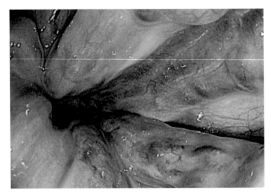

Fig. 21.4 Endoscopic appearance of esophageal varices with cherry red sign suggesting impending variceal rupture.

80% of patients but is associated with high rate of severe adverse events and a mortality rate near 20% [47]. Balloon tampodade should not exceed 24 h.

21.1.5.2 Prevention of Rebleeding of Esophageal Varices

Patients who recover from the first episode of VH have a high rebleeding risk, with a mortality of up to 33%. Therapy to prevent rebleeding is therefore mandatory in these patients and should be instituted before the patients are discharged from the hospital. First-line therapy for patients who received EVL is the combination of non-selective beta blocker (NSBB), either propranolol or nadolol. A recent meta-analysis comparing combination therapy to monotherapy with EVL or drug therapy has demonstrated that combination therapy (EVL + NSBB) is significantly more effective than EVL alone in preventing all-source GI hemorrhage. However, use of NSBB in patients with refractory ascites is not recommended because it might lower patient survival.

21.1.6 Hepatorenal Syndrome

Hepatorenal syndrome (HRS) is defined as a deterioration of kidney function that takes place in the context of severe chronic liver diseases, such as advanced cirrhosis or acute liver failure [48]. It is characterized by functional circulatory changes in the kidneys that overpower physiologic compensatory mechanisms and lead to reduced glomerular filtration rate (GFR). Re-establishment of adequate renal blood flow leads to improvement in renal function and is achieved by liver transplantation or vasoconstrictor drugs. The diagnosis of HRS is essentially one of exclusion of other causes of renal failure. The pathophysiology associated with HRS includes vasodilation in the splanchnic arterial bed and low cardiac output. There are two types of HRS. Type 1 HRS, now termed HRS-acute kidney injury (AKI), is a rapidly progressive acute renal failure that frequently develops in temporal relationship with a precipitating factor for a deterioration of liver function together with deterioration of other organ function. It is characterized by rapid deterioration caused by precipitating events that leads to the failure of one or more organs, aggravating the patient's central hypovolemic state [49]. Conventionally, HRS-AKI is only diagnosed when the serum creatinine increases more than 100% from baseline to a final level of greater than 2.5 mg/dl. Type 2 HRS, now termed HRS-non-AKI (HRS-NAKI), occurs in patients with refractory ascites and there is a steady but moderate degree of functional renal failure, often with avid sodium retention. HRS-NAKI is defined by estimated GFR rather than serum creatinine [48]. NAKI is divided into HRS-acute kidney disease (HRS-AKD) if the eGFR is less than 60 mL/min/1.73 m^2 for less than three months and HRS-chronic kidney disease (HRS-CKD) if it is less than this for more than three months.

21.1.6.1 Drug Therapy

The management of HRS starts with a fluid challenge of 20–25% intravenous albumin at 1 g/kg/day for two days and withdrawal of diuretics. This is not only needed to rule out pre-renal azotemia but also promotes early plasma volume expansion in the setting of reduced effective arterial blood volume. The specific treatment of HRS-AKI comprises vasoconstrictors in combination with albumin infusion and reversal of precipitating factors. Among the vasoconstrictors used, those that have been investigated more extensively are the vasopressin analogues, particularly terlipres-

sin [50]. The rationale for the use of vasopressin analogues in HRS is to improve the markedly impaired circulatory dysfunction by causing a vasoconstriction of the extremely dilated splanchnic vascular bed and increasing arterial pressure [51, 52]. Terlipressin shows greater efficacy in reversal of HRS-AKI in patients with a systemic inflammatory response [53], which may relate to indirect vasopressin mediated anti-inflammatory effects [54]. Response to terlipressin therapy is generally characterized by a slowly progressive reduction in serum creatinine, and an increase in arterial pressure, urine volume, and serum sodium concentration. Median time to response is 14 days and usually depends on pre-treatment serum creatinine, the time being shorter in patients with lower baseline serum creatinine [55]. The most frequent side effects of treatment are cardiovascular or ischemic complications, which have been reported in an average of 12% of patients treated [51].

21.1.6.2 TIPS

Transjugular intrahepatic portosystemic shunt has been reported to improve renal function in patients with HRS-AKI [56]. However, the applicability of TIPS in this setting is very limited because many patients have contraindications to the use of TIPS including portal vein tumor thrombosis. TIPS has also been shown to improve renal function and the control of ascites in patients with HRS-NAKI [57].

21.1.6.3 Renal Replacement Therapy

Renal replacement therapy (RRT) may be indicated for patients with HRS-AKI unresponsive to drug treatment and with volume overload, uremia, or electrolyte derangement. However, RRT does not improve survival in HRS, and it should be reserved for use as a bridge to LT [58, 59]. Short-term mortality in patients with cirrhosis and AKI who are ineligible for transplantation approaches 90% regardless of the cause of AKI [60, 61].

21.1.6.4 Liver Transplantation

The functional nature of HRS means that improvement in renal function is expected with

LT. Accordingly, LT is the treatment of choice for both HRS-AKI and HRS-NAKI, with survival rates of approximately 65% in HRS-AKI [62]. The lower survival rate compared to patients with cirrhosis without HRS is a result of renal failure being a major predictor of poor outcome after transplantation. Kidney recovery is not universal and is dependent of multiple factors, particularly duration of kidney injury [63]. Moreover, patients with HRS-AKI have a high mortality while on the waiting list and ideally should be given priority for transplantation. In patients with liver cancer who underwent radiation therapy and have no or minimal tumor burden (i.e., within Milan criteria), LT should be considered for HRS-AKI and HRS-NAKI.

21.1.7 Hepatic Encephalopathy

Hepatic encephalopathy (HE) is a prevalent complication of portal hypertension and cirrhosis that is seen in 50–70% of patients [64]. It manifests as a wide spectrum of neurological or psychiatric abnormalities ranging from subclinical alterations such as reduced awareness to coma. In patients with liver cancer who underwent radiation therapy, HE may occur because of diminishing functioning hepatocytes or aggravation of portosystemic shunt. The incidence and prevalence of HE are associated with the severity of the underlying liver insufficiency [65, 66]. In its lowest expression, HE is not overt. Instead, there is only abnormal behavior on psychometric tests oriented toward attention, working memory, psychomotor speed [67, 68]. As HE progresses, personality changes, frequent falls, incompetent driving, and fatigue may occur, and obvious alterations in consciousness and motor function occur. Disturbances of the sleep-wake cycle with excessive daytime sleepiness are frequent [69], whereas complete reversal of the sleep-wake cycle is less consistently observed. Patients may develop progressive disorientation to time and space, inappropriate behavior, and an acute state of confusion with agitation or somnolence, stupor, and finally, coma [70]. Asterixis or "flapping tremor" is often present in the early to middle

stages of HE that precede stupor or coma and is not a tremor, but a negative myoclonus consisting of loss of postural tone. It is easily elicited by actions that require postural tone, such as hyperextension of the wrists with separated fingers or the rhythmic squeezing of the examiner's fingers. However, asterixis can be observed in other areas, such as the feet, legs, arms, tongue, and eyelids. Asterixis is not pathognomic of HE because it can be observed in other diseases such as hypercarbia and uremia [71].

21.1.7.1 Diagnosis of HE

Currently, there are no gold-standard laboratory markers that can be used to diagnose HE. Hepatologists have graded the severity of HE according to the West Haven criteria [72]. However, these are subjective tools with limited interobserver reliability, especially for grade I HE, because slight hypokinesia, psychomotor retardation, and a lack of attention can easily be overlooked in clinical examination. Diagnosing cognitive dysfunction is not difficult. It can be established from clinical observation as well as neuropsychological or neurophysiological tests. The difficulty is to assign them to HE. For this reason, HE remains a diagnosis of exclusion in the patient population that is often susceptible to mental status abnormalities resulting from medications, alcohol abuse, drug use, effects of hyponatremia, and psychiatric disease. Thus, as clinically indicated, exclusion of other etiologies by laboratory and radiological assessment for a patient with altered mental status in HE is warranted. Although increased blood ammonia levels often are found in HE in large population studies, in an individual patient it often is not useful as a diagnostic test [73]. On the contrary, a normal ammonia level that occurs in a cirrhotic patient with altered mental status should lead the physician to question the diagnosis of HE [74]. Computed tomography (CT), magnetic resonance (MR), or other modality scans do not contribute diagnostic or grading information. However, the risk of intracerebral hemorrhage is at least five time higher in this patient group [75], and the symptoms may be indistinguishable. A brain scan is usually, therefore, part of the diagnostic workup of first-time HE and on clinical suspicion of other pathology including brain metastasis during or after radiotherapy for liver cancer.

21.1.7.2 Treatment of HE

The goal of therapy for HE episodes are to diagnose and treat the inciting factor because up to 90% of patients will have a precipitant [76]. Lactulose is the most used disaccharide for the treatment of HE. This nonabsorbable disaccharide has laxative effects and change the gut microbiome to non-urase-producing bacteria, reducing intestinal ammonia production [77]. Lactulose is usually administered as an oral syrup with dosages titrated for a goal of 2–4 soft bowel movements a day. Lactulose also can be given rectally (300 mL in 700 mL of saline), which is preferred in patients in whom oral administration is contraindicated [78]. Common side effects of lactulose include flatulence, abdominal discomfort, and diarrhea. There is a danger that overuse of lactulose will lead to complications such as aspiration, dehydration, hypernatremia, and severe perianal skin irritation, and overuse can even precipitate HE [79]. Rifaximin has been used for the therapy of HE in a number of trials comparing it with placebo, other antibiotics, nonabsorbable disaccharides, and in dose-ranging studies [80]. These trials showed that the effect of rifaximin was equivalent or superior to the compared agents with good tolerability. L-ornithine-L-aspartate can reduce blood ammonia levels via stimulating both the urea cycle and glutamine synthesis [81]. Liver transplantation remains the only treatment option for HE that does not improve on any other treatment.

21.1.7.3 Prevention of HE

Data for nonabsorbable disaccharides for the secondary prevention of HE have been sparse. However, it is still widely recommended and practiced. An open-label RCT showed that lactulose was able to prevent recurrent HE in patients with cirrhosis [82]. Another RCT supports lactulose as prevention of HE subsequent to upper gastrointestinal bleeding [83]. Rifaximin added to lactulose is the best-documented agent to maintain remission in patients who have already experienced one or more bouts of HE.

21.2 Conclusions

Patients with liver cancer are regarded to have not one disease, but two: cancer and underlying liver disease. In some patients, even a large or advanced tumor can be cured by treatments including radiotherapy. However, most patients may suffer from hepatic dysfunction resulting in occurrence of ascites, jaundice, or variceal bleeding that requires LT. Fortunately, sophisticated application of radiation therapy with high technology significantly reduced the incidence of liver dysfunction in patients with liver cancer compared to the past. Nevertheless, radiation oncologists and hepatologists must be cautious of possible hepatic dysfunction in these patients.

References

1. Jung BG, Kim YD, Kim SG, et al. Hepatitis B virus reactivation after radiotherapy for hepatocellular carcinoma and efficacy of antiviral treatment: a multicenter study. PLoS One. 2018;13:e0201316.
2. Lawrence TS, Robertson JM, Anscher MS, et al. Hepatic toxicity resulting from cancer treatment. Int J Radiat Oncol Biol Phys. 1995;31:1237–48.
3. Choi SH, Seong J. Strategic application of radiotherapy for hepatocellular carcinoma. Clin Mol Hepatol. 2018;24:114–34.
4. Lee UE, Friedman SL. Mechanisms of hepatic fibrogenesis. Best Pract Res Clin Gastroenterol. 2011;25:195–206.
5. Kim J, Jung Y. Radiation-induced liver disease: current understanding and future perspectives. Exp Mol Med. 2017;49:e359.
6. Dawson LA, Normolle D, Balter JM. Analysis of radiation-induced liver disease using the Lyman NTCP model. Int J Radiat Oncol Biol Phys. 2002;53:810–21.
7. Pan CC, Kavanagh BD, Dawson LA. Radiation-associated liver injury. Int J Radiat Oncol Biol Phys. 2010;76:256–63.
8. Guha C, Kavanagh BD. Hepatic radiation toxicity: avoidance and amelioration. Semin Radiat Oncol. 2011;21:256–63.
9. Munoz-Schuffenegger P, Ng S, Dawson LA. Radiation-induced liver toxicity. Semin Radiat Oncol. 2017;27:350–7.

10. Fortune B, Cardenas A. Ascites, refractory ascites and hyponatremia in cirrhosis. Gastroenterol Rep. 2017;5:104–12.

11. Runyon BA. Care of patients with ascites. New Engl J Med. 1994;330:337–42.

12. Runyon BA. Ascites and spontaneous bacterial peritonitis. In: Feldman M, Friedman LS, Brandt LJ, editors. Sleisenger and Fordtran's gastrointestinal and liver disease. 9th ed. Philadelphia: Saunders Elsevier; 2010. p. 1517–41.

13. Eisenmenger WJ, Ahrens EH, Blondheim SH, et al. The effect of rigid sodium restriction in patients with cirrhosis of the liver and ascites. J Lab Clin Med. 1949;34:1029–38.

14. Sungaila I, Bartle WR, Walker SE, et al. Spironolactone pharmacokinetics and pharmacodynamics in patients with cirrhotic ascites. Gastroenterology. 1992;102:1680–5.

15. Arroyo V. Pathophysiology, diagnosis and treatment of ascites in cirrhosis. Ann Hepatol. 2002;1:72–9.

16. Sola E, Gines P. Renal and circulatory dysfunction in cirrhosis: current management and future perspectives. J Hepatol. 2020;53:1135–45.

17. Serste T, Melot C, Francoz C, et al. Deleterious effects of beta-blockers on survival in patients with cirrhosis and refractory ascites. Hepatology. 2010;52:1017–22.

18. Boyer TD, Zia P, Reynolds TB. Effect of indomethacin and prostaglandin A1 on renal function and plasma renin activity in alcoholic liver disease. Gastroenterology. 1979;77:215–22.

19. Peltekian KM, Wong F, Liu PP, et al. Cardiovascular, renal and neurohumoral responses to single large-volume paracentesis in cirrhotic patients with diuretic-resistant ascites. Am J Gastroenterol. 1997;92:394–9.

20. Tito L, Gines P, Arroyo V, et al. Total paracentesis associated with intravenous albumin management of patients with cirrhosis and ascites. Gastroenterology. 1990;98:146–51.

21. Runyon BA. Introduction to the revised American Association for the Study of Liver Diseases Practice Guideline management of adult patients with ascites due to cirrhosis 2012. Hepatology. 2013;57:1651–3.

22. Arroyo V, Gines P, Gerbes AL, et al. Definition and diagnostic criteria of refractory ascites and hepatorenal syndrome in cirrhosis. Hepatology. 1996;23:164–76.

23. Moreau R, Delegue P, Pessione F, et al. Clinical characteristics and outcomes of patients with cirrhosis and refractory ascites. Liver Int. 2004;24:457–64.

24. Hoefs JC, Canawati HN, Sapico FL, et al. Spontaneous peritoneal peritonitis. Hepatology. 1982;2:399–407.

25. Felisart J, Rimola A, Arroyo V, et al. Randomized comparative study of efficacy and nephrotoxicity of ampicillin plus tobramycin versus cefotaxim in cirrhotics with severe infection. Hepatology. 1985;5:457–62.

26. Navasa M, Follo A, Llovet JM, et al. Randomized, comparative study of oral ofloxacin versus intravenous cefotaxime in spontaneous bacterial peritonitis. Gastroenterology. 1996;111:1011–7.

27. Soriano G, Teixedo M, Guarner C, et al. Selective intestinal decontamination prevents spontaneous bacterial peritonitis. Gastroenterology. 1991;100:477–81.

28. Gines P, Rimola A, Planas R, et al. Norfloxacin prevents spontaneous bacterial peritonitis recurrence in cirrhosis: results of a double-blind, placebo-controlled trial. Hepatology. 1990;12:716–4.

29. Chaudhury P, Barkin A, Barkun J. ACS surgery: principles and practice. 2010. Available from: http://www.slideshare.net/medbookonline/acs0503-jaundice-2006.

30. Moses RA, Grodzki WJ, Starcher BC, et al. Elastin content of the scleral spur, trabecular mesh, and sclera. Invest Ophthalmol Vis Sci. 1978;17:817–8.

31. Blasco A, Forns X, Carrion JA, et al. Hepatic venous pressure gradient identifies patients at risk of severe hepatitis C recurrence after liver transplantation. Hepatology. 2006;43:492–9.

32. Groszmann RJ, Garcia-Tsao G, Bosch J, et al. Beta-blockers to prevent gastroesophageal varices in patients with cirrhosis. N Engl J Med. 2005;353:2254–61.

33. Ripoll C, Groszmann R, Garcia-Tsao G, et al. Hepatic venous pressure gradient predicts clinical decompensation in patients with compensated cirrhosis. Gastroenterology. 2007;133:481–8.

34. Bruix J, Castells A, Bosch J, et al. Surgical resection of hepatocellular carcinoma in cirrhotic patients. Prognostic value of preoperative portal pressure. Gastroenterology. 1996;111:1018–22.

35. Lebrec D, De Fleury P, Rueff B, et al. Portal hypertension, size of esophageal varices, and risk of gastrointestinal bleeding in alcoholic cirrhosis. Gastroenterology. 1980;79:1139–44.

36. Garcia-Tsao G, Groszmann RJ, Fisher RL, et al. Portal pressure, presence of gastroesophageal varices and variceal bleeding. Hepatology. 1985;5:419–24.

37. Bosch J, Groszmann RJ, Shah VH. Evolution in the understanding of the pathophysiological basis of portal hypertension: how changes in paradigm are leading to successful new treatments. J Hepatol. 2015;62(1 Suppl):S121–30.

38. Iwakiri Y, Groszmann RJ. Vascular endothelial dysfunction in cirrhosis. J Hepatol. 2007;46:927–34.

39. Turco L, Garcia-Tsao G. Portal hypertension: pathogenesis and diagnosis. Clin Liver Dis. 2019;23:573–87.

40. D'Amico G, Pasta L, M orabito A, et al. Competing risks and prognostic stages of cirrhosis: a 25-year inception cohort study of 494 patients. Aliment Pharmacol Ther. 2014;39:1180–93.

41. de Franchis R, Baveno V. Faculty. Expanding consensus in portal hypertension. Report of the Baveno VI Consensus Workshop: stratifying risk and individualizing care for portal hypertension. J Hepatol. 2015;63:743–52.

42. Villanueva C, Colombo A, Bosch A, et al. Transfusion strategies for acute upper gastrointestinal bleeding. N Engl J Med. 2013;368:11–21.

43. Bernard B, Grange JD, Khac EN, et al. Antibiotic prophylaxis for the prevention of bacterial infections in cirrhotic patients with gastrointestinal bleeding: a meta-analysis. Hepatology. 1999;29:1655–61.

44. Chavez-Tapia NC, Barrientos-Gutierrez T, Tellez-Avila F, et al. Meta-analysis: antibiotic prophylaxis for cirrhotic patients with upper gastrointestinal bleeding-an updated Cochrane review. Aliment Pharmacol Ther. 2011;34:509–18.

45. Fernandez J, Ruiz dA, Gomez C, et al. Norfloxacin vs ceftriaxone in the prophylaxis of infections in patients with advanced cirrhosis and hemorrhage. Gastroenterology. 2006;131:1049–56.

46. Seo YS, Park SY, Kim MY, et al. Lack of difference among terlipressin, somatostatin, and octreotide in the control of acute gastroesophageal variceal hemorrhage. Hepatology. 2014;60:954–63.

47. Garcia-Tsao G, Sanyal AJ, Grace ND, et al. Prevention and management of gastroesophageal varices and variceal hemorrhage in cirrhosis. Hepatology. 2007;46:922–38.

48. Gines P, Guevara M, Arroyo V, et al. Hepatorenal syndrome. Lancet. 2003;362:1819–27.

49. Busk TM, Bendtsen F, Moller S. Hepatorenal syndrome in cirrhosis: diagnostic, pathophysiological, and therapeutic aspects. Expert Rev Gastroeneterol Hepatol. 2016;10:1153–61.

50. Gines P, Schrier RW. Renal failure in cirrhosis. N Engl J Med. 2009;361:1279–90.

51. Moreau R, Lebrec D. The use of vasoconstrictors in patients with cirrhosis: type 1 HRS and beyond. Hepatology. 2006;43:385–94.

52. Gines P, Guevara M. Therapy with vasoconstrictor drugs in cirrhosis: the time has arrived. Hepatology. 2007;46:1685–7.

53. Wong F, Pappas SC, Boyer TD, et al. Terlipressin improves renal function and reverses hepatorenal syndrome in patients with systemic inflammatory syndrome. Clin Gastroenterol Hepatol. 2017;15:266–73.

54. Russell JA, Walley KR. Vasopressin and its immune effects in septic shock. J Innate Immu. 2010;2:446–60.

55. Nazar A, Pereira GH, Guevara M, et al. Predictors of response to therapy to terlipressin and albumin in patients with cirrhosis and type 1 hepatorenal syndrome. Hepatology. 2010;51:219–26.

56. Guevara M, Gines P, Bandi JC, et al. Transjugular intrahepatic portosystemic shunt in hepatorenal syndrome: effects on renal function and vasoactive systems. Hepatology. 1998;28:416–22.

57. Gines P, Uriz J, Calahorra B, et al. Transjugular intrahepatic portosystemic shunting versus paracentesis plus albumin for refractory ascites in cirrhosis. Gastroenterology. 2002;123:1839–47.

58. Zhang Z, Maddukuri G, Jaipaul N, et al. Role of renal replacement therapy in patients with type 1 hepatorenal syndrome receiving combination treatment of vasoconstrictor plus albumin. J Crit Care. 2015;30:969–74.

59. Lenhart A, Hussain S, Salgia R. Chances of renal recovery of liver transplantation after hospitalization for alcoholic liver disease requiring dialysis. Dig Dis Sci. 2018;63:2800–9.

60. Fraley DS, Burr RT, Bernadini J, et al. Impact of acute renal failure on mortality in end-stage liver disease with or without transplantation. Kidney Int. 1998;54:518–24.

61. Allegretti AS, Parada XV, Eneanya ND, et al. Prognosis of patients with cirrhosis and AKI who initiate RRT. Clin J Am Soc Nephrol. 2018;13:16–25.

62. Gonwa TA, Morris CA, Goldstein RM, et al. Long-term survival and renal function following liver transplantation in patients with and without hepatorenal syndrome – experience in 300 patients. Transplantation. 1991;51:428–30.

63. Israni AK, Xiong H, Liu J, et al. Predicting end-stage renal disease after liver transplant. Am J Transplant. 2013;13:1782–92.

64. Bustamante J, Rimola A, Ventura PJ, et al. Prognostic significance of hepatic encephalopathy in patients with cirrhosis. J Hepatol. 1999;30:890–5.

65. Riggio O, Ridola L, Pasquale C, et al. Evidence of persistent cognitive impairment after resolution of overt hepatic encephalopathy. Clin Gastroenterol Hepatol. 2011;9:181–3.

66. Bajaj JS, Schubert CM, Heuman DM, et al. Persistence of cognitive impairment after resolution of overt hepatic encephalopathy. Gastroenterology. 2020;138:2332–40.

67. Bajaj JS. Current and future diagnosis of hepatic encephalopathy. Metab Brain Dis. 2020;25:107–10.

68. Kappus MR, Bajaj JS. Covert hepatic encephalopathy: not as minimal as you might think. Clin Gastroenterol Hepatol. 2012;10:1208–19.

69. Montagnese S, De Pitta C, De Rui M, et al. Sleep-wake abnormalities in patients with cirrhosis. Hepatology. 2014;59:705–12.

70. Weissenborn K. Diagnosis of encephalopathy. Digestion. 1998;59(Supple 2):22–4.

71. Patidar KR, Bajaj JS. Covert and overt hepatic encephalopathy: diagnosis and management. Clin Gastroenterol Hepatol. 2015;13:2048–61.

72. Wijdicks EE, Rabinstein AA, Bamlet WR, et al. FOUR score and Glasgow Coma Scale in predicting outcome of comatose patients: a pooled analysis. Neurology. 2011;77:84–5.

73. Lockwood AH. Blood ammonia levels and hepatic encephalopathy. Metab Brain Dis. 2004;19:345–9.

74. Vilstrup H, Amodio P, Bajaj JS. Hepatic encephalopathy in chronic liver disease: 2014 Practice Guideline by the American Association for the Study of Liver Diseases and the European Association for the Study of the Liver. Hepatology. 2014;60:715–35.

75. Gronbaek H, Johnson SP, Jepsen P, et al. Liver cirrhosis, other liver diseases, and risk of hospitalization for intracerebral haemorrhage: a Danish population-based case-control study. BMC Gastroenterol. 2008;8:16.

76. Strauss E, Tramote R, Silva EP, et al. Double-blind randomized clinical trial comparing neomycin and placebo in the treatment of exogenous hepatic encephalopathy. Hepato-Gastroenterology. 1992:542–5.

77. Nielsen K, Clemmesen JO, Vassiliadis E, et al. Liver collagen in cirrhosis correlates with portal hypertension and liver dysfunction. APMIS. 2014;122:1213–22.

78. Gerber T, Schomerus H. Hepatic encephalopathy in liver cirrhosis: pathogenesis, diagnosis and management. Drugs. 2000;60:1353–70.

79. Bajaj JS, Sanyal AJ, Bell D, et al. Predictors of the recurrence of hepatic encephalopathy in lactulose-treated patients. Aliment Pharmacol Ther. 2020;31:1012–7.

80. Patidar KR, Bajaj JS. Antibiotics for the treatment of hepatic encephalopathy. Metab Brain Dis. 2013;28:307–12.

81. Sundaram V, Shaikh OS. Hepatic encephalopathy: pathophysiology and emerging therapies. Med Clin North Am 2009;93:819–836, vii.

82. Sharma BC, Sharma P, Agrawal A, et al. Secondary prophylaxis of hepatic encephalopathy: an open-label randomized controlled trial of lactulose versus placebo. Gastroenterology. 2009;137:885–91.

83. Sharma P, Agrawal A, Sharma BC, et al. Prophylaxis of hepatic encephalopathy in acute variceal bleed: a randomized controlled trial of lactulose versus no lactulose. J Gastroenterol Hepatol. 2011;26:996–1003.

Lymphopenia Following Radiotherapy for Hepatocellular Carcinoma

22

Hwa Kyung Byun and Jinsil Seong

Abstract

Lymphocytes are highly radiosensitive cells. A substantial proportion of circulating lymphocytes can be affected by radiation during a course of conventional fractionated radiotherapy. Radiation-induced lymphopenia is a common side effect of radiotherapy. Reduced pretreatment lymphocyte counts and reduced lymphocyte infiltration in pathologically resected specimens have been associated with poor disease-free survival and overall survival in various types of cancer as well as in liver cancer. The advent of immunotherapy has renewed the focus on preserving a pool of functioning lymphocytes in the circulation. A novel strategy is urgently needed to preserve the total lymphocyte count during radiotherapy.

Keywords

Radiation-induced lymphopenia · Lymphocyte · Immunotherapy · Overall survival · Interleukin-7

H. K. Byun · J. Seong (✉)
Department of Radiation Oncology, Yonsei Cancer Center, Yonsei University College of Medicine, Seoul, South Korea
e-mail: jsseong@yuhs.ac

22.1 The Radiosensitivity of Lymphocytes

Lymphocytes are the most radiosensitive cells among cells of erythroid, myeloid, and lymphoid lineages [1]. The lethal dose required to decrease the surviving fraction of lymphocytes by 50% and 90% is 2 Gy and 3 Gy, respectively [2]. The exact mechanism underlying radiosensitivity of lymphocytes is not well known. Decreased DNA repair capacity, possibly related to the active DNA recombination that helps the development of an individual's immunity, may be related to radiosensitivity of lymphocytes. B-lymphocytes are slightly more radiosensitive than T-lymphocytes, and naïve T-lymphocytes seem to be more radiosensitive than memory cells [3]. A preclinical study showed T cell reprogramming in the tumor microenvironment and similarities with tissue-resident memory T cells, which are more radio-resistant than circulating/lymphoid tissue T cells, although the results need to be validated in human subjects [4].

A substantial proportion of circulating lymphocytes can be affected by radiation during a long course of conventional fractionated radiotherapy (RT). Therefore, lymphopenia is a common side effect seen after RT. Radiation-induced lymphopenia has been reported in various types of tumor such as hepatocellular carcinoma, brain tumors, esophageal cancer, and pancreatic cancer [5–11].

© Springer Nature Singapore Pte Ltd. 2021
J. Seong (ed.), *Radiotherapy of Liver Cancer*, https://doi.org/10.1007/978-981-16-1815-4_22

Although radiation is known for local effects, peripheral organ irradiation can result in a substantial proportion of circulating lymphocytes being irradiated during a course multiple fractionation. Radiation-induced lymphopenia can be induced by damaging the bone marrow [8] or lymphoid organs, such as the spleen [12]. However, local RT to non-marrow organs, such as the liver, brain, esophagus, rectum, and pancreas can also induce systemic lymphopenia by irradiating circulating blood [5–11].

22.2 Factors Associated with Radiation-Induced Lymphopenia

The Common Terminology Criteria for Adverse Events is used for grading lymphopenia in many studies: Grade 1 ($<\sim 1000–800/mm^3$), Grade 2 ($<800–500/mm^3$), Grade 3 ($<500–200\ mm^3$), and Grade 4 ($<200/mm^3$). Clinical factors related to lymphopenia and key findings for various cancers are shown below and Table 22.1.

Firstly, large planning target volume (PTV) and multiple fractionation are related to the increased risk of lymphopenia due to a greater chance of circulating blood to receive radiation. The association between RT-related parameters and radiation-induced lymphopenia can be supported by a mathematical computation model [13]. A typical glioblastoma plan (a four-field conformal plan, 8-cm tumor, 60 Gy/30 fractions) was constructed, and radiation doses to circulating cells were analyzed using the model. The result showed that a single radiation fraction delivered 0.5 Gy to 5% of circulating cells; after 30 fractions 99% of circulating blood had received ≥ 0.5 Gy. Moreover, the model examined two different size of PTVs (PTV diameter: 2 cm; PTV volume: 4.2 cm^3 vs. 8 cm; 268 cm^3) and showed a substantial difference in the proportion of irradiated blood. The importance of PTV size and fractionation is also shown in several clinical studies. Rudra et al. [14] reported that a large PTV was associated with increased incidence of acute severe lymphopenia in 210 patients with glioblastoma. Wild et al. [15] reported that stereotactic body radiotherapy

Table 22.1 Factors associated with radiation-induced lymphopenia

Author/Year	Site	Risk factors of lymphopenia
Yovino (2013) [13]	Glioblastoma (mathematical model)	PTV, the number of fractionation
Rudra (2014) [14]	Glioblastoma ($n = 210$)	Large field, Brain V25 Gy
Wild (2015) [15]	Pancreatic cancer ($n = 133$)	Conventional RT (vs. SBRT)
Liu (2017) [16]	Hepatocellular carcinoma ($n = 59$)	Spleen irradiation dose
Chadha (2016) [12]	Pancreatic cancer ($n = 177$)	Spleen irradiation dose
Shiraishi (2018) [17]	Esophgeal cancer ($n = 480$)	Proton (vs. photon) (likely resulted in lower dose to heart and lung)
Lin (2018) [18]	Glioma ($n = 151$)	concurrent and adjuvant chemotherapy
Byun (2019) [10]	hepatocellular carcinoma ($n = 920$)	PTV, the number of fractionation, baseline TLC, concurrent chemotherapy

(SBRT) (5 fractions) was less associated with a decrease in total lymphocyte count (TLC) compared with conventional RT (28 fractions) in 133 patients with pancreatic cancer.

Secondly, if lymphopoietic sites or organs containing large blood volumes are within the PTV, it will contribute to lymphopenia. Several studies have also reported that higher spleen irradiation doses (total dose of 50–60 Gy) were significantly correlated with more patients experiencing lymphopenia during RT for hepatocellular carcinoma, pancreatic cancer, or palliative RT [15]. Based on these results, Liu et al. [16] recommend sparing of the spleen during abdominal irradiation. Furthermore, a lower heart and lung dose resulted in less lymphopenia [19–21].

Thirdly, the use of concurrent chemotherapy is another important factor. As described previously, RT alone can induce or worsen lymphopenia. Combination of RT with systemic treatment may further augment treatment-related lymphopenia. Concurrent chemotherapy has been shown to have an impact on the severity of lymphopenia, whereas adjuvant chemotherapy induced prolongation of the duration of lymphopenia [18]. It is noteworthy that the severity of lymphopenia varies depending on chemotherapy agents.

22.3 Radiation-Induced Lymphopenia and Treatment Outcome

Many studies have shown the association between radiation-induced lymphopenia and treatment outcome in various types of cancer (Table 22.2). Decrease in pretreatment lymphocyte counts as well as in lymphocyte infiltration in pathologically resected specimens have been associated with poor disease-free survival (DFS) and overall survival (OS) in cancer involving breast, rectal, glioblastoma, non-small cell lung cancer, and other tumors. Grossman et al. [5] reported that treatment-related lymphopenia is associated with reduced survival in patients with malignant glioma, pancreatic cancer, and non-small cell lung cancer. Lee et al. [22] reported that treatment-related lymphopenia was associated with poorer OS and DFS while recovery from lymphopenia after treatment was associated with better OS and DFS among the 497 patients with pancreatic cancer who underwent concurrent chemoradiotherapy. Cho et al. [9] reported that peri-immunotherapy lymphopenia was associated with poorer DFS (median, 2.2 vs. 5.9 months) and OS (median, 5.7 vs. 12.1 months) among the patients with non-small cell lung cancer who were treated with immunotherapy. Fang et al. [21] reported that high TLC level during neoadjuvant chemotherapy for esophageal cancer was associated with a higher rate of pathologic complete response (OR, 1.82; 95% CI, 1.08–3.05). Sun et al. [23] conducted a post hoc analysis using the data from 598 patients with breast cancer from a randomized controlled trial comparing postmastectomy conventional and hypofractionated RT. DFS was significantly lower in patients with a nadir-TLC/pre-TLC ratio < 0.8 than in those with ≥0.8, but OS were comparable between the groups. The underlying mechanism explaining association of radiation-induced lymphopenia

Table 22.2 Studies showing the association between radiation-induced lymphopenia and treatment outcomes

Author/Year	Site	Interpretation
Grossman (2015) [5]	Malignant glioma ($n = 96$), resected pancreatic cancer ($n = 53$), unresectable pancreatic cancer ($n = 101$), and non-small cell lung cancer ($n = 47$)	An increased risk for death was attributable to lymphopenia in each cancer cohort
Lee (2020) [22]	Pancreatic cancer ($n = 497$)	Lymphopenia was associated with poorer OS and DFS while recovery after treatment was associated with better OS and DFS
Cho (2019) [9]	Non-small cell lung cancer ($n = 268$)	Peri-immunotherapy lymphopenia was associated with poorer DFS and OS among the patients with non-small cell lung cancer who were treated with immunotherapy
Sun (2020) [23]	Breast cancer ($n = 598$)	DFS was significantly lower in patients with a nadir-TLC/pre-TLC ratio < 0.8 than in those with ≥0.8, but OS were comparable between the groups
Byun (2019) [10]	hepatocellular carcinoma ($n = 920$)	Acute severe lymphopenia was associated with poor OS

and decreased oncologic outcome remains to be understood.

22.4 Radiation-Induced Lymphopenia and Immune System

Since the approval of the immune checkpoint inhibitor ipilimumab, an anti-cytotoxic T lymphocyte-associated protein 4 (CTLA-4) antibody, for the treatment of metastatic melanoma in 2011, immunotherapy has been current hot issue in the management of patients with cancer. Optimism in terms of the potential synergistic effect between RT and immunotherapy has increased the number of clinical trials evaluating immunotherapy–RT combinations.

The advent of immunotherapy and the recognition that the immune system plays a critical role in tumor surveillance has renewed the focus on preserving a pool of functioning circulating lymphocytes. Given that circulating lymphocytes are the cells that eventually infiltrate tumors, it may be reasonable to assume that their depletion might contribute to suboptimal treatment outcomes. RT acts as a double-edged sword on the immune system. It has an immunostimulatory effect via radiation-induced neoantigens, increased expression of heat shock proteins (HSP), increased release of tumor-associated antigens (TAA), release of high mobility group box protein (HMBG) and recruitment of effector cells into the tumor micro-environment. In contrast, it also has an immunosuppressive effect by cytotoxic T lymphocyte antigen-4 (CTLA-4), increasing expression of MHC class molecules, upregulating programmed death domain ligand-1 (PDL-1), and depletion of circulating lymphocytes and lymphoid progenitor cells in lymphoid organs [24].

22.5   Chronicity of Radiation-Induced Lymphopenia

There is a discrepancy between lymphopenia that persists beyond three months in many instances and the half-life of circulating lymphocytes of <100 days, which is a conundrum in radiation-induced lymphopenia. The decrease in TLC usually starts during the course of chemoradiation and recovers marginally post-treatment at three months. However, a significant number of patients have persistent lymphopenia beyond three months, which persists as chronic lymphopenia for years after treatment in a subset

of patients. This is contrary to lymphopenia observed in other clinical situations, such as HIV and sepsis, or those receiving chemotherapy where the lymphopenia tends to recover earlier [25]. It is interesting that patients with RT-induced lymphopenia often lack a feedback mechanism, a classical compensatory increase in homeostatic cytokines IL-7 and IL-15, in contrast to lymphopenia in other situations [26]. Thus, it is suggested that radiation-induced lymphopenia is driven by an acute depletion of lymphocytes that is combined with the inability to mount a robust compensatory surge in IL-7 for clonal expansion of lymphocytes and IL-7 and IL-15 for maturation and formation of memory. This double mechanism probably contributes to the chronicity of lymphopenia seen in patients receiving RT and may reduce the potential synergy achievable with immunotherapeutic agents and RT. Conversely, maintaining and restoring an optimal TLC may have direct clinical implication in improved treatment outcomes or synergy with immunotherapy.

22.6   Liver Cancer and Radiation-Induced Lymphopenia

Like other types of malignancy, liver cancer also presents lymphopenia following RT (Table 22.3). Compared with other types of tumors, HCC is unique with regard to RT-related lymphopenia; it is a hypervascular tumor and its location in the liver harbors a very rich blood circulation. This leads to a greater amount of blood being exposed to radiation, which can maximize the radiation effect and cause lymphopenia. Our group analyzed the TLC of 920 patients who received RT for hepatocellular carcinoma and showed the risk factors of the development of radiation-induced lymphopenia as well as the association between radiation-induced lymphopenia and survival [10]. The median TLCs decreased from 1120 cells/μl to 310 cells/μl in one month after initiation of RT. The TLCs did not fully recover to their initial level during the first year after

Table 22.3 Radiation-induced lymphopenia in hepatocellular carcinoma

Author/Year	N	Site of irradiation	Risk factors of lymphopenia	Lymphopenia development	Interpretation
Byun (2019) [10]	920	Liver	PTV, the number of fractionation, baseline TLC, concurrent chemotherapy	87.4%, <500 cells/μl within 3 months	Acute severe lymphopenia was associated with poor OS
Liu (2017) [16]	59	Liver	Spleen irradiation dose	25.4%, <300 cells/μl during RT	Maximum sparing for spleen irradiation during RT is recommended to
Park (2019) [8]	302	Bone metastases	The percentage of active bone marrow within the RT field	33.4%, <500 cells/μl within 2 months	Acute severe lymphopenia was associated with poor OS

treatment. Overall, 87.4% of patients developed acute severe lymphopenia (ASL; <500 cells/μl). The median overall survival was 13.6 and 46.7 months for patients with and without ASL, respectively ($p < 0.001$). Lymphopenia was independently associated with poor overall survival with a hazard ratio (HR) of 1.40; 95% confidence interval (CI), 1.02–1.91 ($p = 0.035$). In the multivariate analysis, larger PTV (HR, 1.02; 95% CI, 1.01–1.03; $p < 0.001$) and lower baseline TLC (HR, 0.86; 95% CI, 0.82–0.91; $p < 0.001$) were significantly associated with an increased risk of ASL, while hypofractionation (HR, 0.19; 95% CI, 0.07–0.49; $p = 0.001$) was significantly associated with a reduced risk of lymphopenia. Liu et al. [16] showed that higher radiation doses to the spleen were significantly correlated with lower minimum TLC during RT for hepatocellular carcinoma. The authors recommended maximum sparing of spleen irradiation during RT as well as limiting V5 Gy to preserve peripheral blood lymphocytes. Park et al. [8] reported that radiation-induced lymphopenia is associated with poor survival using the clinical data of 302 patients receiving RT for 511 bone metastases from hepatocellular carcinoma. Overall, 33.4% of patients developed severe lymphopenia (<500 cells/mm^3) two months after initiating RT. OS was significantly worse in patients with severe lymphopenia than in those without (median OS: 3.7 vs. 6.5 months, $p < 0.001$). The percentage of active bone marrow within the RT field was the only significant factor associated with severe lymphopenia ($p < 0.001$).

22.7 Recommendations to Reduce the Development of Radiation-Induced Lymphopenia

Since radiation-induced lymphopenia is associated with poor treatment outcome and may have a detrimental effect on anti-tumor immunity, a novel strategy is urgently needed to preserve the TLC during RT. RT-induced lymphopenia can likely be mitigated by modifying RT technique, fractionation, and possibly, modality. Because longer fractionation is associated with the development of lymphopenia, SBRT or hypofractionation are useful approaches. In RT for hepatocellular carcinoma, SBRT was associated with reduced risk of lymphopenia (HR, 0.19; 95% CI, 0.07–0.49; $p = 0.001$) [10]. SBRT for pancreatic cancer over two weeks has been associated with significantly less radiation-induced lymphopenia than standard chemoradiation therapy (CRT) over five weeks [15]. Radiation-induced lymphopenia could be further reduced by the volume of radiation exposure, which is known to be substantially different comparing photon therapy to charged particles. Shiraishi et al. [17] compared IMRT and proton beam therapy in esophageal cancer patients undergoing neoadjuvant chemoradiation therapy. In the matched groups, a greater proportion of the IMRT patients (55/136, 40.4%) developed grade 4 lymphopenia during nCRT compared with the PBT patients (24/136, 17.6%, $P < 0.0001$). Lambin et al. [27] proposed to apply the As Low As Reasonably Achievable

(ALARA) principle to Lymphocyte-related Organs At Risk (LOARs) without compromising irradiation of the planning target volume and keeping the constraints for "conventional" organs at risk, such as lung, heart and spinal cord, as recommended in clinical protocols. The authors suggested that dose, fractionation, dose rate, and mean doses to LOARs be reported as a minimum. Blood can be seen as a "moving OAR", thus long irradiation times needs to be avoided. Instead, high-dose rate irradiation, following the principle of ALARA should be considered, for example, using flattening filter-free irradiation.

22.8 Prospects

Since the role of the immune system is very important for clinical outcomes in cancer patients, current study focuses on explaining the complex interplay between treatment characteristics and the immune system and how to influence this relationship. To preserve the immune system from the effects of radiation and chemotherapy, Campian et al. [28] attempted lymphocyte reinfusion after completion of chemoradiotherapy. Lymphocytes were isolated before the treatment, stored, and administered again to the patient upon treatment completion. Although lymphocyte harvesting/reinfusion was feasible and safe, serial lymphocyte counts looked similar to matched controls without reinfusion. Another interesting approach is immunoadjuvant therapy with interleukin-7 (IL-7). IL-7 is a non-hematopoietic cell-derived cytokine with a central role in the homeostasis of lymphocytes [29, 30]. In patients with lymphopenia, the circulating levels of IL-7 increase, thereby promoting lymphocyte development in the thymus and maintaining the homeostasis of naive and memory T cells in the periphery [31]. The administration of exogenous IL-7 before RT can be a good option to prevent the decline in the TLC during RT, particularly in patients with a high chance of developing acute severe lymphopenia during RT because of a large PTV size, multiple fractionation, or low baseline TLC. The effect of exogenous IL-7 on increasing the number of T lymphocytes has been demonstrated in earlier studies of HIV-infected patients and patients with melanoma or sarcoma [32, 33]. Currently, clinical studies are being conducted regarding the effect of exogenous IL-7 to restore the TLC after RT [34]. Byun et al. examined blood IL-7 levels and TLC of 98 patients with hepatocellular carcinoma treated with RT from a prospective cohort. High pre-RT IL-7 levels was significantly associated with reduced lymphopenia development during RT and high post-RT IL-7 level was significantly positively correlated with the TLC at two months after initiation of RT (unpublished data). They also tested efficacy of exogeneous IL-7 using established mouse models of radiation-induced lymphopenia. Radiation-induced lymphopenia was rapidly recovered up to 373% of the initial level in one week after IL-7 injection, whereas it was gradually recovered to the initial level over three weeks without IL-7 injection. Pathologic specimens of tumor showed more tumor-infiltrated lymphocytes in the group of IL-7 administration. Furthermore, tumor growth was significantly suppressed in the combination of IL-7 and RT group than in the RT alone group (unpublished data). These newer therapeutic approaches to counter RT-induced lymphopenia are expected to have roles in future RT practice.

References

1. Button LN, DeWolf WC, Newburger PE, Jacobson MS, Kevy SV. The effects of irradiation on blood components. Transfusion. 1981;21(4):419–26.
2. Nakamura N, Kusunoki Y, Akiyama M. Radiosensitivity of CD4 or CD8 positive human T-lymphocytes by an in vitro colony formation assay. Radiat Res. 1990;123(2):224–7.
3. Belka C, Ottinger H, Kreuzfelder E, Weinmann M, Lindemann M, Lepple-Wienhues A, et al. Impact of localized radiotherapy on blood immune cells counts and function in humans. Radiother Oncol. 1999;50(2):199–204.
4. Arina A, Beckett M, Fernandez C, Zheng W, Pitroda S, Chmura SJ, et al. Tumor-reprogrammed resident T cells resist radiation to control tumors. Nat Commun. 2019;10(1):3959.
5. Grossman SA, Ellsworth S, Campian J, Wild AT, Herman JM, Laheru D, et al. Survival in patients with severe lymphopenia following treatment with radiation and chemotherapy for newly diagnosed solid tumors. J Natl Compr Cancer Netw. 2015;13(10):1225–31.

6. Deng W, Xu C, Liu A, van Rossum PSN, Deng W, Liao Z, et al. The relationship of lymphocyte recovery and prognosis of esophageal cancer patients with severe radiation-induced lymphopenia after chemoradiation therapy. Radiother Oncol. 2019;133:9–15.

7. Byun HK, Kim N, Yoon HI, Kang SG, Kim SH, Cho J, et al. Clinical predictors of radiation-induced lymphopenia in patients receiving chemoradiation for glioblastoma: clinical usefulness of intensity-modulated radiotherapy in the immuno-oncology era. Radiat Oncol (London, England). 2019;14(1):51.

8. Park S, Byun HK, Seong J. Irradiation-related lymphopenia for bone metastasis from hepatocellular carcinoma. Liver Cancer. 2019;8(6):468–79.

9. Cho Y, Park S, Byun HK, Lee CG, Cho J, Hong MH, et al. Impact of treatment-related lymphopenia on immunotherapy for advanced non-small cell lung cancer. Int J Radiat Oncol Biol Phys. 2019;105(5):1065–73.

10. Byun HK, Kim N, Park S, Seong J. Acute severe lymphopenia by radiotherapy is associated with reduced overall survival in hepatocellular carcinoma. Strahlentherapie und Onkologie: Organ der Deutschen Rontgengesellschaft [et al]. 2019;195(11):1007–17.

11. Liu H, Wang H, Wu J, Wang Y, Zhao L, Li G, et al. Lymphocyte nadir predicts tumor response and survival in locally advanced rectal cancer after neoadjuvant chemoradiotherapy: Immunologic relevance. Radiother Oncol. 2019;131:52–9.

12. Chadha AS, Liu G, Chen HC, Das P, Minsky BD, Mahmood U, et al. Does unintentional splenic radiation predict outcomes after pancreatic cancer radiation therapy? Int J Radiat Oncol Biol Phys. 2017;97(2):323–32.

13. Yovino S, Kleinberg L, Grossman SA, Narayanan M, Ford E. The etiology of treatment-related lymphopenia in patients with malignant gliomas: modeling radiation dose to circulating lymphocytes explains clinical observations and suggests methods of modifying the impact of radiation on immune cells. Cancer Investig. 2013;31(2):140–4.

14. Rudra S, Hui C, Rao YJ, Samson P, Lin AJ, Chang X, et al. Effect of radiation treatment volume reduction on lymphopenia in patients receiving chemoradiotherapy for glioblastoma. Int J Radiat Oncol Biol Phys. 2018;101(1):217–25.

15. Wild AT, Herman JM, Dholakia AS, Moningi S, Lu Y, Rosati LM, et al. Lymphocyte-sparing effect of stereotactic body radiation therapy in patients with unresectable pancreatic cancer. Int J Radiat Oncol Biol Phys. 2016;94(3):571–9.

16. Liu J, Zhao Q, Deng W, Lu J, Xu X, Wang R, et al. Radiation-related lymphopenia is associated with spleen irradiation dose during radiotherapy in patients with hepatocellular carcinoma. Radiat Oncol (London, England). 2017;12(1):90.

17. Shiraishi Y, Fang P, Xu C, Song J, Krishnan S, Koay EJ, et al. Severe lymphopenia during neoadjuvant chemoradiation for esophageal cancer: a propensity matched analysis of the relative risk of proton versus photon-based radiation therapy. Radiother Oncol. 2018;128(1):154–60.

18. Lin AJ, Campian JL, Hui C, Rudra S, Rao YJ, Thotala D, et al. Impact of concurrent versus adjuvant chemotherapy on the severity and duration of lymphopenia in glioma patients treated with radiation therapy. J Neuro-Oncol. 2018;136(2):403–11.

19. Badiyan SN, Robinson CG, Bradley JD. Radiation toxicity in lung cancer patients: the heart of the problem? Int J Radiat Oncol Biol Phys. 2019;104(3):590–2.

20. Fang P, Shiraishi Y, Verma V, Jiang W, Song J, Hobbs BP, et al. Lymphocyte-sparing effect of proton therapy in patients with esophageal cancer treated with definitive chemoradiation. Int J Particle Therapy. 2018;4(3):23–32.

21. Fang P, Jiang W, Davuluri R, Xu C, Krishnan S, Mohan R, et al. High lymphocyte count during neoadjuvant chemoradiotherapy is associated with improved pathologic complete response in esophageal cancer. Radiother Oncol. 2018;128(3):584–90.

22. Lee BM, Byun HK, Seong J. Significance of lymphocyte recovery from treatment-related lymphopenia in locally advanced pancreatic cancer. Radiother Oncol. 2020;151:82–7.

23. Sun GY, Wang SL, Song YW, Jin J, Wang WH, Liu YP, et al. Radiation-induced lymphopenia predicts poorer prognosis in patients with breast cancer: a post hoc analysis of a randomized controlled trial of postmastectomy hypofractionated radiation therapy. Int J Radiat Oncol Biol Phys. 2020;108(1):277–85.

24. Formenti SC, Demaria S. Systemic effects of local radiotherapy. Lancet Oncol. 2009;10(7):718–26.

25. Dean RM, Fry T, Mackall C, Steinberg SM, Hakim F, Fowler D, et al. Association of serum interleukin-7 levels with the development of acute graft-versus-host disease. J Clin Oncol. 2008;26(35):5735–41.

26. Ellsworth S, Balmanoukian A, Kos F, Nirschl CJ, Nirschl TR, Grossman SA, et al. Sustained CD4(+) T cell-driven lymphopenia without a compensatory IL-7/IL-15 response among high-grade glioma patients treated with radiation and temozolomide. Onco Targets Ther. 2014;3(1):e27357.

27. Lambin P, Lieverse RIY, Eckert F, Marcus D, Oberije C, van der Wiel AMA, et al. Lymphocyte-sparing radiotherapy: the rationale for protecting lymphocyte-rich organs when combining radiotherapy with immunotherapy. Semin Radiat Oncol. 2020;30(2):187–93.

28. Campian JL, Ye X, Gladstone DE, Ambady P, Nirschl TR, Borrello I, et al. Pre-radiation lymphocyte harvesting and post-radiation reinfusion in patients with newly diagnosed high grade gliomas. J Neuro-Oncol. 2015;124(2):307–16.

29. Nguyen V, Mendelsohn A, Larrick JW. Interleukin-7 and immunosenescence. J Immunol Res. 2017;2017:4807853.

30. Corfe SA, Paige CJ. The many roles of IL-7 in B cell development; mediator of survival, proliferation and differentiation. Semin Immunol. 2012;24(3):198–208.

31. Ponchel F, Cuthbert RJ, Goeb V. IL-7 and lymphopenia. Clin Chim Acta Int J Clin Chem. 2011;412(1–2):7–16.
32. Levy Y, Sereti I, Tambussi G, Routy JP, Lelievre JD, Delfraissy JF, et al. Effects of recombinant human interleukin 7 on T-cell recovery and thymic output in HIV-infected patients receiving antiretroviral therapy: results of a phase I/IIa randomized, placebo-controlled, multicenter study. Clin Infect Dis. 2012;55(2):291–300.
33. Rosenberg SA, Sportes C, Ahmadzadeh M, Fry TJ, Ngo LT, Schwarz SL, et al. IL-7 administration to humans leads to expansion of CD8+ and CD4+ cells but a relative decrease of CD4+ T-regulatory cells. J Immunother (Hagerstown, Md: 1997). 2006;29(3):313–9.
34. Study of the Effect IL 7/NT-I7 on CD4 Counts in Patients With High Grade Gliomas 2016. Available from: https://clinicaltrials.gov/ct2/show/NCT02659800.

Perspectives of Radiotherapy in Immuno-oncology Era

23

Yvonne Chiung-Fang Hsu
and Jason Chia-Hsien Cheng

Abstract

The liver develops "immune tolerance" for the massive but harmless antigen influx and does not elicit immune responses. Dynamic interactions of immunocytes in the liver help maintain the balance between immunity and tolerance. The dysfunction causes defective immunosurveillance and may lead to the emergence of hepatocellular carcinoma (HCC).

Phase I/II immunotherapy trials on advanced HCC included nivolumab, pembrolizumab, and combined lenvatinib and pembrolizumab. Phase III trial on combined atezolizumab and bevacizumab defeated sorafenib for unresectable or metastatic HCC. However, immunotherapy has the concerns of adverse events and is contraindicated in posttransplant patients.

Radiotherapy (RT) can enhance antitumor immunity. Synergism between RT and immunotherapy was reported in the case series. With various immune reactions of RT, the dose fractionation confounds different responses to the immune modulation.

The multiplicity of the immune environment in the liver may account for the limited efficacy of cancer immunotherapy. The abscopal effect on systemic control could be a potential addition, including activation of the natural killer cell by major histocompatibility complex I chain-related protein A/B, interleukin 12, histone deacetylase inhibitor, personalized peptide vaccination, glucocorticoid-induced tumor necrosis factor receptor, and T cell immunoglobulin and mucin-domain containing molecule-3. The unmet need of RT to HCC urges the integration of immunotherapy for improved outcomes.

Keyword

Hepatocellular carcinoma · Immunotherapy Radiotherapy · Combination · Abscopal Fractionation

Y. C.-F. Hsu
Division of Radiation Oncology, Department of Oncology, National Taiwan University Hospital, Taipei, Taiwan

J. C.-H. Cheng (✉)
Division of Radiation Oncology, Department of Oncology, National Taiwan University Hospital, Taipei, Taiwan

Graduate Institute of Oncology, National Taiwan University College of Medicine, Taipei, Taiwan
e-mail: jasoncheng@ntu.edu.tw

23.1 Immune Environment of Liver

23.1.1 Special Immune Environment of Liver

The liver is an organ to play the role of metabolic and immunological functions. The immunocytes in the liver build up the special immune environment. The enriched natural killer (NK) cells and natural killer T (NKT) cells in the liver recruit the circulatory T cells. The antigen-presenting cells (APCs) can present antigens to T cells and then activate the immune responses. Besides the classic APCs such as dendritic cells dwelling in the liver, there are liver-specific APCs, including Kupffer cells, hepatic stellate cells, and hepatic sinusoidal endothelial cells.

As a systemic filter in the digestive tract, the liver is constantly exposed to massive but harmless antigens from the portal system. Therefore, the liver develops a default "immune tolerance," a status of indifference to the substance that should elicit an immune response normally. The APCs in the liver present CD80/CD86 and programmed cell death ligand 1/2 (PD-L1/PD-L2) on their surface, which can respectively bind the cytotoxic T-lymphocyte antigen 4 (CTLA-4) and programmed cell death protein 1 (PD-1) on the activated T cells and regulatory T cells (Tregs) to downregulate the immune activity.

23.1.2 Immune Dysfunction of HCC

In general, the liver works well under the balance between immunity and tolerance. The immune response is activated toward the pathogens and is downregulated after adequate elicitation. Immune tolerance is induced by exposure to self-antigens or host cells. Dynamic interactions of the numerous immunocytes in the liver are key to maintaining balance.

Sometimes the system just goes wrong. The system crashes in various chronic liver diseases and is responsible for defective immuno-surveillance, leading to the emergence of hepatocellular carcinoma (HCC). Chronic inflammation without infectious stimulation leads to sterile liver injury, tissue damage, and remodeling. The consequent immunodeficiency allows for chronic infection and tumor growth.

The deregulation of immune checkpoints such as CTLA-4 and PD-1 in immune tolerance is involved in the pathogenesis and carcinogenesis of chronic diseases. HCC expresses a higher level of immune markers, including the immune

checkpoint genes CTLA4, PDCD1 (PD-1), and CD274 (PD-L1), compared with tumor-adjacent normal tissues [1]. The recent success of targeted therapies against immune checkpoint genes also proves the interactions between them.

23.1.3 Immune-Related Tumor Microenvironment

Immune-related tumor microenvironment (TME) is a complex and dynamic ecosystem, composed of tumor cells, tumor-supporting cells, and immunocytes, etc.

The decrease of T cells and the increase of Tregs, particularly in tumor-infiltrating lymphocytes (TILs), are found in HCC [2], indicating the suppression of antigen-presenting systems in the tumor environment. The proliferation of tumor-associated macrophages promotes tumor initiation and growth through epithelial-mesenchymal transition [3].

The immune suppressor mechanisms, including the infiltration of immuno-suppressive cells and the inhibition of antigen-presenting systems among tumor cells, prefer tolerance to immunity and thus promote the progression of HCC [4].

HCC is a very complex disease with many driver genes identified [5]. Tumor initiation and progression are partly related to immune tolerance, which fails to detect and destroy tumor cells. Therefore, HCC may be a potential candidate for immunotherapy aiming to restore antitumor immunity.

23.2 Immunotherapy in HCC

23.2.1 The Limitation of Treatment in HCC

The standard treatment of HCC at an early stage is liver-directed locoregional therapy with evidence-based improved survival. In contrast, the treatment options are limited for HCC at an advanced stage. Portal vein tumor thrombosis (PVTT), with hepatic tumor invading the portal vein, accounts for approximately 10–40%

of HCC patients [6]. These patients are histori-cally contraindicated for locoregional therapies. The recommended first-line treatment for HCC patients with PVTT is sorafenib, based on the two phase III randomized controlled trials [7, 8]. However, survival outcomes remain unsatisfac-tory, along with no complete response and few partial responses of tumors to sorafenib (2% and 3.3%, respectively).

The development of targeted therapy in advanced HCC was limited in the past decades, with four failed phase III trials on sunitinib, brivanib, linifanib, and erlotinib plus sorafenib. Success has been made with regorafenib in RESORCE trial (NCT01774344) and cabozan-tinib in CELESTIAL trial (NCT01908426) pro-viding survival benefit for patients with HCC progression after sorafenib [9, 10]. Besides, REFLECT trial (NCT01761266) with lenvatinib demonstrated non-inferiority to sorafenib with a median survival of 13.6 months and 12.3 months, respectively [11].

23.2.2 Evolving Immunotherapy in HCC

Immune checkpoint inhibitors have emerged as promising treatments for some cancer patients at an advanced stage. Immune checkpoints, includ-ing CTLA-4 and PD-1, are surface proteins on immunocytes and mostly provide immuno-suppressive signals. Monoclonal antibodies against CTLA-4 and PD-1 have shown their antitumor activity in a wide spectrum of human cancers.

PD-L1 is a ligand of PD-1 that plays a major role in suppressing the immune system. The engagement of PD-L1 with its receptor PD-1 on T cells transmits the inhibitory signals and sup-presses IL-2 production and T cell proliferation. Anti-PD-L1 antibodies disrupt the interaction between PD-1 and PD-L1, and thereby reverse T cell suppression and enhance antitumor immu-nity. Earlier clinical trials on checkpoint inhibi-tors in HCC included the anti-CTLA-4 agent tremelimumab and anti-PD-1 agent nivolumab [12, 13]. Nivolumab showed in the phase II

trial the potential as a second-line therapy both in terms of tumor response and patient survival. Accordingly, the standard treatment for HCC patients with PVTT is systemic therapy, includ-ing sorafenib approved in the first line, and three other agents, regorafenib, cabozantinib, and nivolumab, approved for the second-line use. Besides, the first-line lenvatinib is non-inferior to sorafenib, but excludes patients with main portal trunk invasion [14, 15].

A few small trials of the therapeutic vaccine on HCC were conducted but showed divergent, unsatisfactory results and limited improved out-comes [16–18]. It is probably because the mul-tifactorial etiology of HCC and very few known HCC-specific tumor-associated antigens (TAAs) are not good enough to elicit an effective immune response [19].

Combinatorial strategies with cancer vaccine could be a possible solution to counter-balance the immuno-suppressive environment. Besides, new TAAs or tumor-associated epitopes can be identified by the integration of omics technology, a methodology aimed at the detection of genes, mRNA, proteins, and metabolites [20]. The investigations on the therapeutic vaccine in HCC patients are ongoing.

23.2.3 Current Status of Immunotherapy in HCC

Early clinical trials on immunotherapy in advanced HCC patients included phase I/II nivolumab (CheckMate 040; NCT01658878) [13] and phase II pembrolizumab (KEYNOTE-224; NCT02702414) [21]. Objective responses of 15–20% by nivolumab and 17% by pembro-lizumab were shown, respectively. Based on CheckMate 040 study, nivolumab was approved in several countries for HCC patients previ-ously treated with sorafenib. This was the first immunotherapy approved for HCC patients and gave rise to the emergence of phase III random-ized study with nivolumab monotherapy versus sorafenib (CheckMate 459; NCT02576509). In addition, the results of KEYNOTE-224 study showed pembrolizumab, an anti-PD-1 agent, was effective and tolerable. The treatment responses and safety for Asian patients were similar to the overall treatment population. Both nivolumab and pembrolizumab exhibit their potential as a treatment for advanced HCC.

Another randomized trial on the integration of targeted drug into immunotherapy was the use of bevacizumab combined with atezolizumab versus sorafenib in patients with unresectable HCC (IMBrave150; NCT03434379) [22]. The combination successfully demonstrated the superior objective response (27.3% vs. 11.9%, $p < 0.001$), median progression-free survival (6.8 months vs. 4.3 months, $p < 0.001$), and 12-month overall survival (67.2% vs. 54.6%, $p < 0.001$), respectively. Atezolizumab in combination with bevacizumab was approved by Food and Drug Administration for patients of unresectable or metastatic HCC without previous systemic therapy. Besides the combinational treatment of bevacizumab and atezolizumab, a phase Ib trial with the use of lenvatinib and pembrolizumab demonstrated promising antitumor activity with an objective response rate of 36% and median overall survival of 22 months in unresectable HCC [23]. This study gave rise to the ongoing randomized controlled phase III study (LEAP-002; NCT03713593) of lenvatinib plus pembrolizumab versus lenvatinib plus placebo in patients with unresectable HCC.

23.2.4 The Concerns of Immunotherapy in HCC

Specific immune-related adverse events (IRAEs) have been reported in patients treated with immunotherapy. The general adverse events related to immune activation include rash, fatigue, and diarrhea. Organ-specific IRAEs are uncommonly reported but at higher risk with anti-PD-1 drugs, including hypothyroidism, pneumonitis, colitis, and hypophysitis [24]. Several studies reported that patients with IRAEs had remarkable improvements in progression-free survival, overall survival, and overall response rate compared to patients with no toxicity [25]. It is hypothesized that those with treatment-responsive immune systems are

likely to have autoimmune toxicities. Notably, one other concern of immunotherapy is that immunotherapeutic drugs may not be suitable for patients with recurrence after liver transplantation, mainly because of the high risk of allograft rejection.

23.3 The Integration of Radiotherapy in Immunotherapy

23.3.1 Radiation and Immune Response

Some preliminary experiments on animals showed the benefit of radiation for tumor control. According to the study by Stone et al., the needed radiation dose in immuno-competent mice for tumor control was 1.67-fold higher than that in immuno-deficient mice [26]. The mice treated with TILs and focused radiotherapy (RT) had fewer metastases compared with either treatment alone in the study by Cameron et al. [27].

Radiation can induce inflammation within the TME and may activate antitumor immunity, as shown by the cytokine productions in the murine models [28, 29]. Radiation enhances the immune responses not only by the release of cytokines after the induced apoptosis but also by upregulating expression of major histocompatibility complex (MHC) I on tumor cells [9].

It is established that radiation can help antigen presentation and activate dendritic cells with the change of composition on the cell surface [30]. Radiation also recruits T cells to the TME with the promotion of chemokines and adhesion molecules [28, 31]. Besides, radiation upregulates the natural killer group 2 member D (NKG2D), an activating receptor on the surface of NK cells, and can enhance the cytolytic activity of NK cells toward tumor cells.

Given the traditional role in DNA damage, RT modulates immune reactions and induces a potential antitumoral immune response. The "reactivation" of antitumor immune response forms the basis of the 6Rs in radiobiology in addition to the original 5Rs (repair, redistribution, reoxygenation, repopulation, and radiosensitivity) [32].

23.3.2 Radiation and Immune-Related TME

Chew et al. found the isolated TILs in HCC patients after yttrium-90 radioembolization (Y90-RE) activated local immune responses [33]. Higher expression of granzyme B and infiltration of immunocytes including CD8+ T cells, CD56+ NK cells, and CD8+ CD56+ NKT cells were also demonstrated. In contrast, Tregs were rich in TILs of the treatment-naïve group. Y90-RE could change the TME to be less immuno-suppressive. The increase of tumor necrosis factor-α (TNF-α) on T cells and the percentage of APCs after Y90-RE indicate a systemic immune activation, particularly in patients with sustained response to Y90-RE.

23.3.3 Abscopal Effect with RT

In general, radiation induces modifications of both innate and adaptive immune responses. RT also has local and systemic effects in the TME. Irradiated tumor releases antigens which could be an in situ vaccine. Tumor regression at a site distant from the primary site treated by RT, known as the abscopal effect, has long been described. The induced tumor cell death is thought to be related to the release of damage-associated molecules. The abscopal effect was reported in 52% of advanced melanoma patients with the associated prolonged survival [34].

However, RT has also been shown with the immuno-suppressive effect by the increased myeloid-derived suppressor cells in organs and tumor-associated macrophages from irradiated tumors, which may restrict the efficacy of anti-tumor response [35, 36]. Radiation upregulates PD-L1 and T cell immuno-receptor with Ig and ITIM domains (TIGIT), a co-inhibitory receptor on T cells and NK cells. Both PD-L1 and TIGIT act as immune checkpoints to limit antitumor immunity. Although such immunosuppression can lead to tumor radioresistance, synergism between RT and immune checkpoint inhibitors was shown in preclinical models of various cancers [37].

23.3.4 The Impact of RT Dose and Fractionation on Immune Modulation

The efficacy of RT depends on the balance between immuno-stimulatory and immuno-suppressive effects, and the dose fractionation of RT should be further optimized for the resultant effects [38].

The degraded DNA in the cytosol can bind to cyclic GMP-AMP synthase (cGAS) and activate the stimulator of interferon genes (STING) [39]. The cGAS-STING pathway leads to the production of interferon β and further recruitment of dendritic cells. In the preliminary study by Vanpouille-Box et al., the threshold doses of 8–10 Gray (Gy) per fraction attained the effective anti-tumor immune response, while the doses above 12–18 Gy attenuated the immunity with the accumulation of degraded cytosolic DNA [40].

Conventional fractionation of solid tumors is given with doses of 1.8–2.0 Gy per day for 3–7 weeks while hypofractionation is given with doses exceeding 2.0 Gy per day. The ultra-short hypofractionated RT, known as SBRT, is typically delivered in 3–10 fractions and has shown improved local control in HCC. It is generally accepted that SBRT or hypofractionated RT is more immunogenic than normal fractionated daily 2-Gy treatment. In the murine model by Lugade et al., the single dose of 15 Gy enhanced the immune response more effectively than the fractional dose of 3 Gy for 5 fractions [41].

The use of a total dose of 3–6 Gy in 2–3 fractions has shown the immuno-suppressive effects to relieve the painful enthesopathies [42], and the doses of 10 Gy in 5 fractions showed the immuno-stimulatory effects with metabolically active macrophages causing DNA damage [43]. In addition, a single-fraction high dose of radiosurgery enhanced the activation of dendritic cells [44]. On the contrary, a very high single dose may attenuate the immune response by the degraded DNA [45]. Of note, the optimal immuno-susceptible radiation dose and fractionation remain to be defined and may be dependent on many factors, such as types of tumor, the immuno-modulation within TME, timing of RT, and the combined use of immunotherapy.

23.3.5 Clinical Trial on Combined RT and Immunotherapy in Non-HCC Cancers

Currently, the only success in the controlled trial comparing the combined RT and immunotherapy with either treatment is in lung cancer but not HCC. The phase III PACIFIC study (NCT02125461) investigated the use of anti-PD-L1 agent durvalumab versus placebo in patients with stage III non-small-cell lung cancer (NSCLC) after platinum-based chemoradiotherapy [46]. The results showed improved median progression-free survival (16.8 months vs. 5.6 months, $p < 0.001$), a higher response rate (28.4% vs. 16.0%, $p < 0.001$), and an improved 3-year overall survival rate (66.3% vs. 43.5%), leading to global approvals of durvalumab in advanced unresectable NSCLC after chemoradiotherapy [47]. It is hypothesized that anti-PD-L1 agents may help restore systemic immune response after chemoradiotherapy, as evidenced by upregulation of PD-L1 expression in tumor cells after RT [48].

23.4 Experimental Model of RT and Immunotherapy in HCC

23.4.1 The Limitation of RT and the Need of Combined RT and Immunotherapy in HCC

RT plays a major role in local tumor control. Although radiation could induce some immune responses and even the abscopal effect in selected patients, it is not effective enough to control the distant metastasis in most situations. In a systemic review by Ohri et al., local control rates with stereotactic body radiation therapy (SBRT) were reported with 93%, 89%, and 86% at 1, 2, and 3 years, respectively, for primary liver tumor [49]. However, out-field recurrence remains the major failure after SBRT, mostly in the untreated liver [50]. With the limited treatment efficacy of RT, the effort to combine immunotherapy with RT has been made.

23.4.2 Preclinical Experiments of RT and Immunotherapy in HCC

Increased expression of PD-L1 was found in murine HCC cells after radiation. It is hypothesized that radiation could upregulate PD-L1 expression on tumor cells through interferon-γ (IFN-γ) or STAT3 signaling, and thus facilitate the therapeutic effect by anti-PD-L1 antibodies. Experiments on HCC-bearing mice treated with radiation and anti-PD-L1 agent showed a significantly suppressed tumor growth and improved 7-week survival rate, compared with the anti-PD-L1 agent alone or radiation alone group [51].

The multiplicity of an immuno-tolerant microenvironment in both tumor and liver may limit the efficacy of cancer immunotherapy. Besides immune checkpoint inhibitors, further enhancement of local and systemic control by targeted therapy or epigenetic drugs may be considered as a potential addition.

23.4.3 NK Cell and MHC I Chain-Related Protein A/B

NK cells, as a component of the innate immune system, can lyse and kill tumor cells without MHC recognition. NK cells have been described in patients with HCC, and loss of the MHC I expression in dysplastic hepatocytes is concomitant with the decrease of NK cells in the murine model [52]. This highlights a critical role of metabolic disorders and innate immunity at the early stages of HCC.

A rare case of an HCC patient with multiple metastases in the right atrium and bilateral lungs attained complete remission on the treatment of RT, transarterial chemoembolization (TACE), and sorafenib [53]. High NK cell activity was observed in the blood of the patient after the multidisciplinary treatments.

MHC I chain-related protein A/B (MICA/B) are ligands binding to NKG2D, an immunoreceptor to activate the cytolytic activity of NK cells. Hypoxia and decreased glucose supply during HCC progression can lead to unfolded protein response (UPR) in the TME. According to Fang et al., UPR is found to downregulate MICA/B expression in HCC [54]. Reducing UPR may cause the upregulation of MICA/B expression and enhancement of cytotoxic immunity of NK cells. NKG2D makes tumor cells more susceptible to the killing effect by NK cells and T cells and is associated with cancer immuno-surveillance [55]. MICA/B could be a possible target to enhance the immunity of NK cells in HCC.

23.4.4 Personalized Peptide Vaccination

Personalized peptide vaccination (PPV) is another type of immunotherapy and is thought to activate cytotoxic lymphocytes (CTLs) with stronger antitumor cytotoxicity. In a case series reported by Shen et al., 9 HCC patients with distant metastasis were treated with RT and PPV composed of four selected HLA 1A-matched peptides and showed the response rate and disease control rate of 33% and 66%, respectively [56]. Besides, these patients could tolerate this regimen well without serious side effects. The findings suggested the potential of using combined RT and CTL-based immune therapy to reduce tumor progression in future clinical trials of advanced HCC.

23.4.5 Interleukin 12

Interleukin 12 (IL-12), a cytokine that can induce immune responses by activating NK cells and T lymphocytes producing TNF-α and IFN-γ with anti-angiogenic effect, is considered as a potential anti-cancer drug. IL-12 has shown an antitumor effect in combination with RT in several animal models [57]. Wu et al. designed the combination therapy of radiation and IL-12, which led to prolonged mean survival, compared with radiation or IL-12 monotherapy (96 $\pm$ 3 days, 61 $\pm$ 2 days, and 61 $\pm$ 3 days, $p < 0.001$) with dramatic tumor regression in animals bearing large subcutaneous HCC and metastatic tumors [58]. Radiation alone induced tumor regression at an early time but most tumors regained exponential growth afterward, while IL-12 monotherapy only delayed tumor growth.

23.4.6 Histone Deacetylase Inhibitor

Epigenetic drugs have immune-mediated anti-tumor effects that may improve the activity of immunotherapy agents. Histone deacetylase inhibitor (HDACi) was shown to sensitize tumor cells to radiation, and protect tumor-specific lymphocytes from radiation by facilitating DNA repair [59]. In murine HCC model, belinostat, an HDACi drug, improves the antitumor activity of anti-CTLA-4 but not of anti-PD-1 therapy [60]. In the study by Armeanu et al., sodium valproate, an HDACi by selectively inducing the degradation of HDAC-2, upregulated the expression of MICA/B in HCC *in vivo* and promoted the recognition of tumor cells by T cells via NKG2D [61].

23.4.7 Glucocorticoid-Induced Tumor Necrosis Factor Receptor

Glucocorticoid-induced tumor necrosis factor receptor (GITR), one of the co-stimulatory receptors in solid malignancies, is considered as a potential agonistic target to enhance the intra-tumoral immunity of T cells. GITR can reinforce the functionality of TILs isolated from HCC. Targeting GITR can be a possible addition to boost the immunity against HCC. The combined treatment with low doses of both GITR-ligation and anti-CTLA-4 antibodies was found to restore antitumor T cell immunity in *ex vivo* liver tumor cells by enhancing T cell proliferation and cytokine production [62]. Combining GITR-ligation with anti-PD1 agent nivolumab also enhanced immune responses of TIL to the tumor in some HCC patients [63].

23.4.8 T Cell Immunoglobulin and Mucin-Domain Containing Molecule-3

T cell immunoglobulin and mucin-domain-containing molecule-3 (TIM-3), a co-inhibitory receptor expressed on IFN-γ-producing T cells, Tregs, and innate immune cells such as NK cells, can suppress the immunity of tumor cells and is proposed to be a potential target for cancer immunotherapy [64, 65]. Combination therapies with blockade of TIM-3 signaling and other inhibitory molecules have shown synergistic effects and the restoration of antitumor immunity in non-HCC preclinical experiments [66–68]. Although TIM-3 is a marker for mature and activated NK cells, the engagement of TIM-3 has shown opposing effects on NK cells. The stimulation of TIM-3 with agonistic antibodies decreased the cytotoxicity of NK cells but selectively enhanced the production of IFN-γ by NK cells via galectin-9 (Gal-9), the ligand of TIM-3 [69, 70]. Interestingly, Gal-9 can inhibit the function of human and murine NK cells independent of TIM-3 [71]. It is hypothesized that upregulated expression of TIM-3 initially enhances the cytotoxicity of NK cells, but the overexpressed TIM-3 leads to the dysfunction of NK cells [72]. The combination therapy with anti-TIM-3 agent and radiation delayed tumor growth and improved median survival compared to monotherapy of anti-TIM-3 agent or radiation in a murine HCC model. The antitumor effect was associated with increased apoptosis, decreased proliferation of tumor cells, and activation of T cells.

23.5 Perspectives in the Combination of RT and Immunotherapy to HCC

23.5.1 Completed, Ongoing, and Upcoming Clinical Studies on the Use of Combined RT and Immunotherapy in HCC Patients

Several clinical reports have shown the promising results of local RT in combination with immune checkpoint inhibitors in patients with advanced HCC [51, 73–76]. A patient with angioinvasive HCC undergoing Y90-RE and combined treatment with nivolumab reported by Wehrenberg-Klee et al. achieved a successful bridging effect to hepatectomy with pathological complete response [77].

In the study by Yu et al., the combination of nivolumab with previous or concurrent RT in patients with advanced HCC showed superior outcomes to nivolumab monotherapy. Improved progression-free/overall survival rates were 51.8%/22.0% at 6 months ($P = 0.008$) and 46.2%/19.1% at 12 months ($P = 0.007$), respectively [78]. The limited but encouraging experiences suggest the effect of radiation should be more than a simple increase of the released cytokines and the changes of TME. A variety of immune responses, including local microenvironment to radiation and systemic inflammatory reactions to immunotherapy, are to be investigated for both the irradiated tumor control and abscopal effect outside the radiation region.

Phase I studies investigating the combinational treatment of RT or Y90-RE and immunotherapy include NCT02837029 on Y90-RE and nivolumab in advanced HCC patients, NCT03099564 on Y90-RE and pembrolizumab in HCC patients with poor prognosis and preserved liver function, NCT03203304 on 40-Gy SBRT and either nivolumab or ipilimumab in HCC, and NCT03812562 on Y90-RE and nivolumab in HCC patients undergoing surgical resection.

There are several ongoing or upcoming phase II studies with the use of combined RT or Y90-RE and immunotherapy in HCC. The studies include NCT03033446 on Y90-RE and nivolumab in Asian patients with advanced HCC, NCT03316872 on 5-fraction high-dose SBRT and pembrolizumab in patients with advanced HCC after sorafenib, NCT03380130 on Y90-RE and nivolumab in patients with unresectable HCC, NCT03482102 on RT combined with

Table 23.1 Summary of ongoing or upcoming clinical trials in hepatocellular carcinoma (HCC) patients treated with external-beam radiotherapy (RT) and immunotherapy

NCT number	Intervention	Phase
NCT03199807	RT (5 Gy/10 fr) and neoantigen-reactive T cell	Ib/II
NCT03203304	SBRT (40 Gy/5 fr) with either nivolumab or ipilimumab	I
NCT03316872	SBRT (high doses/5 fr) and pembrolizumab	II
NCT03482102	RT with tremelimumab and durvalumab	II
NCT03817736	Sequential TACE and SBRT with immune checkpoint inhibitors	II
NCT04167293	SBRT and sintilimab versus SBRT alone	II/III
NCT04193696	IMRT or SBRT (40 Gy/10 fr, 30 Gy/10 fr, and 20 Gy/10 fr) and carelizumab	II
NCT04430452	Hypofractionated RT and durvalumab with or without tremelimumab	II

SBRT stereotactic body radiation therapy, *TACE* transarterial chemoembolization, *IMRT* intensity-modulated radiation therapy

tremelimumab and durvalumab for HCC and biliary tract cancer, NCT03817736 on sequential TACE and SBRT combined with the selected immune checkpoint inhibitors in HCC patients to the downstage tumor for hepatectomy, and NCT04430452 on hypofractionated RT followed by durvalumab with or without tremelimumab in HCC patients with progression after prior anti-PD-1 agent.

The other upcoming studies include NCT03199807, a phase Ib/II trial on personalized neoantigen reactive T cells and RT with doses of 5 Gy in 10 fractions in patients with advanced HCC, NCT04124991, a phase I/II trial on Y90-RE and durvalumab in patients with locally advanced and unresectable HCC, NCT04167293, a phase II/III trial investigating the efficacy of

SBRT followed by sintilimab (an anti-PD-1 agent) versus SBRT alone in HCC patients with portal vein invasion, NCT04193696 on the combined treatment of carelizumab (an anti-PD-1 agent) and intensity-modulated radiation therapy or SBRT in patients with advanced HCC, and NCT04522544 on combined durvalumab and tremelimumab with either Y90-RE or TACE for intermediate-stage HCC.

A summary of clinical trials with combined RT and immunotherapy in HCC patients is listed in Table 23.1.

23.5.2 A Future Scope of RT in Immuno-oncology Era for HCC

Combination therapy has become one of the major approaches in cancer therapy nowadays. The rationale is to block more than one pathway for the synergistic or additive effects. However, fewer than 5% of the combinations were superior to monotherapy in progression-free survival [79]. In light of the special immune environment in the liver, several immune checkpoint inhibitors have shown promising effects on HCC. With the proposed interactions between RT and immune responses (Fig. 23.1), the preclinical experiments with animal models showed encouraging results and implied the potential efficacy of the combinational treatment of RT and immunotherapy. Given the unsatisfactory response of PVTT and the out-field recurrence/metastasis as the main patterns of failure after RT to HCC, there is an unmet need for the combined treatment of RT and immunotherapy with both target and abscopal effects. Future clinical investigations may be designed on the basis of the selected immune cells and/or target proteins.

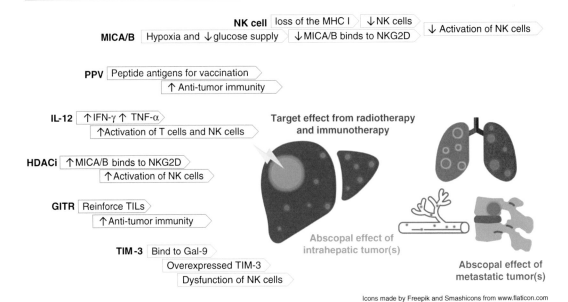

Fig. 23.1 A proposed role of combined immunotherapy and radiotherapy in hepatocellular carcinoma with multiple liver tumors and systemic metastasis includes the target effect on the irradiated liver tumor(s) and the abscopal effect on nonirradiated metastases via the multidimensional mechanisms. Abbreviation: *GITR* glucocorticoid-induced tumor necrosis factor receptor, *HDACi* histone deacetylase inhibitor, *IFN-γ* interferon-γ, *IL-12* interleukin 12, *MHC* major histocompatibility complex, *MICA/B* MHC I chain-related protein A/B, *NK* natural killer, *NKG2D* natural killer group 2 member D, *PPV* personalized peptide vaccination, *TIL* tumor-infiltrating lymphocyte, *TIM-3* T cell immunoglobulin and mucin-domain containing molecule-3, *TNF-α* tumor necrosis factor-α

References

1. Comprehensive and Integrative Genomic Characterization of Hepatocellular Carcinoma. Cell. 2017;169(7):1327–41.e23.
2. Unitt E, Rushbrook SM, Marshall A, Davies S, Gibbs P, Morris LS, et al. Compromised lymphocytes infiltrate hepatocellular carcinoma: the role of T-regulatory cells. Hepatology. 2005;41(4):722–30.
3. Yeung OW, Lo CM, Ling CC, Qi X, Geng W, Li CX, et al. Alternatively activated (M2) macrophages promote tumour growth and invasiveness in hepatocellular carcinoma. J Hepatol. 2015;62(3):607–16.
4. Zhang HH, Mei MH, Fei R, Liu F, Wang JH, Liao WJ, et al. Regulatory T cells in chronic hepatitis B patients affect the immunopathogenesis of hepatocellular carcinoma by suppressing the anti-tumour immune responses. J Viral Hepat. 2010;17(Suppl 1):34–43.
5. Ding X, He M, Chan AWH, Song QX, Sze SC, Chen H, et al. Genomic and epigenomic features of primary and recurrent hepatocellular carcinomas. Gastroenterology. 2019;157(6):1630–45.e6.
6. Llovet JM, Bustamante J, Castells A, Vilana R, Ayuso Mdel C, Sala M, et al. Natural history of untreated nonsurgical hepatocellular carcinoma: rationale for the design and evaluation of therapeutic trials. Hepatology. 1999;29(1):62–7.
7. Llovet JM, Ricci S, Mazzaferro V, Hilgard P, Gane E, Blanc JF, et al. Sorafenib in advanced hepatocellular carcinoma. N Engl J Med. 2008;359(4):378–90.
8. Cheng AL, Kang YK, Chen Z, Tsao CJ, Qin S, Kim JS, et al. Efficacy and safety of sorafenib in patients in the Asia-Pacific region with advanced hepatocellular carcinoma: a phase III randomised, double-blind, placebo-controlled trial. Lancet Oncol. 2009;10(1):25–34.
9. Bruix J, Qin S, Merle P, Granito A, Huang YH, Bodoky G, et al. Regorafenib for patients with hepatocellular carcinoma who progressed on sorafenib treatment (RESORCE): a randomised, double-blind, placebo-controlled, phase 3 trial. Lancet (London, England). 2017;389(10064):56–66.
10. Abou-Alfa GK, Meyer T, Cheng AL, El-Khoueiry AB, Rimassa L, Ryoo BY, et al. Cabozantinib in patients with advanced and progressing hepatocellular carcinoma. N Engl J Med. 2018;379(1):54–63.
11. Kudo M, Finn RS, Qin S, Han KH, Ikeda K, Piscaglia F, et al. Lenvatinib versus sorafenib in first-line treatment of patients with unresectable hepatocellular carcinoma: a randomised phase 3 non-inferiority trial. Lancet (London, England). 2018;391(10126):1163–73.
12. Sangro B, Gomez-Martin C, de la Mata M, Iñarrairaegui M, Garralda E, Barrera P, et al. A clinical trial of CTLA-4 blockade with tremelimumab in

patients with hepatocellular carcinoma and chronic hepatitis C. J Hepatol. 2013;59(1):81–8.

13. El-Khoueiry AB, Sangro B, Yau T, Crocenzi TS, Kudo M, Hsu C, et al. Nivolumab in patients with advanced hepatocellular carcinoma (CheckMate 040): an open-label, non-comparative, phase 1/2 dose escalation and expansion trial. Lancet (London, England). 2017;389(10088):2492–502.

14. Marrero JA, Kulik LM, Sirlin CB, Zhu AX, Finn RS, Abecassis MM, et al. Diagnosis, staging, and management of hepatocellular carcinoma: 2018 Practice Guidance by the American Association for the Study of Liver Diseases. Hepatology. 2018;68(2):723–50.

15. EASL Clinical Practice Guidelines: management of hepatocellular carcinoma. J Hepatol. 2018;69(1):182–236.

16. Lee WC, Wang HC, Hung CF, Huang PF, Lia CR, Chen MF. Vaccination of advanced hepatocellular carcinoma patients with tumor lysate-pulsed dendritic cells: a clinical trial. J Immunother. 2005;28(5):496–504.

17. El Ansary M, Mogawer S, Elhamid SA, Alwakil S, Aboelkasem F, Sabaawy HE, et al. Immunotherapy by autologous dendritic cell vaccine in patients with advanced HCC. J Cancer Res Clin Oncol. 2013;139(1):39–48.

18. Sawada Y, Yoshikawa T, Nobuoka D, Shirakawa H, Kuronuma T, Motomura Y, et al. Phase I trial of a glypican-3-derived peptide vaccine for advanced hepatocellular carcinoma: immunologic evidence and potential for improving overall survival. Clin Cancer Res. 2012;18(13):3686–96.

19. Buonaguro L. Developments in cancer vaccines for hepatocellular carcinoma. Cancer Immunol Immunother. 2016;65(1):93–9.

20. Sharma M, Krammer F, García-Sastre A, Tripathi S. Moving from empirical to rational vaccine design in the 'omics' era. Vaccines (Basel). 2019;7(3).

21. Zhu AX, Finn RS, Edeline J, Cattan S, Ogasawara S, Palmer D, et al. Pembrolizumab in patients with advanced hepatocellular carcinoma previously treated with sorafenib (KEYNOTE-224): a non-randomised, open-label phase 2 trial. Lancet Oncol. 2018;19(7):940–52.

22. Finn RS, Qin S, Ikeda M, Galle PR, Ducreux M, Kim TY, et al. Atezolizumab plus Bevacizumab in unresectable hepatocellular carcinoma. N Engl J Med. 2020;382(20):1894–905.

23. Finn RS, Ikeda M, Zhu AX, Sung MW, Baron AD, Kudo M, et al. Phase Ib study of lenvatinib plus pembrolizumab in patients with unresectable hepatocellular carcinoma. J Clin Oncol Off J Am Soc Clin Oncol. 2020;38(26):2960–70.

24. Baxi S, Yang A, Gennarelli RL, Khan N, Wang Z, Boyce L, et al. Immune-related adverse events for anti-PD-1 and anti-PD-L1 drugs: systematic review and meta-analysis. BMJ. 2018;360:k793.

25. Das S, Johnson DB. Immune-related adverse events and anti-tumor efficacy of immune checkpoint inhibitors. J Immunother Cancer. 2019;7(1):306.

26. Stone HB, Peters LJ, Milas L. Effect of host immune capability on radiocurability and subsequent transplantability of a murine fibrosarcoma. J Natl Cancer Inst. 1979;63(5):1229–35.

27. Cameron RB, Spiess PJ, Rosenberg SA. Synergistic antitumor activity of tumor-infiltrating lymphocytes, interleukin 2, and local tumor irradiation. Studies on the mechanism of action. J Exp Med. 1990;171(1):249–63.

28. Matsumura S, Wang B, Kawashima N, Braunstein S, Badura M, Cameron TO, et al. Radiation-induced CXCL16 release by breast cancer cells attracts effector T cells. J Immunol (Baltimore, Md: 1950). 2008;181(5):3099–107.

29. Lugade AA, Sorensen EW, Gerber SA, Moran JP, Frelinger JG, Lord EM. Radiation-induced IFN-gamma production within the tumor microenvironment influences antitumor immunity. J Immunol (Baltimore, Md: 1950). 2008;180(5):3132–9.

30. Kroemer G, Galluzzi L, Kepp O, Zitvogel L. Immunogenic cell death in cancer therapy. Annu Rev Immunol. 2013;31:51–72.

31. Hallahan D, Kuchibhotla J, Wyble C. Cell adhesion molecules mediate radiation-induced leukocyte adhesion to the vascular endothelium. Cancer Res. 1996;56(22):5150–5.

32. Boustani J, Grapin M, Laurent PA, Apetoh L, Mirjolet C. The 6th R of radiobiology: reactivation of antitumor immune response. Cancers (Basel). 2019;11(6).

33. Chew V, Lee YH, Pan L, Nasir NJM, Lim CJ, Chua C, et al. Immune activation underlies a sustained clinical response to Yttrium-90 radioembolisation in hepatocellular carcinoma. Gut. 2019;68(2):335–46.

34. Grimaldi AM, Simeone E, Giannarelli D, Muto P, Falivene S, Borzillo V, et al. Abscopal effects of radiotherapy on advanced melanoma patients who progressed after ipilimumab immunotherapy. Onco Targets Ther. 2014;3:e28780.

35. Xu J, Escamilla J, Mok S, David J, Priceman S, West B, et al. CSF1R signaling blockade stanches tumor-infiltrating myeloid cells and improves the efficacy of radiotherapy in prostate cancer. Cancer Res. 2013;73(9):2782–94.

36. Tsai CS, Chen FH, Wang CC, Huang HL, Jung SM, Wu CJ, et al. Macrophages from irradiated tumors express higher levels of iNOS, arginase-I and COX-2, and promote tumor growth. Int J Radiat Oncol Biol Phys. 2007;68(2):499–507.

37. Twyman-Saint Victor C, Rech AJ, Maity A, Rengan R, Pauken KE, Stelekati E, et al. Radiation and dual checkpoint blockade activate non-redundant immune mechanisms in cancer. Nature. 2015;520(7547):373–7.

38. Hader M, Frey B, Fietkau R, Hecht M, Gaipl US. Immune biological rationales for the design of combined radio- and immunotherapies. Cancer Immunol Immunother. 2020;69(2):293–306.

39. Cai X, Chiu YH, Chen ZJ. The cGAS-cGAMP-STING pathway of cytosolic DNA sensing and signaling. Mol Cell. 2014;54(2):289–96.

40. Vanpouille-Box C, Alard A, Aryankalayil MJ, Sarfraz Y, Diamond JM, Schneider RJ, et al. DNA exonuclease Trex1 regulates radiotherapy-induced tumour immunogenicity. Nat Commun. 2017;8:15618.

41. Lugade AA, Moran JP, Gerber SA, Rose RC, Frelinger JG, Lord EM. Local radiation therapy of B16 melanoma tumors increases the generation of tumor antigen-specific effector cells that traffic to the tumor. J Immunol (Baltimore, Md: 1950). 2005;174(12):7516–23.

42. Seegenschmiedt MH, Micke O, Muecke R. Radiotherapy for non-malignant disorders: state of the art and update of the evidence-based practice guidelines. Br J Radiol. 2015;88(1051):20150080.

43. Teresa Pinto A, Laranjeiro Pinto M, Patrícia Cardoso A, Monteiro C, Teixeira Pinto M, Filipe Maia A, et al. Ionizing radiation modulates human macrophages towards a pro-inflammatory phenotype preserving their pro-invasive and pro-angiogenic capacities. Sci Rep. 2016;6:18765.

44. Lee Y, Auh SL, Wang Y, Burnette B, Wang Y, Meng Y, et al. Therapeutic effects of ablative radiation on local tumor require CD8+ T cells: changing strategies for cancer treatment. Blood. 2009;114(3):589–95.

45. Vanpouille-Box C, Alard A, Aryankalayil MJ, Sarfraz Y, Diamond JM, Schneider RJ, et al. DNA exonuclease Trex1 regulates radiotherapy-induced tumour immunogenicity. Nat Commun. 2017;8(1):15618.

46. Antonia SJ, Villegas A, Daniel D, Vicente D, Murakami S, Hui R, et al. Durvalumab after chemoradiotherapy in stage III non-small-cell lung cancer. N Engl J Med. 2017;377(20):1919–29.

47. Gray JE, Villegas A, Daniel D, Vicente D, Murakami S, Hui R, et al. Three-year overall survival with Durvalumab after chemoradiotherapy in stage III NSCLC-update from PACIFIC. J Thorac Oncol. 2020;15(2):288–93.

48. Gong X, Li X, Jiang T, Xie H, Zhu Z, Zhou F, et al. Combined radiotherapy and anti-PD-L1 antibody synergistically enhances antitumor effect in non-small cell lung cancer. J Thorac Oncol. 2017;12(7):1085–97.

49. Ohri N, Jackson A, Mendez Romero A, Miften M, Ten Haken RK, Dawson LA, et al. Local control following stereotactic body radiotherapy for liver tumors: a preliminary report of the AAPM Working Group for SBRT. Int J Radiat Oncol Biol Phys. 2014;90(1):S52.

50. Huang WY, Jen YM, Lee MS, Chang LP, Chen CM, Ko KH, et al. Stereotactic body radiation therapy in recurrent hepatocellular carcinoma. Int J Radiat Oncol Biol Phys. 2012;84(2):355–61.

51. Kim KJ, Kim JH, Lee SJ, Lee EJ, Shin EC, Seong J. Radiation improves antitumor effect of immune checkpoint inhibitor in murine hepatocellular carcinoma model. Oncotarget. 2017;8(25):41242–55.

52. Coulouarn C, Factor VM, Conner EA, Thorgeirsson SS. Genomic modeling of tumor onset and progression in a mouse model of aggressive human liver cancer. Carcinogenesis. 2011;32(10):1434–40.

53. Kim DH, Cho E, Cho SB, Choi SK, Kim S, Yu J, et al. Complete response of hepatocellular carcinoma with

54. Fang L, Gong J, Wang Y, Liu R, Li Z, Wang Z, et al. MICA/B expression is inhibited by unfolded protein response and associated with poor prognosis in human hepatocellular carcinoma. J Exp Clin Cancer Res. 2014;33(1):76.

55. López-Soto A, Huergo-Zapico L, Acebes-Huerta A, Villa-Alvarez M, Gonzalez S. NKG2D signaling in cancer immunosurveillance. Int J Cancer. 2015;136(8):1741–50.

56. Shen J, Wang LF, Zou ZY, Kong WW, Yan J, Meng FY, et al. Phase I clinical study of personalized peptide vaccination combined with radiotherapy for advanced hepatocellular carcinoma. World J Gastroenterol. 2017;23(29):5395–404.

57. Palata O, Hradilova Podzimkova N, Nedvedova E, Umprecht A, Sadilkova L, Palova Jelinkova L, et al. Radiotherapy in combination with cytokine treatment. Front Oncol. 2019;9:367.

58. Wu CJ, Tsai YT, Lee IJ, Wu PY, Lu LS, Tsao WS, et al. Combination of radiation and interleukin 12 eradicates large orthotopic hepatocellular carcinoma through immunomodulation of tumor microenvironment. Onco Targets Ther. 2018;7(9):e1477459.

59. Pugh JL, Sukhina AS, Seed TM, Manley NR, Sempowski GD, van den Brink MR, et al. Histone deacetylation critically determines T cell subset radiosensitivity. J Immunol (Baltimore, Md: 1950). 2014;193(3):1451–8.

60. Llopiz D, Ruiz M, Villanueva L, Iglesias T, Silva L, Egea J, et al. Enhanced anti-tumor efficacy of checkpoint inhibitors in combination with the histone deacetylase inhibitor Belinostat in a murine hepatocellular carcinoma model. Cancer Immunol Immunother. 2019;68(3):379–93.

61. Armeanu S, Bitzer M, Lauer UM, Venturelli S, Pathil A, Krusch M, et al. Natural killer cell-mediated lysis of hepatoma cells via specific induction of NKG2D ligands by the histone deacetylase inhibitor sodium valproate. Cancer Res. 2005;65(14):6321–9.

62. Pedroza-Gonzalez A, Zhou G, Singh SP, Boor PP, Pan Q, Grunhagen D, et al. GITR engagement in combination with CTLA-4 blockade completely abrogates immunosuppression mediated by human liver tumor-derived regulatory T cells ex vivo. Onco Targets Ther. 2015;4(12):e1051297.

63. van Beek AA, Zhou G, Doukas M, Boor PPC, Noordam L, Mancham S, et al. GITR ligation enhances functionality of tumor-infiltrating T cells in hepatocellular carcinoma. Int J Cancer. 2019;145(4):1111–24.

64. He Y, Cao J, Zhao C, Li X, Zhou C, Hirsch FR. TIM-3, a promising target for cancer immunotherapy. Onco Targets Ther. 2018;11:7005–9.

65. Friedlaender A, Addeo A, Banna G. New emerging targets in cancer immunotherapy: the role of TIM3. ESMO Open. 2019;4(Suppl 3):e000497.

66. Sakuishi K, Apetoh L, Sullivan JM, Blazar BR, Kuchroo VK, Anderson AC. Targeting Tim-3

and PD-1 pathways to reverse T cell exhaustion and restore anti-tumor immunity. J Exp Med. 2010;207(10):2187–94.

67. Huang YH, Zhu C, Kondo Y, Anderson AC, Gandhi A, Russell A, et al. CEACAM1 regulates TIM-3-mediated tolerance and exhaustion. Nature. 2015;517(7534):386–90.

68. Kurtulus S, Sakuishi K, Ngiow SF, Joller N, Tan DJ, Teng MW, et al. TIGIT predominantly regulates the immune response via regulatory T cells. J Clin Invest. 2015;125(11):4053–62.

69. Ndhlovu LC, Lopez-Vergès S, Barbour JD, Jones RB, Jha AR, Long BR, et al. Tim-3 marks human natural killer cell maturation and suppresses cell-mediated cytotoxicity. Blood. 2012;119(16):3734–43.

70. Gleason MK, Lenvik TR, McCullar V, Felices M, O'Brien MS, Cooley SA, et al. Tim-3 is an inducible human natural killer cell receptor that enhances interferon gamma production in response to galectin-9. Blood. 2012;119(13):3064–72.

71. Golden-Mason L, McMahan RH, Strong M, Reisdorph R, Mahaffey S, Palmer BE, et al. Galectin-9 functionally impairs natural killer cells in humans and mice. J Virol. 2013;87(9):4835–45.

72. Khan M, Arooj S, Wang H. NK cell-based immune checkpoint inhibition. Front Immunol. 2020;11:167.

73. Dovedi SJ, Adlard AL, Lipowska-Bhalla G, McKenna C, Jones S, Cheadle EJ, et al. Acquired resistance to fractionated radiotherapy can be overcome by concurrent PD-L1 blockade. Cancer Res. 2014;74(19):5458–68.

74. Postow MA, Callahan MK, Barker CA, Yamada Y, Yuan J, Kitano S, et al. Immunologic correlates of the abscopal effect in a patient with melanoma. N Engl J Med. 2012;366(10):925–31.

75. Shaverdian N, Lisberg AE, Bornazyan K, Veruttipong D, Goldman JW, Formenti SC, et al. Previous radiotherapy and the clinical activity and toxicity of pembrolizumab in the treatment of non-small-cell lung cancer: a secondary analysis of the KEYNOTE-001 phase 1 trial. Lancet Oncol. 2017;18(7):895–903.

76. Choi C, Yoo GS, Cho WK, Park HC. Optimizing radiotherapy with immune checkpoint blockade in hepatocellular carcinoma. World J Gastroenterol. 2019;25(20):2416–29.

77. Wehrenberg-Klee E, Goyal L, Dugan M, Zhu AX, Ganguli S. Y-90 radioembolization combined with a PD-1 inhibitor for advanced hepatocellular carcinoma. Cardiovasc Intervent Radiol. 2018;41(11):1799–802.

78. Yu JI, Lee SJ, Lee J, Lim HY, Paik SW, Yoo GS, et al. Clinical significance of radiotherapy before and/or during nivolumab treatment in hepatocellular carcinoma. Cancer Med. 2019;8(16):6986–94.

79. Gao H, Korn JM, Ferretti S, Monahan JE, Wang Y, Singh M, et al. High-throughput screening using patient-derived tumor xenografts to predict clinical trial drug response. Nat Med. 2015;21(11):1318–25.

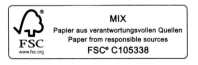

Printed by Books on Demand, Germany